HANDBOOK OF CLINICAL NEUROEPIDEMIOLOGY

Handbook of Clinical Neuroepidemiology

Valery L. Feigin

and

Derrick A. Bennett

Editors

Nova Science Publishers, Inc.

New York

NOTICE TO THE READER

The Publisher has taken reasonable care in the preparation of this book, but makes no expressed or implied warranty of any kind and assumes no responsibility for any errors or omissions. No liability is assumed for incidental or consequential damages in connection with or arising out of information contained in this book. The Publisher shall not be liable for any special, consequential, or exemplary damages resulting, in whole or in part, from the readers' use of, or reliance upon, this material.

Independent verification should be sought for any data, advice or recommendations contained in this book. In addition, no responsibility is assumed by the publisher for any injury and/or damage to persons or property arising from any methods, products, instructions, ideas or otherwise contained in this publication.

This publication is designed to provide accurate and authoritative information with regard to the subject matter covered herein. It is sold with the clear understanding that the Publisher is not engaged in rendering legal or any other professional services. If legal or any other expert assistance is required, the services of a competent person should be sought. FROM A DECLARATION OF PARTICIPANTS JOINTLY ADOPTED BY A COMMITTEE OF THE AMERICAN BAR ASSOCIATION AND A COMMITTEE OF PUBLISHERS.

LIBRARY OF CONGRESS CATALOGING-IN-PUBLICATION DATA

Handbook of clinical neuroepidemiology / Valery L. Feigin and D.A. Bennett, editors.
    p. ; cm.
  Includes bibliographical references and index.
  ISBN 13: 978-1-60021-511-7
  ISBN 10: 1-60021-511-4
  1.Nervous system- -Diseases- -Epidemiology. I. Feigin, Valery L. II. Bennett, D.A. (Derrick A.)
  [DNLM:1. Nervous System Diseases- -epidemiology. 2. Epidemiologic Methods.
WL 140 H2349 2006]
RA645.N48H358 2006
614.5--dc22
                    2006039485

Published by Nova Science Publishers, Inc. ✦ New York

CONTENTS

INTRODUCTION

Valery L. Feigin and Derrick A. Bennett

In the recent years there has been significant advance in our knowledge of risk factors, gene-environment interactions, incidence, prevalence, outcomes, and prevention strategies of many neurological disorders. These advances have been accompanied by developments in study design methodologies and statistical analysis procedures. This book is primarily aimed at neurologists, internists, health policy decision makers and other health professionals with limited experience of epidemiological and statistical methods. Most medical researchers will have received some form of statistical training, but it may have been far too brief, many years ago, and long forgotten by now. The aims of the first chapter of this book are threefold (a) to reacquaint the reader with some of the fundamental statistical concepts that are needed to conduct research (b) to introduce aspects of epidemiological study designs and to incorporate the role played by statistics in analysing and interpreting the results of such study designs (c) outline the rationale and results of some case-studies in recent neuroepidemiological research literature which have employed these study designs and analytical methods.

We were motivated to write this book by the belief that the introductory texts currently available in neuroepidemiology were rather long, aimed at specialist rather than at a wider epidemiological audience, and were therefore more useful as an occasional reference. We have aimed to produce a text that the general health professional with the interest in neuroepidemiology can refer to on a daily basis. Written by leading world experts in neuroepidemiology and clinical neurology this handbook this book aims to bridge the gap between current neuroepidemiological knowledge and its evidence-based application in everyday practice

We have assumed that most researchers have access to a computer but not necessarily a statistical software package. A CD has been provided that contains a document which outlines how to download the free statistical software package R and how to perform some simple analyses that have been described in Chapter 1. In addition, a detailed description of a real dataset and a selection of documented programs written in the R (version 2.4.0) syntax are provided in order to encourage the reader to try some of these standard analyses themselves. The aim is to give the reader a taste of the types of analyses that can be conducted and how to present the results in a clear and concise manner.

BASICS OF NEUROEPIDEMIOLOGY

In: Handbook of Clinical Neuroepidemiology
Editors: V. L. Feigin and D. A. Bennett, pp. 3-64

ISBN 978-1-60021-511-7
© 2007 Nova Science Publishers, Inc.

Chapter 1

FUNDAMENTAL STATISTICAL AND EPIDEMIOLOGICAL CONCEPTS

Derrick A. Bennett[1] and Valery L. Feigin[2]

[1]Clinical Trial Service Unit and Epidemiological Studies Unit, University of Oxford,
Richard Doll Building, Old Road Campus, Roosevelt Drive,
Oxford, OX3 7LF, United Kingdom;
[2]Clinical Trials Research Unit, School of Population Health, The University of Auckland,
Private Bag 92019, Auckland, New Zealand

ABSTRACT

This chapter aims to introduce various stages of the epidemiological research process with illustrative examples from the neurological literature. We begin by introducing some fundamental statistical concepts including sampling schemes, hypothesis testing, confidence intervals, and sample size estimation. Different epidemiological study designs with their corresponding strengths and weaknesses and the main measures of effect are then discussed. Some common and more advanced statistical tests are then introduced along with the role of correlation and regression in epidemiology. Finally, the interpretation of the results of individual studies and meta-analyses of such studies, for different study designs are discussed.

INTRODUCTION

Statistics is a key discipline that needs to be considered throughout the research process. Knowledge of statistics is relevant from defining the research question, design of the study, data collection, processing and analysis through to interpretation and presentation of the results. In order to be as effective as possible, clinicians and other health professionals need to be able to read and evaluate the findings produced by research in their chosen field. There has been a dramatic increase in the use of statistics in research over recent decades. Thus a good grasp of the key concepts behind statistics is crucial for understanding and critically appraising medical research. This chapter aims to provide the reader with the basic tools in order to improve their abilities to design, conduct and interpret the results of epidemiological studies in relation to neuroepidemiology.

FUNDAMENTALS OF STATISTICS

Sampling

A population is the totality of the measurements or counts obtainable from all objects possessing some common specified characteristic. Some examples are all males living in the U.K. (a count) or the height of all U.K. females (a measurement). It is up to the investigator to define the population that they are interested in. However, a population can vary markedly in size, and usually it is not possible to measure or count the entire population. So we have to take a sample from the population and make inferences about the population from the sample. A sample is a set of measurements which constitutes part of a population. We can have a random sample which is a sample in which any one measurement in the population is as likely to occur as any other. We can also have a biased sample where some individual measurements have a greater chance of being included than others. Common types of sampling methodology are:

1. *Random sampling:* each person has the same chance of being selected for the study.
2. *Stratified sampling:* the population is divided into strata with the characteristics of interest. Individuals are then selected randomly from within each stratum.
3. *Cluster-sampling*: this involves sampling groups of individuals such as schools or cities instead of sampling each individual separately.
4. *Multi-stage sampling*: this involves taking samples at different stages. The primary sampling unit could be city, the secondary sampling unit is suburb, the tertiary sampling unit is street and the final sampling unit could be within a household.

Estimation

A parameter is a numerical descriptive measure of a population and is calculated from the data in the entire population. A sample statistic is a numerical descriptive measure of a sample and is calculated from the observations in the sample. Population parameters are fixed so long as the population itself does not change. Sample statistics vary from sample to sample even though samples may be random and the population does not change.

Types of Data, Presentation of Data

Any quantity that varies is called a variable. Variables and parameters are sometimes confused by non-statisticians and Altman and Bland give a useful description of the distinction [1]. Variables can be qualitative or quantitative. Qualitative (also known as categorical) variables can be further described as nominal or ordinal and quantitative variables can be described as discrete or continuous. Nominal variables take attributes that simply classify the units into categories (such as ethnicity). Ordinal variables are attributes that enable the units to be ordered with respect to the variable of interest (such as disease severity). Quantitative variables are measurements that enable the determination of how much more or less of the characteristic being measured is possessed by one unit than another (such as blood pressure). Altman and Bland give a useful introduction to the typical types of data that a researcher would encounter in most medical applications [2]. When it comes to analysing your data, the first stage is to describe the data. It is essential that the variable type is correctly identified for the appropriate numerical summaries to be applied to the data. Tables 1a and 1b gives some examples of the different types of variable encountered in many epidemiological studies.

Table 1a: Example of different types of variables encountered in medical research

Type of variable	*Scale of measurement*
Binary	Two alternatives only
Categorical (nominal)	More than two alternatives
Ordered categorical (ordinal)	More than two alternatives with natural ordering
Quantitative	Discrete (counts)
	Continuous

Table 1b: Examples of different types of quantitative variables encountered in epidemiological research

Variable name	Categories/ Scale of measurement	Type
Sex	Male or Female	Discrete(Binary)
Age	Less than 75, 75+ years	Discrete (Binary)
Ethnicity	Caucasian, Black, Chinese, Indian	Categorical(Nominal)
Disease state	Mild, Moderate, Severe	Categorical (Ordinal)
Systolic Blood Pressure (SBP)	mmHg	Continuous
Homocysteine (tHcy)	μmol/L	Continuous

SUMMARISING CONTINUOUS DATA

The Mean, Median and Mode

The most popular summary measure of quantitative data set is the arithmetic mean or simply the mean of a data set. The mean of a set of quantitative data is equal to the sum of the measurements divided by the number of measurements contained in the data set. The sample mean is denoted by $\bar{x}$ (pronounced x bar) and the population mean is denoted by μ (the Greek letter mu). The median is useful if there are some very large or very small observations. The median is the middle number when the measurements in a dataset are arranged in ascending (or descending) order. To calculate the median we arrange the n measurements from the smallest to the largest. If n is odd, the median is the middle number. If n is even, the median is the average of the two middle numbers. The mode is the measurement that occurs most frequently in the dataset.

Measures of Variation

The sample variance is basically a measure which determines how much each individual observation in the sample deviates from the arithmetic mean of the sample. The larger the deviations from the arithmetic mean the greater the variability of the observations. The sample variance is conventionally denoted by s2. The population variance is denoted by σ2 (the Greek letter sigma). The sample standard deviation is the square root of the sample variance and is denoted by s or SD. Quantiles are observations which divide the distribution such that there are a given proportion of observations below the quantile. The median is the central value of the distribution such that half the points or less than or equal to it and half are greater than or equal to it. Quartiles divide the distribution into four equal parts. The second quartile is the median. Percentiles divide the distribution into 100 equal parts. The median is the 50th percentile. The interquartile range (IQR) is upper quartile minus the lower quartile. The lower quartile is the 25th percentile of a dataset. The middle quartile (50th percentile) is the median and the upper quartile is the 75th percentile. In order to gain some further insight into the types of data that an investigator is likely to encounter and how to summarise these data the reader is referred to the website http://www.stat.berkeley.edu/users/stark/SticiGui/ Text/index.htm for some useful examples.

Summarising Categorical Data

Proportions are summary measures for qualitative data. The population is classified into two or more categories. For example people can be classified as male or female, exposed or unexposed, and as smokers or non-smokers. Both the sex and the smoking category are then binary variables (with only two possible values). If the non-smokers were further split into ex-smokers and those who had never smoked, the variable 'smoking' would have three possible values (smokers, ex-smokers and non-smokers). We can then count how many individuals are in each category in a given sample or population. Dividing this by the total number of individuals in the sample gives the proportion in each category. One proportion is sufficient to describe a binary variable (if you know that 43% of the sample is male, it follows that the rest (57%) must be female), two proportions are needed if there are three categories, etc.

Frequency Distributions

When examining a set of data, it is useful to have a visual summary picture or graph. This enables the investigator to know how the data are distributed. For example, such a pictorial display can enable the researcher to see whether all observations are very close together or whether or they vary a lot. A simple graphical way of depicting or summarising data graphically is by using a histogram in which the number or frequency of observations is plotted for different values or groups of values.

For binary or categorical variables this would be the number (or percentage) of individuals falling into each category (e.g. percent male, percent female; percent in each ethic group Caucasian, Black, Chinese, Indian). For quantitative variables, values are usually grouped into a finite number of categories (e.g. height in cm: less than 160cm, 160-164cm, 165-169cm etc.). The number (or percentage) in each category can then be calculated.

The Normal Distribution and Sampling Distributions

The distributions of many medical measurements approximate to the Normal distribution in terms of its symmetric, bell-shape (e.g. blood pressure levels). The Normal distribution plays a very important role in statistical inference. Figure 1 show the shape of a Normal distribution and indicates that for data that follow a Normal distribution 68% of the data fall within ±1 SD of the mean.

Figure 2 shows the "normal range" (also known as a reference range) in which 95% of the data from a Normal distribution falls within ±1.96 SD of the mean.

Standard Normal Distribution

The Normal distribution with a mean of 0 and a standard deviation of 1 is very important and is referred to as the *standard Normal distribution*. For the standard Normal distribution the area under the curve represents a probability with the mean at its centre. For the standard Normal distribution, most of the area is between -3 and +3 and it is possible to use tables to find these probabilities via tables or via a statistical computer package.

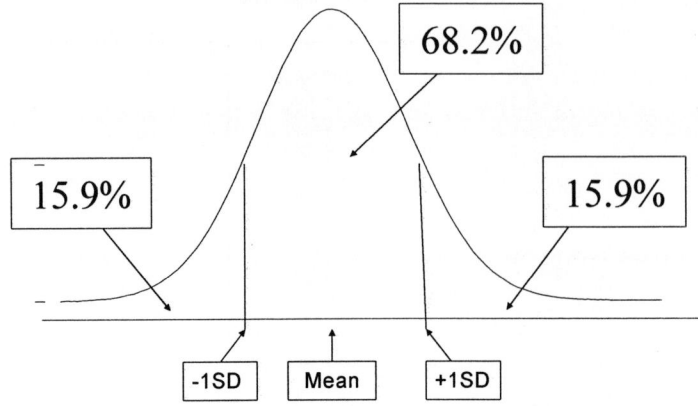

Figure 1. The Normal distribution

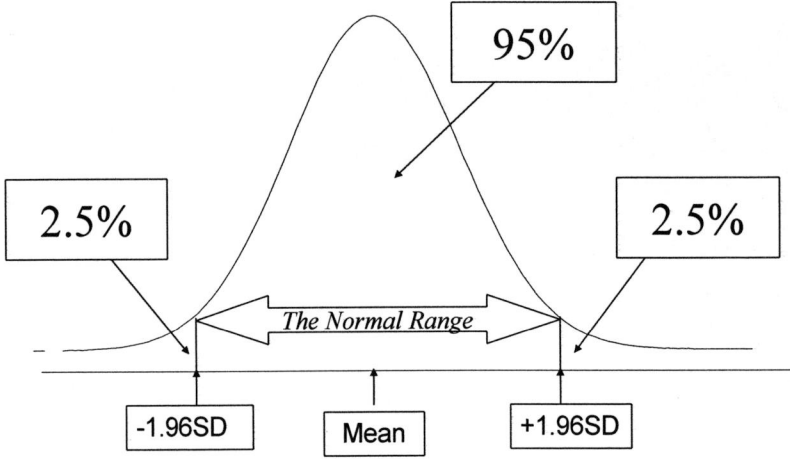

Figure 2. The "Normal range" or "reference range"

Standardising

Given a set of data which is known to be from a Normal distribution it is possible to produce what is known as a Z-score which basically quantifies the number of standard deviations between the designated measurement level of interest and the group average. It is fairly straightforward to compute the Z-score as follows:

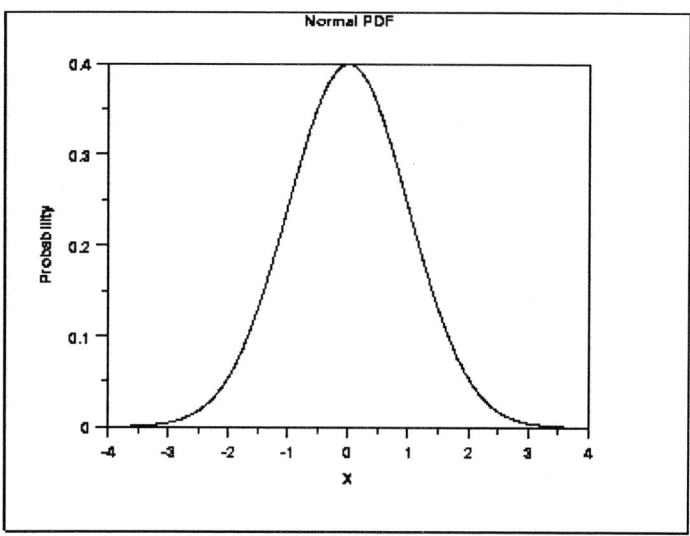

Figure 3. Histogram data from a standard Normal distribution

$$Z \equiv \frac{X - \mu}{\sigma}$$

where X is our variable of interest (e.g. blood pressure), μ (represents the mean or group average) and σ represents the standard deviation. Figures 4a and 4b show the three steps involved in computing a Z score and the effect on the Normal distribution. Figure 4c shows 1000 systolic blood pressure data generated from a Normal distribution with a mean of 170mmHg and a standard deviation of 29 mmHg.

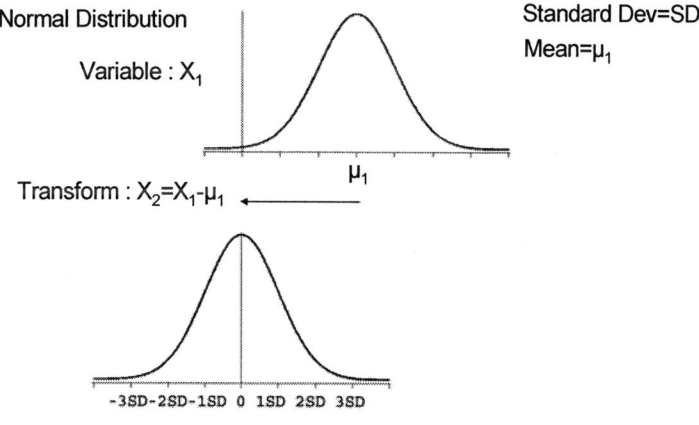

Figure 4a. Transforming Normal distributions

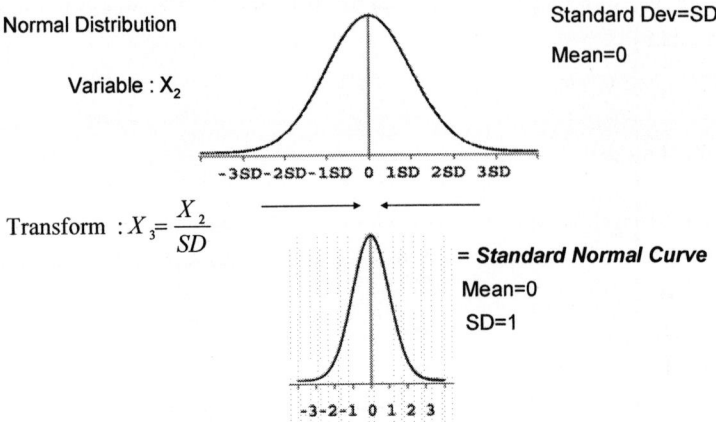

Figure 4b. Transforming Normal distributions

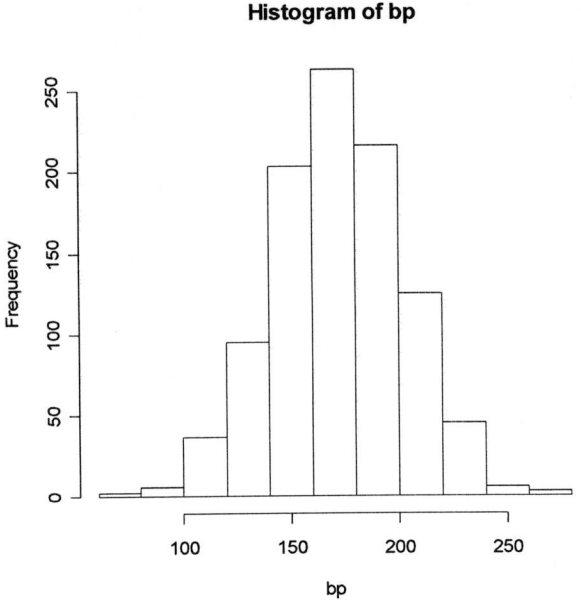

Figure 4c. Histogram artificial blood pressure data from a Normal distribution

If we took an individual measurement from this Normal distribution and found its value was 190mmHg we could compute a Z score thus:

$$Z = (190-170)/29 = 0.70 \text{ standard deviations above the mean}$$

Computing a Z-score is known as standardising the data. Once the Z-score is formed it is possible to use the standard Normal distribution calculate the probability of finding a difference of this size in the individual measurement under consideration. Some background reading on the Normal distribution and its importance in medical applications can be found in Altman and Bland [3].

Statistical Inference

Statistical inference, drawing conclusions about the population on the basis of a sample, can take the form of estimation or hypothesis testing (which we shall discuss later. The simplest type of statistic used to make inferences about a population parameter is a point estimator such as the mean, median or mode (see Figure 5).

However, the sample may not be representative of the population – i.e. it is biased. We expect each sample to give a different result because of sampling variation. When investigators conduct studies in different settings and in different countries, for example, there will be differences in the results due to sampling variation.

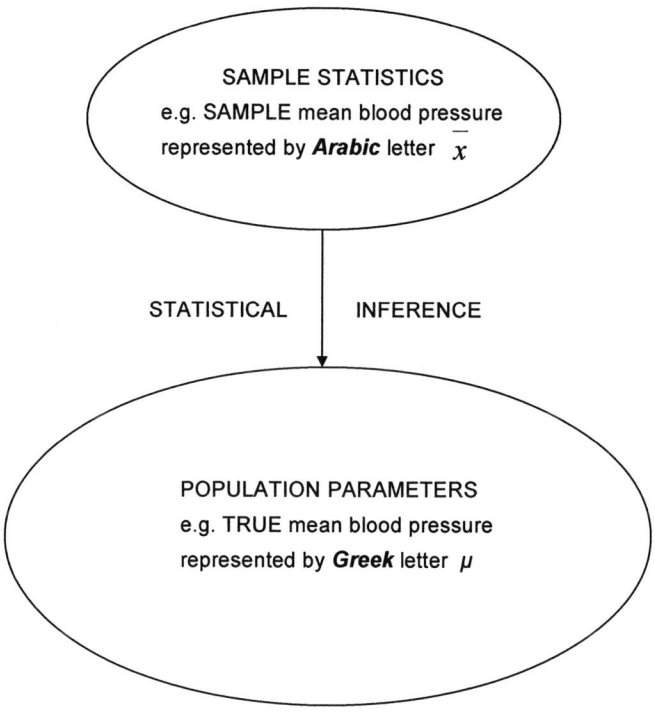

Figure 5. Populations and samples

Sampling Distributions

It is not feasible to conduct an infinite number of studies so it is necessary to take into account the **degree of statistical uncertainty** associated with the results of a single study. The **sampling distribution** of a sample statistic calculated from a sample of measurements is the frequency distribution of the statistic (such as the mean). The most common point estimator used is the mean and most methods of statistical inference are based on the properties of the sampling distribution of the mean. Figure 6 shows schematic of how the sampling distribution of the mean is derived. In actual practice, the sampling distribution of a statistic is obtained mathematically or (at least approximately) by simulating the sample on a computer.

By examining the sampling distribution, we can determine how large the difference between an estimate and the true value of the parameter (*called the error of estimation*) is likely to be. The *standard deviation of the sampling distribution of a statistic* is called *the standard error* of the statistic.

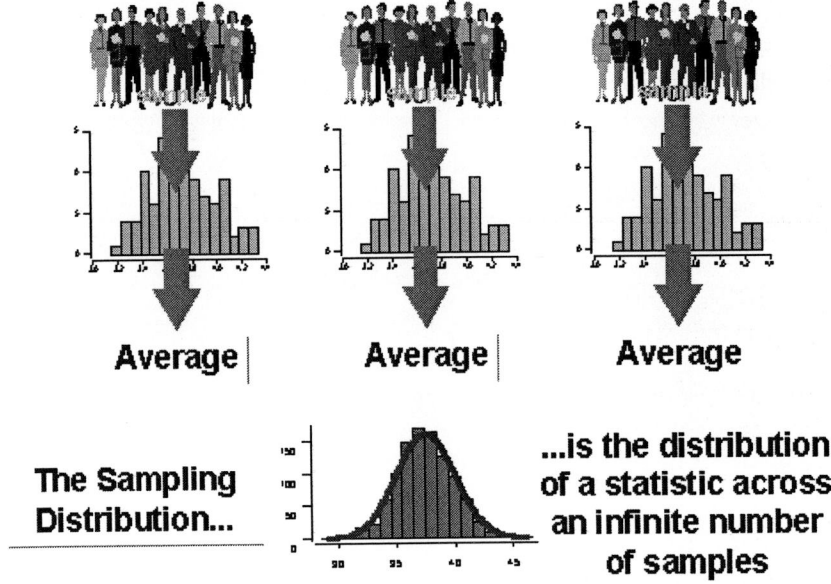

Figure 6. Sampling variation

Properties of the Sampling Distribution of the Mean

PANEL 1

1. Mean of sampling distribution = Mean of population distribution
2. Standard deviation of a sampling distribution of the mean is often referred to as the *standard error*

$$\text{Standard error} = \frac{\text{population standard deviation}}{\text{square root of the sample size}}$$

3 The standard error gives an estimate of *sampling error* or *precision.*
4. The sampling distribution of the mean is approximately Normal for large sample sizes.

The Central Limit Theorem

If a random variable of n observations is selected from a population (even if the population is non-Normal), then when n is sufficiently large, the sampling distribution of $\bar{x}$ (i.e. the mean) will be approximately a Normal distribution. The larger the sample size, the better will be the approximation to Normal distribution, for the sampling distribution of $\bar{x}$ (the mean).

Confidence Interval for a Mean

For data that follows a Normal distribution it is known that 95% of the observed data lies within 2 standard deviations of the mean. Usually the population standard deviation, σ is not known, however s, (the sample standard deviation) can be used instead as it is a reliable estimator of σ .

PANEL 2

Using the sampling distribution of the mean, it follows that $\bar{x}$ (mean) ± 2*standard error is likely to contain the unknown population mean for a sample of size n.

This interval is called **the 95% confidence interval for the population mean** and $\bar{x}$ (mean) ± 2*standard error are the lower and upper 95% confidence limits for the population mean respectively.

For large samples 95% C.I. = $\bar{x}$ (mean) ± (2 x s/$\sqrt{n}$)

For **smaller samples** two aspects may alter:

1. The sample standard deviation, s, which is also subject to sampling variation, may not be a reliable estimate of σ population standard deviation.

2. When the distribution of the population is non-Normal, the distribution of the sample mean may also be non-Normal.

For more information, the reader is referred to the website http://www.ruf.rice.edu/~lane/stat_sim/ sampling_dist/index.html for useful demonstrations of sampling distributions, standard error and the central limit theorem.

Confidence Interval for a Categorical Variable

For data that is categorical it is possible to compute a variety of summary statistics (such as the odds ratio or relative risk) as well as a standard error for these summary statistics (see section on epidemiological study designs for more details). Due to the Central Limit Theorem if the sample is large enough even the natural logarithm of relative risk or odds ratio follows a Normal distribution. As a consequence 95% confidence intervals can be computed in a similar manner to the confidence interval for a mean.

Interpretation of Confidence Intervals

When we calculate confidence limits it is hoped that they will include the true population parameter. To clarify, consider obtaining an infinite number of random samples of size n from a Normally distributed population and computing $\overline{x}$ (mean) for each sample. It is possible to construct a confidence interval based on each computed $\overline{x}$ (mean). If we are calculating 95% confidence limits then *95% of samples from the population will include the true population parameter whilst 5% of samples from the population will not include the true population parameter*. Figure 7 shows 95% CI computed for a 100 studies. The 95% CI for the studies marked XX do not contain the "truth". Note, that for 95 out of 100 studies, the CI contains the truth (and 5 times out of 100 it does not).

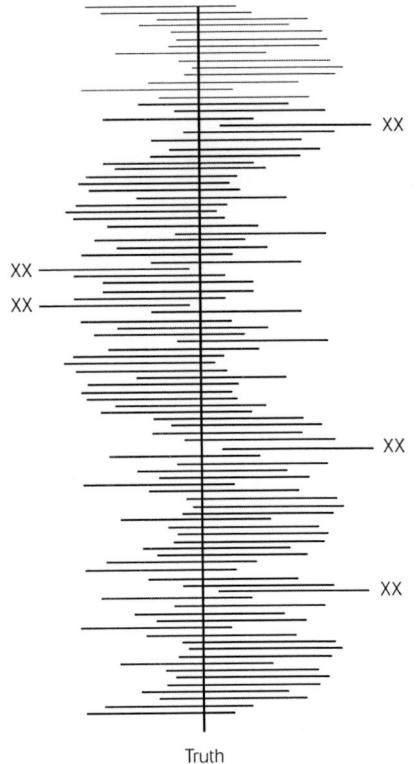

Truth

Reproduced from "Primer on 95% Confidence Intervals" *Effective Clinical Practice,* September/October 2001. 4:229-231. with permission from the American College of Physicians

Figure 7. Interpreting 95% confidence intervals

In other words the probability that a randomly selected interval from this infinite set will contain μ is 0.95. A similar thought process can be used for summary measures for categorical data. Key points to remember about confidence intervals are:

a. Raising the confidence level from 95% to 99% increases the assurance that the confidence interval contains the population mean but it makes the estimate less precise.
b. Any confidence level can be chosen but 95% and 99% are the most common.

For a useful demonstration of confidence intervals the reader is referred to http://www.ruf.rice.edu/~lane/stat_sim/conf_interval/index.html .

Hypothesis Testing

Statistical inference, drawing conclusions about the population on the basis of a sample, can take the form of estimation (confidence intervals) or hypothesis testing. This section concentrates on the hypothesis testing form of statistical inference. Hypothesis testing and significance testing are synonymous terms. Hypothesis testing allows us to measure the strength of evidence which the sample data supply concerning some research question of interest. Before setting up the steps involved in hypothesis testing it is important to consider the research question of interest. Hypothesis tests can be used for a wide variety of research questions such as:

1. Is there a difference in the true risk for brain tumours in people who use cellular phones compared to those who do not?
2. Is fish consumption associated with a true reduced risk of all-cause mortality?

A hypothesis is some testable belief or opinion, and hypothesis testing is the process by which the belief is tested by statistical methods.

Steps of hypothesis testing:

Decide on a null hypothesis, H_0
Decide on an alternative hypothesis, H_1
Calculate the appropriate test statistic
Refer the test statistic to a known distribution it would follow, if the null hypothesis were true
Calculate the probability of obtaining a value as, or more, extreme than the test statistic observed, if the null hypothesis were true
Decide whether the data are consistent or inconsistent with the null hypothesis
State the conclusion in terms of the original research question
In general a statistical package will be employed to implement steps 3-5.

The *null hypothesis* (denoted H_0) is often the negation of the research question that generated the data. In medical research, where comparisons are being made between treatments or different groups of patients, the (null hypothesis) true effect of interest in the population is often zero or unity. The *alternative hypothesis* is usually the opposite of the null hypothesis e.g. that the true effect of interest in the population is not zero. The *alternative hypothesis* (denoted H_1 or H_a) can on occasion specify that the true effect in the population falls in one direction e.g. that the true effect is greater than zero or unity that the true effect is not equal to a certain value. This will result in either a *one sided or two sided alternative hypothesis* respectively.

Example

Research Question: To assess whether the fish consumption is associated with a true reduced risk of all cause mortality.

H_0: fish consumption does not reduce the true risk of all cause mortality
(i.e. true risk = 1)

H_1: fish consumption does reduce risk of all cause mortality (i.e. risk < 1)

One sided alternative hypothesis as this relates to *one-tailed* tests as the *direction of effect is specified.*

Two-sided alternative hypothesis

H_1: fish consumption is associated with all cause mortality (true risk $\neq$ 1). This leads to a *two-tailed* test as *no direction of effect is specified.*

The *test statistic* is calculated from the observed value of the quantity of interest and the value expected if the null hypothesis were true. Most test statistics take the form of

$$\text{test statistic} = \frac{\text{observed value - hypothesised value}}{\text{standard error of observed value}}$$

As mentioned above, in many cases in medical research the hypothesised value will be equal to zero (if continuous) or 1 (if we are investigating a ratio). Therefore the test statistic will be the ratio of the observed value to its standard error. The test statistic should follow a Normal distribution with a mean of zero and with a standard deviation of 1 if the null hypothesis is true (i.e. it represents a Z score).

Results of Hypothesis Testing

PANEL 3

There are only four possible results when we test a given hypothesis.

a. We accept a true hypothesis - a correct decision.
b. We reject a false hypothesis - a correct decision.
c. We reject a true null hypothesis - an incorrect decision. (**Type I error**)
d. We accept a false null hypothesis - an incorrect decision. (**Type II error**).

Type I and Type II Errors

Efforts are made to avoid any type of error but it is not possible to make a correct decision with a 100% certainty when a hypothesis is tested by sampling, there is always the possibility of Type I or Type II errors. The errors are mutually exclusive; an error can be Type I or Type II but not both. The errors are split into two types because there are situations where it is much more important to avoid one type of error than the other. In the statistical literature the probability (Type I error) = α (alpha) and the probability (Type II error) = β (beta). The **power** of a test is **1-probability (Type II error) = 1- β**.

Significance Levels

When a sample is taken to test some hypothesis it is likely that the information gleaned from the sample data (e.g. the sample mean or sample standard deviation) does not completely support the hypothesis. The comparison of the test statistic with the appropriate distribution will return a P-value, which will indicate the probability of obtaining a value as large as or more extreme than the test statistic when the null hypothesis is true. The P value will then be compared to a cut off point, known as a significance level. The cut off level for statistical significance is usually taken as 0.05 (5% significance level) or 0.01 (1% significance level). If the P value is less than the stated cut off, the null hypothesis is not supported. The significance level is the cut off point for the probability that the effect is not due to chance factors. A significance level is the risk that we take in rejecting the null hypothesis in favour of the alternative hypothesis when in reality the null hypothesis is the correct hypothesis (Type I error). The reason why the sample data does not support the hypothesis could be due to either; the original hypothesis being wrong or the sample being slightly unrepresentative (which virtually all samples are to a greater or lesser extent). Hypothesis testing and confidence interval approaches to statistical inference are complementary as shown in Figure 8.

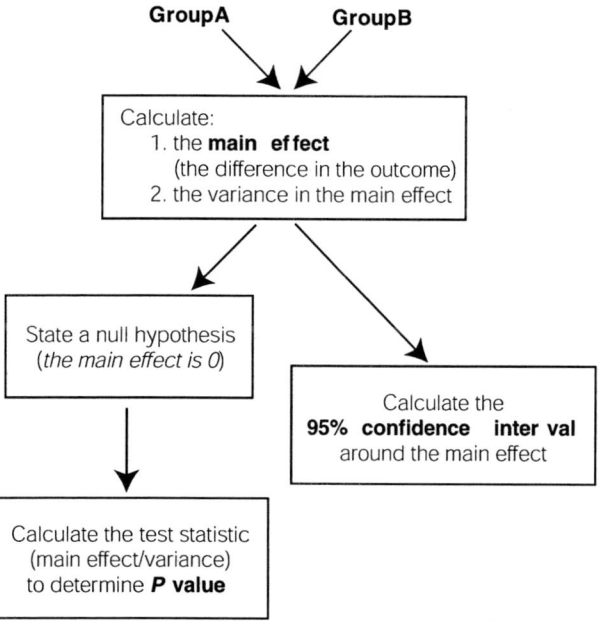

Reproduced from "Primer on 95% Confidence Intervals" *Effective Clinical Practice,* September/October 2001. 4:229-231. with permission from the American College of Physicians.

Figure 8. Comparing hypothesis testing and confidence intervals

The hypothesis tests will show whether the difference, between the hypothesis and the sample data, can be attributed to random (chance) factors or not. If the hypothesis test indicates that the effect is *probably not due to chance factors then the null hypothesis can be rejected and the result is said to be statistically significant.* It is important to note that if we fail to reject the null hypothesis it does not mean that the effect does not exist only that there is *an absence of evidence* that the effect exists. Altman and Bland [4] outline this important concept in terms of interpreting the results of epidemiological studies. Figure 9 shows the general relationship between 95% CI and p-values.

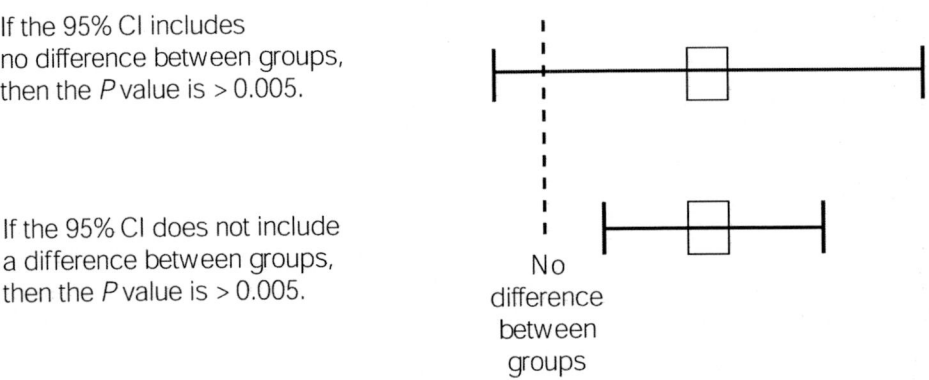

If the 95% CI includes
no difference between groups,
then the *P* value is > 0.005.

If the 95% CI does not include
a difference between groups,
then the *P* value is > 0.005.

No difference between groups

Reproduced from "Primer on 95% Confidence Intervals" *Effective Clinical Practice,* September/October 2001. 4:229-231. with permission from the American College of Physicians.

Figure 9. Relationship between P-value and 95% confidence interval

Summary

In statistical analyses the sample should be representative of the overall population. The main aim to estimate population parameters from our sample and it is important to remember that in the statistical literature Greek letters denote population parameters; Arabic letters denote sample estimates of the population parameters. When dealing with continuous data the standard deviation should be used to describe the degree of variability in the data that has been collected. In contrast the standard error describes the precision of the estimate that has been chosen to summarise the data (usually the mean). In general a large standard error indicates that the *estimate is imprecise.* In terms of confidence intervals a wide confidence interval suggests that the estimate is imprecise whilst a narrow confidence interval suggests that the estimate is precise. When looking at a confidence interval the upper and lower limits can be used to assess the clinical importance of the results. It is thus preferable when presenting study results to give confidence intervals rather than p-values alone as confidence intervals give the reader more information about the evidence presented. It is extremely important to note that in hypothesis testing if we fail to reject the null hypothesis it does not mean that the effect does not exist only that there is an *absence of evidence* that the effect exists.

EPIDEMIOLOGICAL STUDY DESIGNS

There are several study designs that are commonly used in epidemiological investigations (Figure 10). Each of these designs has there own strengths and weaknesses. The aim of this section is to outline the most common study designs encountered in epidemiological research and highlight the aforementioned strengths and weaknesses.

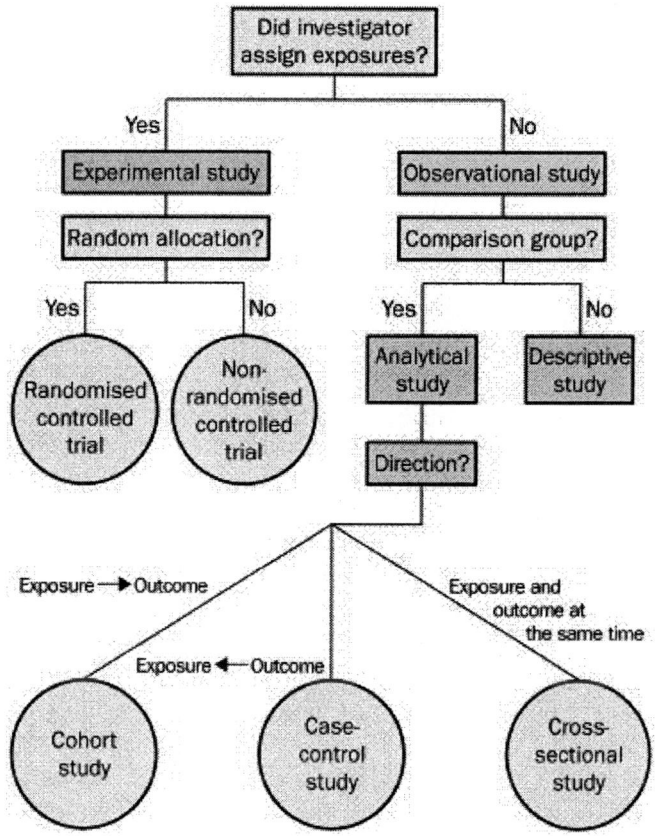

Grimes DA and Schulz K Lancet 2002 (359) 56-61 reproduced with permission.

Figure 10. Different types of epidemiological study

Experimental Studies

Experimental studies refer to epidemiologic studies in which the investigator has complete control over the conditions of the experiment and subjects are randomly assigned to the specific interventions which have been pre-defined. Usually there will be a "control" group where the participants receive either "usual care" or an inactive intervention known as a placebo. The control group is then used in order to compare the effects of the new intervention with "usual care" or the inactive intervention. This type of study design is called randomized controlled trial (RCT). The "uncertainty principle" suggests that if the investigator has sufficient **belief** to expose ½ the subjects and sufficient **doubt** to withhold (not expose) ½ study subjects then the investigator can allocate (by randomisation) which subjects get exposed and which do not. [5]

Parallel versus Crossover Randomized Controlled Trials

There are two main types of trial design, the ***parallel groups*** design (each subject receives only one treatment) and the ***crossover*** design (each subject receives all treatments in random order, often with a washout period between treatments).

Crossover trials are only suitable for chronic reversible diseases i.e. the type of treatments used are palliative rather than curative (giving short term relief only). This sort of design has been used in trials of asthma, hypertension and arthritis. The primary strength of crossover trials is increased efficiency as each subject serves as his or her own control which enables treatment comparisons to be made within subject rather than between subjects. This allows the treatment effect to be estimated with greater precision. The typical data structure for a crossover trial is shown below:

Outcome on Treatment B   ***Outcome on Treatment A***

	Failure	Success	Total
Failure	w	Y	w+y
Success	x	Z	x+z
Total	w+x	y+z	w+x+y+z = n

Rate of failure with treatment A   = (w+x)/(w+x+y+z)
Rate of failure with treatment B   = (w+y)/(w+x+y+z)

Particular interest focuses on the numbers of patients with discordant findings (x and y).

Parallel trials trials are used to compare two groups. Figure 11 shows the design of a typical parallel trial.

Parallel trials can take several difference forms:

Therapeutic clinical trials: These studies are used when a therapeutic agent (usually a drug) or procedure is given in an attempt to cure the disease, relieve the symptoms, or prolong the survival of the subjects involved in the study. The simplest of these types of study may evaluate a new agent or procedure against an existing agent or procedure.

Preventive or prophylactic trials: These studies differ from therapeutic trials in that the subjects are healthy with no existing disease or condition.

Community intervention trials: In some trials it may not be possible to keep experimental and control subjects separated. This is quite common in trials which are trying to implement a behavioral intervention and randomization of individuals is not feasible. In this type of study the intervention (or exposure) under investigation is assigned to groups of healthy subjects on a community-wide basis will all individuals in a community receiving the same intervention.

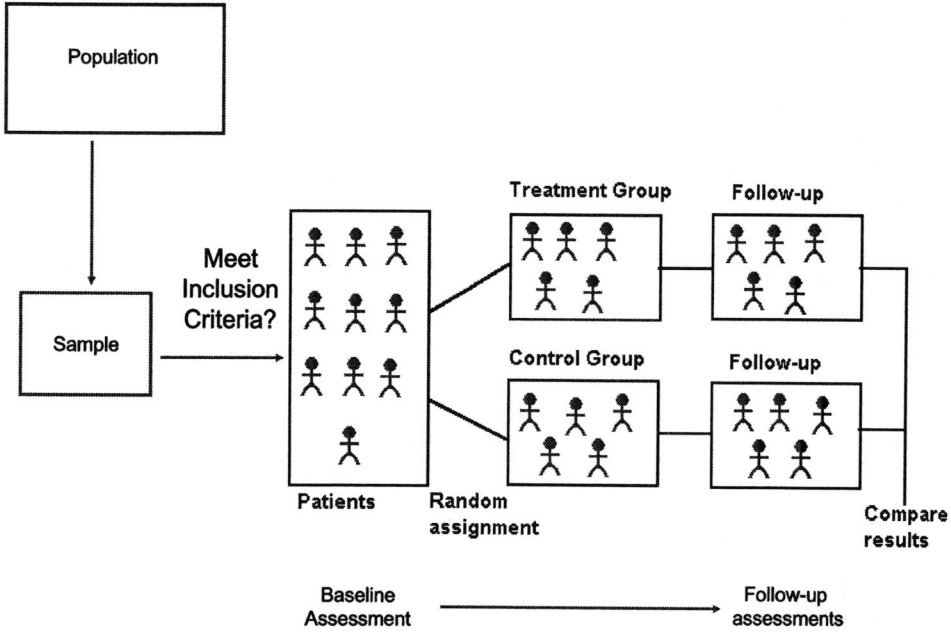

Adapted from SUNY Downstate EBM Tutorial http://library.downstate.edu/EBM2/2200.htm

Figure 11. Diagrammatic representation of parallel trial

The data structure for a typical parallel trial is shown below:

Treatment	*Outcome*		
	Failure	Success	Total
A	A	c	n_A
B	B	d	n_B

Rate of failure with treatment A, R_A = a/(a+c) = a/n_A
Odds on failure with treatment A = a/c
Rate of failure with treatment B, R_B = b/(b+d) = b/n_B
Odds on failure with treatment B = b/d

In parallel trials the ***risk difference*** **(RD)**, the difference in rates between the control group and the treated group, is the most often used measure

$$\text{Risk difference} = b/(b+d) - a/(a+c)$$
$$= R_A - R_B$$

For the difference between two risks ($R_A - R_B$) in a sample size of n_A and n_B, the standard error is calculated as $\sqrt{(R_A(1-R_A)/n_A) + (R_B(1-R_B)/n_B)}$.

The reciprocal of the RD is the ***number needed to treat***, the number of patients who need to be treated to prevent one endpoint (e.g. in a placebo-controlled trial of a drug for stroke it could be the number of patients who must be treated with the drug to prevent one stroke). It is a useful measure in balancing the costs and benefits of treatments.

Experimental studies can give a clear answer to many research questions in epidemiology. For example, despite decades of accumulated non-experimental evidence, the balance of risk and benefits for hormone use in healthy postmenopausal women remained uncertain. The Women's Health Initiative [6] was devised to answer this research question. The study recruited 16,608 postmenopausal women whose uterus was intact at baseline from 40 centres around the US. Participants received either conjugated equine estrogens plus medroxyprogesterone (8506) acetate in 1 tablet or placebo (8102). The trial was intended to run for 8.5 years but was stopped after 5.2 years of follow-up because the overall health risks exceeded the benefits from use of the combined estrogen plus progestin. We shall return to this example later on in this chapter.

Non-Experimental (Observational) Studies

A question which is often posed in medicine is "Does exposure A cause disease B?" It may not be feasible to randomise subjects to these exposures, so instead we must use recording information which is available to us. For example, some people choose to smoke, so we can compare the rates of disease in those who smoke with those who don't. However there may well be other differences in characteristics between smokers and non-smokers. Non-experimental studies are the studies when changes or differences in one characteristic are studied in relation to changes in other(s), without the intervention of the investigator. These studies are commonly used to study *risk factors* (associations between exposure and outcome), assess incidence, prevalence, prognosis, and survival rate in a population.

Rates, Ratios, Numerator and Denominator

Rates: These measure the change in an event over time in a population that is at risk. Rates are the most accurate measure of risk because they measure a population without disease but at risk for a disease in the beginning of the time period and the rate of disease that occurs during the time period.

Ratios: Ratios do not measure the change over time and are used as summary measures and approximations of risk.

To make accurate conclusions about the distributions of disease in a population, it is important to define the *numerator* and *denominator*. This includes knowing whether one or both numbers measures time. It should be defined whether the *numerator is measuring cases or events* and *what population the denominator represents.* Usually the denominator will represent the *person-time* (which is the multiple of the number of individuals over the time period of concern) and could be in years or months (i.e. person-years or person-months). Figure 12 shows a schematic diagram which illustrates the differences between rates and ratios.

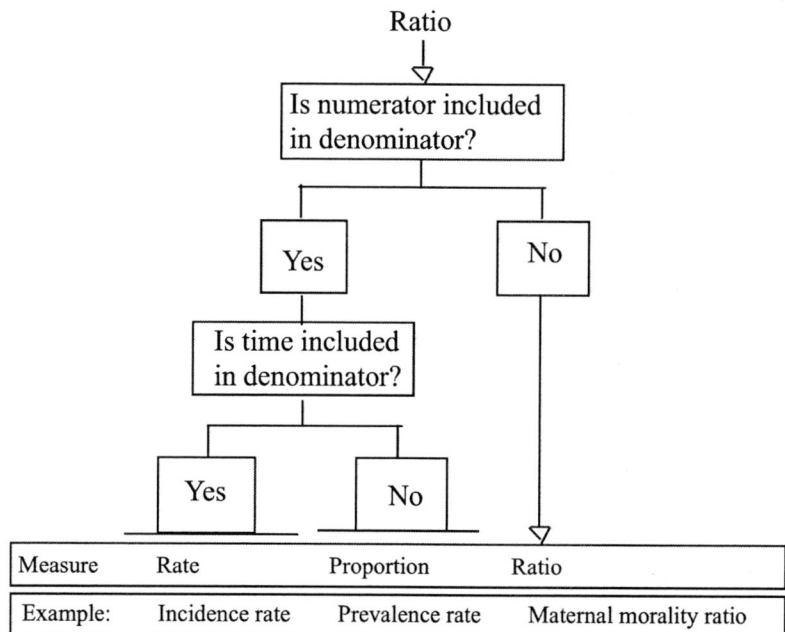

Grimes DA and Schulz K Lancet 2002 (359) 56-61 reproduced with permission from Lancet

Figure 12. Rates, ratios and proportions

Incidence and Prevalence

Non-experimental studies are particularly useful for assessing *prevalence* or *incidence*. *Prevalence* represents the proportion (usually as a percentage) of people with new and old cases of a given disease or condition among the population at risk. *Point prevalence* is the number of people with disease at a point in time. *Period prevalence* is the number of people with disease during a specified time period. *Incidence* is measured by first identifying a population free of the event of interest, and then following them through time with periodic examinations for occurrences of the event.

An *incidence rate* is the number of new cases per unit time i.e.

$$\text{Incidence rate} = \frac{\text{number of new cases of a disease during a given period of time}}{\text{total person-time(years) of observation}}$$

Cumulative incidence is the number of new cases per total population at risk i.e.

$$\text{Cumulative incidence} = \frac{\text{number of new cases of a disease during a given period of time}}{\text{total population at risk}}$$

Mortality rate is number of deaths per unit time i.e.

$$\text{Mortality} = \frac{\text{number of deaths from a disease during a given period of time}}{\text{total person-time(years) of observation}}$$

Case-fatality is number of deaths from a disease as a percentage of all cases of the disease i.e.

$$\text{Case fatality} = \frac{\text{number of deaths from a disease during a given period of time}}{\text{total number of cases of the disease (fatal and non-fatal)}}$$

Attributable risk is a measure of the absolute difference in incidence rates between a group that is exposed to a factor and the incidence rate of a group not exposed to the factor. This is measure enable a researcher to quantify the risk attributed to a particular exposure.

There are three major types of non-experimental studies each of them can be used to compare exposed and unexposed groups: cohort studies (or follow-up studies), cross-sectional studies and case-control studies. These shall now be described in turn.

Cohort Studies

Cohort studies are not as reliable as experimental studies, however, when experimentation to study risk factors of the disease is not possible these types of study are a good way of establishing incidence [i.e. absolute risk] directly. In a cohort study we define a subgroup of the population to follow-up over a period of time. Exposures in the participants are measured at the outset of the study and their disease experience during follow-up is recorded.

Although certain exposures may be measured on a continuous scale (e.g. daily cigarette consumption) it is usual in epidemiological studies to form categories (e.g. <20 per day, $\geq$20 per day). They are then compared with respect to incidence of the disease in each of the groups. There are three approaches to defining the unexposed group in a cohort study (the procedures used to identify new cases of the disease should be similar for the exposed and unexposed groups):

1. *internal comparison*: a single "population" is identified that contains a sufficient number of exposed and unexposed subjects;
2. *external comparison* : an exposed "population" is identified and efforts are made to find another "population" that is unexposed but is similar in other respects to the exposed cohort;
3. *a comparison with the "general" population*: an exposed "population" is identified and comparisons are made with the disease incidence in, for example, the total population of a defined geographic region considered as "unexposed".

Rochon et al [7] give an example of choice of comparison group in a cohort study in order to investigate whether patients who received an atypical antipsychotic drug were at an increased risk of hip fracture. People taking atypical antipsychotic drugs could be compared with either people taking an alternative antipsychotic drug or those not prescribed antipsychotic drugs. These comparisons could then be made in a general population such as all people $\geq$ 55 years of age or in a restricted population (internal or external) such as all people $\geq$ 55 years of age with dementia.

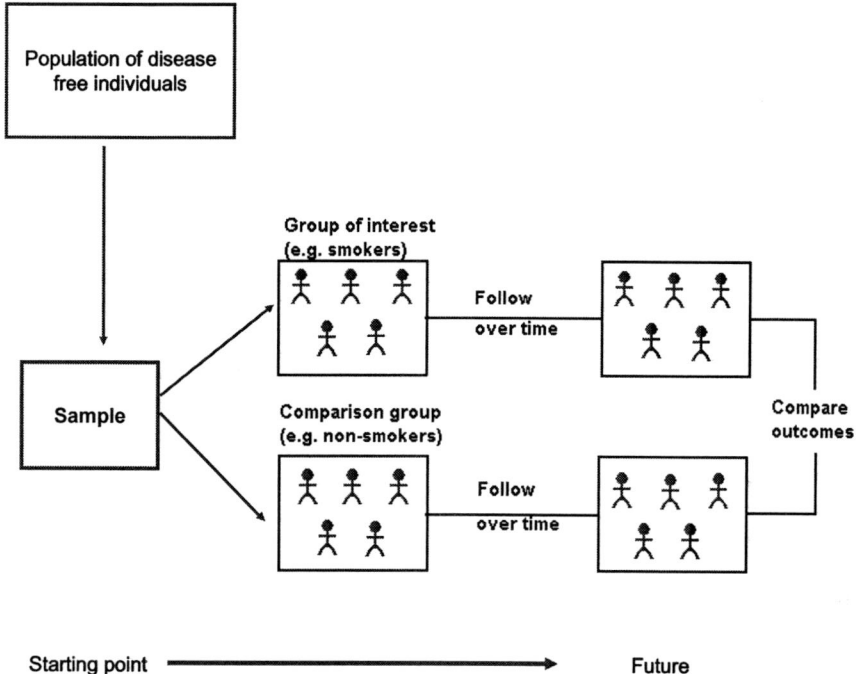

Starting point   ⟶   Future

Adapted from SUNY Downstate EBM Tutorial http://library.downstate.edu/EBM2/2400.htm

Figure 13. Diagrammatic representation of cohort study

In term of timing, cohort studies are generally prospective or longitudinal in nature and can include incidence or mortality studies. When existing records alone are used to conduct the study, this is known as an *historical cohort study* or *retrospective cohort study*. Unfortunately most types of cohort studies are usually time consuming and expensive and such studies that follow-up (or trace less) than 80% of subjects are generally regarded with scepticism. The data structure for a cohort study is below:

Exposure status	**Disease incidence**		Total
	Yes	No	
Exposed	a	c	$n_{Exposed}$
Unexposed	b	d	$n_{Unexposed}$

Risk of disease in exposed $= a/(a+c) = a/n_{Exposed}$
Risk of disease in unexposed $= b/(b+d) = b/n_{Unexposed}$

In cohort studies the **relative risk** is most often used as a measure of effect size. It is the risk of disease in the exposed group relative to the risk of disease in the unexposed group and is sometimes referred to as the **rate ratio**

Relative risk $= \{a/(a+c)\} / \{b/(b+d)\}$

For a natural logarithm of the relative risk ($\log_e$ RR) (a, b, c, and d are table 2 x 2 entries), the standard error is calculated as $\sqrt{1/a - 1/(a+b) + 1/c - 1/(c+d)}$.

An example of a well designed cohort study is the Rotterdam Study [8]. This was a community based prospective cohort study of individuals aged 55 or over. All of the 10,275 residents of a Rotterdam suburb who were over 55 years of age were eligible. 78% of residents agreed to take part and gave consent for the investigators to obtain medical information from their family doctor. Baseline assessments took place between 1990 and 1993 which involved an interview and a medical examination. This took place at the study centre or at the home of the individual whichever was more convenient. 6070 participants with complete data who were free of dementia at baseline were followed up for 2 years. During the mean follow-up of 2.1 years there were 146 incident cases of dementia detected of which 105 were Alzheimer's disease.

Some cohort studies follow-up individuals at equally or unequally spaced intervals and collect repeat measurements on these individuals over time. This enables the individual change or development of a certain outcome variable to be ascertained and whether this change can be related to the changes in other risk factors or exposures can be investigated. One such study was conducted by Meyer and colleagues [9] in order to investigate cognitive performance in women going through menopause. The authors conducted a population-based study with annual follow-up interviews beginning January 1996 through to November 2001.

Cross-Sectional and Survey Studies

Cross-sectional studies measure both the exposure and disease in an individual at some specific point in time. Cross-sectional studies provide information on the frequency of disease in a population at one point in time. Unfortunately, they do not provide direct evidence of the sequence of events and as a consequence only prevalence can be reliably estimated.

Surveys collect information of interest at a particular point in time. They are reliant on questionnaires which can be administered in a variety of ways including by mail or telephone. The type of questions included on the questionnaires can be closed or open ended and the choice is dependent on the nature of the research question of interest. New and insufficiently validated questionnaires should usually be piloted in order to assess how easy the questionnaire is to complete, if all relevant questions have been asked, and if the respondent may have difficulty with particular questions. The sampling scheme is also important for a valid study as the investigator needs to ensure that a representative sample is obtained. Unfortunately surveys can suffer from low response rates which can affect the validity of the results. Lau and colleagues report on a cross-sectional survey of Multiple Sclerosis (MS) patients in Hong Kong among all neurologists between January and June 1999 [10]. The questionnaire covered patients' demographic and clinical characteristics, and details on whether the patients had received computed tomography (CT), MRI or lumbar puncture (involving cerebrospinal fluid [CSF] oligoclonal banding) were recorded. Patient's degree of neurological impairment was assessed by use of the Kurtzke's Expanded Disability Status Scale (EDSS). The number of relapse patients experienced over a two year period

(1997-1998) was recorded as well as past and present treatment. Patients remained anonymous throughout the data collection process and in order to ensure that questionnaires were fully completed, the participants were followed-up by telephone.

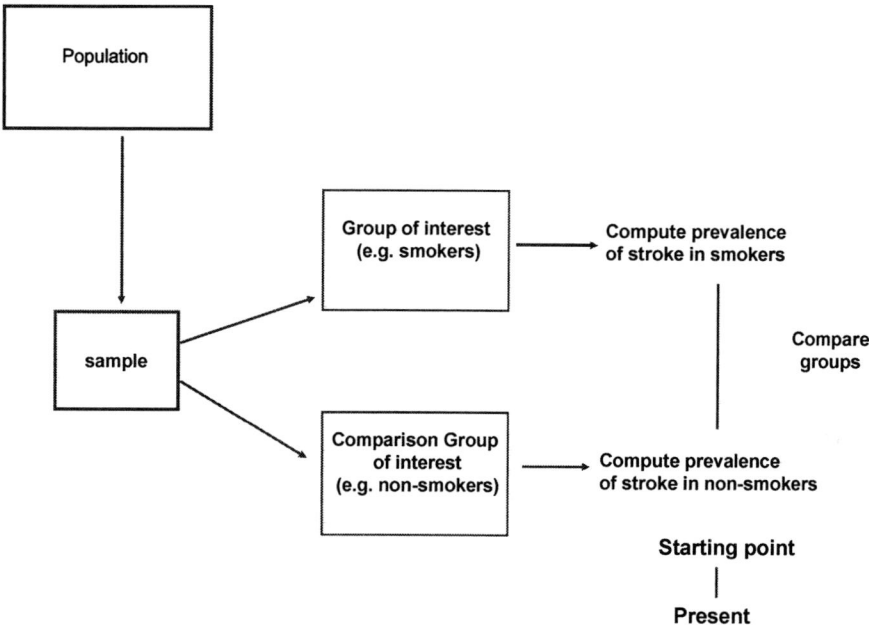

Figure 14. Diagrammatic representation of cross-sectional study

Ecological Studies

The ecological study focuses on the characteristics of population groups rather than their individual members. The unit of analysis is not an individual but a group defined by time (calendar period, birth cohort), geography (country, city), or socio-demographic characteristics (ethnicity, religion). Ecological studies are frequently the first stage of constructing an epidemiological picture of the differential distribution of diseases among people with different risk profiles. Variations in disease risk between different categories of persons can indicate differences in genetic composition, differences in environmental exposures, differences in both genes and environment, or interaction between the two. The kinds of comparisons usually take advantage of routinely collected data and are therefore inexpensive. A note of caution is that a phenomenon known as the *ecological fallacy* occurs when associations seen in the population under study is assumed to be also occurring at the individual level.

Maheswaran and Elliot [11] investigated the hypothesis that living near main roads increases the risk of stroke mortality. They used an ecological study design with 1991 census enumeration districts (CED) as the unit of analysis based on nearly 113.5 thousand CED's in England and Wales. Stroke mortality was based on ICD-9 codes 430-438 from 1990-1992 for men (and women) ≥ 45 years of age. Exposure was calculated as the distance between each

CED population centroid to the nearest main road. A main road was defined as a motorway, primary or A-road. The distance was from each CED centroid to each type of road was computed and the shortest of the three distances was used for analysis. The authors adjusted for socioeconomic deprivation using the Carstairs Index (a widely used scale in the UK) calculated at the CED level. The authors also adjusted for regional variation in stroke mortality using 9 standard regions in England and Wales. The findings were that after adjustment for potential confounding factors men living less than 200m away from a main road were at a 7%; 95%CI: (4%-9%) higher risk of stroke death than men living greater than 1000m away from a main road. A similar finding was found for women 4%; 95%CI: (2%-6%) and men and women combined 5%; 95% CI: (4%-7%).

Case-Control Studies

In a **case-control study** we identify a group of subjects with the disease (the cases) and a second group without the disease (the controls). The frequency of an exposure is then determined in both groups, most usually by retrospective recall by the subjects involved. If more cases are exposed than controls then this is an indication that the exposure may be a risk factor for the disease. These types of study usually estimate the odds of disease but they can be used to estimate relative risk of a rare disease (i.e., arbitrarily, prevalence $\leq$ 5-10%). Case-control studies are sometimes called retrospective studies because they usually start after the onset of disease and look back over time from the outcome at potential exposures [12].

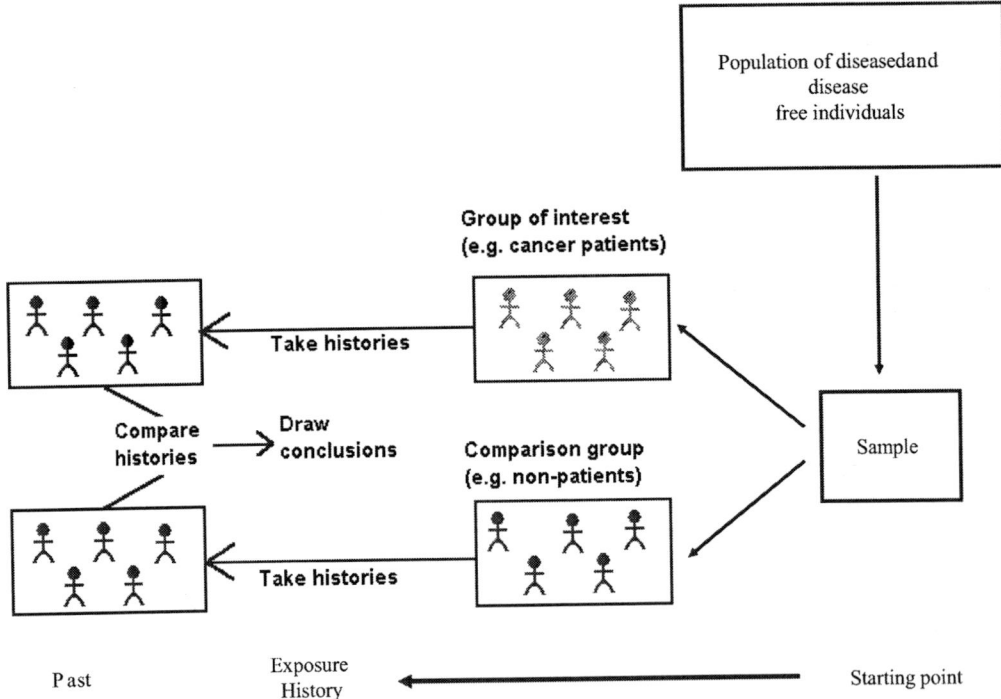

Adapted from SUNY Downstate EBM Tutorial http://library.downstate.edu/EBM2/2500.htm

Figure 15. Diagrammatic representation of case-control study

In case-control studies the *odds ratio* is most often used as the measure of effect. The odds ratio is the ratio of the odds on exposure in those with disease relative to the odds on exposure in those without. The data structure of a case-control study is shown below:

Exposure status	Disease status	
	Case	Control
Exposed	a	c
Unexposed	b	d
Total	n_{Case}	$n_{Control}$

$$\text{Odds ratio} \quad = \{a/b\} \; / \; \{c/d\} \quad = ad \; / \; bc$$

For the natural logarithm of the odds ratio (loge OR) (a, b, c, and d are table 2 x 2 entries), the standard error is calculated as $\sqrt{1/a + 1/b + 1/c + 1/d}$.

For rare diseases the odds ratio calculated from a case control study provides a good estimate of the relative risk as defined in a cohort study. Case-control studies are notorious for many forms of bias. The choice of a suitable control group can be difficult [13] and sometimes controls are individually *matched* with cases to reduce biases. In a *matched* case-control study the most common design is one control matches to each case (ideally the control group reflects the exposure distribution in the entire study population and when it is defined as a random sample of the study population). The data structure for a matched case-control study is shown below:

Exposure status among cases	Exposure status among controls		
	Exposed	Unexposed	Total
Exposed	A	B	A+B
Unexposed	C	D	C+D
Total	A+C	B+D	A+B+C+D = n

Interest is focused on the number of discordant pairs of each type (B and C) and the Odds ratio (OR) is given by:

$$OR = B \; / \; C$$

Choosing two or three controls for each case can be employed for rare diseases to increase the precision of cause-effect estimates. An example of a well designed case-control study is the one performed by Christenson and colleagues [14] to assess the association between cellular telephone use and brain tumours. The authors report on a population-based case control study on 252 people with gliomas and 175 with meingioma compared 822 randomly sampled controls in Denmark. Tumours were differentiated into gliomas and meningioma as they are regarded as two separate diseases. The diagnoses of glioma and meningioma cases were confirmed by histological examination. Controls were a random sample from the Danish Central Population Register and were frequency matched on age (within 5 year ranges) and sex. Face to face interviews were conducted either by a study nurse or a trained medical student and respondents were asked if they had ever used a cellular telephone. If they responded positively to this question they were then asked if they were regular users and how many different types of cellular phone had they used regularly. Start and stop dates of each cellular phones that was used regularly were recorded. The interviewer also asked questions about the number and duration of calls made as well as the pattern of usage over a 6 month period. This information was used to estimate lifetime number of calls and lifetime hours of telephone use. The information recorded for cases and controls on frequency and duration was validated by using the most recently reported cellular telephone information from the two largest networks operators in Denmark. No statistical associations were found between glioma odds ratio (OR):1.08; 95% CI: (0.58-2.00) and meningioma OR: 1.00 95% CI: (0.54-1.28) and the authors concluded that the evidence did not support the hypothesis that cellular telephone use increased the risk of brain tumour.

Case-Reports or Case-Series

Case reports are individual reports on a single patient who may have a rare disease or unusual medical outcome (Figure 16). This type of study is usually reported to promote discussion of ideas and hypotheses about disease frequency, risk, mechanism, prognosis, and possible treatment. They are potentially useful as they could be reporting new and novel clinical results for the first time.

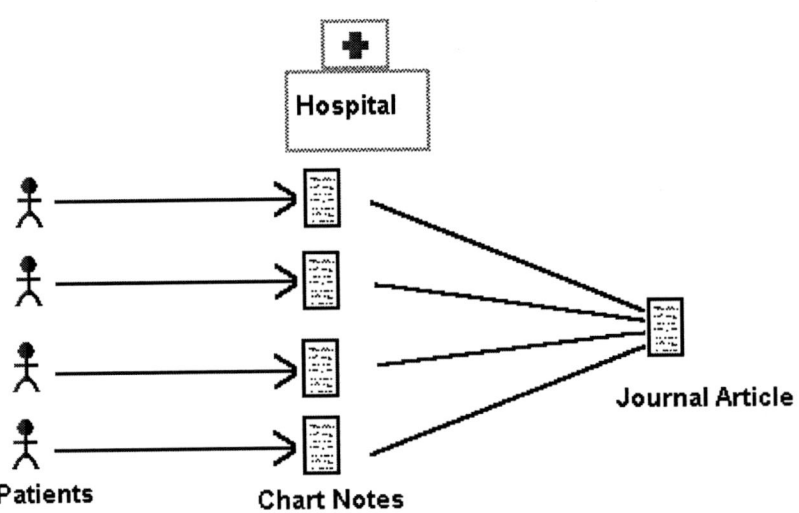

Source: SUNY Downstate EBM Tutorial http://library.downstate.edu/EBM2/2600.htm

Figure 16. Diagrammatic representation of a cse report/series

An example of such as case-study was reported by Finelli [15]. The author reported on a 44-year old man with a 6-week history of progressive left-sided weakness and an 18kg weight loss over several months. A CT scan and a MRI scan showed an area of abnormality consistent with cerebral infarction. The results of routine laboratory tests were normal whilst neurobiological examinations showed a lethargic patient with impaired comprehension. The patient was diagnosed as having progressive multifocal leukoencephalopathy (PML) by the findings of a brain biopsy and cerebrospinal fluid polymerase chain reaction.

A case-series is a report of several cases of the same unusual disease or outcome and may be more useful to the medical community than a single case-report as it may display patterns or tends of interest. Kang and colleagues [16] describe patients with a syndrome combining a variety of symptoms including peripheral neuropathy, visceromegaly, endocrinopathy, monoclonal gammopathy, and skin changes (known as POEMS syndrome). Three patients with acute cerebral infarction associated with POEMS syndrome underwent a structured interview, MRI scan, diffusion-weighted imaging, magnetic resonance angiography, transcranial Doppler ultrasonography, and serum fibrinogen level and C-reactive protein level analysis. The serum fibrinogen before stroke was collected retrospectively from the hospital medical records. There was an elevated fibrinogen level in all patients. The serum fibrinogen level prior to stroke was high in two patients and unilateral or bilateral end artery border-zone infarcts were observed on the brain MRI scan. The authors concluded that elevated fibrinogen might play a role in the pathogenesis of stroke.

INTERPRETING EPIDEMIOLOGICAL STUDIES

When reading the results of an epidemiological study the reader will need to consider the point estimate and confidence interval reported in the manuscript. Figure 17 shows the hypothetical results of three intervention studies.

Study A suggests that the intervention has no effect (i.e. the true relative risk is 1) and is very precise (i.e., the confidence interval is narrow). You can be confident that it is not missing an important difference.

Study B suggests that the intervention has no effect (i.e., the true RR is 1) but is very imprecise (i.e., the confidence interval is wide). This study may be missing an important difference. An investigator should be worried about type II error, but this study is just as likely to be missing an important harmful effect as an important beneficial one.

Study C suggests that the intervention has a clinically important beneficial effect (i.e., the true RR is much less than 1) and is also very imprecise. A large part of the confidence interval includes clinically important beneficial effects. As a consequence of this an investigator might be concerned that a type II error is very likely. This is a study that should be repeated using a larger sample.

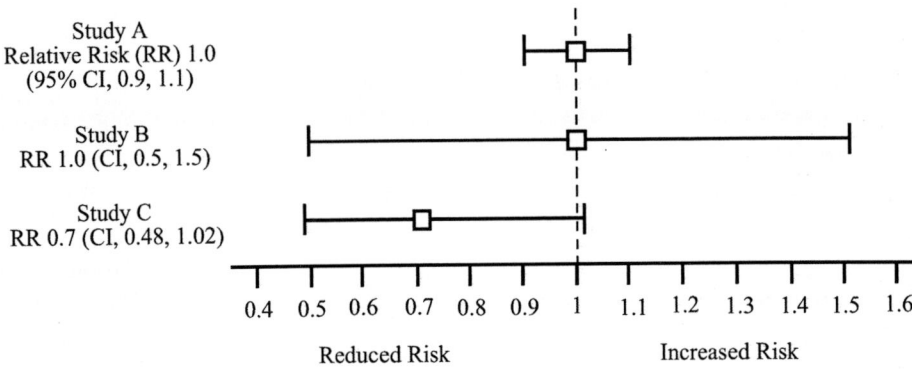

Figure 17. Role of 95% CIs in assessing type II errors

Sample Size

Sample size of a study is extremely important because if a study is too small then it is unlikely that the investigators will be able to detect small but clinically important difference. Conversely, if a study is too large then time and resources will be wasted. Prior to the commencement of a study the investigators should therefore spend a reasonable length of time deciding on a feasible sample size required in order to meet the goals of the study. The required sample size for a study depends on four criteria:

- The minimum clinically relevant effect size that you wish to detect for the endpoint of interest.
- The required power of the study (usually set at 80% or 90%).
- The required significance level (usually set at 5%).
- The variance of the endpoint or outcome of interest.

There are many different formulae for computing the required sample size which depend on the design of the study (e.g. case-control or cohort) and the nature of the endpoint under study (e.g. time to event or dead or alive). There are many free computer software programs that compute sample size for the most common endpoints and study designs and these are available at http://members.aol.com/johnp71/javasta2.html#Biostatistics. Some other software packages that can compute sample size for more complex endpoints such as survival have been reviewed by Iwane and colleagues [17]. For both standard errors and confidence intervals it is possible to increase precision by collecting a larger sample.

Ethical Issues

Since the investigator is actively intervening rather than just observing, ethical considerations are more important in experimental studies than other types of epidemiological study. Ensuring that the study is ethical is primarily the responsibility of the investigator(s). However, whether a study is judged to be ethical or unethical is a subjectively based on cultural norms, which vary greatly between countries, groups within countries, and over time. When conducting experimental studies it is usual to obtain approval from a research ethics committee (also known as Institutional Review Boards) who will be concerned with informed consent (do participants in the study fully understand the risks as well as the benefits of the study), autonomy (are participants physically and mentally capable of deciding what they will allow to be done to them), and whether there is sufficient uncertainty to justify randomization. It is unethical to conduct a study that has not been properly planned and inadequate attention to sample size is considered a serious issue.

Summary

Different study designs can be performed in epidemiology and are more appropriate in some situations than others. Ecological studies aim to assess exposures at a community level rather than at an individual level. Case-control studies are more appropriate when the investigator wishes to determine the risk of a disease in a group of individuals with a disease compared to those without. Cross-sectional studies are useful for estimating the prevalence of a disease but cannot make firm conclusions about risk. Cohort studies are more appropriate when the investigator wishes to obtain the incidence of a disease. Randomised controlled trials are the gold standard designs to study effectiveness of the intervention under investigation.

BIAS IN EPIDEMIOLOGICAL STUDY DESIGNS

Bias is a systematic error that leads to a systematic difference between groups. There are several types of biases:

Selection bias: This type of bias occurs when the selection of the study participants for a case-control or cohort study are somehow related to the exposure of interest.

Information bias: This occurs when the information that has been collected is incomplete or incorrect for some reason. This can lead to misclassification bias where subjects are incorrectly assigned to one group when they should be in another. *Non-differential misclassification bias* applies to the situation when the degree of misclassification in the groups is of the same magnitude and can lead to underestimation of the effect. *Differential-misclassification* is much more serious as the degree of misclassification differs between the groups and can lead to either over- or under-estimation of the effect. *Recall bias* can occur in case-control studies when there is a difference between cases and controls in the accuracy and completeness of exposure information.

Measurement bias: This occurs when the methods of measurements are consistently dissimilar among groups of participants, or if the presence of the outcome directly affects one of the following: [a]the exposure, [b] the subject's recollection of the exposure, and [c] the measurement or recording of the exposure;

Confounding bias: A confounding factor must be a risk factor for the disease among the non-exposed, and be associated with the exposure variable in the population from which the cases derive (see figure 18a). The example of a confounder is taken from Kahn and Sempos [18] which shows that grey hair is related to any disease such as stroke which is also age-related. However, this does not imply that grey hair is a risk factor for stroke, as grey hair is caused by the aging. A confounder must not be an intermediate variable in the casual path between the exposure and the disease (figure 18b). In the example smoking and fibrinogen are risk factors for stroke but smoking increases fibrinogen which in turn increase the risk of stroke [19]. Controlling for fibrinogen as well as smoking would mean that an overcorrection would be performed. Confounding bias occurs when two factors of processes are interrelated and it has been incorrectly concluded that one of the factors is the causal factor.

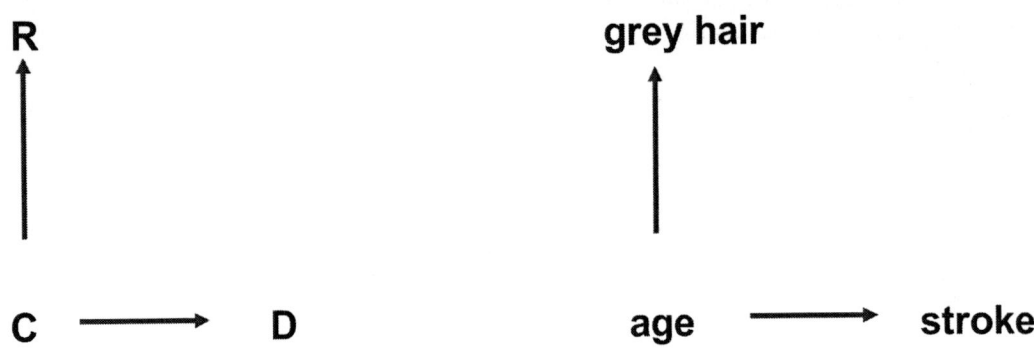

Figure 18a. C is a confounding factor, R is a risk factor and D is the disease

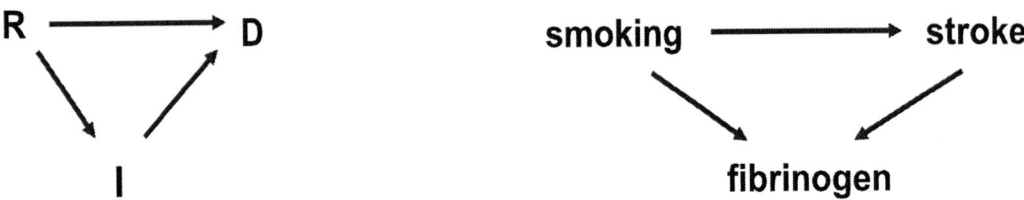

Figure 18b. I is an intermediate factor, R is a risk factor and D is the disease

Practical Ways to Control for Bias in Non-Experimental Studies

For any non-experimental study bias can be reduced at the design stage or the analysis stage (minimising bias at the design stage of the study is the best approach, and not all biases can be dealt with at the analysis stage). At the design stage of a non-experimental study bias can controlled by two strategies: (1) *Restriction* – strict inclusion and exclusion criteria can be applied in order to produce homogeneous groups; (2) *Matching* - for each patient in one group (individual matching) or for groups of patients (frequency matching) with a particular disease (outcome) in the index series, one or more disease-free subjects (unexposed people in a cohort study or controls in a case-control study) with the same characteristics and potential confounding factors are selected for a comparison group. At the analysis stage the following three approaches are common to assess whether bias is present or to control for bias. *Stratification* can be used which compare rates within subgroups [strata] of subjects with otherwise similar risk.

Standardization is used to give equal weight of crude rates to strata to be compared; standardization is a procedure that exemplifies one type of stratified analysis. Standardization of rates is commonly used when comparing mortality rates or incidence rates across populations. Examples include comparing geographical regions (such as cities or counties) or certain groups (such as different occupations or ethnicities). There are two forms of standardisation procedure known as *direct standardization* and *indirect standardization*.

Direct standardization is used to compare category-specific rates observed in two or more populations for each of which the category-specific rates are known; it's defined as a sum of weighted average of the category-specific rates according to the weights distribution taken from the standard population (sum of the category-specific rates in the study population multiplied by their observed category-specific weights of the standard population).

Example

Since age is positively correlated with most chronic diseases and risk of death, and since most populations have different age structures, age adjusted rates need to be computed in order to make fair comparisons across populations. This is a fictional example that gives the death rates from stroke in two cities City X and City Y. The combined city X and Y data will be used as the standard population in this example.

Table 2a: Death Rates from stroke in two cities X and Y

Age	CITY X			CITY Y		
	Population	Number of deaths	Death Rate	Population	Number of deaths	Death Rate
50-69	20000	250	0.0125	5000	50	0.01
70-79	10000	250	0.025	10000	500	0.05
80+	5000	250	0.05	20000	800	0.04
Total	35000	750		35000	1350	

Table 2b: Combined death rates of cities X and Y

COMBINED CITY X AND Y		
AGE	*POPULATION*	*DEATHS*
50-69	*25000*	*300*
70-79	*20000*	*750*
80+	*25000*	*1050*
TOTAL	*70000*	*2100*

Table 3: Expected deaths in cities X and Y

Age	Expected deaths for City X and City Y	
	City X expected deaths	City Y expected deaths
50-69	312.5	250
70-79	500	1000
80+	1250	1000
Total	2062.5/70000=0.0295	2250/70000=0.0321

The 0.0295 and 0.0321 are the standardized incidence rates for City X and City Y respectively. The ratio of the two standardized incidence rates is 0.0295/0.032=0.91. This suggests that individuals in City X have approximately 9% less chance of having a stroke compared to those in city Y.

Indirect standardization is used to compare two populations in one of which the specific rates are not known or, if known, are unreliable due to a small number of events. This method, instead of supplying the weighted distribution, supplies a standard set of rates, which are then weighted to the distribution of the population under study to obtain an "expected" rate in the study population (the expected number is obtained by multiplying the category-specific rates of the standard population by the denominators in each category of the study population; the total of category-specific expected rates is the overall number of expected rates in the study population). A common way to express the results is the standardized morbidity or mortality ratio (SMR) which is the ratio of the number of overall observed rates in the study population to the number of the overall expected rates in the study population (the SMR of the standard population is always 1, since the expected number of cases in this population is the same as the observed number; the SMR of the study population may take on any value).

Example

If we want to compare the same two cities but some of the information about one of the cities was missing we can employ indirect standardisation.

Table 4: Death rates for city X unknown, death rates for city Y available

AGE	CITY X			CITY Y		
	POPULATION	NUMBER OF DEATHS	DEATH RATE	POPULATION	NUMBER OF DEATHS	DEATH RATE
50-69	20000	?	?	5000	50	0.01
70-79	10000	?	?	10000	500	0.05
80+	5000	?	?	20000	800	0.04
TOTAL	35000	750		35000	1350	

Table 5: City X expected deaths assuming city Y death rates

AGE	CITY X EXPECTED DEATHS
50-69	200
70-79	500
80+	200
TOTAL	900

Standardised Mortality Ratio =observed deaths/expected deaths

SMR =750/900=0.833

This suggests that individuals in City X have 17% less risk of developing stroke than those in city Y.

Finally, **statistical adjustment** can be employed in which a number of potential confounders are identified and these are included in a multivariable statistical model (such as a regression analysis, discussed later). . Grimes and Schulz give a thorough overview of biases and how to control for them in epidemiological studies [20]

Practical Ways to Control for Bias in Experimental Studies

For an experimental study there are several ways to reduce the problem of bias. These are:

(1) **Randomization:** assign patients to groups in a way that gives each patient an equal chance of falling into one or the other group this should ensure that all factors are balanced between groups. Altman and Bland outline some common methods of randomisation used in experimental studies [21]. Commonly accepted methods of administering the randomisation include: centralised randomization by computer or telephone, randomization scheme controlled by pharmacy, numbered or coded containers administered sequentially to enrolled participants, on site computer system which can only be accessed after entering the characteristics of an enrolled participant, and sequentially numbered sealed opaque envelopes. Commonly unaccepted methods of administering randomisation are: via sealed envelopes but not sequentially numbered or opaque, alternation, date of birth, day of week, or open list of random numbers.

(2) **Having a comparison group:** In a controlled trial one of the treatments is included in the trial as a basis for comparison. It may be either an **active** treatment or a **placebo**. A true placebo is an inert or inactive treatment otherwise identical to the treatment (intervention) under investigation in term of appearance, taste, frequency and mode of administration (e.g. oral), for example a pill containing an inactive substance. Placebos are often used when the trial is to be conducted in a **blinded** fashion.

(3) **Blinding or masking:** Blinding (or masking) is necessary so that there is no risk of knowledge of the treatment received can influence the assessment of the patient. Blinding (or masking) can be single, double or triple in a clinical trial setting. In a single-blind study only the investigators are aware of the treatment the participant is receiving. In a double-blind

study neither the participant nor the investigators know the treatment assigned. Finally, in a triple-blind study the investigators, participants and the data analyst/data monitoring committee do not know the identity of the treatment groups. Day and Altman discuss practical ways to blind an RCT and other studies [22].

*(4) **Have a high compliance (adherence) rate:*** Compliance (adherence) is defined as the extent to which patients follow the treatment or medical advice under investigation. The efficacy of an intervention is the benefit of among patients who actually receive the treatment (i.e. these people follow the trial protocol exactly). Therapeutic effectiveness is the benefit of intervention being studied under the usual clinical practice among patients who are offered the treatment (i.e. the participants do not necessarily follow the trial protocol exactly and is thus considered a more accurate reflection of "real life"). In the PROGRESS trial [23] which had a mean duration of follow-up of 3.9 years in 6105 patients randomised treatment was continued for 86% among those assigned active and 87% assigned placebo

*(5) **Employ an intention-to-treat analysis:*** All patients randomly allocated to one of the treatments in a trial should be analyzed together as representing that treatment, whether or not they completed, or indeed received that treatment [24]. A *** per protocol analysis*** (where participants are only included in the final analysis if they follow the trial protocol exactly) can also be used as a sensitivity analyses. As a consequence the advantages of randomization are diminished based on the proportion of patients who were lost to follow-up or were excluded from the final analysis for other reasons.

Mendelian Randomisation Studies

"Mendelian randomization" refers to the random assortment of genes transferred from parent to offspring at the time of gamete formation and has been compared to a randomized control trial of genetic variants (see figure 19).

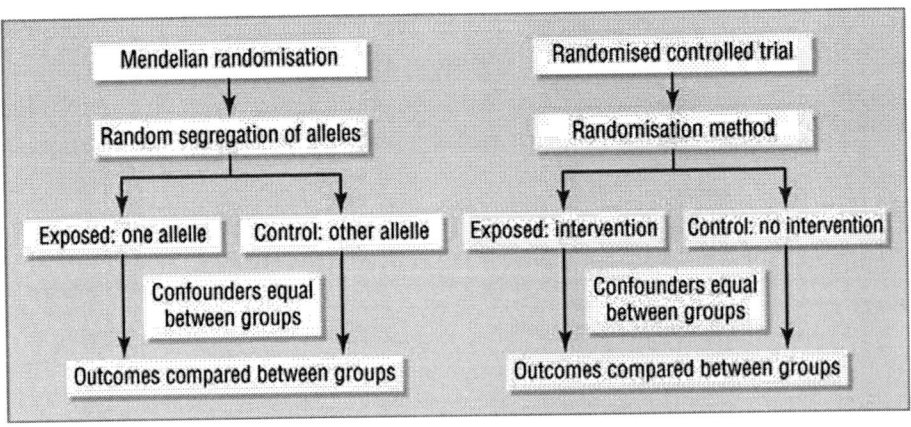

Figure 19. Comparison of design of Mendelian randomisation studies and randomised controlled trials Davey Smith, G. et al. BMJ 2005;330:1076-1079 reproduced with permission from the BMJ Publishing Group

In a genetic association study if a particular polymorphism is known to affect the levels but not the function of a potential risk factor then differences in this potential risk factor due to genotype will have been established from birth. With adequate control for population structure the opportunity for bias and confounding due to environmental factors is greatly reduced [25] Davey-Smith and Ebrahim [26] have outlined some of the potential benefits of investigating epidemiological associations using this approach (panel 4).

Elevated plasma total homocysteine concentrations have been associated with risk of stroke, but it is uncertain if these associations are causal [27]. Several studies have investigated the relationship between the 677 C→T polymorphism for the methylenetetrahydrofolate reductase (*MTHFR*) gene (that is associated with elevated homocysteine concentrations) and stroke using Mendelian randomisation approach to the analysis. One such study by Alluri et al [28] found that the prevalence of CT and TT genotypes in patients with arterial stroke were 30% and 1.4% compared to 2.4% and 0% in controls. Patients with arterial stroke had homocysteine values almost twice as large as controls. The authors suggested that MTHFR evaluation may help in preventing or reducing the morbidity caused by stroke. However, studies using "Mendelian randomization" should be interpreted with caution due to several issues (see panel 5).

**Panel 4: Problems in observational epidemiology
where Mendelian randomization may help**

Confounding
Reverse causation
Biological
through exposure assignment
Due to reporting bias
Associative selection bias (Berkson's bias)
Attenuation by errors (regression dilution bias)

Davey-Smith,G and Ebrahim S.(2004), Mendelian randomization: prospects, potentials, and limitations. International Journal of Epidemiology, 33: 30 - 42. Reproduced with permission from Oxford University Press.

Panel 5: Limitations of Mendelian randomization

Failure to establish reliable genotype—intermediate phenotype or genotype—disease associations

---

Confounding of genotype—intermediate phenotype—disease associations

Pleiotropy and the multi-function of genes

Canalization and developmental compensation

Lack of suitable polymorphisms for studying modifiable exposures of interest

---

Davey-Smith,G and Ebrahim S.(2004), Mendelian randomization: prospects, potentials, and limitations. International Journal of Epidemiology, 33: 30 - 42. Reproduced with permission from Oxford University Press.

Summary

For simplicity, we have only concentrated on the most common epidemiological study designs. However, there are several other designs such as case-crossover, nested case-control, case-cohort and record linkage studies that are described in the recommended reading list (see reference 15, Essential Epidemiology). There are several biases that are present in non-experimental epidemiological studies. The most serious of these is confounding. While matching can prevent confounding in a cohort study, it has some disadvantages in a case-control study because (a) it may introduce confounding if the matching factor is unrelated to disease in the study population but is correlated with the exposure; (b) if a factor has been matched, it is no longer possible to estimate the effect of that factor, since its distribution is forced to be identical for cases and controls, and (c) it adds analytic complexity requiring multivariable analysis to control confounding by factors that have not been matched. Greenhalgh has produced a very readable article which outlines some of the methodological issues that should be considered when interpreting the results of different study designs [29]. Mendelian randomization is emerging as a promising new epidemiological technique to remove the effects of confounding. However, it is not without limitations and the results of such studies still need to be interpreted with caution.

SOME COMMON STATISTICAL TESTS

The statistical tests which that will be described are used when the variable of interest is *continuous and Normally distributed*. Tests which assume the data follows a Normal distribution are called *parametric tests.* When there are more than one group of observations it is essential to distinguish the case where the data are *paired* (dependent) from that where the groups are *independent.*

Comparison of Means in Two Related (Paired) Samples - Paired T-Test (One-Sample T-Test)

This test is used when we have ***related data (dependent)*** i.e. when the same individuals are studied more than once, or when two different groups of subjects have been individually matched (as in a matched case-control study).

Examples

Barber et al.[30] conducted a matched case-control study to determine whether prior drug treatment (with anticoagulant or antiplatelet agents) or early adverse physiological features (such as hypoxia) were associated with progression of ischemic stroke. 196 cases of progressing ischemic stroke were matched with 196 controls by age and stroke type. The Normally distributed characteristics of the cases and controls such as blood pressure (systolic and diastolic) were compared via a paired t-test. Statistically significant differences were found between SBP on admission between cases and controls (mean difference =10mmHg $p=0.003$), no differences were found between DBP and mean arterial blood pressure (MABP).

Comparison of the Means of Two Independent Groups – Independent T-Test (2-Sample T-Test)

Examples

Research Question: A new drug to treat hypertension has been discovered. How does this new drug (Drug A) compare to the conventional antihypertensive agent (Drug B) for the treatment of hypertension in the adult population in controlling blood pressure? Patients were randomly allocated to receive either Drug A or Drug B.

When we have two independent samples we would use the unpaired t -test to assess whether there is a significant difference between the two samples. If this P value is small (<0.05) then it is unlikely that the effect observed is due to random (chance) factors. The P value will indicate whether there is sufficient evidence to reject the null hypothesis and conclude that in the population there does appear to be a difference in the effectiveness of the two drugs in controlling blood pressure. The t-test is demonstrated at the following website http://www.kuleuven.ac.be/ucs/java/ using both a paired t-test (one-sample) and an unpaired t-test (two-sample).

Comparison of Categorical Data

Sample proportions may be used to draw inferences about the equivalent proportions in the population from which the sample was taken. As with continuous variables, these inferences may be expressed as confidence intervals or hypothesis tests. Lau and colleagues report on a cross-sectional survey of Multiple Sclerosis (MS) patients in Hong Kong among all neurologists between January and June 1999 [10]. The questionnaire covered patients' demographic and clinical characteristics, and details on whether the patients had received computed tomography (CT), MRI or lumbar puncture (involving cerebrospinal fluid [CSF] oligoclonal banding) were recorded. Patient's degree of neurological impairment was assessed by use of the Kurtzke's Expanded Disability Status Scale (EDSS). The number of relapse patients experienced over a two year period (1997-1998) was recorded as well as past and present treatment. Fifty-three Chinese MS patients were identified, of whom 48 were women and 5 were men. Fifty-one patients had already been diagnosed by neurologists, while the two other patients were diagnosed after reviewing their hospital records. Fifty-two of the 53 patients had MRI and/or CT scans of the brain/spinal cord. Of these, 46 had abnormalities that were consistent with MS. It was noted that only 25 of the 53 patients had their CSF sent for oligoclonal banding, a test that helps confirm the diagnosis of MS. The overall prevalence rate was estimated to be 0.77 per 100,000 people. The authors concluded that MS in Hong Kong Chinese has a low prevalence, a high female to male ratio, and a low cerebrospinal fluid oligoclonal banding presence.

Comparison of Proportions from Two Independent Groups

Chi Squared Test

Research question: Is there a difference between the true proportion of men who are current smokers with the true proportion of women who are current smokers?

Another way of expressing this question is whether the two variables are **associated** or not; is there *an association* between gender and smoking status. A contingency table of the two categorical variables can be constructed.

	Male	Female	Total
Current smoker	40	42	82
Non smoker	80	110	190
Total	120	152	272

To test the null hypothesis of no association, we could construct a table similar to the one above which contains the values we would expect to see if the null hypothesis were true (i.e. if the two variables were not associated). A test of the null hypothesis could reasonably be based on the difference between the observed and expected values (approximated by $(40*110)/(80*42)$); such a test, is known as the *chi-squared test.* The value of the test statistic will then be compared with the appropriate Chi squared distribution. For general two-dimensional tables the *degrees of freedom* are derived from the formula $(r-1) \times (c-1)$, where r is the number of rows and c the number of columns. The larger the observed chi-squared statistic is, the more evidence there is that the two variables are associated, and the less likely it is that they are really independent. In this example the chi-squared statistic $=1.31$ and is not statistically significant at the conventional 5% level of significance. Thus there is no evidence of an association in this example (i.e. we cannot reject the null hypothesis that the true proportion of male and female smokers is the same). For very small sample sizes can use *Fisher Exact test* for association as an alternative.

Comparison of Proportions from Two Related Groups

If we want to conduct a case-control study of disease and an exposure in which cases and controls are closely matched on potential confounders. For analysis we must take into account the matching. Matched pairs are classified as follows:

Exposure status among cases	*Exposure status among controls*		
	Exposed	Unexposed	Total
Exposed	A	B	A+B
Unexposed	C	D	C+D
Total	A+C	B+D	A+B+C+D = n

In this table, cells A and D contain counts of the **concordant pairs** (case-control pairs-members are same with respect to exposure status) and cells *B* and *C* contain counts of **discordant pairs** (case-control pairs-members are different with respect to exposure status). The **odds ratio** estimate is the ratio of case-positive to case-negative matched pairs:

$OR = B / C$

This matched pairs test is formally known as **McNemar test**. Suppose that in studying 50 matched-pairs (100 people total) we find:

	Control pair-member is E+	Control pair-member is E-
Case pair-member is E+	5	30
Case pair-member is E-	10	10

Therefore, $OR = 30 / 10 = 3$.

The chi-square statistic = $(B-C)^2/(B+C) = (30-10)^2/40 = 10$ on 1 degree of freedom; this is statistically significant at the conventional 5% level of significance. So there is evidence to suggest that there is an increased odds of disease for the exposure of interest.

Summary

Statistical tests are extremely common in epidemiological research. The investigator should state clearly the research question they are trying to answer as well as choosing the correct statistical test to analyse the data. It is important to note that if we fail to reject the null hypothesis it does not mean that the effect does not exist only that there is *an absence of evidence that the effect exists*. The fact that an investigator has not found any evidence to reject the null hypothesis could be due to an inadequate sample size. In a case-control or cohort study one way to decide whether there are confounding factors is to compare baseline characteristics between study groups using statistical tests such as the t-test (for example to compare age) or chi-square tests (for example to compare smoking history) with statistically significant differences being taken as an indicator of potential confounding.

SOME MORE ADVANCED STATISTICAL TESTS

Comparison of More Than Two Means (ANOVA)

The independent samples t-test compares the means across two groups. It would be incorrect to use this t-test to compare each pair of groups. If there are three groups this would involve 3 individual t-tests, 4 groups will result in 7 individual t-tests etc. As the number of groups increases so does the number of tests that require to be applied to the data, this increases the chance that a significant difference will be detected between one of the pairs when in fact the null hypothesis is true (increases chance of Type I error). The appropriate statistical test for when there are more than two groups is **Analysis of Variance (ANOVA)**.

Assumptions of Analysis of Variance

There are two assumptions of analysis of variance which are required to be satisfied. The data should come from Normal distributions within the groups and the variances of these distributions should be the same (homoscedasticity assumption). Muir et al [31] report a dose finding trial of the sodium channel blocker sipatrigine in patients who had been clinically diagnosed within 12 hours of stroke. Twenty –seven patients were assigned to either placebo or four different doses of sipatrigine and their outcome at 30 days or three months was assessed via Barthel or Rankin scores as well as recording routine laboratory measurements. The authors compared blood pressure and heart rate for the 5 groups using ANOVA and found no statistically significant cardiovascular effects for blood pressure (p=0.89) and heart rate (p=0.20).

Transformations

Most of the statistical methods that have been described make some assumptions about the data and these assumptions need to be checked in order to ascertain whether the results are robust. If the assumptions of the methods are not met then it may be necessary to transform the data. There are three reasons why a transformation may be necessary:

1. To Normalise distributions
2. To eliminate heterogeneity of variance
3. To linearise relationships

The advantage of a transformation is that it may allow the use of **parametric methods (i.e. methods that make some assumtptions about the distribution of the data)**. The disadvantage is that the units of the transformed variable usually mean interpretation is less convenient as well as extra computation being required. The most common transformations are:

Logarithmic y = Loge (x) (x> 0)

Square root y = √x   (x > 0)

Logit (or logistic) y = loge (p/(1-p)) which is the log of the odds ratio   (0 < p < 1)

Inverse y=1/x (x>0)

Transformations to Normalise Distributions

Skewness is a measure of the asymmetry of a distribution. The Normal distribution is symmetric, centred around the mean and therefore has no skewness. *Positively skewed* distributions have a long right tail (figure 20a) and the median is a better measure centrality than the mean. An investigator could try the logarithmic, reciprocal, or square root transformations depending on the extent of the positive skewness to Normalise the data. *Negatively skewed* distributions have a long left tail (figure 20b) and once again the median is better measure of centrality than the mean. The investigator could try the square or cubic transformations depending on the extent of the negative skewness to Normalise the data. These transformations are useful when the assumptions of the t-test or ANOVA are not met [32].

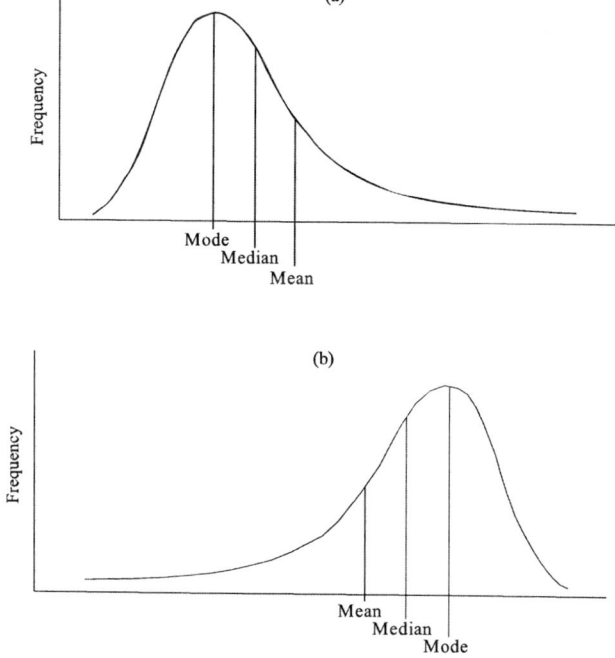

Figure 20. Illustration of skewness (a) positive; (b) negative

Transformations to Eliminate Heterogeneity of Variance

If we have unequal variation can try logarithmic, reciprocal, or square root transformations in order to remedy the situation. These transformations are most common when this particular assumption of the t-test, ANOVA or regression based methods (discussed later) are not met.

Non-Parametric Tests

If the assumptions of parametric tests it is possible to transform the data prior to performing one of the standard tests outlined. However, an alternative is to perform a non-parametric test (i.e. tests that do not make any assumptions about the distribution of the data). There are non-parametric equivalents to the unpaired t-test (Mann-Whitney test), paired t-test (Wilcoxon test), ANOVA (Kruskal-Wallis test). The details are beyond the scope of this book, however, the interested reader is referred to the recommended reading list for more details.

Summary

Transformations of data can be useful when the assumptions of common tests are not met. The analysis of transformed data does not affect the statistical interpretation of the analyses. The investigator should choose transformation carefully as the units of analyses may not be meaningful if a complex transformation is used.

CORRELATION

Correlation measures the strength of the linear association between two continuous variables X and Y such as height and weight.

Pearson Product Moment Correlation Coefficient

R = -1	Strong negative linear relationship. Negative correlation implies that as the value of X increases the value of Y decreases.
R = 0	No **linear** relationship between X and Y
R = +1	Strong positive relationship. Positive correlation implies that as the value of X increases the value of Y increases.

The correlation coefficient is always a number between -1 and +1. It is important that the data is plotted in addition to calculating the correlation coefficient as there may be a relationship between the variables, which is not linear. Figure 21 depicts perfect positive (R=+1) and perfect negative (R=-1) correlations. For an R=0 the data would be simply a random scatter on the plot.

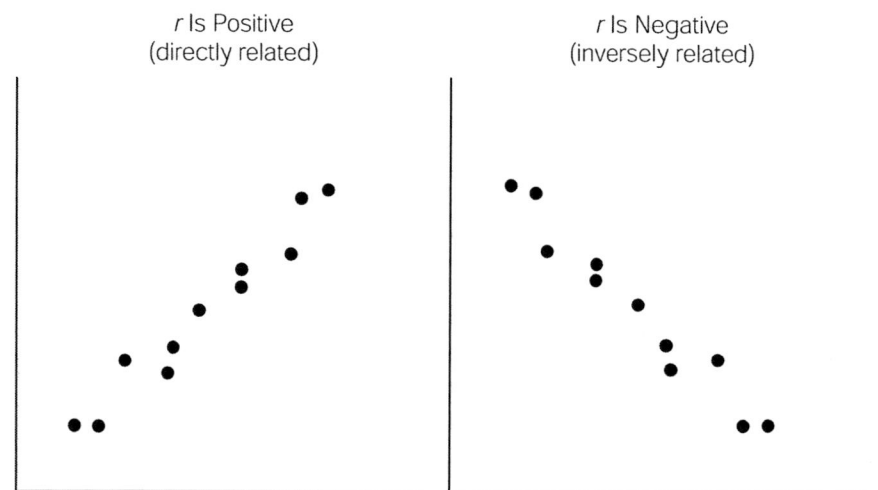

"Primer on Correlation Coefficients" *Effective Clinical Practice*, May/June 2001. 4:305-306. Reproduced with permission from the American College of Physicians

Figure 21. Illustration of correlation using artificial data

Significance Test for Correlation Coefficient

A t-test is used to test whether the sample correlation, r, is significantly different from zero, or in other words whether the observed sample correlation could simply be due to chance.

H_0: $\rho = 0$ (i.e. the true population correlation coefficient is equal to zero)
H_1: $\rho \neq 0$ (i.e. the true population correlation coefficient is not equal to zero)

The significance of the correlation will depend on the size of the correlation coefficient and the number of observations. For small samples a large correlation is required before the null hypothesis can be rejected whereas with large samples a very small correlation can be deemed to be statistically significant. The *assumption of the test* requires that *at least one* of the variables needs to be Normally distributed.

Spearman's Rank Correlation Coefficient

Spearman's rank correlation is the non-parametric equivalent of the product moment correlation coefficient. Spearman's correlation coefficient is calculated if one or more of the following conditions are present:

(a) Neither X nor Y follow a Normal distribution
(b) The sample size is small
(c) Either X or Y is measured on an ordinal scale
(d) The investigator needs to compute a measure of association between two continuous variables which appears to be non-linear.

As with the product moment correlation, Spearman's correlation coefficient is always a number between -1 and +1.

Summary

It is important that the data is plotted in addition to calculating a correlation coefficient as there may be a relationship between the variables, which is not linear. It should be noted that an observed correlation between two variables does not indicate a causal association between the two variables.

REGRESSION BASED METHODS

Regression based methods are extremely common in epidemiological research as they allow the investigator to explore relationships between a measured exposure(s) and measured outcome(s) of interest. In addition these methods allow the investigator to simultaneously adjust for potential confounding factors. These most common of these types of approaches will now be described in more detail.

Linear Regression

Linear regression is used to describe the straight line relationship that exists between two variables. Often it is of interest to predict the value of one variable (dependent) from a given value of another (independent).

1. y is called the dependent variable
2. x is called the independent or explanatory variable.

Linear regression gives the equation of the straight line that describes how the y-variable increases (or decreases) with an increase in the x-variable. The researcher should choose carefully which variable to call the dependent variable because, unlike correlation, the two alternative regressions do not give the same conclusions.

The equation, $y' = a + bx + \epsilon$ is the regression equation of Y on X, where a is the intercept and b is the slope. The intercept (a) is the point where the regression line crosses the y-axis (vertical axis) and gives the value of y for when x=0. The slope (b) is the increase in y corresponding to one unit increase in x. The slope b is sometimes called the regression coefficient. It has the same sign as the correlation coefficient. When there is no correlation between the x and y variables then, b equals zero corresponding to a horizontal line at height y.

The values of a and b are calculated so as to minimise the sum of the squares of the vertical distances from the line. This is called the least squares fit. The term ϵ is known as the residual or error of estimation term.

Multiple Linear Regression

Situations frequently occur when we are interested in the dependency of a variable on several independent (such as exposures or risk factors) variables not just one. The joint influence of the variables taking into account possible correlations among them may be investigated using multiple regression. Consider the situation where we have two groups of patients have been receiving different treatments for their hypertension. One group has been prescribed drug A and the other group drug B. After 6 months of treatment a comparison of the effectiveness of the two drugs is made. On inspection of the data it is apparent that the group of patients on drug A are older than the group of patients receiving drug B. It is known that blood pressure is related to age. Comparing the effectiveness of the two drugs using a t-test on blood pressure at 6 months would not be appropriate since any difference in blood pressure could be due to a difference in effectiveness of the drugs or it could be due to the different age distribution in the two groups (i.e. age is a confounder). Regression analysis can be used to remove any variation in blood pressure that is due to variation in age, before comparing the two cohorts of patients for a difference in blood pressure. This is also known as adjusting blood pressure for age.

When there are two independent variables the regression equation is

$$y' = a + b_1 x_1 + b_2 x_2$$

When there are more than two independent variables, say k, the regression equation becomes

$$y' = a + b_1 x_1 + b_2 x_2 + ... + b_k x_k$$

Multiple Correlation

The correlation between the dependent variable (y) and the combined predictors x_1, x_2, ...x_k is called the *coefficient of multiple correlation* and is denoted by R. The proportion of variance in y accounted for by the combined predictors x_1, x_2, ...,x_k is obtained by squaring the multiple correlation coefficient and is called the *coefficient of multiple determination, R².*

Assumptions of Multiple Linear Regression

1. To apply multiple linear regression analysis the relationship between the dependent variable and each of the independent variables must be linear. Two additional

assumptions are required for testing the significance of regression coefficients and constructing confidence intervals

2. For any value of x, the distribution of the predicted y values, y', should be Normally distributed.

3. The standard deviations of the predicted y values, y', are the same for all values of x. This is referred to as the homoscedasticity assumption.

Checking the Assumptions

After the regression model has been fitted to the data, it is essential to check that the assumptions of multiple linear regression have not been violated.

1. Plots of the dependent variable against all the independent variables entered in the model to check that the relationships are linear. This assumption can also be checked by plotting the residuals against the predicted values to check that there is no curvature in the plot.

2. Normally distributed residuals can be tested using a histogram or a normal probability plot of the residuals. The histogram should look symmetrical and the normal probability plot should display a straight line relationship.

3. The residuals have a constant variance can be assessed by plotting residuals against predicted values. There should be an even spread of residuals around zero and 'equal' variation in the spread of residuals for the predicted values.

The Relationship between Multiple Regression and ANOVA

There is a large overlap between multiple regression and ANOVA. A multiple regression where all the independent variables are discrete (i.e. categorical) is in fact the same as an ANOVA with several factors. The two approaches give identical results and in fact most statistical software will display both forms of results.

Analysis of Covariance (ANCOVA)

An extension to the Analysis of Variance (ANOVA) which allows the comparison of the endpoint of interest between groups is Analysis of Covariance (ANCOVA). Such data can be analyzed using multiple regression techniques by creating one or more binary variables to differentiate between the groups. So if an investigator wishes to compare the average values of y in two treatment groups, while controlling (or adjusting) for the effect of several other variables such as age and sex. So if binary variable x_1 coded as 1 for treatment A and 0 for treatment B was fitted in a multiple regression along with age and sex the estimate b_1 obtained from the multiple regression would be the estimated difference in the response y between treatment A and B after adjustment for age and sex.

Logistic Regression

Logistic regression is very similar to linear regression except that it is used when the response is a binary variable (such as the presence or absence of disease) and we have a number of explanatory variables (exposures or risk factors) of interest. We can model the data using the probability that a person will be classified into a particular category. To overcome mathematical difficulties we use the logistic transformation the logit (p) is equivalent to the natural logarithm of the odds ratio i.e. Logit (p) =ln(p/1-p).

When there are two independent variables the logistic regression equation is

$$\log it(p) = a + b_1 x_1 + b_2 x_2$$

When there are more than two independent variables, say k, the regression equation becomes

$$\log it(p) = a + b_1 x_1 + b_2 x_2 + \dots + b_k x_k$$

The b_1, b_2,....., b_k are the logistic regression coefficient and the exponential of one of these coefficients say e^{b1} give the odds of disease when x_1 takes a particular value relative to the odds of disease for a 1 unit change x_1 whilst adjusting for x_2 ....., x_k . The x's can be continuous or categorical variables depending on the risk factors and exposures that have been collected during the study. An *odds ratio in excess of 1 implies an increased risk of disease* for that exposure or risk factor after adjustment for the other factors in the model. An *odds ratio less than unity implies that the exposure or risk factor may have a protective effect* on disease after the adjustment of other factors in the model. Recall the example of the case-control study to assess the association between brain tumours and cellular telephone use. Christensen and colleagues [14] report on a population-based case control study on 252 people with gliomas and 175 with meingioma compared 822 randomly sampled controls in Denmark. Tumours were differentiated into gliomas and meningioma as they are regarded as two separate diseases. The diagnosis of glioma and meningioma cases was confirmed by histological examination. Controls a random sample from the Danish Central Population Register and were frequency matched on age (within 5 year ranges) and sex. In order to assess whether there was an association with cellular phone use and case-control status the data were analysed by logistic regression with all analyses stratified by age and sex and additionally adjusted for education level, region of residence and marital status (i.e. potential confounding factors were adjusted for in the statistical analysis). The authors found that gliomas were not associated with regular use of cellular telephones OR 0.71 95% CI (0.50, 1.01) and similarly meningiomas were not associated with regular cellular phone use OR 0.83 (0.54, 1.24).

Survival Times and Cox Regression

Survival times are concerned with the time it takes for an individual to reach an endpoint of interest (usually but not always death). Some common "times to event" time to hospital discharge or time spent on treatment before non-fatal or fatal stroke. Censoring may occur - if the event does not happen within the study period. There are several types of censoring that can be encountered with survival times. **Right censoring** is when the event time was greater than some amount but we do not know the exact time. **Left censoring** this is when we observe the presence of the state or condition but do not know when it began. **Interval censoring** is when the individuals come in and out of observation (maybe because they are in a disease screening program) and they develop the state or condition within some interval but we do not know the exact time. The term censoring usually refers to right censoring as this is the most common form.

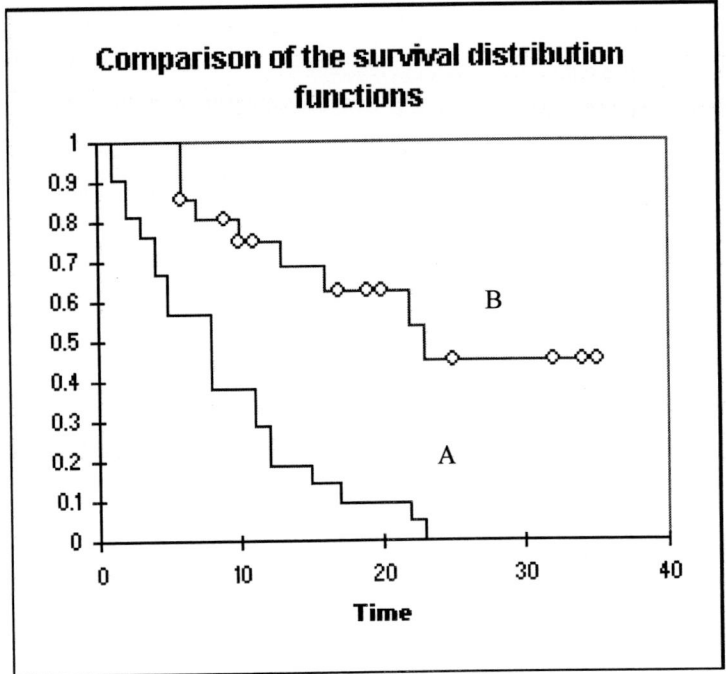

Figure 22. Example of Kaplan-Meir graph for two groups in a fictitious clinical trial

Displaying Survival Times

Survival times can be displayed using Kaplan-Meier graphs. The K-M graph displays the cumulative probability of an individual not experiencing the endpoint at any time after the start of the study. The survival curve changes in steps when a group of individuals experience the endpoint of interest. Figure 22 depicts the results of a randomized clinical trial investigating the effect of a drug A survival time (in weeks) of patients with a life threatening illness.

The aim of the study is to ascertain whether the drug influences the survival time, by comparing the survival curves for two groups of 21 patients, the first being treated, and the second being a control group. All 21 patients of the control group (line A) died from the disease. Only 9 of the drug treated patients (line B) died, while the 11 others were right censored (denoted by open diamonds). Survival probabilities can also be displayed using *a life table* approach and both these methods are implemented in standard statistical software. For further reading and details on some of these basic concepts with illustrations the reader is referred to the work of Clark et al [33].

Cox Proportional Hazards Regression

In most studies the investigators will wish to asses the role played by a number of risk factors or exposures on survival time. However, in most situations we would like to assess the role of several factors simultaneously. We can use the *Cox proportional hazards regression* model (usually called *Cox regression*) when we wish to estimate the *hazard* of experiencing a particular endpoint (given that the individual has been free of the endpoint up until that point in time) based a several factors of interest.

When there are more than two independent variables, say k, the regression equation becomes

$$\lambda(t) = \lambda_0(t)\exp(\beta_1 x_1 + \beta_2 x_2 + \ldots + \beta_k x_k)$$

λ (t) is the hazard for individual i at time t, $\lambda_0(t)$ is an arbitrary baseline hazard, $x_1,\ldots\ldots,x_k$ are explanatory variables (i.e. risk factors or exposures) and β_1, β_2,....., β_k are the Cox regression coefficients. For example in a clinical trial we may wish to know whether the hazard is reduced in individuals receiving an active treatment versus those individuals receiving a placebo after taking into account of age, sex and disease severity. The β_1, β_2,....., β_k are the Cox regression coefficients and the exponential of one of these coefficients say eβ_1 give the hazard ratio of reaching the endpoint for a unit change in x1 whilst adjusting for x2 ....., xk . As with logistic regression the x's can be continuous or categorical variables depending on the risk factors and exposures that have been collected during the study. Also in common with logistic regression a hazard ratio greater than in 1 implies an increased risk of experiencing the endpoint after adjustment for the other factors in the model. A hazard ratio less than 1 implies that the exposure or risk factor may have a protective effect on the hazard of experiencing the endpoint after the adjustment of other factors in the model.

Recall the example of the Women's Health Initiative study [6] which recruited 16,608 postmenopausal women whose uterus was intact at baseline from 40 centres around the United States of America. Participants received either conjugated equine estrogens plus medroxyprogesterone (8506) acetate in 1 tablet or placebo (8102). The trial was intended to run for 8.5 years but was stopped after 5.2 years of follow-up because the overall health risks exceeded the benefits from use of the combined estrogen plus progestin. The primary outcome was coronary heart disease (CHD) which was nonfatal myocardial infarction and

CHD death, with invasive breast cancer as the adverse outcome. Hazard ratios computed via Cox regression analyses indicated that participants were at increased risk of CHD 1.29; 95%CI: [1.02-1.63] with 286 cases; breast cancer 1.26; 95%CI: [1.00-1.59] with 290 cases and stroke 1.41; 95%CI: [1.07-1.85] with 212 cases.

Poisson Regression and Mixed Model Regression

Poisson regression is used to model count data. In an epidemiological setting an investigator may wish to employ Poisson regression when assessing which risk factors influence the incidence of a particular disease. It is not as common as logistic and Cox regression so we shall not go into more detail here. The interested reader is referred to the general statistical texts in the recommended reading list. Mixed model regression methods have been used to analyze cohort studies that have collected repeated measurements over time in a group of individuals. Common types of mixed model regression are generalized estimating equations, random coefficient models in which the exposures or risk factors in the model are modeled simultaneously so that the regression coefficient β represents the relationship between longitudinal development of the outcome variable and the corresponding exposures. The exposures can be continuous or categorical and the methods can also handle missing data. The interested reader should consult the book by Twisk for a detailed overview of these approaches (as well as some simpler analyses) and a description of available statistical software [34]. An example of such an analysis is the study conducted by Meyer et al [9] described earlier in this chapter (see section on cohort studies) which investigated the role of cognitive performance in women progressing through the menopause at yearly intervals between 1996 and 2001. The authors used random coefficients models to assess whether cognitive performance showed a consistent rate of change over time, with incremental changes as women passed from one menopausal status to another after adjustment for other covariates. They also assessed whether the rate of change in cognitive performance differed by menopausal status. The authors found small increases in working memory and perceptual speed which were unaffected after adjustment for chronological age, education, family income, ethnicity or baseline self-reported health.

Effect Modification

Where the effect of one variable (for example treatment in a randomised controlled trial) depends on the value of another variable (for example sex), we call the second variable (sex) an "effect modifier" because it modifies the effect of the first variable (treatment). Effect modification is not the same thing as confounding. Confounders influence the effect of a variable in the same way for everyone and the confounders can be adjusted for by being included in our multiple, logistic or Cox regression analyses.

We allow for effect modification in our model by fitting an "interaction" term. We should only fit an interaction term if it makes clinical or biological sense - i.e. there is a good reason why the effect may be different in each group. Cox proportional hazards regression methods with an illustration of some of these and other issues can be found in Bradburn et al. 2003a [35] and Bradburn et al 2003b [36].

Summary

Regression methods use the data collected in order to take into account the effects of confounders in the analysis in order to produce an adjusted estimate. The choice of regression method is based on the type of outcome variable of interest (i.e. continuous, binary, time to an event). The main advantage of regression based methods over simpler methods (such as stratification) is that: they use all of the data; can adjust for several confounders simultaneously; they can investigate for effect modification by the inclusion of interaction terms. However, the validity of regression based methods are dependent on certain assumptions being satisfied and these assumptions should be checked as a matter of routine before reporting results of such analyses. Finally, regression based analyses can be extended to any number of variables although it is recommended that the number be kept reasonably small, as with larger numbers the interpretation becomes increasingly more complex.

CAUSALITY AND CRITICAL APPRAISAL

An association is simply a relationship between two variables but the presence of an association does not mean that the relationship is causal. Causation is the ability of a factor to produce an effect or change in the disease. Causality is that relationship between the cause and effect. Determining the cause of disease is a complex and inter-related process. It is rare to find a single exposure or factor that will directly cause one disease. Hill [37] described several criteria for causation which have been used by epidemiologists as a guide in order to enhance the understanding of the disease process.

Criteria for Causation

The criteria for causation involve assessing the strength of the association, consistency of effect, biological plausibility, dose response, temporal sequence and specificity of effect. *Strength of association* determines how important a specific exposure or factor is in the disease process. The effect of the exposure can be quantified by computing some useful statistic which measures the strength of association (such as an odds ratio). *Consistency of effect* is important as it can be used to corroborate the results of epidemiological studies with other studies. Observing similar associations in different populations and different study designs can increase the confidence in the results. *Biological plausibility* is required as a statistical association in isolation could be a chance finding and is thus insufficient evidence of causation. The association should make sense in terms of the biological mechanisms leading to the disease outcome of interest. The discovery of a *dose-response* relationship is important as it informs the investigator that as the frequency or duration of the exposure increases the strength of the disease association also increases thus improving the possibility of the exposure or risk factor being causal. The **temporal sequence** must be ascertained as an exposure cannot be deemed to be causal if it did not occur before the effect. The time period between the exposure and the disease must make biological sense and can only be determined via prospective studies. Finally, most diseases are caused by multiple factors or exposures. If a **specificity of effect** is observed i.e. a specific factor or exposure causes a specific disease, this is good evidence of causality. A strong association with disease of a particular factor in the presence of other known risk factors is evidence of specificity. The removal of an exposure or risk factor which leads to decreased risk of disease is also evidence of specificity.

Strength of Evidence for Causality

The best way to study cause-and-effect relationships are via an RCT. In this respect, well-conducted cohort studies are the next best thing to experimental studies, because they can be conducted to minimize the effects of selection and measurement biases, as well as known confounding biases.

It is customary to grade clinical evidence for a cause-and-effect relationship into three groups: **strong** (this evidence comes from RCT, cohort study), **moderate** (this evidence is based on large relative risks or odds ratios, dose-response relationship, reversible association, case-control studies), and **weak** (this type of evidence is based on correct temporal sequence, cross-sectional studies, small relative risks or odds ratios, biologic plausibility, and consistency of results). Levels of evidence based on the study designs discussed so far are in increasing order of evidence:

1. Case report: demonstrates that some event of clinical interest is possible
2. Case series: demonstrates certain possibly related clinical events but subject to large selection biases
3. Observational study: "natural" exposures or treatment selection and comparison group chosen by design
4. Randomised Controlled clinical trial: treatment assignment by design. Endpoint rigorously ascertainment performed and analysis planned prior to study.
5. Replicated clinical trials: independent verification of treatment efficacy.

In order to suspect that an exposure is a causal risk factor the investigator has to demonstrate that the association cannot be explained by chance, methodological flaws, or by confounding. Doll [38] suggests that the essential criterion for causality is temporal sequence as in some circumstances the strength of association may be so great (as with some occupational risk factors), and other evidence is lacking, that other criteria such as plausibility and consistency are irrelevant.

Critical Appraisal

When reading the epidemiological literature the reader needs to be able interpret the findings of the study based on the study design employed, the potential biases inherent in the study design and how the study was analysed statistically. There are several critical appraisal tools which are available for evaluating the quality of different study designs such as the Consolidated Standards of Reporting Trials (CONSORT)[39] and Tooth and colleagues have devised a checklist that assesses the quality of reporting of observational longitudinal research [40]. The reader of the epidemiological literature can then use checklists such as these as guidelines in order to decide whether the findings of a particular study are sound, and also how do they apply to their own clinical/research work. An extremely useful article by Greenhalgh [41] describes how to read and interpret a paper that has published in a medical journal as well as pitfalls to avoid.

Summary

There are now many epidemiological studies that demonstrate large relative risks or odds ratios, with evidence of dose-response relationships which cannot be disregarded due chance and methodological weaknesses. However, there also exist many studies where the results show much weaker effects of association which are also challenged by problems of eliminating bias and confounding. As a consequence large datasets are required in order to confirm whether the associations observed are causal. This has led to the formation of collaborative groups in order pool their resources and combining their data sets in order to investigate some unanswered questions.

META-ANALYSIS

There are now thousands of research articles produced every year in most fields of medicine which makes it difficult for researchers to keep abreast of developments. In the past reviews of research in a particular field have been mainly narrative and included articles that author decided to include, sometimes with no explanation why other were omitted. It is now more common that reviews are performed systematically with rigorous inclusion and exclusion criteria for studies and may contain a narrative component as well as a quantitative synthesis of the evidence known as "meta-analysis". The studies involved are usually randomized controlled trials (particularly useful as there are a large number of similar trials being conducted at any one time and trials provide the "gold standard" of evidence), but epidemiological studies and other non-randomised studies can also be considered for pooling in this manner. The words "meta-analysis", "systematic review" and "overview" are in common use and are usually treated as synonymous in the medical literature. A systematic review does not necessarily have to contain a quantitative pooling of the results and basically refers to any review that has been prepared using strict criteria to reduce the risk of bias. The term systematic review is the one used by the Cochrane Collaboration (a worldwide network of clinicians, epidemiologists and other health professionals that produces such reviews). Figure 23 displays the hierarchy of evidence which shows that systematic reviews or meta-analyses are considered the highest level of evidence.

A meta-analysis or systematic review should be conducted like a real study and therefore involves formulating the problem, evaluating the retrieved studies, combining the studies (if possible), writing up the findings, dissemination of the findings as widely as possible through publication, conference presentations etc [42]. Panel 6 briefly summarises the main aims of a meta-analysis.

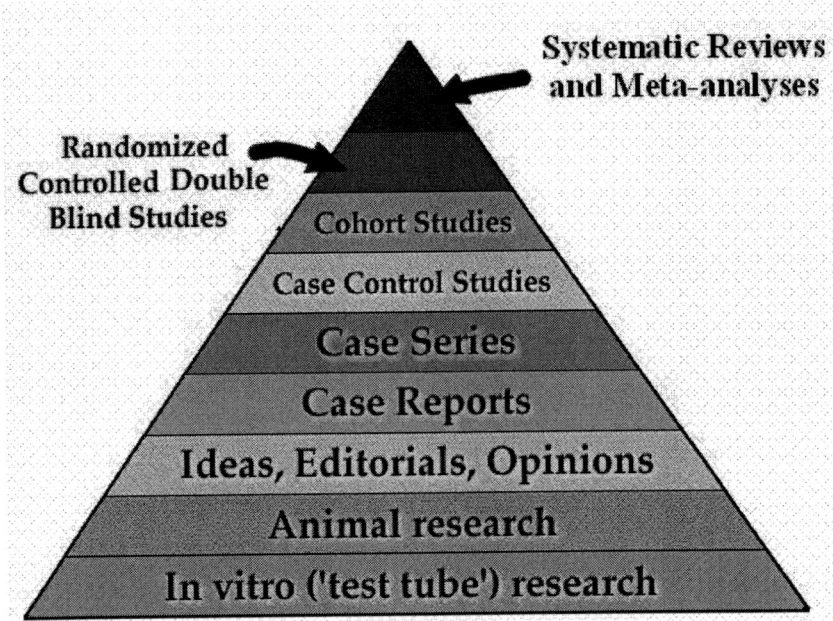

Source: SUNY Downstate EBM Tutorial http://library.downstate.edu/EBM2/2100.htm

Figure 23. Diagrammatic representation of the hierarchy of evidence

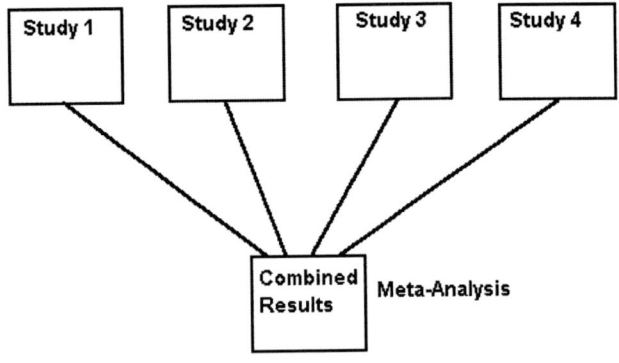

Source: SUNY Downstate EBM Tutorial http://library.downstate.edu/EBM2/2700.htm

Figure 24. Diagrammatic representation of meta-analysis

PANEL 6

Aims of meta-analysis
- To test the null hypothesis relative to the effect size
- To obtain an accurate and precise estimate of the effect size
- To enable investigators to perform sub-group analyses
- To produce offer the methodological reliable generalizations of the findings whose power is very low if carried out on individual studies
- To guide other researchers in planning new studies and suggesting new research questions.

Meta-Analysis of Randomised Controlled Trials

Meta-analyses of randomized trials are usually considered to be the gold standard of evidence. One such example is reported by McIntyre and colleagues in JAMA [43] and focused on the effects of hypothermia on mortality and neurological outcome in adults after traumatic brain injury (TBI.) The authors aimed to ascertain if the depth, duration, and rate of re-warming from hypothermia influenced mortality and neurological outcome. Inclusion criteria specified study design (RCT), target population (adults with TBI), therapeutic intervention and comparison ($\geq$ 24 hours of therapeutic hypothermia at any time after sustaining TBI vs. normothermia), and primary and secondary outcomes (all-cause mortality and neurological outcome). The selection process was thorough and included a variety of Medical Subject Headings (MeSH) terms and text words were used to perform electronic searches in medical databases such MEDLINE. Additional searches were performed using other less known databases such as EMBASE and Current Contents, as well as the Cochrane Library. Conference proceedings and hand searching were also performed in addition to contacting authors of studies in order to ascertain whether there were unpublished or ongoing trials in the pipeline. Searches were not restricted to the English language.

12 RCTs were included in the meta-analysis, representing a total of 1,069 patients - 543 patients in the therapeutic hypothermia group, and 526 patients in the normothermia or control group. In addition to pooled relative risks, the authors examined RR according to (1) depth of cooling (33.5-34.5 vs. 32-33°C,) (2) duration of cooling (24 hrs vs. 48 hrs vs. > 48 hrs,) (3) rates of re-warming ($\leq$ 24 hrs vs. > 24 hrs,) and (4) trial quality (concealment of outcome and randomization scheme).

The authors appraised the methodologies of the included studies individually by focusing on whether or not the trials performed "allocation concealment" and "blinding of the outcome assessment." The blinding assessment here was of neurological outcome. Methodological quality was stratified into "high" (allocation concealed, outcome blinded), "moderate" (allocation concealment unclear, outcome blinded), and "low" (allocation concealment unclear, outcome not blinded). Analyses according to trial quality did not detect significant differences in outcome.

Meta-Analysis of Non-Randomised Studies

It is not always possible to conduct meta-analyses on randomised controlled trials and recently overviews of observational data have become more frequent. An example of one such overview is the European Studies of Dementia (EURODEM) published in Neurology, [44]. In 1988, investigators formed the EURODEM network in order to harmonise the protocols used in their newly initiated, population based studies on newly demented diseases. The analyses were based on 528 incident dementia patients and 28,768 person-years of follow-up. The studies included Odense study (Denmark), the PAQUID study (France), The Rotterdam study (The Netherlands) and the MRC-ALPHA study (United Kingdom). The individual studies included a population based sample of individuals who were either 65 years of age or older and living in the community and in the nursing homes. Data on risk factors were collected on all subjects at baseline when they were dementia free and all questions were administered by interviewers in the home of participants. Diagnostic data on dementia was reviewed by the EURODEM panel of experts which included neurologists, psychiatrists and neuro-epidemiologists. Investigators from the individual studies recoded their own data into a standardized format developed collaboratively by the EURODEM data managers. Data for the entire EURODEM cohort was checked by the co-ordinating centre and queries were sent back to individual centres if required. The final database was analysed as one large dataset in order to obtain the combined results.

Summary

Meta-analyses and systematic reviews have become extremely popular over the last decade or so. Mulrow outlines in the detail the rationale for conducting systematic reviews [45]. Although such studies are considered to be extremely useful they are not without problems. Two key issues are publication bias (where only published studies are located), statistical heterogeneity (how to combine studies that are statistically different after taking into account differences in study characteristics). Egger et al describe some of the problems and limitations of systematic reviews [46]. It is important for authors of such reviews to describe in detail how they have dealt with these issues when reporting their findings. The standards of reporting for meta-analyses of randomized trials have been addressed in the Quality of Reporting of Meta-analyses (QUOROM) [47]. Greenhalgh has described in detail what to look for when reading a meta-analytical paper [48]. Many meta-analyses use summary data reported in published or unpublished papers. However, it is becoming more common for collaborative groups (such as EURODEM) to collect individual participant data from several studies to perform more detailed analyses. Sometimes there is very little evidence available and authors have chosen to perform a best evidence synthesis which uses evidence from a number of different sources (and across different study designs) in order to come up with a conclusion. This partcular approach is becoming more common in health services research and economic decision modelling.

CONCLUSION

This chapter has aimed to describe some of the fundamental concepts of statistics, epidemiological study design, and interpretation of study results. We have concentrated on the most commonly used statistical tests so the tests described here are not exhaustive and the reader should explore the recommended reading list for a more comprehensive overview of statistical tests. We have emphasized good study design and how to reduce the biases that can occur in such studies. The ability to critically appraise research findings has become crucial in the last decade or so and is vital for clinicians, researchers and epidemiologists who wish to apply the results of other studies to their own patients. We have emphasized good practice by referring to guidelines on how to read and review a paper and to determine how reliable the evidence from a particular study design is. We hope that this will facilitate understanding and appreciation of subsequent chapters.

REFERENCES

[1]   Altman DG, Bland JM. Statistics notes: variables and parameters. *BMJ* 1999; 318(7199):1667.

[2]   Altman DG, Bland JM. Statistics Notes: Presentation of numerical data. *BMJ* 1996; 312(7030):572.

[3]   Altman DG, Bland JM. Statistics notes: the normal distribution. *BMJ* 1995; 310(6975):298.

[4]   Altman DG, Bland JM. Statistics notes: Absence of evidence is not evidence of absence. *BMJ* 1995; 311(7003):485.

[5]   Altman DG, Bland JM. Statistics notes. Treatment allocation in controlled trials: why randomise? *BMJ* 1999; 318(7192):1209.

[6]   Rossouw JE, Anderson GL, Prentice RL *et al.* Risks and benefits of estrogen plus progestin in healthy postmenopausal women: principal results From the Women's Health Initiative randomized controlled trial. *JAMA* 2002; 288(3):321-33.

[7]   Rochon PA, Gurwitz JH, Sykora K *et al.* Reader's guide to critical appraisal of cohort studies: 1. Role and design. *BMJ* 2005; 330(7496):895-7.

[8]   Ott A, Slooter AJ, Hofman A *et al.* Smoking and risk of dementia and Alzheimer's disease in a population-based cohort study: the Rotterdam Study. *Lancet* 1998; 351(9119):1840-3.

[9]   Meyer PM, Powell LH, Wilson RS *et al.* A population-based longitudinal study of cognitive functioning in the menopausal transition. *Neurology* 2003; 61(6):801-6.

[10]   Lau KK, Wong LK, Li LS, Chan YW, Li HL, Wong V. Epidemiological study of multiple sclerosis in Hong Kong Chinese: questionnaire survey. *Hong Kong Med J* 2002; 8(2):77-80.

[11]   Maheswaran R, Elliott P. Stroke mortality associated with living near main roads in England and wales: a geographical study. *Stroke* 2003; 34(12):2776-80.

[12]   Schulz KF, Grimes DA. Case-control studies: research in reverse. *Lancet* 2002; 359(9304):431-4.

[13] Grimes DA, Schulz KF. Compared to what? Finding controls for case-control studies. *Lancet* 2005; 365(9468):1429-33.

[14] Christensen HC, Schuz J, Kosteljanetz M *et al.* Cellular telephones and risk for brain tumors: a population-based, incident case-control study. *Neurology* 2005; 64(7):1189-95.

[15] Finelli PF. Images in neurology. Mass effect in progressive multifocal leukoencephalopathy. *Arch Neurol* 1998; 55(8):1148-9.

[16] Kang K, Chu K, Kim DE, Jeong SW, Lee JW, Roh JK. POEMS syndrome associated with ischemic stroke. *Arch Neurol* 2003; 60(5):745-9.

[17] Iwane M, Palensky J, Plante K. A user's review of commercial sample size software for design of biomedical studies using survival data. *Control Clin Trials* 1997; 18(1):65-83.

[18] Kahn H.A. and Sempos CT. Statistical Methods in Epidemiology. New York: Oxford University Press, 1989.

[19] Wilhelmsen L, Svardsudd K, Korsan-Bengtsen K, Larsson B, Welin L, Tibblin G. Fibrinogen as a risk factor for stroke and myocardial infarction. *N Engl J Med* 1984; 311(8):501-5.

[20] Grimes DA, Schulz KF. Bias and causal associations in observational research. *Lancet* 2002; 359(9302):248-52.

[21] Altman DG, Bland JM. Statistics notes: How to randomise. *BMJ* 1999; 319(7211):703-4.

[22] Day SJ, Altman DG. Statistics Notes: Blinding in clinical trials and other studies. *BMJ* 2000; 321(7259):504.

[23] PROGRESS Collaborative Group. Randomised trial of a perindopril-based blood-pressure-lowering regimen among 6,105 individuals with previous stroke or transient ischaemic attack. *Lancet* 2001; 358(9287):1033-41.

[24] Newell DJ. Intention-to-treat analysis: implications for quantitative and qualitative research. *Int J Epidemiol* 1992; 21(5):837-41.

[25] Davey Smith G, Ebrahim S. What can mendelian randomisation tell us about modifiable behavioural and environmental exposures? *BMJ* 2005; 330(7499):1076-9.

[26] Davey Smith G, Ebrahim S. 'Mendelian randomization': can genetic epidemiology contribute to understanding environmental determinants of disease? *Int J Epidemiol* 2003; 32(1):1-22.

[27] Verhoef P, Hennekens C, Malinow M, Kok F, Willett W, Stampfer M. A prospective study of plasma homocyst(e)ine and risk of ischemic stroke. *Stroke* 1994; 25(10):1924-30.

[28] Alluri RV, Mohan V, Komandur S, Chawda K, Chaudhuri JR, Hasan Q. MTHFR C677T gene mutation as a risk factor for arterial stroke: a hospital based study. *Eur J Neurol* 2005; 12(1):40-4.

[29] Greenhalgh T. How to read a paper: Assessing the methodological quality of published papers. *BMJ* 1997; 315(7103):305-8.

[30] Barber M, Wright F, Stott DJ, Langhorne P. Predictors of early neurological deterioration after ischaemic stroke: a case-control study. *Gerontology* 2004; 50(2):102-9.

[31] Muir KW, Holzapfel L, Lees KR. Phase II clinical trial of sipatrigine (619C89) by continuous infusion in acute stroke. *Cerebrovasc Dis* 2000; 10(6):431-6.

[32] Altman DG, Bland JM. Statistics Notes: Comparing several groups using analysis of variance. *BMJ* 1996; 312(7044):1472-3.

[33] Clark TG, Bradburn MJ, Love SB, Altman DG. Survival analysis part I: basic concepts and first analyses. *Br J Cancer* 2003; 89(2):232-8.

[34] Twisk JRW. *Applied Longitudinal Data Analysis for Epidemiology: A practical guide.* Cambrdige, UK: Cambridge University Press, 2003.

[35] Bradburn MJ, Clark TG, Love SB, Altman DG. Survival analysis part II: multivariate data analysis--an introduction to concepts and methods. *Br J Cancer* 2003; 89(3):431-6.

[36] Bradburn MJ, Clark TG, Love SB, Altman DG. Survival analysis Part III: multivariate data analysis -- choosing a model and assessing its adequacy and fit. *Br J Cancer* 2003; 89(4):605-11.

[37] Hill AB. The Environment And Disease: Association Or Causation? *Proc R Soc Med* 1965; 58:295-300.

[38] Doll R. Proof of causality: deduction from epidemiological observation. *Perspect Biol Med* 2002; 45(4):499-515.

[39] Begg C, Cho M, Eastwood S *et al.* Improving the Quality of Reporting of Randomized Controlled Trials: The CONSORT Statement. *JAMA* 1996; 276(8):637-9.

[40] Tooth L, Ware R, Bain C, Purdie DM, Dobson A. Quality of Reporting of Observational Longitudinal Research. *Am. J. Epidemiol.* 2005; 161(3):280-8.

[41] Greenhalgh T. How to read a paper: Statistics for the non-statistician. II: "Significant" relations and their pitfalls. *BMJ* 1997; 315(7105):422-5.

[42] Normand ST. Meta analysis: formulating, evaluating, combining and reporting. *Stat Med* 1999; 18:321-59.

[43] McIntyre LA, Fergusson DA, Hebert PC, Moher D, Hutchison JS. Prolonged therapeutic hypothermia after traumatic brain injury in adults: a systematic review. *JAMA* 2003; 289(22):2992-9.

[44] Launer LJ, Andersen K, Dewey ME *et al.* Rates and risk factors for dementia and Alzheimer's disease: results from EURODEM pooled analyses. EURODEM Incidence Research Group and Work Groups. European Studies of Dementia. *Neurology* 1999; 52(1):78-84.

[45] Mulrow CD. *Rationale for systematic reviews.* Chalmers I, Altman DG London: BMJ Publishing, 1995.

[46] Egger M, Dickersin K, Davey Smith G. *Problems and limitations in conducting systematic reviews.* 2nd edition. London: BMJ Books, 2001.

[47] Moher D, Cook DJ, Eastwood S, Olkin I, Rennie D, Stroup DF. Improving the quality of reports of meta-analyses of randomised controlled trials: the QUOROM statement. Quality of Reporting of Meta-analyses. *Lancet* 1999; 354(9193):1896-900.

[48] Greenhalgh T. How to read a paper: Papers that summarise other papers (systematic reviews and meta-analyses). *BMJ* 1997; 315(7109):672-5.

RECOMMENDED FURTHER READING

1. Mary E. *Understanding Epidemiology,* Torrance, Mosby, 1997
2. *Clinical Trials: A Methodological Perspective.* Steven Piantadosi. Wiley, 1997.
3. Hedges LV & Olkin I. *Statistical methods for meta-analysis.* New York: Academic Press, 1985.
4. Chalmers I and Altman DG. *Systematic Reviews,* London BMJ Publishing, 1995.
5. Sterne JAC, Egger M and Davey-Smith G. Systematic reviews in health care: Investigating and dealing with publication and other biases in meta-analysis. *BMJ* 2001;323: 101 - 105.
6. Bland JM and Altman DG. Statistics Notes: The odds ratio. *BMJ*, 2000; 320: 1468.
7. Bland JM and Altman DG. Statistics Notes: One and two sided tests of significance *BMJ*, Jul 1994; 309: 248.
8. Bland JM. *An Introduction to Medical Statistics* (2nd Edition). OUP, 1995.
9. Altman DG. *Practical Statistics for Medical Investigations.* Chapman & Hall/CRC, 1991.
10. Bower D. *Statistics from Scratch: A guide for health professionals.* Wiley, 1997.
11. Bower D. *Further Statistics from Scratch: A guide for health professionals.* Wiley, 1997.
12. Petrie A and Sabin C. *Medical Statistics: At a Glance.* Blackwell, 2000.
13. Rowntree, D. *Statistics without Tears.* Pelican, 1981.
14. Greenhalgh T. *How to Read a Paper: The Basics of Evidence Based Medicine.* BMJ Publications, 2001.
15. Webb, P., Bain, C., Pirozzo, S. *Essential Epidemiology: an introduction for students and health professionals.* Cambridge University Press, 2005.

CLINICAL DISORDERS

In: Handbook of Clinical Neuroepidemiology

Editors: V. L. Feigin and D. A. Bennett, pp. 67-103

ISBN 978-1-60021-511-7

© 2007 Nova Science Publishers, Inc.

Chapter 2

CEREBROVASCULAR DISORDERS

Valery L. Feigin[1], David O. Wiebers[2] and Derrick A. Bennett[3]

[1]Clinical Trials Research Unit, School of Population Health, The University of Auckland, Auckland, New Zealand;

[2]Department of Neurology, Mayo Clinic, SW Rochester, MN, USA;

[3]Clinical Trial Service Unit and Epidemiological Studies Unit, University of Oxford, Oxford, UK.

ABSTRACT

Cerebrovascular disorders represent one of the most prevalent and devastating diseases of adults. One in every ten deaths worldwide is due to stroke and more than half of stroke survivors are left dependent on others for everyday activities. The epidemiology and management of cerebrovascular disorders are evolving quickly. There is evidence of noticeable ethnic and geographical differences in stroke incidence, prevalence and outcomes. While incidence of stroke tends to decrease in some developed countries, it increases in others and takes epidemic proportions in developing countries. The overall prevalence and socioeconomic burden of stroke tend to increase due to worldwide aging of the population. There is a lack of good quality comparable epidemiological data on stroke incidence and prevalence, especially from developing countries and over a long period of follow-up. Nor are there are many stroke management strategies of proven effectiveness and much research remains to be done in these areas. The purpose of this chapter is to provide a brief overview of the current knowledge in incidence, prevalence, risk factors, medical and socioeconomic outcomes, and management strategies of cerebrovascular disorders, with the emphasis on population-based studies in stroke and transient ischemic attack.

INTRODUCTION

Cerebrovascular disease is a heterogeneous disorder. It comprises of a number of distinct pathologies, including transient ischemic attack, stroke pathological types (ischemic stroke, intracerebral hemorrhage, subarachnoid hemorrhage) and etiological subtypes (e.g. cardioembolic, atherothrombotic, lacunar ischemic strokes, aneurysmal subarachnoid hemorrhage), and other intracranial vascular disorders (e.g. vascular malformations, unruptured aneurysms), each of which has different epidemiological and management features.

Stroke is the second commonest cause of death worldwide [1] and the most frequent cause of disability in adults in many countries [2]. It also has an enormous physical, psychological and financial impact on patients, families, the health care system, and society. The lifetime costs per stroke patient in various countries are estimated to range from US$59,800 to US$230,000 [3]. Moreover, stroke burden on families and societies is projected to rise from around 38 million disability-adjusted life years (DALYs) lost globally in 1990 to 61 million DALYs in 2020 [4] largely due to ageing of the populations. Although stroke mortality in Western populations has declined steadily over the last few decades, stroke incidence trends differ between the countries and the overall number of stroke survivors tends to increase. The best management strategy to reduce burden of stroke is its prevention on both individual and population levels. Given that over half of survivors remain dependent on others for everyday activities, often with significant adverse effects on caregivers [5,6], reducing the impact of stroke, on caregivers as well as patients, is key to the maintenance of independence, quality of life and burden on health services in populations.

INCIDENCE AND PREVALENCE

Stroke

In epidemiological research, stroke is commonly defined using the WHO definition of stroke, "rapidly developing signs of focal (or global) disturbance of cerebral function, leading to death or lasting longer than 24 hours, with no apparent cause other than vascular" [7]. Despite a continuous decrease of stroke mortality rates observed in many developed countries over the last few decades, globally stroke as a cause of death has moved from third to second place in the world and is now the leading cause of physical disability in adults aged 65 years and older. In recent years, there has been an unprecedented increase of stroke burden in developing countries (Figure 1). Although causes of the changing epidemiology of stroke are not fully understood, importance of ageing of the population has been postulated.

Good quality stroke incidence studies are essential for evidence-based health care planning and resource allocation in stroke, and they are also important for quantifying the burden of stroke. Monitoring trends in stroke incidence and outcomes allows projection of future stroke burden as well as an evaluation of effectiveness of various stroke prevention and management strategies. A physician who knows age- and sex-specific incidence rates of stroke in his/her area is able to tell their patients an exact probability (absolute risk) that an individual will have a stroke during a specified period of time (usually a year). For example, Table 1 shows age- and sex-specific incidence rates of stroke types derived from a population-based study in Auckland, New Zealand in 2002-2003 [8]. As shown in the table, the absolute risk of having an ischemic stroke during one year for any man within 65-74 years age band is about 0.6% (95% CI 0.5% to 0.7%).[1] In other words, one can say with 95% confidence that approximately 10 to 14 of 200 men of this age group would have an ischemic stroke during a year.

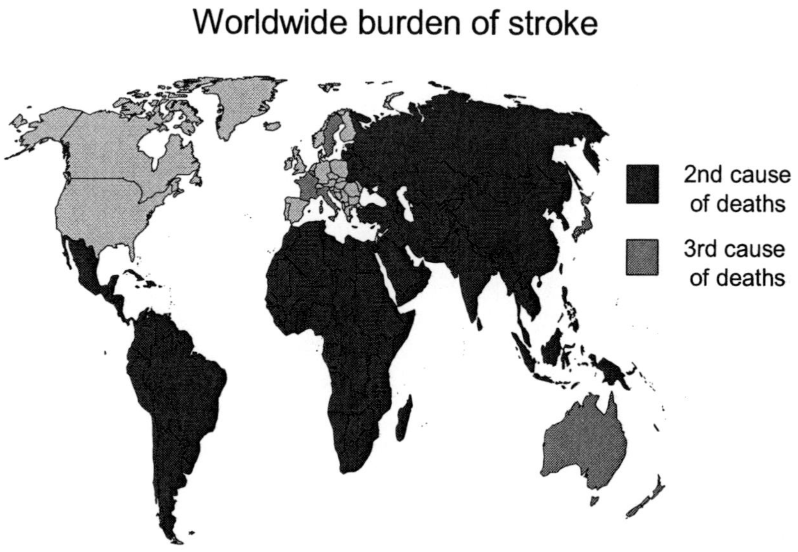

Worldwide burden of stroke

Figure 1. Worldwide stroke mortality.

Table 1. Age- and sex-specific incidence rates of major pathological types of stroke per 100,000 population per year*

Sex, age group, yrs	Total population	n	Ischemic stroke Rate (95% CI)	n	Intracerebral hemorrhage Rate (95% CI)	n	Subarachnoid hemorrhage Rate (95% CI)
Men							
15-64	380139	152	40 (34-47)	31	8 (6-12)	30	7.9 (6-11)
65-74	28173	160	568 (486-663)	23	82 (54-123)	6	21 (10-47)
75-84	15210	154	1013 (865-1186)	24	158 (106-235)	3	20 (6-61)
85+	3633	42	1156 (854-1564)	2	55 (14-220)	2	55 (14-220)
Women							
15-64	407967	116	28 (24-34)	25	6 (4-9)	31	8 (5-11)
65-74	31281	104	333 (274-403)	22	70 (46-107)	4	13 (5-34)
75-84	22605	188	832 (721-959)	34	150 (108-211)	8	35 (18-71)
85+	8874	116	1307 (1090-1568)	16	180 (111-294)	3	34 (11-105)

*Modified from Feigin et al. [8] with permission from *the Lancet Neurology*

---

[1] 568 new ischemic stroke cases per 100,000 population equals approximately 0.6 per 100 population or 0.6% (confidence intervals are computed in the same way).

Of course, this absolute risk does not take into account other risk factors for stroke (for more information on absolute risk of stroke see Risk Factor section in this chapter). This information can be used by doctors and patients for some decision-making (e.g. weighing up the benefits and risks of carotid endarterectomy against the background risk of stroke). Another useful utilization of good quality stroke incidence data is for health care planning. For example, if one would know the total stroke incidence rate in the population served, it could be calculated how many hospital beds are needed for acute stroke patients in the population. For example, if stroke incidence rate in a given population is 1.5 per 1000 people per year (it is an average stroke incidence rate in developed countries), the total population is 200,000 residents, the expected or desirable percentage of hospitalization with acute stroke is between 80% and 95% with the average length of hospital stay in Acute Stroke Unit (ASU) of 6 days (bed turnover of 50 during a year), then one would need approximately 5-6 beds in the ASU to serve acute stroke patients in the population.[2] Similar calculations can be used to compute an expected workload for CT/MRI head scanning of admitted stroke patients, number of staff members, medications and diagnostic procedures that would be required for the hospitalized stroke patients per year. Knowing the total number of acute stroke patients in the population served and assuming that approximately 20% of acute stroke patients die within a month after stroke onset, 20% survivors live in rest homes or private hospitals, 50% survivors are discharged home, and only 30% survivors remain independent in their activities of daily living (these figures are common in many developed countries), one can also approximate the number out-patient services and stroke-associated costs needed in the community.

Stroke incidence data are commonly reported together with stroke mortality and/or stroke case-fatality data obtained in the same population-based study. While high mortality rates may be a reflection of high stroke incidence rates in the population (especially if incidence rates parallel mortality rates), high stroke case-fatality is suggestive of either greater severity of stroke (e.g. high proportion of hemorrhagic strokes of large cerebral infarcts) and/or poor management of stroke patients in the population. These data have clear practical implications. Finally, incidence rates by stroke subtypes may provide some information on the etiology of the stroke subtypes. For example, high incidence of intracerebral haemorrhage is suggestive of high prevalence and/or poor control of hypertension in the population; high incidence of large anterior circulation infarctions (atherothrombotic strokes) is suggestive of high prevalence and/or poor control of carotid artery stenosis in the population etc. Data on incidence of various pathological types of stroke and its subtypes can also be used for more specific health care planning and resource allocation (e.g. number of acute atherothrombotic strokes in the population can be used to calculate the expected number of emergency interventional procedures on carotid arteries; number of patients with aneurysmal subarachnoid hemorrhage can be used to calculate the required number of neurosurgical services for these patients etc).

However, validity and generalisability of information about stroke incidence rates largely depends on validity of methods used to collect the data. Commonly used in the past stroke mortality and hospitalization data, while providing important information for trends and

---

[2] $(1.5 \times 200 \times 0.8) / 50 = 4.8$ beds; $(1.5 \times 200 \times 0.95)/50 = 5.7$ beds

patterns of stroke mortality and hospitalization, can not be generalized to the whole population, suffer from selection (hospital data) and classification (mortality data) biases and, therefore, are of limited scientific value. Analyses limited to hospital cases, incomplete mortality data or cases with varying criteria and definitions, may distort results due to non-standardised measures and non-representative study populations.

It is well recognized that good quality population-based studies are the most reliable source of information about stroke incidence on a population-level. However, identifying all new stroke events in a population is particularly challenging, so such epidemiological studies are relatively rare compared with studies using mortality data, hospital-based stroke registers, or incidence studies in younger age groups only [9,10].

Panel 1. Gold standards for an "ideal" stroke incidence study

Domains	Core criteria	Supplementary criteria
Standard definitions	• World Health Organization definition of stroke • At least 80% CT/MRI verification of the diagnosis of ischaemic stroke, intracerebral haemorrhage, and subarachnoid haemorrhage* • First-ever-in-a-lifetime stroke	• Classification of ischaemic stroke into subtypes (e.g. large artery disease, cardioembolic, small artery disease, other)* • Recurrent stroke*
Standard methods	• Complete, population-based case ascertainment, based on multiple overlapping sources of information (hospitals, outpatient clinics, general practitioners, death certificates)[†] • Prospective study design • Large, well-defined and stable population, allowing at least 100,000 person-years of observation[†] • Follow-up of patients' vital status for at least 1 month* • Reliable method for estimating denominator (not more than 5 years old census data)[†]	• Ascertainment of patients with TIA, recurrent strokes and those referred for brain, carotid or cerebral vascular imaging* • "Hot pursuit" of cases • Direct assessment of under-ascertainment* by regular checking of general practitioners' databases and hospital admissions for acute vascular problems and cerebrovascular imaging studies and/or interventions
Standard data presentation	• Complete calendar years of data; not more than 5 years of data averaged together[†] • Men and women presented separately • Mid-decade age bands (e.g., 55-64 years) used in publications, including ≥85 years old[†] • 95% confidence interval around rates	• Unpublished 5-year age bands available for comparison with other studies

*New criteria; [†]Updated and modified by Feigin & Carter [14] from Sudlow and Warlow [15], with permission from *Stroke*.

In 1987, Malmgren et al [11] published a list of 12 core criteria for "ideal" stroke incidence studies that were related to definitions, methods and mode of data presentation, by which the quality of population-based studies of stroke could be judged. These criteria have been updated by Bonita (1995) [12], Sudlow and Warlow (1996) [13], and, most recently (2004), by Feigin et al (Panel 1) [10]. Even among published population-based stroke incidence studies there are differences in the methodologies used to ensure completeness of case ascertainment and some studies, although claiming to be population or community based, did not meet all of the criteria for a population-based study.

Although developed primarily for affluent developed countries, these criteria for an "ideal" stroke incidence study have been successfully utilized in recent stroke incidence studies in Chile [16] and Georgia [17], suggesting that they can be of use in some less affluent countries. However, these criteria may not be practical for stroke studies undertaken in other developing countries, where most strokes occur and resources are limited. To address the problem of accurate and comparable data in these countries, a stepwise approach to increasing detail in the data to be collected for stroke surveillance has recently been proposed by the WHO [18]. This flexible and sustainable system includes three steps: standard (hospital-based case-ascertainment for calculating hospital admission due to stroke), expanded population coverage (ascertainment of death certificates or verbal autopsy in the whole community to calculate mortality rates), and comprehensive population-based (additional ascertainment of non-fatal events to calculate incidence and case-fatality in the community). These steps could provide vital basic epidemiological estimates of the burden of stroke in many countries around the world.

The first most reliable single-center population-based data on stroke incidence and outcomes came from the Rochester, MN, USA [19]. In this important study, stroke registration on the population level started in 1935 and continues to the present day, providing one of the most reliable sources of information on stroke incidence, outcomes and risk factors, including trends data. The first international multi-center study on stroke incidence was carried out under the auspices of the WHO in 17 centers representing 12 countries in 1971-1974 [7]. It is noteworthy that in this study registration of stroke cases was not restricted by age of stroke patients. This study demonstrated a relatively low stroke incidence in developing countries and rather moderate geographical differences in stroke incidence worldwide. Noticeable geographical variations in stroke incidence were also demonstrated in the WHO MONICA Project (1985-1987) [20], but this study registered stroke in people 25-74 years old only (in majority of centers, only people aged 25-64 were registered). Interestingly, substantial geographical differences in the incidence of subarachnoid haemorrhage were also noted in this age group of the population at the study period [21].

In 1997, Sudlow and Warlow published a comprehensive overview of 11 (available at that time) population-based stroke incidence studies from Europe (Oxfordshire, UK; Dijon, France; Umbria and Valle d'Aosta, Italy; Frederiksberg, Denmark; Söderhamn, Sweden; Warsaw, Poland), Novosibirsk (Russia), Perth (Australia), Auckland (New Zealand) and Rochester, MN (USA) [22]. Age- and sex-standardized annual incidence rates for subjects aged 45 to 84 years were similar (between approximately 300/100,000) and 500/100,000) in most places but were significantly lower in Dijon, France (238/100,000), and higher in

Novosibirsk, Russia (627/100,000) [23]. The distribution of pathological types, when these were reliably distinguished, did not differ significantly between studies. Our recent overview of population-based stroke incidence studies [10] included 17 new studies (9 new stroke incidence studies published since 1990 and 8 new studies on secular trends in stroke incidence) and confirmed Sudlow and Warlow findings [24] of modest geographical variations in the incidence of total stroke and stroke pathological types. As shown on Figures 2-6, towards the end of the 20th century and early in the 21st century, the incidence of all strokes combined, age-specific incidence, proportions of stroke subtypes, prevalence, and one month case-fatality exhibit, with a few exceptions, rather modest geographical variation between the studies included in the analyses, as compared to that observed in the MONICA Project [25,26].

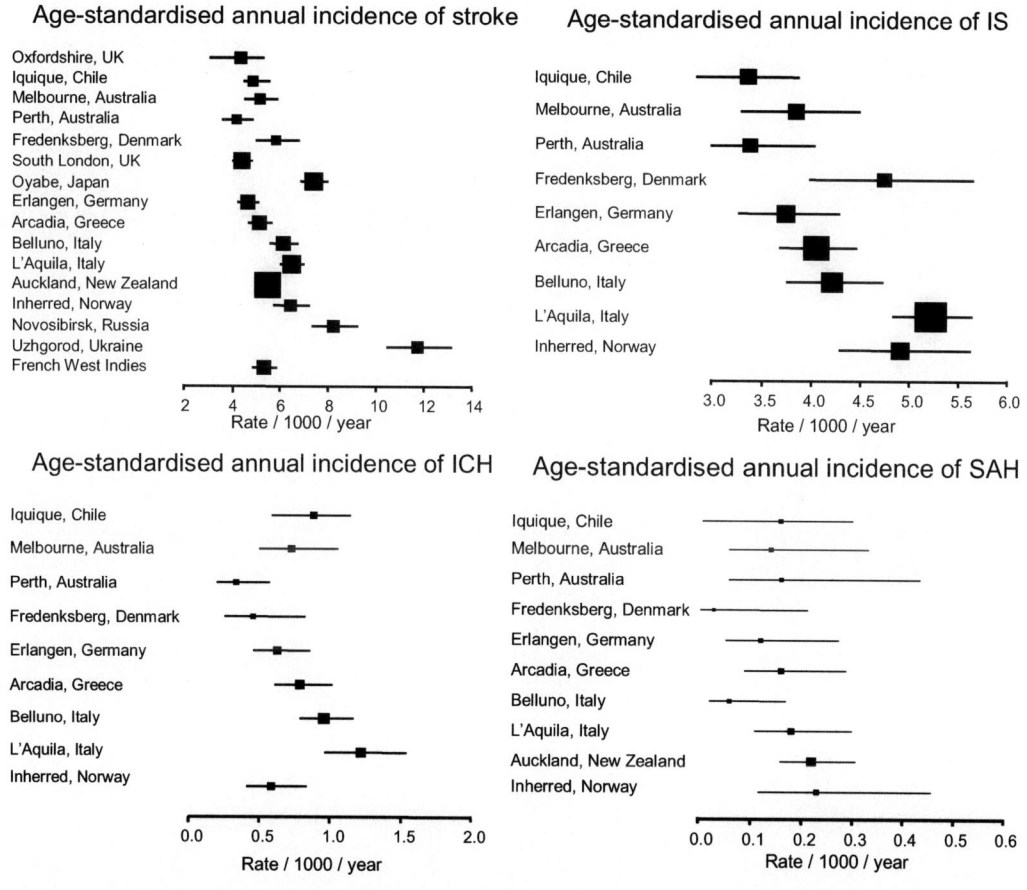

Figure 2. Age-standardized annual incidence per 1000 population of all strokes combined and by pathological type in people aged ≥ 55 years.*

It has been suggested that highest stroke incidence in Russia and Ukraine may be attributed to well-known social and economic changes that have occurred in these countries over the last decade, including changes in medical care, in access to vascular prevention strategies among those at high risk, and in the prevalence of risk factors [10]. Reasons for the relatively high stroke incidence in Japan compared to other developed countries, are not clear but may be related to genetic and environmental (e.g. diet, prevalence of cardiovascular risk factors etc.) parameters. In this overview, hospitalization rate of acute stroke patients ranged from 41% in Japan to 95% in Germany, averaging 81%, one month case-fatality averaged 23%, and the prevalence of stroke per 1000 population in 9 studies published after 1990 ranged from 5 to 11.

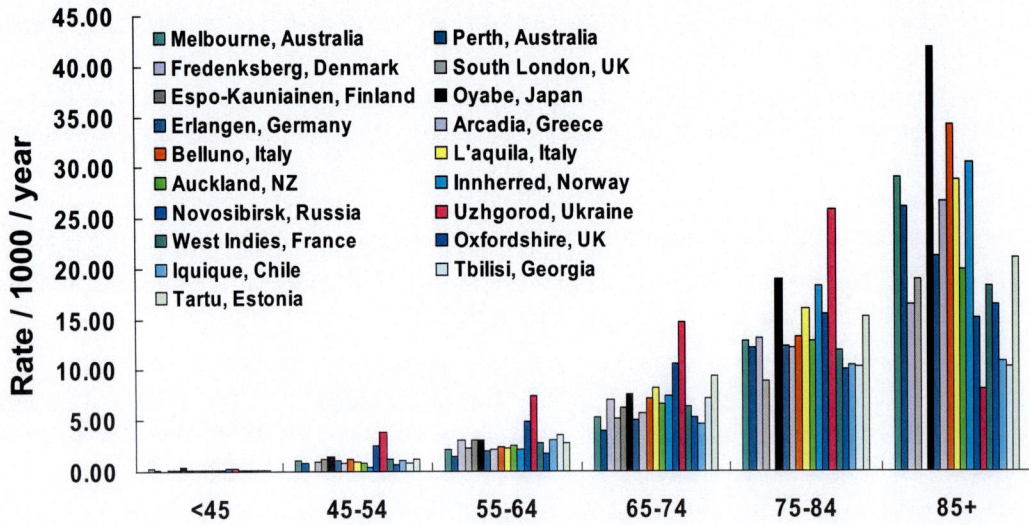

Figure 3. Age-specific annual incidence per 1000 population of all strokes combined in selected populations.*

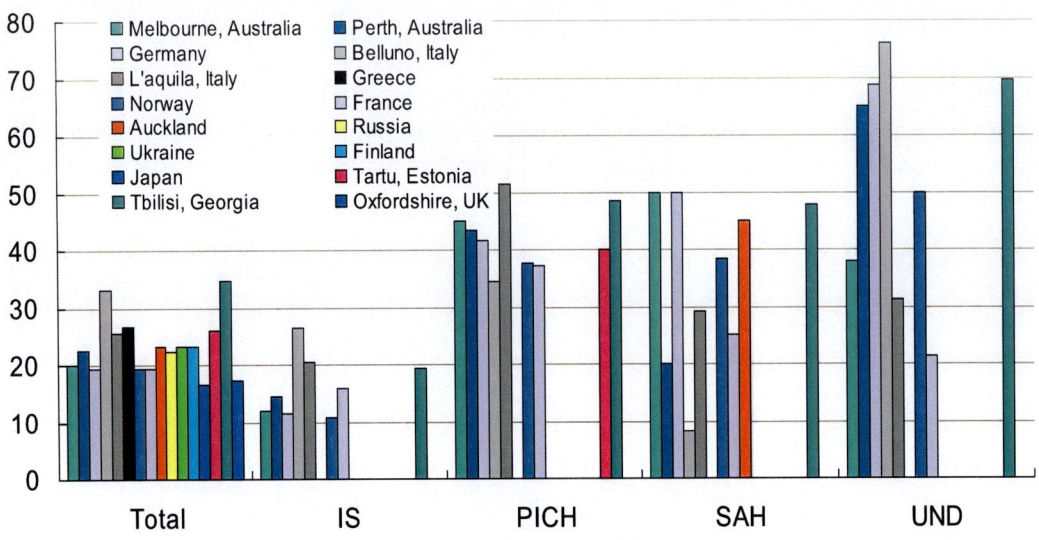

Figure 4. Case-fatality within 1 month of stroke onset by stroke type in selected populations.*

Over the last few years, data from new reviews and population-based stroke incidence studies have become available [17,27-30]. Overall proportional frequency of pathological types of stroke and of ischemic stroke subtypes in white populations was reviewed by

Warlow and colleagues [31]. According to their review, atherothromboembolism accounts for half of all ischemic strokes, while intracranial small vessel disease and cardioembolism account for 25% and 20% ischemic strokes, respectively (Figure 7).

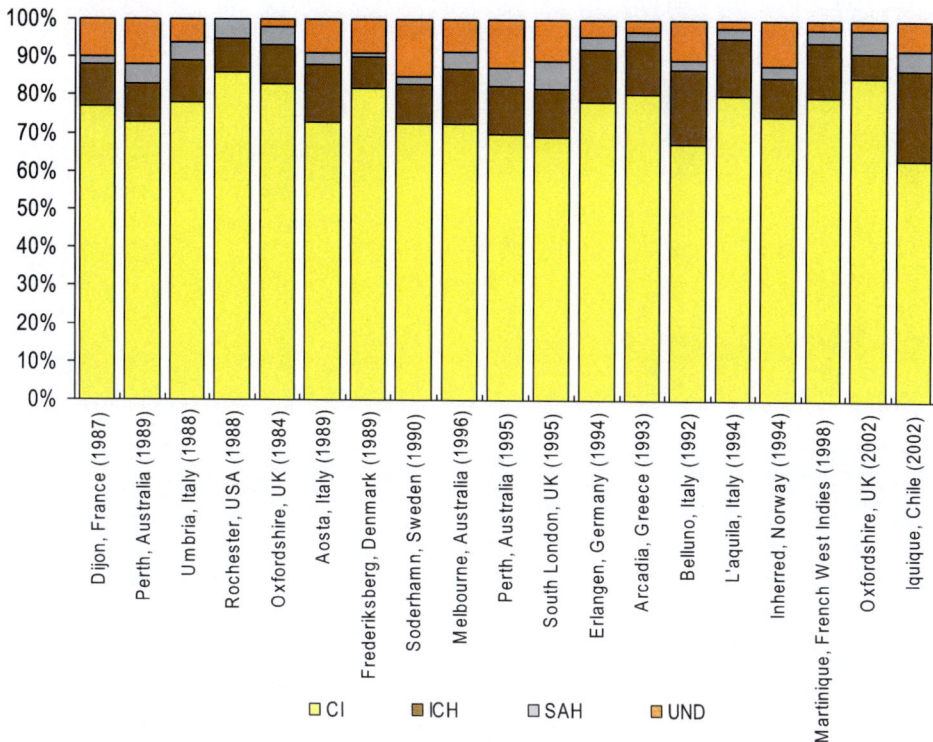

Figure 5. Proportional frequency of stroke pathological types in selected populations.*

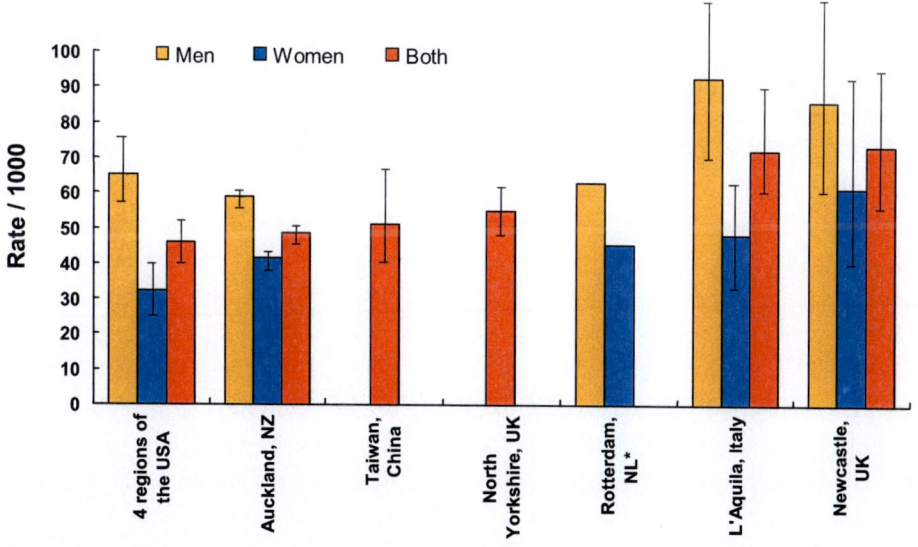

Figure 6. Age-standardized prevalence of stroke per 1000 people aged ≥65 years in selected populations.*

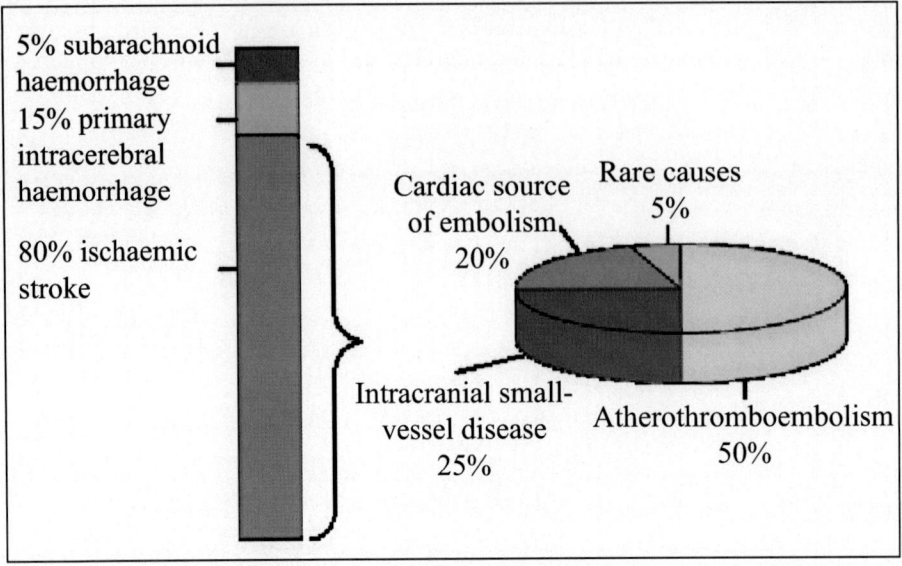

Figure 7. Overall proportional frequency of pathological types of stroke and of ischemic stroke subtypes in white populations (Warlow et al. reproduced from *the Lancet* by permission).

Rothwell and colleagues [27] recently reported results of a population-based TIA/stroke incidence study that analyzed changes in TIA/stroke rates, outcomes and risk factors in Oxfordshire, UK over the period of 20 years (1981-2004). This was the first 'ideal' population-based study that showed a significant reduction in stroke incidence (particularly for ischaemic stroke and intracerebral haemorrhage) and mortality (but not case-fatality) over the last 20 years, thus providing evidence that preventive strategies do actually reduce the incidence of stroke on the community level. It was also the first population-based study to document the predominance of acute cerebrovascular incidence (stroke and transient ischemic attack combined) over the incidence of acute coronary events (myocardial infarction and unstable angina combined) (relative incidence 1.2; 95% confidence interval 1.1-1.3). Anderson and colleagues have recently completed the largest Auckland Regional Community Stroke (ARCOS) 2002-2003 stroke incidence and outcomes study in Auckland, New Zealand, 2002-2003 [28] and compared its results with 2 similar stroke population-based studies in Auckland carried out in 1981-1982 and 1991-1992. This study showed modest declines in overall stroke incidence and attack rates in Auckland over the two decades. Two other recent publications based on the ARCOS 2002-2003 study demonstrated substantial ethnic differences in trends and stroke subtype incidence rates in New Zealand [8,32], with non-white populations (particularly Pacific and Maori people) having experienced a high and increased incidence rate and a greater risk of stroke (especially ischemic stroke and intracerebral hemorrhage) compared with New Zealand European people. A decrease in stroke incidence rates was also recently observed in Tartu, Estonia [29]. These and other 'ideal' population-based studies [10] published after 1990 showed a decline in stroke incidence, as summarized in Table 2. A stroke incidence and outcomes study by Lavados and colleagues [30] in Iquique, Chile (the PISCIS Project) was the first population-based stroke incidence study in Latin America that met not only the standard [33] but also the most rigorous criteria for an 'ideal' stroke incidence study [14]. The key findings of this study were that stroke outcomes and incidence rates in a predominantly Hispanic-mestizo population of the city of Iquique, Chile, are similar to those in other populations, but the proportion of intracerebral haemorrhage is somewhat higher. Another population-based stroke incidence study in a less affluent country was recently carried out in Tbilisi, Georgia [17]. This study demonstrated overall stroke incidence rates comparable to those reported in developed countries, but the proportion of hemorrhagic strokes and one-month case-fatality were greater than those in developed countries.

Table 2. Secular trends in stroke incidence rates in 'ideal' population-based studies

Study region (city, country)	Period of study	Change in stroke incidence
Rochester, MN, USA [37]	1955-1989	30% decline
Fredericksburg, Denmark [38]	1972-1990	15% increase
Copenhagen, Denmark [39]	1982-1991	3% decline
Espoo-Kauniainen, Finland [40]	1972-1991	20% decline
Oyabe, Japan [41]	1977-1991	30% decline
Novosibirsk, Russia [42]	1982-1992	22% decline
Perth, Australia [43]	1989-1996	23% decline
Tartu, Estonia [29]	1991-2003	18% decline
Auckland, NZ [28]	1981-2003	11% decline
Oxfordshire, UK [27]	1981-2004	29% decline

The age-standardized prevalence of stroke in 65+ years old people ranges from 4.6% to 7.3% (6-9% in men and 3-6% in women) [10]. Similar to incidence rates, prevalence of stroke increases with age with moderate geographical differences in prevalence (Figure 6) and there is evidence that stroke prevalence over the last few decades tends to increase. For example, age-, race-, and sex-adjusted stroke prevalence in the USA among 25-74 years old people increased from 1.41% to 1.87% from 1971-1975 to 1988-1994 [34]. The recent increase in stroke prevalence is likely to be associated with improved management of stroke patients and aging of the population. Only few studies reported prevalence of both total strokes and strokes with associated disability and impairment, with the latter varying from 55% of all strokes in New Zealand [35] to 99% in the UK [36]. Common acute impairments in stroke survivors include limb weakness (ranges in different studies from 72% to 99%), urinary incontinence (32-79%), dysphagia (28-51%), cognitive impairment (14-41%) [36]. There is also evidence that prevalence of impairment and disability profiles varies between pathological types of stroke and ischemic stroke subtypes and ethnic groups [36]. These prevalence data are important for evidence-based planning of community and rehabilitation services for stroke survivors.

Panel 2 summarizes key features of modern stroke incidence and prevalence.

Panel 2. Key features of modern stroke incidence and prevalence research*

- The overall age-standardised incidence of stroke in people aged ≥55 years ranges from 4.2 to 11.7 per 1000 person-years. The proportion of ischemic stroke ranges from 67 to 81%, intracerebral hemorrhage – 7 to 20% and subarachnoid hemorrhage – 1 to 7%. The risk of ischemic stroke (including ischemic stroke subtypes) and intracerebral hemorrhage and the proportion of intracerebral hemorrhage in non-white populations is about two times greater than that in white populations.
- Two third of stroke-related deaths occur in developing countries and there is some evidence that, at least in developed countries, acute cerebrovascular events (stroke and transient ischemic attack) become more common events than acute coronary events (myocardial infarction and unstable angina).
- Stroke incidence, prevalence, stroke-subtype structure, one month case-fatality and mortality rates show modest geographical variations, with the exception of Ukraine, Russia and Japan, where incidence rates are highest, and Italy and the UK where prevalence rates are highest.
- The average age of patients affected by stroke is 70 years in men and 75 years in women, but it is substantially younger in non-white populations and developing countries. In developed countries, more than half of all strokes occur in people over 75 years of age. Approximately 25% of all strokes occur in people younger than 65 years, and 5% in people younger than 45 years.
- The age-standardised prevalence rate of stroke in people aged ≥65 years ranges from 5 to 7% and it tends to increase due to aging of the population and improved survival, therefore the overall burden of stroke is likely to continue increase.
- In developed countries, overall case-fatality within 1 month of stroke onset is approximately 23% and is higher for intracerebral haemorrhage (42%) and subarachnoid haemorrhage (32%) than for ischemic stroke (16%). Early stroke-related case-fatality in developing countries is substantially greater than that in developed countries.
- Overall, there is a trend towards stabilizing or decreasing stroke incidence in some developed countries, but there is suggestive evidence that incidence of stroke is increasing in developing countries.

*Modified from Feigin et al [10].

Transient Ischemic Attack

Transient ischemic attack (TIA) is commonly diagnosed on the basis of presence of focal neurological symptoms relating to focal cerebral, brain stem, or retinal ischemia with abrupt onset and complete resolution within 24 hours (usually within minutes). Although this definition of TIA is commonly used in epidemiologic research, it should be noted that structural lesions in the brain relevant to TIA can be found in 30 to 67% of the patients [44]. TIA constitutes approximately 10 to 50% of stroke incidence but population-based data on TIA are scarce and inconsistent [45-50]. The highest incidence rates of TIA (approximately 70 cases per 100000 people per year) were reported in Rochester, MN, USA [49] and Northern Portugal [51], the lowest (approximately 30 cases per 100000 people per year) in

Tartu, Estonia [52] and Novosibirsk, Russia [53]. Overall, 80% of all TIA occur in carotid artery and 20% in vertebrobasilar distribution, with incidence rates increasing with age.

RISK FACTORS

Medical and Environmental Risk Factors

A number of stroke risk factors have been identified [54-67] and commonly described as well documented and less well documented, modifiable and non-modifiable. The major established risk factors for stroke that can be addressed therapeutically are elevated blood pressure, cardiac disease, TIA, asymptomatic carotid stenosis, cigarette smoking, and diabetes mellitus. Less well-documented but also potentially controllable risk factors include low socioeconomic status, unhealthy diet/nutrition, excessive alcohol intake, obesity, diabetes mellitus, physical inactivity, some blood disorders and lipid abnormalities, migraine, hormone replacement therapy, oral contraceptives, drug abuse, inflammatory processes, elevated plasma fibrinogen level, and low personal and environmental temperature. Non-modifiable but well documented risk factors for stroke are increasing age (almost doubling for each successive decade), sex (men are at greater risk of stroke than women until the age of 65 years but women are at greater risk of stroke than men at older age). Some studies suggest that a parental history of stroke and genetic predisposition are also important risk factors for stroke [55,67]. Current evidence suggests that stroke and vascular risk factors have similar relative effects across the world, with modest interaction with race/ethnicity and nation [68,69]. Table 3 summarises evidence from systematic reviews (meta-analyses) of the literature concerning risk factors for stroke.

Although some risk factors are similar for various stroke pathological types and subtypes (e.g. elevated blood pressure, cigarette smoking), some are more specific for particular types of stroke (e.g. unruptured intracranial aneurysms for SAH, atrial fibrillation for cardioembolic stroke etc.). Several systematic and narrative reviews [93-95] identified the following major risk factors for ischemic stroke: age, gender, non-white ethnicity, heredity, elevated blood pressure, cardiac disease (particularly atrial fibrillation), diabetes mellitus, hypercholesterolemia, cigarette smoking, and alcohol excess. There is also evidence of differences in risk factor profiles by ischemic stroke etiological subtypes [96]. For example, male sex and elevated cholesterol level appear to be significant risk factors for large vessel ischemic stroke (OR 1.8; 95% CI 1.1-2.8 and 1.6; 95% CI 1.3-1.9, respectively) but male sex is protective for small vessel ischemic stroke (OR 0.5; 95% CI 0.3-0.7) and elevated cholesterol level is protective for cardioembolic stroke (OR 0.6; 95% CI 0.5-0.8. No association between lacunar stroke (small vessel ischemic stroke) and diabetes or hypertension have been found in some population-based studies [8,97]. People with cardioembolic stroke often found to be older or have a history of cardiac disease than people with other subtypes of ischemic stroke, a finding largely explained by the increasing prevalence of atrial fibrillation with older age. There is evidence that people with large vessel (atherothrombotic) ischemic stroke more likely to have a smoking history or elevated lipid levels [8,98,99]. Table 4 summarises current evidence concerning risk factors for ischemic stroke.

Table 3. Cause-effect associations of selected risk factors with stroke (systematic reviews)*

Risk factor [reference study]	Summary risk estimates	Notes
Elevated blood pressure [70-72]	Each 10 mm Hg lower systolic BP is associated with a decrease in risk of stroke of approximately one third. The association is continuous down to levels of at least 115/75 mm Hg and is consistent across sexes, regions, and stroke subtypes and for fatal and nonfatal events.	The proportional association is age dependent but is still strong and positive in those aged 80 years.
Total blood cholesterol level [72-74]	Each 1-mmol/l higher level of total cholesterol was associated with 35% (95% CI 26-44%) increased risk of fatal or non-fatal ischaemic stroke, and 20% (95% CI 8-30%) decreased risk of fatal haemorrhagic stroke.	Statin therapy can safely reduce the 5-year incidence of stroke by about one fifth per mmol/L reduction in LDL cholesterol.
Cigarette smoking [75-77]	Cigarette smoking independently increases the RR of stroke about three-fold. The risk is dependent upon the amount of cigarettes smoked, is consistent for all subtypes of stroke, and is strongest for subarachnoid haemorrhage and cortical ischaemic stroke caused by arterial atherothromboembolism	Up to one quarter of all strokes are directly attributable to cigarette smoking.
Alcohol intake [78]	Compared with abstainers, consumption of more than 60 g of alcohol/day was associated with an increased RR of total stroke, 1.6 (95% CI 1.4-1.9); ischemic stroke, 1.7 (95% CI 1.3-2.2); and hemorrhagic stroke, 2.2 (95% CI 1.5-3.2), while consumption of less than 12 g/d was associated with a reduced RR of total stroke, 0.8 (95%, CI 0.8-0.9) and ischemic stroke, 0.8 (95% CI 0.7-1.0), and consumption of 12 to 24 g/d was associated with a reduced RR of ischemic stroke, 0.7 (95% CI 0.6-0.9).	Heavy alcohol consumption increases the relative risk of stroke while light or moderate alcohol consumption may be protective against total and ischemic stroke
Fish consumption [79]	Compared with those who never consumed fish or ate fish less than once per month, the pooled RRs for total stroke were 0.9 (95% CI 0.8-1.1) for individuals with fish intake 1 to 3 times per month, 0.8 (95% CI 0.7-0.9) for 2 to 4 times per week, and 0.7 (95% CI 0.5-0.9) for ≥5 times per week	Fish consumption as seldom as 1 to 3 times per month may protect against the incidence of ischemic stroke
Physical activity [80;81]	Moderately intense physical activity compared with inactivity, showed a protective effect on total stroke for both occupational (RR = 0.6, 95% CI 0.5-0.9) and leisure time physical activity (RR = 0.9, 95% CI 0.8-0.9). Highly active individuals had a 27% lower risk of stroke incidence or mortality (RR=0.7; 95% CI 0.7-0.8) than did low-active individuals.	Moderately intense physical activity is sufficient to achieve risk reduction. Moderate and high levels of physical activity are associated with reduced risk of total, ischemic, and hemorrhagic strokes.
C-reactive protein (CRP) [82]	RR for stroke when persons with the highest quartile of CRP concentration were compared to the lowest quartile was 1·68 (95% CI 1.4–2.0)	High levels of CRP were also predictive of cognitive decline & dementia

Table 3. (Continued)

Risk factor [reference study]	Summary risk estimates	Notes
Chronic infection [83]	OR of H. pylori seropositivity and stroke was 1.5 (95% CI 1.2-1.8), for the association between stroke and anti-CagA positivity was 2.2 (95% CI 1.5-3.4)	Association between H. pylori positivity, anti-CagA positivity and stroke seemed higher with stroke due to large vessel disease
Oral contraceptives (OC) [84]	RR of ischemic stroke associated with current use of low dose combined OC was 2.1 (95% CI 1.6-2.9), and 2.5 (95% CI 2.0-3.3) for second generation OC	A hazardous effect was also shown for third generation OC
Hormone replacement therapy (HRT) [85]	Total stroke: OR 1.3 (95% CI 1.1-1.5). Ischemic stroke: OR 1.3 (1.1-1.6). Hemorrhagic stroke or TIA: OR 1.1 (95% CI 0.7-1.8) and 1.0 (95% CI 0.8-1.3).	HRT was also associated with worse outcomes in stroke survivors
Plasma fibrinogen [86]	HR for total stroke for 1 g/L increase in usual fibrinogen level was 2.1 (95% CI 1.8-2.3)	Causal relevance remains to be researched
Homocysteine [87]	Evidence is emerging that homocysteine may be a marker for stroke but may not be causal. The OR of stroke for a 5 micromol/l increase in serum homocysteine was 1.6 (95% CI 1.3 to 2.0) in prospective studies.	Lowering homocysteine concentrations by 3 micromol/l from current levels (achievable by increasing folic acid intake) would reduce the risk of stroke by 24% (15% to 33%). There is also a continuous, inverse linear relation between plasma homocysteine concentrations and cognitive performance in older persons.
Migraine [88]	RR for ischemic stroke in migraine with aura was 2.3 (95% CI 1.6-3.2), in migraine without aura – 1.8 (95% CI 1.1-3.2)	Mechanism of the associations should be studied
Low socioeconomic status [89;90]	Stroke incidence is higher in low socioeconomic groups (RR 1.7; 95% CI 1.2-2.2)	The mechanisms through which socioeconomic status affects stroke risk remain unclear.
Genes [91]	OR for factor V Leiden Arg506Gln was 1.3 (95% CI 1.1-1.6); methylenetetrahydrofolate reductase C677T - 1.2 (95% CI 1.1-1.4); prothrombin G20210A - 1.4 (95% CI 1.1-1.9); angiotensin-converting enzyme insertion/deletion - 1.2 (95% CI 1.1-1.4)	Only studies of ischemic stroke in white adults were analyzed. No single gene with major effect was identified; rather, common variants in several genes, each exerting a modest effect, contribute to the risk of stroke
Family history of stroke [92]	Monozygotic twins were more likely to be concordant than dizygotic twins (OR, 1.7; 95% CI 1.2-2.3). A positive family history was a risk factor for stroke in both case-control (OR, 1.8; 95% CI 1.7-1.9) and cohort (OR, 1.3; 95% CI 1.2-1.5) studies.	Reliable interpretation of published family history studies is undermined by major heterogeneity, insufficient detail, and potential publication and reporting bias.

*HR - hazard ratio; RR – relative risk; OR – odds ratio; CI – confidence interval

For intracerebral hemorrhage, risk factors appeared to be age, male sex, hypertension, and high alcohol intake [103]. High cholesterol tends to be associated with a lower risk of intracerebral hemorrhage [103]. Smoking, hypertension, and excessive alcohol are the most important risk factors for subarachnoid hemorrhage [104]. It has also been shown that unruptured intracranial aneurysms more than 7 mm in diameter have a high risk of rupture

[105] and, therefore, are the risk factors for SAH. Pooled risk estimates of intracerebral hemorrhage and subarachnoid hemorrhage for selected risk factors in two recent meta-analyses of case-control and cohort studies [103,104] are presented in Table 5.

Table 4. Risk factors for ischemic stroke by level of evidence [54;60;100-102]

Well documented	Less well documented
Modifiable	Modifiable
Elevated blood pressure	Obesity
Hyperlipidemia	Physical inactivity
Cardiac disease (atrial fibrillation,	Poor diet/nutrition
infective endocarditis, valvular heart	Alcohol abuse (≥30 g/day)
disease, recent large myocardial	Hyperhomocysteinemia
infarction, intracardiac congenital	Drug abuse
defects)	Hypercoagulability
Cigarette smoking	Hormone replacement therapy
Asymptomatic carotid stenosis	Oral contraceptive use
Sickle-cell disease	High serum lipoprotein (a) level
Transient ischemic attack	Potentially modifiable
Potentially modifiable	Reduced HDL cholesterol
Diabetes mellitus	Migraine
Left ventricular hypertrophy	Inflammatory processes
Non-modifiable	Anticardiolipin antibodies
Advancing age	Low socioeconomic status
Sex (M > W)	Factors operating during fetal and early neonatal
Race/ethnicity (Non-Whites > Whites)	life (including low birth weight)
Hereditary/genetic factors	Cold weather

Table 5. The most significant risk factors for either intracerebral hemorrhage or subarachnoid hemorrhage (OR – odds ratio estimated from case-control studies; RR – relative risk estimated from cohort studies; CI – confidence interval; NS – statistically nonsignificant) [103;104]

Risk factor	Intracerebral hemorrhage [103]		Subarachnoid hemorrhage [104]	
	RR (95% CI)	OR (95% CI)	RR (95% CI)	OR (95% CI)
Age (every 10-year increase)	2 (1.8-2.2)	not estimated	not estimated	not estimated
Male sex	3.7 (3.3-4.3)	not estimated	not estimated	not estimated
Current smoking	1.3 (1.1-1.6)	NS	2.2 (1.3-3.6)	3.1 (2.7-3.5)
Diabetes mellitus	1.3 (1.0-1.7)	NS	NS	NS
High alcohol intake	NS	3.4 (2.2-5.1)	2.1 (1.5-2.8)	1.5 (1.3-1.8)
Hypertension	2.2-33 (1.5-49)	3.7 (2.5-5.4)	2.5 (2.0-3.1)	2.6 (2.0-3.1)

Hereditary/Genetic Risk Factors

Although twin and family history studies support a role for genetic factors in stroke risk, data on genetic epidemiology of stroke are scarce and not consistent [55,67,92,106,107]. Genome-wide scanning in both human and animal models has led to the identification of regions of the genome that contain genes for stroke susceptibility and sensitivity. In a landmark Icelandic study, linkage was established between stroke and a locus on chromosome 5q12 designated STRK1 [108]. A recent meta-analysis of all candidate gene association studies in ischemic stroke (18,000 cases and 58,000 controls) revealed statistically significant associations of ischemic stroke with factor V Leiden Arg506Gln (OR, 1.33; 95% CI, 1.12-1.58), methylenetetrahydrofolate reductase C677T (OR, 1.24; 95% CI, 1.08-1.42), prothrombin G20210A (OR, 1.44; 95% CI, 1.11-1.86), and angiotensin-converting enzyme insertion/deletion (OR, 1.21; 95% CI, 1.08-1.35). These were also the most investigated candidate genes, including 4588, 3387, 3028, and 2990 cases, respectively. No statistically significant association with ischemic stroke was detected for the 3 next most investigated genes (factor XIII, apolipoprotein E, and human platelet antigen type 1). This comprehensive meta-analysis confirmed a genetic component to ischemic stroke and suggested that no single gene has a major effect but rather, common variants in several genes, each exerting a modest effect, contribute to the risk of ischemic stroke. Moreover, it has been suggested that specific genetic variants interact with specific environmental factors to elevate an individual's risk of intermediate vascular phenotypes and subsequently of traits such as intimal-medial wall thickness (IMT), which leads to risk of stroke and myocardial infarction (Figure 8) [55].

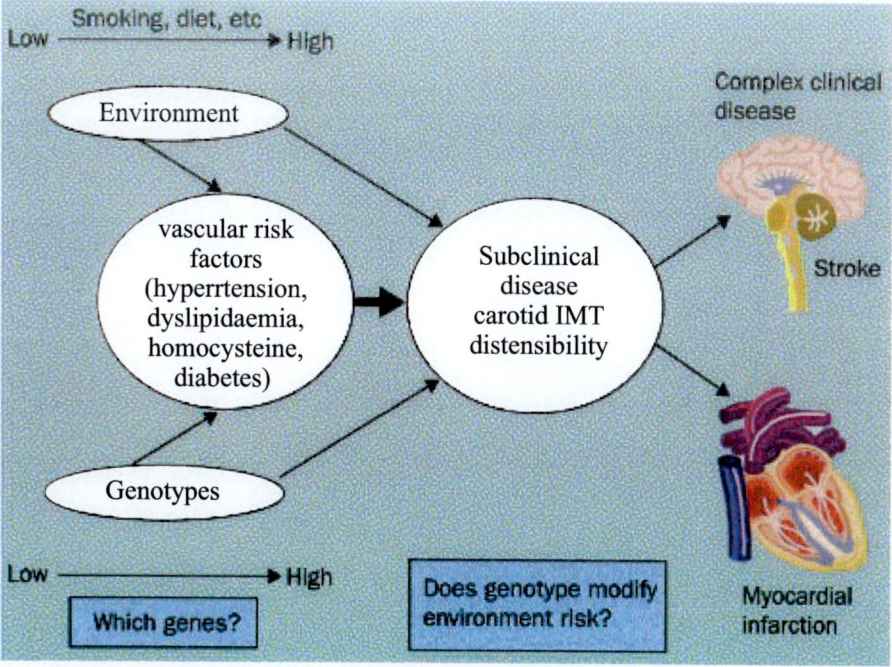

Figure 8. Gene-environment interaction in stroke and risk of myocardial infarction (Reproduced from the Lancet Neurology [55], with permission).

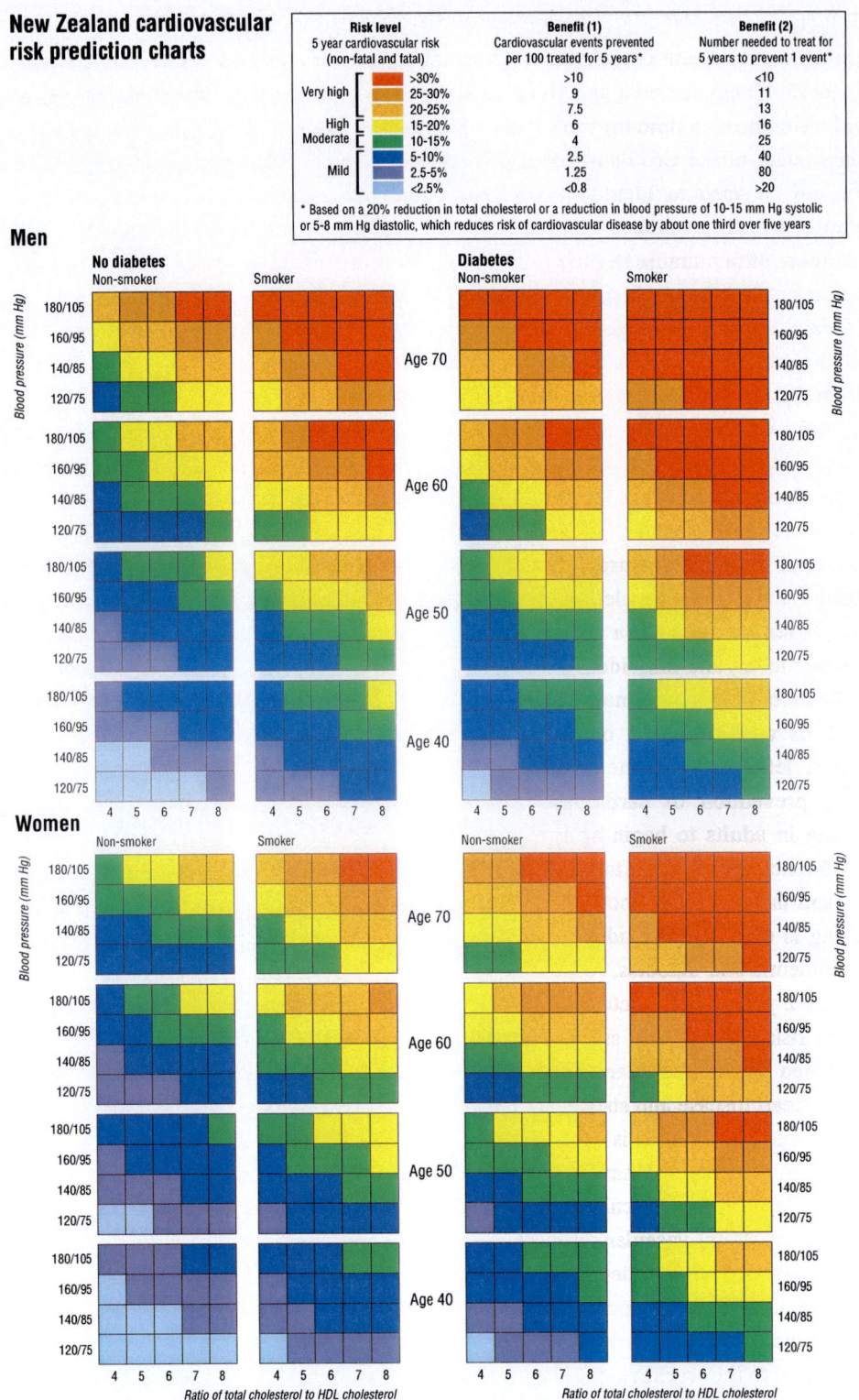

Figure 9. Absolute 5-year risk of developing cardiovascular disease and stroke (adopted from Jackson [114], with permission).

In a recent review of genetic risk factors for stroke and atherosclerosis, Humphries & Morgan [55] demonstrated that high expression of the deletion-allele ACE in plasma or tissue, differences in lipid profile caused by *APOE* ε4 allele, and high homocysteine owing to homozygosity of the C677T *MTHFR* T allele genotype are associated with the risk of IMT, and could be used to identify people with high stroke risk who need earlier and more aggressive control of other modifiable risk factors. It has been suggested that co-occurrence of common, unfavourable genetic mutations has a role in the development of different stroke subtypes [109]. Genes involved in inflammation, including genes that encode for the interleukin-1 receptor antagonist and paraoxonase-1 are currently under investigation [108]. Data on genetic risk factors and gene-environment interactions can be used for refining and individualizing primary and secondary prevention of stroke.

Stroke Prevention Strategies

At least two thirds of strokes are explained by identifiable risk factors [110] and there is suggestive evidence that at least 80% of strokes can be prevented [111]. Modern approach to stroke prevention includes a combination of population-based (control of risk factors on the population level) and individual-based or high-risk strategies. The high-risk strategy includes identification and management of individuals with high risk of stroke or even pre-clinical individuals with high risk of developing of some stroke risk factors (e.g. subjects with increased left atrial volume [112]). Current American Heart Association Guidelines for primary prevention of cardiovascular disease and stroke [113] recommend risk factor screening in adults to begin at age 20 years, with blood pressure, body mass index, waist circumference, and pulse (to screen for atrial fibrillation) to be recorded at least every 2 years; and fasting serum lipoprotein profile (or total and high density lipoprotein cholesterol if fasting is unavailable) and fasting blood glucose measured according to person's risk for hyperlipidemia and diabetes, respectively (at least every 5 years if no risk factors are present, and every 2 years if risk factors are present). For all adults ≥40 years of age or people with 2 or more risk factors (e.g. smoking, elevated blood pressure, total/LDL cholesterol, ECG documented left ventricular hypertrophy, or diabetes) the absolute risk of developing coronary heart disease and stroke can be calculated. Evidence is emerging that apolipoprotein B /apolipoprotein A1 ratio is a better predictor of stroke and MI than total/LDL or LDL/HDL ratios. Prediction charts have also been developed [114] for selecting people with an increased risk of cardiovascular disease (stroke, TIA, coronary heart disease, congestive heart failure or peripheral vascular disease) (Figure 9). Control of risk factors should be aimed to lower the absolute risk of developing coronary heart disease and stroke as much as possible. A stepwise implementation of evidence-based interventions with comprehensive and integrated action at country level have recently been suggested by the WHO [115,116] as the major means to the worldwide prevention and control of chronic diseases including stroke.

STROKE OUTCOMES

Clinical outcomes in stroke can be classified into survival (death), impairment (signs and symptoms of the underlying pathology), disability (limitation in functional activities), handicap (disadvantage to the individual resulting from impairment and disability) [117], and quality of life (patient's general well-being resulting from physical, psychological, and social aspects of life that may be affected by changes in health states) [118,119]. Recent International Classification of Functioning (ICF), Disability and Health (2001) describes outcomes in terms of body functioning, activities (related to tasks and actions by an individual) and participation (involvement in a life situation), and environment.

**Table 6. International Classification of Functioning,
Disability and Health Definitions (2001)**

Old terminology	New terminology	Definition	Examples (selected)
Impairment	Body function / structure	Physiological functions of body systems including psychological. Structures are anatomical parts or regions of their bodies and their components. Impairments are problems in body function or structure.	Beck depression Inventory, Mini-Mental State Examination, Modified Ashworth, Motor-free Visual perception Test
Disability	Activity	The execution of a task by an individual. Limitations in activity are defined as difficulties an individual might experience in completing a given activity.	Barthel Index, Rankin Scale, Berg balance Scale, Functional Independence Measure, Frenchay Activities Index, Modified Rankin Handicap Scale
Handicap	Participation	Involvement of an individual in a life situation. Restrictions to participation describe difficulties experienced by the individual in a life situation or role.	Euroqol-5D, Medical Outcomes Study Short Form 36 (SF-36), Nottingham Health Profile, Stroke Impact Scale, Stroke Specific Quality of Life

Accurate information about short-term and long-term stroke outcomes is important to the patients, their families and health care providers for setting up appropriate goals and expectations and developing appropriate management options (e.g. discharge plan, interventions).

Survival

On the average, about one quarter of stroke patients die within the first month after stroke onset, one third within first 6-12 months, and one half within first two years after stroke, with the average case-fatality of 5% between years 1 and 10 and about 2% between years 10 and 21 after stroke [120-125], with older patients having the worse prognosis. Based on these and other similar population-based studies, cumulative case-fatalities have been estimated at 40 to 60% at 5 years, approximately 80% at 10 years, 90% at 15 years and 93% at 21 years. Stroke patients have nearly twice the mortality rates of the general population. The most important prognostic factors for death are increasing age, urinary incontinence, stroke severity, pre-stroke disability, and the presence of cardiovascular risk factors. While approximately two thirds of deaths within first month after the stroke onset are due to the direct effects of the brain lesion and another one sixth due to recurrent stroke, among one month stroke survivors one fifths of subsequent deaths between 30 day – 1 year, 1-5 year and 5-10 year periods are due to recurrent strokes and about one thirds due to cardiovascular causes [124].

Functional Outcomes

Since stroke often results in activity limitations across multiple domains of functioning and some outcomes may have independent prognostic implications [126,127], it is important to exercise a multifocal approach to studying stroke outcomes and include patient-centred measures that evaluate different functions [127] so that the impact of stroke on the patient as a whole can be understood and quantified. Although a relationship between impairment, disability, handicap and quality of life has been documented [128,129], these relationships are not simple [127,128,130,131].

While the number of studies of outcomes (especially death, disability and neurological impairments) in stroke survivors is substantial [120,132], there have only been three population-based studies evaluating medium to long-term functional outcomes in stroke survivors [133-136]. Two early population-based stroke incidence studies in Auckland (1981-82 and 1991-92) showed that approximately 55% of 3-year stroke survivors have incomplete recovery, and one third of them require assistance in at least one self-care activity [35]. In the 1991-1992 study [133], health-related quality of life (HRQoL) measured using the SF-36 questionnaire, and basic activities of daily living were assessed in stroke survivors 6 years after stroke (n=639) and compared to an age- and sex-matched general population (n=310). The authors found that although the majority of stroke survivors (77%) were living at home, 42% of the patients were dependent in at least 1 aspects of (basic care) activities of daily living, and they had lower scores for the physical health, general health, vitality, and social function components of HRQoL compared with the general population. In the Perth Community Stroke Study (Australia, 1989-1994) [135], 152 stroke patients (41% of acute stroke patients) survived to 5 years. Of survivors who were neither institutionalised nor disabled at the time of their initial stroke, 21 (14%) were institutionalized in a nursing home, and 47 (36%) were disabled at 5 years after stroke. In a larger and more recent population-based study in South London (UK 1995-2000) [134,136], of 639 registered stroke patients, 392 without previous disability survived and were assessed for disability at 3 months, of whom 34 (9%) were severely disabled and 60 (15%) moderately disabled. Of 225 survivors (35%) at 12-month after stroke 11% had moderate or severe disability (Barthel Index <15). Gaze paresis, dysphagia, cognitive impairment (MMSE <24), urinary incontinence, and coma at stroke onset were shown to be independently associated with death and severe disability at three months [36].

As noted above, stroke is a heterogeneous disorder that consists of three major pathological types, each of which has differing short to medium-term outcomes [137-142]. However, data on the long-term functional outcomes and costs in survivors of different stroke subtypes are scarce, limited to one year follow-up and are often inconsistent. There is good evidence that cost of stroke differs in different stroke subtypes, but there was only one population-based study that addressed this issue. In the population-based study in Australia, the total lifetime costs of all new strokes was estimated to be A$1.3 billion a year, of which ischemic stroke (IS) costs constituted 72% (A$937 million), intracerebral hemorrhage (ICH) 26% (A$334 million), and unclassified stroke 2% (A$30 million), with the average cost per case of A$44,428 [143,144]. The lifetime cost per person of first strokes occurring in the USA was estimated to be $228,030 for subarachnoid hemorrhage (SAH), $123,565 for ICH, $90,981 for IS, and $103,576 averaged across all stroke sub-types, and indirect costs accounted for 58% of lifetime costs [145].

To our knowledge, there are only three population-based studies that investigated health outcomes by stroke subtype [131,136,146]. In the study in Perth (Australia) [131], handicap (measured by the London Handicap Scale) differed significantly with severity of disability (measured by the Barthel Index) in ischaemic stroke subtypes (defined by the Oxfordshire stroke classification) at 12 months. In the Australasian study [146], incomplete recovery at 1 year after subarachnoid haemorrhage (SAH) was found in 46% of survivors, of which ongoing memory problems were recorded in 50%, mood abnormalities in 39%, and speech problems in 14%, while a substantial proportion of survivors had diminished level of HRQoL. No association between cognitive impairment and the Oxfordshire Community Stroke Project classification of stroke subtypes was found in the South London population-based study [127].

Although prognostic factors of stroke outcomes have been the subject of much discussion in the literature [140,147-160], there have been only a few studies that addressed some aspects of this issue in the population-based setting [127,134,135,146]. In a population-based study in Perth, Australia (n=152), factors found to be associated with poor outcome (death or disability) at 5 years included increasing age, baseline disability, hemiparesis, and recurrent stroke [135]. No predictors of complete recovery from SAH were determined in a population-based study of SAH in Australasia [146], but the follow-up period was restricted to 1 year and no other measures of disability and handicap were undertaken in this report. In a population-based study in the UK [127,134], initial incontinence was found to be the best predictor of moderate or severe disability (Barthel Index <15) at 1 year after stroke, however it remains unclear whether this association holds true in the long term. A useful model for predicting ipsilateral ischemic stroke after TIA has recently been developed by Rothwell and colleagues [161] (Figure 10). These models allow clinicians to take into account the many characteristics of an individual patient and their interactions, to consider the risks and benefits of interventions (e.g. carotid endarterectomy for stroke prevention) separately if needed, and to provide patients with personalised estimates of their likelihood of benefit. Although stroke incidence and mortality are known to be inversely related to socioeconomic status (SES) [162-165], data on the relationship between SES and stroke functional outcomes are scarce. In a recent UK hospital-based study [166], social deprivation was found to be strongly and inversely related to disability after stroke. Overall, about half of the patients who survive for 6 months after stroke are partially or totally dependent in their activities of daily living such as bathing, dressing, feeding, and mobility (10% need long-term nursing care). About one-third of patients surviving stroke for 1 year are unable to remain independent, and this proportion remains relatively unchanged in survivors followed for up to 5 years. However, functional recovery (lessening of disability or handicap) often continues long after specific neurologic deficits have ceased to change. Therefore patients and their families should never give up their fight for recovery and greater independence.

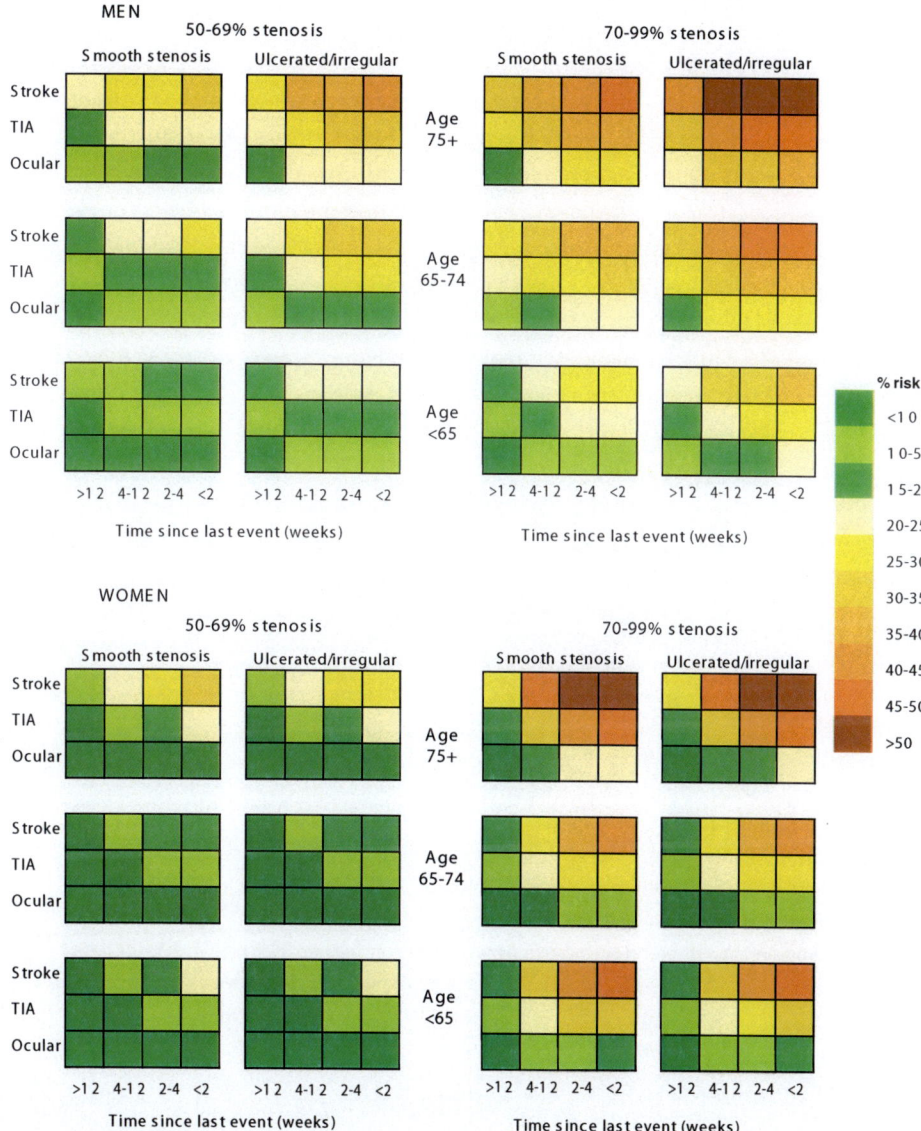

Figure 10. Predicted absolute risk of ipsilateral ischemic stroke on medical treatment in patients with recently symptomatic carotid stenosis by level and characteristics of stenosis (from article by Rothwell et al [161]. The graph is reproduced with permission from *the Lancet*).

MANAGEMENT STRATEGIES

Any acute stroke patient should be admitted to a hospital stroke unit as soon as possible (Panel 3). There is robust evidence that stroke patients who receive organised inpatient care in a geographically defined acute stroke unit (ASU) are more likely to be alive, independent, and living at home one year after the stroke [167]. All patients with acute stroke or TIA, irrespective of age or stroke severity or any other considerations, should be admitted to the ASU for initial evaluation and management. There are 3 major types of stroke units: (1) ASU unit for acute care only (the average length of staying in such units is usually a few days); (2) comprehensive stroke unit that provides both acute care and rehabilitation (the average length of staying in such units is usually from several days to few weeks); and (3) mobile stroke team. Current evidence shows superiority of the first two types of acute stroke units over mobile stroke team. The key elements of acute stroke units are the co-ordinated expert interdisciplinary team working in a geographically-based setting with regular team meetings (at least weekly). The tasks of the team are to establish an accurate diagnosis, observe vital signs, maintain homeostasis, provide acute treatment, prevent complications, implement early rehabilitation, initiate secondary prevention strategies, and develop the most appropriate discharge and rehabilitation plan. There is no evidence that extensive (and expensive!) laboratory monitoring of acute stroke patients is more effective than conventional management in ASU. Current recommendations for management and rehabilitation of acute stroke patients are summarised in Panels 3-6 (modified from *New Zealand Family Physician* 2005 [168], with permission).

Panel 3. Acute Stroke Treatment

	Level of evidence*
All patients with suspected stroke/TIA should be referred to, and assessed by, the ASU team as soon as possible after the patient is considered for admission to hospital.	1
All patients should have a CT head scan ASAP to confirm the diagnosis of stroke and stroke subtype.	2
Unless there is absolute contraindication, or the patient has agreed to thrombolysis with Alteplace or an experimental hyper-acute treatment, all patients with ischaemic stroke should be given aspirin (150-300 mg) as soon as possible after onset.	1
All patients with subarachnoid haemorrhage (SAH), potentially due to intracranial aneurysm rupture, should be urgently evaluated by neurosurgeon for possible neurosurgical intervention.	1
All patients should be closely monitored for hyperglycaemia and hyperthermia ($\geq 37.5°C$); those with diabetes or raised blood-glucose concentration should receive insulin; in patients with hyperthermia, an antipyretic such as paracetamol or cooling devices such as cooling blankets or compresses may be considered to maintain body temperature in the normal range.	2
All patients with deteriorating clinical state due to cerebellar haemorrhage should be considered for neurosurgical referral for possible intervention.	2

Panel 4. Prevention and management of complications of acute stroke

	Level of evidence*
Each stroke patient should undergo swallowing assessment.	2
Urinary catheters should be used with caution and alternative methods for the management of continence explored.	3
All those involved in moving stroke patients should receive training in lifting, transferring, and moving and handling of the upper limb.	3
In patients at high risk of deep vein thrombosis (DVT) and/or pulmonary embolism (PE), external compression stockings or intermittent pneumatic compression devices should be used where heparin/Clexane is contraindicated.	3
Awareness of the possibility of depression and other related mood disorders should lead to prompt evaluation and treatment.	3

Panel 5. Rehabilitation following acute stroke

	Level of evidence*
Rehabilitation should be started as soon as the patient's condition permits	2
Rehabilitation aims, with short and long-term rehabilitation objectives, should be established and agreed by all parties including the patient and carers.	3
Physiotherapy should aim to promote recovery of motor control, independence in functional tasks, optimise sensory stimulation, and prevent secondary complications such as soft tissue shortening and chest infections.	3
The broad role of occupational therapy in the rehabilitation of stroke patients should be recognised. Early referral for assessment is appropriate.	3
All patients with a communication problem resulting from stroke should be referred for speech and language therapy assessment and treatment.	1
Intensive speech and language therapy should be initiated as soon as the patient's condition is stable and may be required to continue over the long term.	2
Where intelligible speech is not a reasonable goal, the speech and language therapist should augment speech attempts and enable communication through means other than spoken language.	2
Speech and language therapist should play a key role in swallowing assessment.	3
Patients with diabetes, high blood cholesterol levels, poor oral intake or who are significantly underweight should be referred to dietician.	3
Active bowel and bladder management should be implemented. Catheters should be used only after full assessment. It is important to have regular bowel movements with at least one bowel empting every 2-3 days. Continence services can be approached when required.	3
Screening for depression and anxiety should be provided. Persistently (>6 weeks) depressed patients should be given antidepressant treatment.	2

It is commonly accepted that all patients should have a follow up plan at discharge from hospital. Follow up may involve different community services. The patients should be reviewed at stroke (neurovascular) clinic, or have a domiciliary visit. At follow up the caregiver should be interviewed, and attempt made to minimise caregiver stress.

Although the duration of rehabilitation therapy is generally determined by the rate of functional recovery, the probability of improvement of movement in paralyzed limbs is maximal during the first month after stroke and decreases significantly after 6 months, whereas improvement of speech, domestic and working skills, and unsteadiness can continue for up to 2 years. Recovery of arm movement is usually less complete than that of leg movement, and complete lack of any movement at onset of stroke, or no measurable grip strength by 4 weeks, is associated with a poor prognosis for return of useful arm function.

Panel 6. Secondary prevention of vascular events

	Level of evidence*
All patients with ischaemic stroke or TIA should be given long-term aspirin (100-150 mg) for prevention of future vascular disease, unless contraindication to aspirin or warfarin is considered more appropriate. Other antiplatelet therapies (dypiridamol) should be used as an adjunct therapy in situations of "aspirin failure".	1
All post-acute patients with either ischaemic stroke or primary intracerebral haemorrhage (when the patient is medically stable, which usually within the first 5-10 days after stroke onset) should receive blood pressure lowering therapy (preferably ACE inhibitor-diuretic combination) irrespective of initial blood pressure (hypertensive or non-hypertensive), age and gender.	1
Warfarin anticoagulation (INR 2-3) should be used where the stroke resulted from a cardiac source (e.g. atrial fibrillation) and the patient has a good understanding of the treatment and they are at low risk of haemorrhagic complications (e.g. low risk of falls, no alcohol abuse).	1
Carotid ultrasound should be organised in patients with severe ipsilateral disease who have no major comorbidities that reduce life expectancy and are prepared to accept the real early risk of surgery.	1
Carotid endarterectomy for patients with high grade carotid artery stenosis should be considered.	1
Post-stroke or TIA patients who have a persistent elevation of cholesterol despite dietary modification and two fasting levels above 5 mmol/L should be considered for statin therapy to reduce the risk of further stroke.	1
Secondary prevention of stroke should include adequate control of stroke risk factors, including lifestyle modifications (e.g. diet low in saturated fat, salt, and cholesterol; smoking abstinence; reasonable physical activity etc).	2

*1 - at least one randomised controlled trial as part of the body of literature of overall good quality and consistency addressing specific recommendation; 2 - availability of well conducted clinical studies but no randomised clinical trials on the topic of recommendation; 3 - evidence obtained from expert committee reports or opinions and/or clinical experiences of respected authorities.

CONCLUSION

Epidemiology of stroke, like any other non-communicable disorders is changing over time. Reliable data on stroke incidence, prevalence and risk factors are essential for evidence-based health care, therefore more good quality stroke incidence, prevalence, outcomes and risk factor studies in various regions and populations (especially in developing countries) are warranted. Despite a continuous decrease of stroke mortality rates observed in many developed countries over the last few decades, globally stroke as a cause of death has moved from third to second place in the world and is now the leading cause of physical disability in adults aged 65 years and older. Recent advances in stroke prevention and management offer an opportunity to reduce the burden of stroke. Urgent and practicable preventive measures, such as those recommended by the WHO, need to be implemented to the stop epidemic of stroke in developing countries.

REFERENCES

[1]   The World Health Report 1997--conquering suffering, enriching humanity. *World Health Forum* 1997;18(3-4):248-60.

[2]   Kaste M, Fogelholm R, Rissanen A. Economic burden of stroke and the evaluation of new therapies. *Public Health* 1998;112:103-12.

[3]   Caro JJ, Huybrechts KF, Duchesne I. Management Patterns and Costs of Acute Ischemic Stroke : An International Study. *Stroke* 2000 Mar 1;31(3):582-90.

[4]   Mackay J, Mensah GA. The Atlas of Heart Disease and Stroke. Geneva: World Health Organization; 2004.

[5]   Anderson CS, Linto J, Stewart-Wynne EG. A population-based assessment of the impact and burden of caregiving for long-term stroke survivors. *Stroke* 1995 May;26(5):843-9.

[6]   WHO. The world health report 2000: Health systems - improving performance. Geneva: *WHO*; 2000.

[7]   Aho K, Harmsen P, Hatano S, Marquardsen J, Smirnov VE, Strasser T. Cerebrovascular disease in the community: results of a WHO collaborative study. *Bulletin of the World Health Organization* 1980;58(1):113-30.

[8]   Feigin V, Carter K, Hackett M, Barber PA, McNaughton H, Dyall L, et al. Ethnic disparities in incidence of stroke subtypes: Auckland Regional Community Stroke Study, 2002-2003. *The Lancet Neurology* 2006 Feb;5(2):130-9.

[9]   Sudlow CLM, Warlow CP. Comparing Stroke Incidence Worldwide: What Makes Studies Comparable? *Stroke* 1996 Mar 1;27(3):550-8.

[10]   Feigin VL, Lawes CM, Bennett DA, Anderson CS. Stroke epidemiology: a review of population-based studies of incidence, prevalence, and case-fatality in the late 20th century. *Lancet Neurology* 2003 Jan;2(1):43-53.

[11]   Malmgren R, Warlow C, Bamford J, Sandercock P. Geographical and secular trends in stroke incidence. *Lancet* 1987 Nov 21;2(8569):1196-200.

[12]   Bonita R, Broad JB, Anderson NE, Beaglehole R. Approaches to the problems of measuring the incidence of stroke: the Auckland Stroke Study, 1991-1992. *International Journal of Epidemiology* 1995 Jun;24(3):535-42.

[13]   Sudlow CLM, Warlow CP. Comparing Stroke Incidence Worldwide : What Makes Studies Comparable? *Stroke* 1996 Mar 1;27(3):550-8.

[14] Feigin V, Carter K. Editorial: Stroke Incidence Studies: One Step Closer to the Elusive Gold Standard? *Stroke* 2004;35:2045-7.

[15] Sudlow CLM, Warlow CP. Comparing Stroke Incidence Worldwide: What Makes Studies Comparable? *Stroke* 1996 Mar 1;27(3):550-8.

[16] Lavados PM, Sacks C, Prina L, Escobar A, Tossi C, Araya F, et al. Incidence, 30-day case-fatality rate, and prognosis of stroke in Iquique, Chile: a 2-year community-based prospective study (PISCIS project). *The Lancet* 2005;365(9478):2206-15.

[17] Tsiskaridze A, Djibuti M, van MG, Lomidze G, Apridonidze S, Gauarashvili I, et al. Stroke incidence and 30-day case-fatality in a suburb of Tbilisi: results of the first prospective population-based study in Georgia. *Stroke* 2004 Nov;35(11):2523-8.

[18] Truelsen T, Bonita R, Jamrozik K. Surveillance of stroke: a global perspective. *International Journal of Epidemiology* 2001;30(Suppl):S11-S16.

[19] Homer D, Whisnant JP, Schoenberg BS. Trends in the incidence rates of stroke in Rochester, Minnesota, since 1935. *Annals of Neurology* 1987 Aug;22(2):245-51.

[20] Thorvaldsen P, Asplund K, Kuulasmaa K, Rajakangas AM, Schroll M. Stroke incidence, case fatality, and mortality in the WHO MONICA project. *Stroke* 1995 Mar;26(3):361-7.

[21] Ingall T, Asplund K, Mahonen M, Bonita R. A multinational comparison of subarachnoid hemorrhage epidemiology in the WHO MONICA stroke study. *Stroke* 2000 May;31(5):1054-61.

[22] Sudlow CL, Warlow CP. Comparable studies of the incidence of stroke and its pathological types: results from an international collaboration. International Stroke Incidence Collaboration. *Stroke* 1997 Mar;28(3):491-9.

[23] Sudlow CL, Warlow CP. Comparable studies of the incidence of stroke and its pathological types: results from an international collaboration. International Stroke Incidence Collaboration. *Stroke* 1997 Mar;28(3):491-9.

[24] Sudlow CL, Warlow CP. Comparable studies of the incidence of stroke and its pathological types: results from an international collaboration. International Stroke Incidence Collaboration. *Stroke* 1997 Mar;28(3):491-9.

[25] Thorvaldsen P, Asplund K, Kuulasmaa K, Rajakangas A-M, Schroll M. Stroke incidence, case fatality, and mortality in the WHO MONICA Project. *Stroke 26*, 361-367. 1995. Ref Type: Journal (Full)

[26] Ingall T, Asplund K, Mahonen M, Bonita R. A Multinational Comparison of Subarachnoid Hemorrhage Epidemiology in the WHO MONICA Stroke Study. *Stroke* 2000 May 1;31(5):1054-61.

[27] Rothwell PM, Coull AJ, Giles MF, Howard SC, Silver LE, Bull LM, et al. Change in stroke incidence, mortality, case-fatality, severity, and risk factors in Oxfordshire, UK from 1981 to 2004 (Oxford Vascular Study). *Lancet* 2004 Jun 12;363(9425):1925-33.

[28] Anderson C, Carter KN, Hackett ML, Feigin VL, Barber PA, Broad JB, et al. Trends in stroke incidence in Auckland, New Zealand, during 1981 to 2003. *Stroke* 2005;36(10):2087-93.

[29] Vibo RM, Korv JM, Roose MM. The Third Stroke Registry in Tartu, Estonia: Decline of Stroke Incidence and 28-Day Case-Fatality Rate Since 1991. [Article]. *Stroke* 2005 Dec;36(12):2544-8.

[30] Lavados PM, Sacks C, Prina L, Escobar A, Tossi C, Araya F, et al. The PISCIS Project. Incidence, 30 day case-fatality rate and prognosis of stroke in Iquique, Chile: results of a two year community based prospective study. *The Lancet* 2005.

[31] Warlow C, Sudlow C, Dennis M, Sandercock P. Stroke. *Lancet* 2003;362:1211-24.

[32] Carter KM, Anderson CP, Hacket MM, Feigin VM, Barber PAP, Broad JBM, et al. Trends in Ethnic Disparities in Stroke Incidence in Auckland, New Zealand, During 1981 to 2003. *Stroke* 2006 Jan;37(1):56-62.

[33] Sudlow CL, Warlow CP. Comparable studies of the incidence of stroke and its pathological types: results from an international collaboration. International Stroke Incidence Collaboration. *Stroke* 1997 Mar;28(3):491-9.

[34] Muntner P, Garrett E, Klag MJ, Coresh J. Trends in stroke prevalence between 1973 and 1991 in the US population 25 to 74 years of age. *Stroke* 2002 May;33(5):1209-13.

[35] Bonita R, Solomon N, Broad JB. Prevalence of stroke and stroke-related disability. Estimates from the Auckland stroke studies. *Stroke* 1997 Oct;28(10):1898-902.

[36] Lawrence ES, Coshall C, Dundas R, Stewart J, Rudd AG, Howard R, et al. Estimates of the prevalence of acute stroke impairments and disability in a multiethnic population. *Stroke* 2001 Jun;32(6):1279-84.

[37] Brown RD, Whisnant JP, Sicks JD, O'Fallon WM, Wiebers DO. Stroke incidence, prevalence, and survival: secular trends in Rochester, Minnesota, through 1989. *Stroke* 1996 Mar;27(3):373-80.

[38] Jorgensen HS, Plesner AM, Hubbe P, Larsen K. Marked increase of stroke incidence in men between 1972 and 1990 in Frederiksberg, Denmark. *Stroke* 1992 Dec;23(12):1701-4.

[39] Thorvaldsen P, Davidsen M, Bronnum-Hansen H, Schroll M. Stable Stroke Occurrence Despite Incidence Reduction in an Aging Population: Stroke Trends in the Danish Monitoring Trends and Determinants in Cardiovascular Disease (MONICA) Population. *Stroke* 1999 Dec 1;30(12):2529-34.

[40] Numminen H, Kotila M, Waltimo O, Aho K, Kaste M. Declining Incidence and Mortality Rates of Stroke in Finland From 1972 to 1991: Results of Three Population-Based Stroke Registers. *Stroke* 1996 Sep 1;27(9):1487-91.

[41] Morikawa Y, Nakagawa H, Naruse Y, Nishijo M, Miura K, Tabata M, et al. Trends in Stroke Incidence and Acute Case Fatality in a Japanese Rural Area: The Oyabe Study. *Stroke* 2000 Jul 1;31(7):1583-7.

[42] Feigin VL, Wiebers DO, Whisnant JP, O'Fallon WM. Stroke incidence and 30-day case-fatality rates in Novosibirsk, Russia, 1982 through 1992. *Stroke* 1995;26:924-9.

[43] Jamrozik K, Broadhurst RJ, Lai N, Hankey GJ, Burvill PW, Anderson CS. Trends in the Incidence, Severity, and Short-Term Outcome of Stroke in Perth, Western Australia. *Stroke* 1999 Oct 1;30(10):2105-11.

[44] Winbeck KM, Bruckmaier K, Etgen TM, von Einsiedel HGM, Rottinger MM, Sander DM. Transient Ischemic Attack and Stroke Can Be Differentiated by Analyzing Early Diffusion-Weighted Imaging Signal Intensity Changes. [Article]. *Stroke* 2004 May;35(5):1095-9.

[45] Ricci S, Celani MG, La Rosa F, Vitali R, Duca E, Ferraguzzi R, et al. A community-based study of incidence, risk factors and outcome of transient ischaemic attacks in Umbria, Italy: the SEPIVAC study. *Journal of Neurology* 1991 Apr;238(2):87-90.

[46] Lemesle M, Madinier G, Menassa M, Billiar T, Becker F, Giroud M. Incidence of transient ischemic attacks in Dijon, France. A 5-year community-based study. *Neuroepidemiology* 1998;17(2):74-9.

[47] Sempere AP, Duarte J, Cabezas C, Claveria LE. Incidence of transient ischemic attacks and minor ischemic strokes in Segovia, Spain. *Stroke* 1996;27:667-71.

[48] Dennis MS, Bamford JM, Sandercock PA, Warlow CP. Incidence of transient ischemic attacks in Oxfordshire, England. *Stroke* 1989 Mar;20(3):333-9.

[49] Brown RD, Jr., Petty GW, O'Fallon WM, Wiebers DO, Whisnant JP. Incidence of transient ischemic attack in Rochester, Minnesota, 1985-1989. *Stroke* 1998;29:2109-13.

[50] Feigin VL, Shishkin SV, Tzirkin GM, Vinogradova TE, Tarasov AV, Vinogradov SP, et al. A population-based study of transient ischemic attack incidence in Novosibirsk, Russia, 1987-1988 and 1996-1997. *Stroke* 2000 Jan;31(1):9-13.

[51] Correia MM, Silva MRM, Magalhaes RB, Guimaraes LP, Silva MCP. Transient Ischemic Attacks in Rural and Urban Northern Portugal: Incidence and Short-Term Prognosis. [Article]. *Stroke* 2006 Jan;37(1):50-5.

[52] Zupping R, Roose M. Epidemiology of cerebrovascular disease in Tartu, Estonia, USSR, 1970 through 1973. *Stroke* 1976 Mar;7(2):187-90.

[53] Feigin VL, Shishkin SV, Tzirkin GM, Vinogradova TE, Tarasov AV, Vinogradov SP, et al. A population-based study of transient ischemic attack incidence in Novosibirsk, Russia, 1987-1988 and 1996-1997. *Stroke* 2000 Jan;31(1):9-13.

[54] Flemming KD, Brown RD, Jr. Secondary prevention strategies in ischemic stroke: identification and optimal management of modifiable risk factors. [Review] [119 refs]. *Mayo Clinic Proceedings* 2004 Oct;79(10):1330-40.

[55] Humphries SE, Morgan L. Genetic risk factors for stroke and carotid atherosclerosis: insights into pathophysiology from candidate gene approaches. [Review] [134 refs]. *Lancet Neurology* 2004 Apr;3(4):227-35.

[56] Lindsberg PJ, Grau AJ. Inflammation and infections as risk factors for ischemic stroke. [Review] [216 refs]. *Stroke* 2003 Oct;34(10):2518-32.

[57] Rothwell PM. Incidence, risk factors and prognosis of stroke and TIA: the need for high-quality, large-scale epidemiological studies and meta-analyses. [Review] [99 refs]. *Cerebrovascular Diseases* 2003;16 Suppl 3:2-10, 2003.:-10.

[58] Leys D, Deplanque D, Mounier-Vehier C, kowiak-Cordoliani MA, Lucas C, Bordet R. Stroke prevention: management of modifiable vascular risk factors.[see comment]. [Review] [101 refs]. *Journal of Neurology* 2002 May;249(5):507-17.

[59] Feigin VL, Anderson CS, Mhurchu CN. Systemic inflammation, endothelial dysfunction, dietary fatty acids and micronutrients as risk factors for stroke: a selective review. [Review] [87 refs]. *Cerebrovascular Diseases* 2002;13(4):219-24.

[60] Sacco RL. Newer risk factors for stroke. [Review] [12 refs]. *Neurology* 2001;57(5 Suppl 2):S31-S34.

[61] Goldstein LB. Novel risk factors for stroke: homocysteine, inflammation, and infection. [Review] [54 refs]. *Current Atherosclerosis Reports* 2000 Mar;2(2):110-4.

[62] Wannamethee SG. Risk factors for stroke: overview. [Review] [10 refs]. *Journal of Cardiovascular Risk* 1999 Aug;6(4):199-202.

[63] Phillips S. Risk factors for stroke. [Review] [49 refs]. *Canadian Journal of Cardiology* 1999 Dec;15 Suppl G:102G-5G, 1999 Dec.:-5G.

[64] Gillum RF. Risk factors for stroke in blacks: a critical review. [Review] [109 refs]. *American Journal of Epidemiology* 1999 Dec 15;150(12):1266-74.

[65] Sacco RL, Wolf PA, Gorelick PB. Risk factors and their management for stroke prevention: outlook for 1999 and beyond. [Review] [65 refs]. *Neurology* 1999;53(7 Suppl 4):S15-S24.

[66] Elkind MS, Sacco RL. Stroke risk factors and stroke prevention. [Review] [134 refs]. *Seminars in Neurology* 1998;18(4):429-40.

[67] Pullicino P, Greenberg S, Trevisan M. Genetic stroke risk factors. [Review] [72 refs]. *Current Opinion in Neurology* 1997 Feb;10(1):58-63.

[68] Feigin VL, Rodgers A. Editorial Comment--Ethnic Disparities in Risk Factors for Stroke: What Are the Implications? *Stroke* 2004 Jul 1;35(7):1568-9.

[69] Pearce N, Foliaki S, Sporle A, Cunningham C. Genetics, race, ethnicity, and health. *BMJ* 2004 May 1;328(7447):1070-2.

[70] Lawes CMM, Bennett DA, Feigin VL, Rodgers A. Blood Pressure and Stroke: An Overview of Published Reviews. [Review]. *Stroke* 2004 Mar;35(3):776-85.

[71] Asia Pacific Cohort Studies Collaboration. Joint Effects of Systolic Blood Pressure and Serum Cholesterol on Cardiovascular Disease in the Asia Pacific Region. [Article]. *Circulation* 2005 Nov 29;112(22):3384-90.

[72] Prospective Studies Collaboration. Cholesterol, diastolic blood pressure, and stroke: 13,000 strokes in 450,000 people in 45 prospective cohorts. Prospective studies collaboration. *Lancet* 1995 Dec 23;346(8991-8992):1647-53.

[73] Asia Pacific Cohort Studies Collaboration. Cholesterol, coronary heart disease, and stroke in the Asia Pacific region. *International Journal of Epidemiology* 2003 Aug;32(4):563-72.

[74] Baigent C, Keech A, Kearney PM, Blackwell L, Buck G, Pollicino C, et al. Efficacy and safety of cholesterol-lowering treatment: prospective meta-analysis of data from 90,056 participants in 14 randomised trials of statins.[erratum appears in Lancet. 2005 Oct 15-21;366(9494):1358]. *Lancet* 2005 Oct 8;366(9493):1267-78.

[75] Hankey GJ. Smoking and risk of stroke. *Journal of Cardiovascular Risk* 1999 Aug;6(4):207-11.

[76] Feigin V, Parag V, Lawes CMM, Rodgers A, Suh I, Woodward M, et al. Smoking and Elevated Blood Pressure Are the Most Important Risk Factors for Subarachnoid Hemorrhage in the Asia-Pacific Region: An Overview of 26 Cohorts Involving 306 620 Participants. *Stroke* 2005 Jul 1;36(7):1360-5.

[77] Shinton R, Beevers G. Meta-analysis of relation between cigarette smoking and stroke. *British Medical Journal* 1989 Mar 25;298(6676):789-94.

[78] Reynolds K, Lewis B, Nolen JD, Kinney GL, Sathya B, He J. Alcohol consumption and risk of stroke: a meta-analysis. *JAMA* 2003 Feb 5;289(5):579-88.

[79] He K, Song Y, Daviglus ML, Liu K, Van HL, Dyer AR, et al. Fish consumption and incidence of stroke: a meta-analysis of cohort studies. *Stroke* 2004 Jul;35(7):1538-42.

[80] Wendel-Vos GC, Schuit AJ, Feskens EJ, Boshuizen HC, Verschuren WM, Saris WH, et al. Physical activity and stroke. A meta-analysis of observational data. [Review] [55 refs]. *International Journal of Epidemiology* 2004 Aug;33(4):787-98.

[81] Lee CD, Folsom AR, Blair SN. Physical activity and stroke risk: a meta-analysis.[see comment]. *Stroke* 2003 Oct;34(10):2475-81.

[82] Kuo HK, Yen CJ, Chang CH, Kuo CK, Chen JH, Sorond F. Relation of C-reactive protein to stroke, cognitive disorders, and depression in the general population: systematic review and meta-analysis. [Review] [84 refs]. *Lancet Neurology* 2005 Jun;4(6):371-80.

[83] Cremonini F, Gabrielli M, Gasbarrini G, Pola P, Gasbarrini A. The relationship between chronic H. pylori infection, CagA seropositivity and stroke: meta-analysis. *Atherosclerosis* 2004 Apr;173(2):253-9.

[84] Baillargeon JP, McClish DK, Essah PA, Nestler JE. Association between the current use of low-dose oral contraceptives and cardiovascular arterial disease: a meta-analysis. *Journal of Clinical Endocrinology & Metabolism* 2005 Jul;90(7):3863-70.

[85] Bath PM, Gray LJ. Association between hormone replacement therapy and subsequent stroke: a meta-analysis.[see comment]. [Review] [15 refs]. *BMJ* 2005 Feb 12;330(7487):342.

[86] Danesh J, Lewington S, Thompson SG, Lowe GD, Collins R, Kostis JB, et al. Plasma fibrinogen level and the risk of major cardiovascular diseases and nonvascular mortality: an individual participant meta-analysis.[erratum appears in JAMA. 2005 Dec 14;294(22):2848]. *JAMA* 2005 Oct 12;294(14):1799-809.

[87] Wald DS, Law M, Morris JK. Homocysteine and cardiovascular disease: evidence on causality from a meta-analysis. *BMJ* 2002 Nov 23;325(7374):1202.

[88] Etminan M, Takkouche B, Isorna FC, Samii A. Risk of ischaemic stroke in people with migraine: systematic review and meta-analysis of observational studies.[see comment][erratum appears in BMJ. 2005 Feb 12;330(7487):345]. [Review] [28 refs]. *BMJ* 2005 Jan 8;330(7482):63.

[89] Cox AM, McKevitt C, Rudd AG, Wolfe CD. Socioeconomic status and stroke. The *Lancet Neurology* 2006 Feb;5(2):181-8.

[90] Wolfe CD, Rudd AG, Howard R, Coshall C, Stewart J, Lawrence E, et al. Incidence and case fatality rates of stroke subtypes in a multiethnic population: the South London Stroke Register. *Journal of Neurology, Neurosurgery & Psychiatry* 2002 Feb;72(2):211-6.

[91] Casas JP, Hingorani AD, Bautista LE, Sharma P. Meta-analysis of genetic studies in ischemic stroke: thirty-two genes involving approximately 18,000 cases and 58,000 controls. *Archives of Neurology* 2004 Nov;61(11):1652-61.

[92] Flossmann E, Schulz UG, Rothwell PM. Systematic review of methods and results of studies of the genetic epidemiology of ischemic stroke. [Review] [87 refs]. *Stroke* 2004 Jan;35(1):212-27.

[93] Weih M, Muller-Nordhorn J, Amberger N, Masuhr F, Lurtzing F, Dreier JP, et al. [Risk factors in ischemic stroke. Review of evidence in primary prevention]. [Review] [41 refs] [German]. *Nervenarzt* 2004 Apr;75(4):324-35.

[94] Gil de CR, Gil-Nunez AC. Risk factors for ischemic stroke. I. Conventional risk factors. *Revista de Neurologia* 2000 Aug 16;31(4):314-23.

[95] Sacco RL. Risk factors and outcomes for ischemic stroke. *Neurology* 1995 Feb;45(2 Suppl 1):S10-S14.

[96] Schulz UGR, Rothwell PM. Differences in Vascular Risk Factors Between Etiological Subtypes of Ischemic Stroke: Importance of Population-Based Studies. *Stroke* 2003 Aug 1;34(8):2050-9.

[97] Lodder J, Bamford JM, Sandercock PA, Jones LN, Warlow CP. Are hypertension or cardiac embolism likely causes of lacunar infarction? *Stroke* 1990 Mar;21(3):375-81.

[98] Whisnant JP, Homer D, Ingall TJ, Baker HLJ, O'Fallon WM, Wievers DO. Duration of cigarette smoking is the strongest predictor of severe extracranial carotid artery atherosclerosis. *Stroke* 1990 May;21(5):707-14.

[99] Steinberg D. Thematic review series: the pathogenesis of atherosclerosis. An interpretive history of the cholesterol controversy: part II: the early evidence linking hypercholesterolemia to coronary disease in humans. *Journal of Lipid Research* 2005 Feb;46(2):179-90.

[100] Sacco RL. Risk factors, outcomes, and stroke subtypes for ischemic stroke. [Review] [37 refs]. *Neurology* 1997 Nov;49(5 Suppl 4):S39-S44.

[101] Goldstein LB, Adams R, Becker K, Furberg CD, Gorelick PB, Hademenos G, et al. Primary prevention of ischemic stroke: A statement for healthcare professionals from the Stroke Council of the American Heart Association.[see comment]. *Stroke* 2001 Jan;32(1):280-99.

[102] Sacco RL, Benjamin EJ, Broderick JP, Dyken M, Easton JD, Feinberg WM, et al. American Heart Association Prevention Conference. IV. Prevention and Rehabilitation of Stroke. Risk factors.[see comment]. *Stroke* 1997 Jul;28(7):1507-17.

[103] Ariesen MJ, Claus SP, Rinkel GJ, Algra A. Risk factors for intracerebral hemorrhage in the general population: a systematic review.[see comment]. [Review] [38 refs]. *Stroke* 2003 Aug;34(8):2060-5.

[104] Feigin VL, Rinkel GJE, Lawes CMM, Algra A, Bennett DA, van Gijn J, et al. Risk Factors for Subarachnoid Hemorrhage: An Updated Systematic Review of Epidemiological Studies. *Stroke* 2005;36(12):2773-80.

[105] Wiebers DO, Piepgras DG, Meyer FB, Kallmes DF, Meissner I, Atkinson JL, et al. Pathogenesis, natural history, and treatment of unruptured intracranial aneurysms. *Mayo Clinic Proceedings* 2004 Dec;79(12):1572-83.

[106] Bak S, Gaist D, Sindrup SH, Skytthe A, Christensen K. Genetic liability in stroke: a long-term follow-up study of Danish twins. *Stroke* 2002 Mar;33(3):769-74.

[107] Jerrard-Dunne P, Cloud G, Hassan A, Markus HS. Evaluating the genetic component of ischemic stroke subtypes: a family history study. *Stroke* 2003 Jun;34(6):1364-9.

[108] Meschia JF, Worrall BB. New advances in identifying genetic anomalies in stroke-prone probands. *Current Neurology & Neuroscience Reports* 2004 Sep;4(5):420-6.

[109] Szolnoki Z, Somogyvari F, Kondacs A, Szabo M, Fodor L. Evaluation of the interactions of common genetic mutations in stroke subtypes. *Journal of Neurology* 2002 Oct;249(10):1391-7.

[110] Ionita CC, Xavier AR, Kirmani JF, Dash S, Divani AA, Qureshi AI. What proportion of stroke is not explained by classic risk factors?. [Review] [49 refs]. *Preventive Cardiology* 2005;8(1):41-6.

[111] Wald NJ, Law MR. A strategy to reduce cardiovascular disease by more than 80%. *BMJ* 2003 Jun 28;326(7404):1419.

[112] Barnes ME, Miyasaka Y, Seward JB, Gersh BJ, Rosales AG, Bailey KR, et al. Left atrial volume in the prediction of first ischemic stroke in an elderly cohort without atrial fibrillation. *Mayo Clinic Proceedings* 2004 Aug;79(8):1008-14.

[113] Pearson TA, Blair SN, Daniels SR, Eckel RH, Fair JM, Fortmann SP, et al. AHA Guidelines for Primary Prevention of Cardiovascular Disease and Stroke: 2002 Update: Consensus Panel Guide to Comprehensive Risk Reduction for Adult Patients Without Coronary or Other Atherosclerotic Vascular Diseases. American Heart Association Science Advisory and Coordinating Committee. [Review] [37 refs]. *Circulation* 2002 Jul 16;106(3):388-91.

[114] Jackson R. Updated New Zealand cardiovascular disease risk-benefit prediction guide. *BMJ* 2000 Mar 11;320(7236):709-10.

[115] Epping-Jordan JE, Galea G, Tukuitonga C, Beaglehole R. Preventing chronic diseases: taking stepwise action. *Lancet* 2005 Nov 5;366(9497):1667-71.

[116] Strong K, Mathers C, Leeder S, Beaglehole R. Preventing chronic diseases: how many lives can we save? *Lancet* 2005 Oct 29;366(9496):1578-82.

[117] International Classification of Impairments, Disabilities and Handicaps. Geneva, Switzerland: World Health Organization; 1980.

[118] de HR, Aaronson N, Limburg M, Hewer RL, van CH. Measuring quality of life in stroke. *Stroke* 1993 Feb;24(2):320-7.

[119] Tengs TO, Yu M, Luistro E. Health-related quality of life after stroke a comprehensive review. Stroke 2001 Apr;32(4):964-72.

[120] Anderson CS, Carter KN, Brownlee WJ, Hackett ML, Broad JB, Bonita R. Very long-term outcome after stroke in Auckland, New Zealand. *Stroke* 2004 Aug;35(8):1920-4.

[121] Dennis MS, Burn JP, Sandercock PA, Bamford JM, Wade DT, Warlow CP. Long-term survival after first-ever stroke: the Oxfordshire Community Stroke Project. *Stroke* 1993 Jun;24(6):796-800.

[122] Petty GW, Brown RDJ, Whisnant JP, Sicks JD, O'Fallon WM, Wiebers DO. Survival and recurrence after first cerebral infarction: a population-based study in Rochester, Minnesota, 1975 through 1989. *Neurology* 1998 Jan;50(1):208-16.

[123] Sacco RL, Wolf PA, Kannel WB, McNamara PM. Survival and recurrence following stroke. The Framingham study. *Stroke* 1982 May;13(3):290-5.

[124] Hardie K, Hankey GJ, Jamrozik K, Broadhurst RJ, Anderson C. Ten-year survival after first-ever stroke in the perth community stroke study. *Stroke* 2003 Aug;34(8):1842-6.

[125] Hankey GJ, Jamrozik K, Broadhurst RJ, Forbes S, Burvill PW, Anderson CS, et al. Five-year survival after first-ever stroke and related prognostic factors in the Perth Community Stroke Study. *Stroke* 2000 Sep;31(9):2080-6.

[126] Doyle PJ. Measuring health outcomes in stroke survivors. *Archives of Physical Medicine & Rehabilitation* 2002 Dec;83(12 Suppl 2):S39-S43.

[127] Patel MD, Coshall C, Rudd AG, Wolfe CD. Cognitive impairment after stroke: clinical determinants and its associations with long-term stroke outcomes. *Journal of the American Geriatrics Society* 2002 Apr;50(4):700-6.

[128] de HR, Horn J, Limburg M, Van Der MJ, Bossuyt P. A comparison of five stroke scales with measures of disability, handicap, and quality of life. *Stroke* 1993 Aug;24(8):1178-81.

[129] Wolfe CD, Taub NA, Woodrow EJ, Burney PG. Assessment of scales of disability and handicap for stroke patients. *Stroke* 1991 Oct;22(10):1242-4.

[130] Rothwell PM, McDowell Z, Wong CK, Dorman PJ. Doctors and patients don't agree: cross sectional study of patients' and doctors' perceptions and assessments of disability in multiple sclerosis. *BMJ* 1997 May 31;314(7094):1580-3.

[131] Sturm JW, Dewey HM, Donnan GA, Macdonell RA, McNeil JJ, Thrift AG. Handicap after stroke: how does it relate to disability, perception of recovery, and stroke subtype? The north North East Melbourne Stroke Incidence Study (NEMESIS). *Stroke* 2002 Mar;33(3):762-8.

[132] Kwakkel G, Wagenaar RC, Kollen BJ, Lankhorst GJ. Predicting disability in stroke--a critical review of the literature. *Age & Ageing* 1996 Nov;25(6):479-89.

[133] Hackett ML, Duncan JR, Anderson CS, Broad JB, Bonita R. Health-related quality of life among long-term survivors of stroke : results from the Auckland Stroke Study, 1991-1992. *Stroke* 2000 Feb;31(3):440-7.

[134] Taub NA, Wolfe CD, Richardson E, Burney PG. Predicting the disability of first-time stroke sufferers at 1 year. 12-month follow-up of a population-based cohort in southeast England. *Stroke* 1994 Feb;25(2):352-7.

[135] Hankey GJ, Jamrozik K, Broadhurst RJ, Forbes S, Anderson CS. Long-term disability after first-ever stroke and related prognostic factors in the Perth Community Stroke Study, 1989-1990. *Stroke* 2002 Apr;33(4):1034-40.

[136] Patel AT. Disability evaluation following stroke. Physical Medicine & Rehabilitation *Clinics of North America* 2001 Aug;12(3):613-9.

[137] Longstreth WT, Nelson LM, Koepsell TD, van Belle G. Clinical course of spontaneous subarachnoid hemorrhage: a population-based study in King County, Washington. *Neurology* 1993 Apr;43(4):712-8.

[138] Anderson CS, Jamrozik KD, Burvill PW, Chakera TM, Johnson GA, Stewart-Wynne EG. Determining the incidence of different subtypes of stroke: results from the Perth Community Stroke Study, 1989-1990. *Medical Journal of Australia* 1993 Jan 18;158(2):85-9.

[139] Brown RD, Whisnant JP, Sicks JD, O'Fallon WM, Wiebers DO. Stroke incidence, prevalence, and survival: secular trends in Rochester, Minnesota, through 1989. *Stroke* 1996 Mar;27(3):373-80.

[140] Petty GW, Brown RD, Jr., Whisnant JP, Sicks JD, O'Fallon WM, Wiebers DO. Ischemic stroke subtypes: a population-based study of functional outcome, survival, and recurrence. *Stroke* 2000 May;31(5):1062-8.

[141] Bamford J, Sandercock P, Dennis M, Burn J, Warlow C. Classification and natural history of clinically identifiable subtypes of cerebral infarction. *Lancet* 1991 Jun 22;337(8756):1521-6.

[142] Thrift AG, Dewey HM, Macdonell RA, McNeil JJ, Donnan GA. Stroke incidence on the east coast of Australia: the North East Melbourne Stroke Incidence Study (NEMESIS). *Stroke* 2000 Sep;31(9):2087-92.

[143] Dewey HM, Thrift AG, Mihalopoulos C, Carter R, Macdonell RA, McNeil JJ, et al. Cost of stroke in Australia from a societal perspective: results from the North East Melbourne Stroke Incidence Study (NEMESIS). *Stroke* 2001 Oct;32(10):2409-16.

[144] Dewey HM, Thrift AG, Mihalopoulos C, Carter R, Macdonell RA, McNeil JJ, et al. Lifetime cost of stroke subtypes in Australia: findings from the North East Melbourne Stroke Incidence Study (NEMESIS). *Stroke* 2003 Oct;34(10):2502-7.

[145] Taylor TN, Davis PH, Torner JC, Holmes J, Meyer JW, Jacobson MF. Lifetime cost of stroke in the United States. *Stroke* 1996 Sep;27(9):1459-66.

[146] Hackett ML, Anderson CS. Health outcomes 1 year after subarachnoid hemorrhage: An international population-based study. The Australian Cooperative Research on Subarachnoid Hemorrhage Study Group. *Neurology* 2000 Sep 12;55(5):658-62.

[147] Adams HP, Jr., Davis PH, Leira EC, Chang KC, Bendixen BH, Clarke WR, et al. Baseline NIH Stroke Scale score strongly predicts outcome after stroke: A report of the Trial of Org 10172 in Acute Stroke Treatment (TOAST). *Neurology* 1999 Jul 13;53(1):126-31.

[148] Anderson TP. Studies up to 1980 on stroke rehabilitation outcomes. *Stroke* 1990 Sep;21(9 Suppl):II43-II45.

[149] DeLisa JA, Miller RM, Melnick RR, Mikulic MA. Stroke rehabilitation: part I. Cognitive deficits and prediction of outcome. *American Family Physician* 1982 Nov;26(5):207-14.

[150] Evans RL, Bishop DS, Matlock AL, Stranahan S, Halar EM, Noonan WC. Prestroke family interaction as a predictor of stroke outcome. *Archives of Physical Medicine & Rehabilitation* 1987 Aug;68(8):508-12.

[151] Fiorelli M, Alperovitch A, Argentino C, Sacchetti ML, Toni D, Sette G, et al. Prediction of long-term outcome in the early hours following acute ischemic stroke. Italian Acute Stroke Study Group. *Archives of Neurology* 1995 Mar;52(3):250-5.

[152] Freed MM, Wainapel SF. Predictors of stroke outcome. *American Family Physician* 1983 Nov;28(5):119-23.

[153] Galski T, Bruno RL, Zorowitz R, Walker J. Predicting length of stay, functional outcome, and aftercare in the rehabilitation of stroke patients. The dominant role of higher-order cognition. *Stroke* 1993 Dec;24(12):1794-800.

[154] Kalra L, Smith DH, Crome P. Stroke in patients aged over 75 years: outcome and predictors. *Postgraduate Medical Journal* 1993 Jan;69(807):33-6.

[155] Lehmann JF, DeLateur BJ, Fowler RSJ, Warren CG, Arnhold R, Schertzer G, et al. Stroke rehabilitation: Outcome and prediction. *Archives of Physical Medicine & Rehabilitation* 1975 Sep;56(9):383-9.

[156] Loewen SC, Anderson BA. Predictors of stroke outcome using objective measurement scales. *Stroke* 1990 Jan;21(1):78-81.

[157] Olsen TS. Arm and leg paresis as outcome predictors in stroke rehabilitation. *Stroke* 1990 Feb;21(2):247-51.

[158] Paolucci S, Antonucci G, Gialloreti LE, Traballesi M, Lubich S, Pratesi L, et al. Predicting stroke inpatient rehabilitation outcome: the prominent role of neuropsychological disorders. *European Neurology* 1996;36(6):385-90.

[159] Reith J, Jørgensen HS, Pedersen PM, Nakayama H, Raaschou HO, Jeppesen, et al. Body temperature in acute stroke: relation to stroke severity, infarct size, mortality, and outcome. *Lancet* 1996 Feb 17;347(8999):422-5.

[160] Vanclay F. Functional outcome measures in stroke rehabilitation. *Stroke* 1991 Jan;22(1):105-8.

[161] Rothwell PM, Mehta Z, Howard SC, Gutnikov SA, Warlow CP. From subgroups to individuals: general principles and the example of carotid endarterectomy. *The Lancet* 2005 Jan 15;365(9455):256-65.

[162] Avendano M, Kunst AE, van LF, Bos V, Costa G, Valkonen T, et al. Trends in socioeconomic disparities in stroke mortality in six european countries between 1981-1985 and 1991-1995. *American Journal of Epidemiology* 2005 Jan 1;161(1):52-61.

[163] Boden-Albala B, Sacco RL. Socioeconomic status and stroke mortality: refining the relationship.[comment]. *Stroke* 2002 Jan;33(1):274-5.

[164] Engstrom G, Jerntorp I, Pessah-Rasmussen H, Hedblad B, Berglund G, Janzon L. Geographic distribution of stroke incidence within an urban population: relations to socioeconomic circumstances and prevalence of cardiovascular risk factors. *Stroke* 2001 May;32(5):1098-103.

[165] Bennett S. Socioeconomic inequalities in coronary heart disease and stroke mortality among Australian men, 1979-1993. *International Journal of Epidemiology* 1996 Apr;25(2):266-75.

[166] Weir NU, Gunkel A, McDowall M, Dennis MS. Study of the Relationship Between Social Deprivation and Outcome After Stroke. *Stroke* 2005 Apr 1;36(4):815-9.

[167] Stroke Unit Trialists' Collaboration. Organised inpatient (stroke unit) care for stroke. *Cochrane Database of Systematic Reviews* 2001;Issue 2, 2001.

[168] Feigin VL. Managing stroke: key principles and updates. *New Zealand Family Physician* 2005;32(4):241-6.

RECOMMENDED FURTHER READING

1. Wiebers DO, Feigin VL, Brown RD,Jr. *'Handbook of Stroke'*. Lippencott Williams & Wilkins © Mayo Foundation, Rochester, Minnesota, USA, Second edition, 2006

2. Feigin VL. *'When Lightning Strikes. An Illustrated Guide to Stroke Prevention and Recovery'*. Auckland, New Zealand, HarperCollinsPublishers Ltd, 2004

3. Feigin VL. *'Stroke Prevention and Recovery: The Ultimate Video Guide"* (a set of 3 DVDs). Auckland, New Zealand, Stroke Education Ltd, 2006

4. Hankey G. *'Stroke Treatment and Prevention: An Evidence-based Approach'*. Cambridge, Cambridge University Press, 2005

5. Warlow CP, Dennis MS, Jan Van Gijn, Hankey GJ, Sandercock PAG, Bamford JM, Wardlaw JM. *'Stroke: A Practical Guide to Management'*. Oxford, Blackwell Publishing Limited; 2 edition, 2001

In: Handbook of Clinical Neuroepidemiology ISBN 978-1-60021-511-7
Editors: V. L. Feigin and D. A. Bennett, pp. 105-122 © 2007 Nova Science Publishers, Inc.

Chapter 3

MIGRAINE

Sandra W. Hamelsky[1], Walter F. Stewart[2] and Richard B. Lipton[3]

[1]Department of Neurology, Albert Einstein College of Medicine,
Bronx, New York, USA;
[2]Geisinger Health System, Danville, PA, USA;
[3]Departments of Neurology, Epidemiology and Population Health, Albert Einstein
College of Medicine and Montefiore Headache Unit, Bronx, New York, USA.

ABSTRACT

Migraine is a chronic neurological disorder characterized by recurrent headache attacks that include both pain and associated symptoms in various combinations, including nausea as well as sensitivity to light and sound. Migraine has an enormous impact on the individual and society, affecting approximately 11% of the population in Western countries. The societal impact of migraine is usually measured through direct costs such as healthcare utilization figures or indirect costs such as work loss (i.e., absenteeism) and reduced productivity while at work due to migraine. The individual impact is often measured by examining attack frequency and severity, as well as the global impact of repeated attacks. Studies of the family members of migraine sufferers provide insight into how the disease affects those around them. This chapter reviews the epidemiology of and risk factors for migraine, as well as the impact the disease has on the individual and society.

INTRODUCTION

Recent epidemiologic evidence suggests that migraine affects approximately 11% of the population in Western countries [1]. Migraine has an enormous impact on the individual and society. The individual impact is measured by the frequency and severity of attacks, while the societal burden is measured in terms of lost workdays and healthcare utilization. In this chapter, we will review the epidemiology of and risk factors for migraine, as well as the impact the disease has on the individual and society.

Table 1. ICHD-2 Categories for Migraine

Migraine without aura
Migraine with aura • Typical aura with migraine headache • Typical aura with non-migraine headache • Typical aura without headache • Familial hemiplegic migraine (FHM) • Sporadic hemiplegic migraine • Basilar-type migraine
Childhood periodic syndromes that are commonly precursors of migraine • Cyclical vomiting • Abdominal migraine • Benign paroxysmal vertigo of childhood
Retinal migraine
Complications of migraine • Chronic migraine • Status migrainosus • Persistent aura without infarction • Migrainous infarction • Migraine-triggered seizure
Probable migraine • Probable migraine without aura • Probable migraine with aura • Probable chronic migraine

CASE DEFINITION

Standard case definitions are provided by the first and second editions of the International Classification of Headache Disorders (ICHD-1, ICHD-2). Developed through an expert consensus and written in uncomplicated, operational terms, the criteria have greatly facilitated the study of headache by standardizing diagnosis. The International Classification of Headache Disorders (ICHD-2) was published in 2004 [2]. The new criteria reflect improved understanding of some disorders and the identification of new disorders.

Further, ICHD-2 is similar in structure to ICHD-1, in that headaches are divided into primary or secondary disorders. However, the new classification has been updated in ways that will affect neurologic practice, clinical trials and epidemiologic research.

The ICHD-2 provides a restructuring of the criteria for migraine, classifying it into 5 major categories (Table 1). The two most important categories, migraine without aura and migraine with aura, remain largely unchanged [3]. The diagnostic criteria for migraine without aura are presented in Table 2, and are unchanged from the 1988 classification. They require at least five lifetime attacks, lasting 4 to 72 hours, with at least 2 of the four pain features, and at least one of the two sets of associated symptoms. Although the diagnostic criteria are unchanged, some additional notes are provided. For example, childhood attacks of migraine without aura may be shorter, between 1 and 72 hours, and photophobia and phonophobia may be inferred from behavior rather than reported.

Table 2. ICHD-2 diagnostic criteria for 1.1 Migraine without aura [2]

A	At least 5 attacks fulfilling criteria B-D
B	Headache attacks lasting 4-72 hours (untreated or unsuccessfully treated)
C	Headache has at least two of the following characteristics: • unilateral location • pulsating quality • moderate or severe pain intensity • aggravation by or causing avoidance of routine physical activity (e.g., walking or climbing stairs)
D	During headache at least one of the following: • nausea and/or vomiting • photophobia and phonophobia
E	Not attributed to another disorder

The criteria for migraine with aura have been restructured. Migraine with typical aura is defined in Table 3. The aura of migraine is characterized by focal neurologic features that usually precede migraine headache, but may accompany it or occur in the absence of headache. Aura symptoms usually develop over less than five minutes, and last no more than 60 minutes. While visual aura is the most common [4], sensory symptoms occur in about one-third of patients who have migraine with aura [5]. Sensory aura usually consists of negative symptoms such as numbness, and positive symptoms like tingling or paresthesia. These symptoms usually occur in the faces and hands.

Perhaps the most important change in the classification is the inclusion of chronic migraine (1.5.1), a condition defined by migraine without aura 15 or more days per month. This condition was intended to capture the large number of individuals who have chronic daily headache (headache ≥15 days per month, lasting ≥24 hours) with migraine features, a condition also sometimes called transformed migraine (TM). In a clinic-based study of 170 adolescents between the ages of 13 and 17 years, 69 people were classified as having transformed migraine without medication overuse according to the Silberstein-Lipton criteria [6,7]. Of those, 71% met the criteria for chronic migraine as defined by the ICHD-2. Of the patients with transformed migraine with medication overuse, only 39.6% met the criteria for probable chronic migraine with probable medication overuse. Revisions of ICHD-2 criteria are currently being contemplated.

Table 3. ICHD-2 criteria for 1.2.1 Typical aura with migraine headache [2]

A	At least 2 attacks fulfilling criteria B-D
B	Aura consisting of at least one of the following, but no motor weakness: • fully reversible visual symptoms including positive features (e.g., flickering lights, spots, or lines) and/or negative features (i.e., loss of vision) • fully reversible sensory symptoms including positive feature (i.e., pins and needles) and/or negative features (i.e., numbness) • fully reversible dysphasic speech disturbance
C	At least two of the following: • homonymous visual symptoms and/or unilateral sensory symptoms • at least one aura symptom develops gradually over ≥5 minutes and/or different aura symptoms occur in succession over ≥5 minutes • each symptom lasts ≥5 and ≤60 minutes
D	Headache fulfilling criteria B-D for 1.1 Migraine without aura begins during the aura or follows aura within 60 minutes
E	Not attributed to another disorder

EPIDEMIOLOGY

Epidemiologic studies are used to estimate the frequency, distribution and burden of disease in the population. Widely used measures of disease frequency include incidence and prevalence. Incidence quantifies the number of new events or cases of disease that develop in a population over a defined period of time. Prevalence refers to the proportion of a population that has the disease over a given period of time. Prevalence is an important measure of the burden of disease.

Incidence

Migraine incidence is best studied in cohort studies of people at risk for the disease. However, few such studies have been reported. The studies that have been published report varying results probably because of differences in study populations (e.g., age, geographic area), as well as study methodology.

Breslau et al. [8] estimated the incidence of migraine in a random sample of 21 to 30 year old members of a large Health Maintenance Organization. A total of 1,007 participants were initially interviewed. The five year incidence of migraine was estimated among the 848 people who did not meet the criteria for migraine at baseline. A total of 71 (8.4%) cases of migraine were identified (female 60 (12%); male 11(3.2%)). This study is likely to have underestimated the incidence of migraine because it included subjects from a very narrow age range, older than the age of suspected peak risk for incident migraine.

Stewart et al. [9] reported a higher incidence based on results from a population-based study that used the reported age of migraine onset to estimate the incidence of migraine. Telephone interviews were conducted among 10,169 residents of Washington County, Maryland who were between the ages of 12 and 29. In total, 392 males and 1,018 females were identified as migraine sufferers. While this study included a broader age range than Breslau et al., the generalizability of the results are also limited because only individuals between the ages of 12 and 29 were interviewed.

Below the age of ten, the incidence of migraine, especially migraine without aura, was higher among males than females. For example, among females between six and seven years old, the incidence rate was 6.3 per 1,000 person years for migraine with aura and 5.4 per 1,000 person years for migraine without aura. For males in the same age group, the incidence rate for migraine with aura was 5.6 per 1,000 and migraine without aura was 8.3 per 1,000. However, during the adolescent years, the incidence of migraine is higher in females than males. For example, among females between 12 and 13 years old, the incidence rate was 14.1 for migraine with aura and 17.3 for migraine without aura per 1,000. The corresponding percentages for males were 3.5 and 9.9 per 1,000. Most of the new onset cases among females were cases of migraine without aura. In addition, the peak incidence of migraine per 1,000 was higher among females (migraine without aura: females 18.9, males 10.1; migraine with aura: females 14.1, males 6.6), but occurred earlier in males (migraine without aura: females 14 to 17 years, males 10 to 11 years; migraine with aura: females 12 to 13 years, males 4 to 5 years).

Stang et al. [10] used linked medical records to estimate the incidence of migraine in Olmstead County, Minnesota. Of the 6,400 patient records reviewed, 629 fulfilled the IHS criteria for migraine. Among females, the incidence of migraine peaked between 20 to 24 years, at 6.9 per 1,000 person years. In males, the highest incidence rate, 2.5 per 1,000 person years, occurred between ten and 14 years. The decreased incidence rates and later peaks in incidence relative to Stewart et al. and Breslau et al. may have occurred because only individuals who consulted a health care provider for headache were identified.

More recently, Lyngberg et al. [11] published a population-based study of the incidence of migraine in a Danish population. This study was a follow-up to a cross-sectional epidemiology study from 1989. Of the 453 subjects ranging in age from 25 to 64 years who did not have migraine in 1989, 42 developed migraine during the study period, resulting in an annual incidence of 0.8%. The annual incidence in females was 1.5% and in males 0.3%. The study was too small to provide age specific estimates of incidence.

Prevalence

Many studies have estimated the prevalence of migraine. Prevalence estimates from studies conducted prior to publication of the 1988 IHS diagnostic criteria vary widely, largely due to differences in case definitions. However, once case definitions were standardized, the variation in prevalence was greatly reduced. For adult populations, the estimates of migraine prevalence range from 3.3% to 21.9% for women and 0.7% to 16.1% for men [1].

In the United States, these large scale, methodologically similar population-based epidemiology studies of migraine were conducted in 1989 [12], 1999 [13] and 2005 [14], in samples selected to be representative of the US population. In the first study (American Migraine Study I), Stewart et al. sent a self-administered questionnaire to 15,000 households [12]. Each household member with severe headache was asked to respond to detailed questions about symptoms, frequency, and severity of headaches. After a single mailing, 20,468 subjects between 12 and 80 years of age responded to the survey. The prevalence of migraine was 17.6% in females and 5.7% in males.

Approximately 10 years later, some of the same researchers conducted a second large scale, population-based prevalence study (American Migraine Study II); in this study questionnaires were mailed to 20,000 households generating some 30,000 respondents.[13] Results were virtually identical to the previous study [15]. Other studies using telephone interviews confirmed and extended the results of the American Migraine Studies I and II. For further reviews about the prevalence of migraine, see Scher et al. [1] and Bigal et al. [16].

Prevalence by Age and Gender

Most studies of migraine prevalence have reported variation by age. Figure 1 displays data from the American migraine study [12,17] demonstrating that migraine prevalence is generally highest between 25 and 55 years, typically the most productive years of life. Migraine prevalence peaks in the late 30s to early 40s, and declines during the fifth decade.

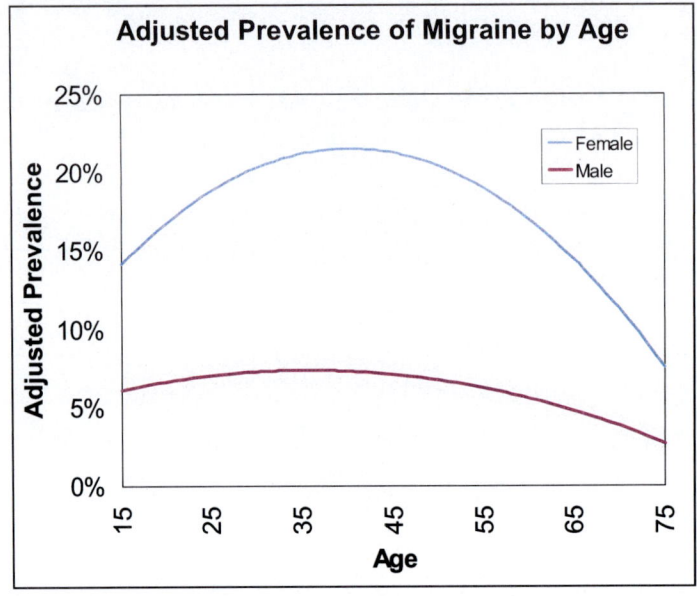

Figure 1. Adjusted prevalence of migraine by age from a meta-analysis of studies using IHS criteria. (from Scher et al., 2001).

Several studies indicate that prior to puberty, the prevalence of migraine is slightly higher in boys than girls [18-21]. For example, a study by Mortimer et al. [20] in the UK reported that migraine prevalence was greater in boys between the ages of 3 to 5 years of age and also 5 to 7 years of age. For the years between 7 and 11, prevalence was approximately equal between the genders. However, as adolescence approaches, migraine becomes more prevalent among females. For example, both Mortimer et al. and Raieli et al. [21] found that after age 11, prevalence was higher in girls than boys.

In the adult population, migraine is more prevalent among females than males. For example, in the American migraine study I [12], a study of individuals 12 years of age and older, the average female to male migraine prevalence ratio was 2.8, with a peak of 3.3 between 40 to 45 years. The ratio remains above 2.0 even after the age of menopause.

Prevalence by Race and Geographic Region

Several studies indicate that migraine prevalence varies by race and geographic region. Stewart et al. [22] conducted a population-based study in the United States, and reported that the lowest prevalence was observed among Asian Americans, intermediate estimates were reported in African-Americans, and the highest prevalence estimates were observed among Caucasians, before and after adjusting for demographic covariates. A more recent meta-analysis confirmed these findings: prevalence was lowest in Africa and Asia, and higher in Europe and Central/South America. The highest estimates were found in North America [1]. Figure 2 presents a figure of the age adjusted migraine prevalence by geographic region.

Since migraine prevalence is low in Africa and Asia, and remains low among African-Americans and Asians in the United States, it has been hypothesized that there are race-related differences in genetic susceptibility to migraine. However, since prevalence in Asia is even lower than in the United States, other variables such as environmental risk factors, or culturally determined differences in symptom reporting may further explain the international variation.

Prevalence by Socioeconomic Status

In the United States, several population-based studies have demonstrated that in the community, migraine prevalence is inversely related to household income [17, 22]. As income or education increased, migraine prevalence declined.

The National Health Interview Survey (NHIS) also demonstrated lower prevalence in the low compared with middle income group; however prevalence was highest among the highest income group [23]. Since this study relied on self-reported medical diagnosis of migraine, and medical diagnosis of migraine rises with income, differential ascertainment by income may explain the association in the highest income group.

Studies conducted outside the United States have not consistently supported the inverse relationship between migraine prevalence and household income. For example, European population-based data from the Genetic Epidemiology of Migraine (GEM) Study indicate that there is no association between migraine and socioeconomic status [24]. In addition, in a population-based study conducted in England, there was no association between migraine and socioeconomic status [25]. The reasons for the international variation are unclear.

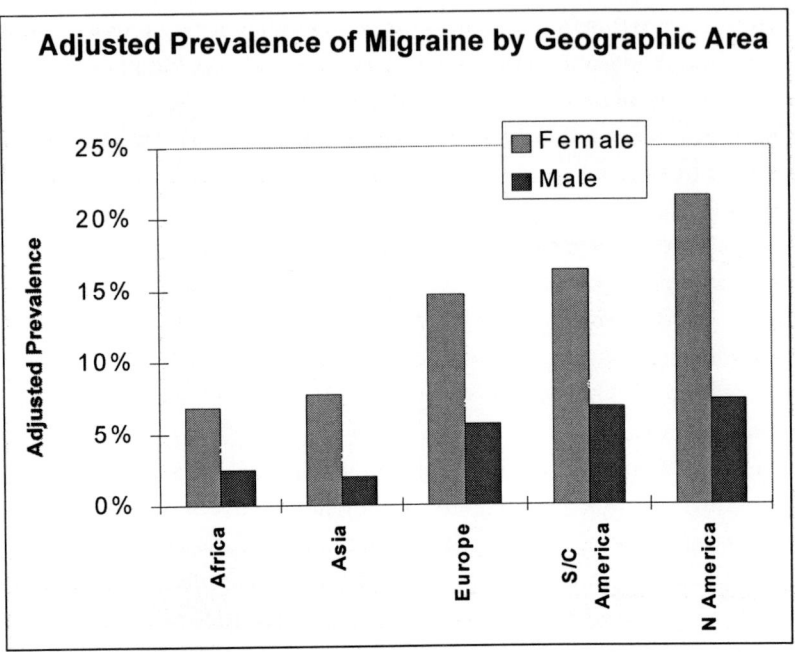

Figure 2. Adjusted prevalence of migraine by geographic area and gender in a meta-analysis of studies using IHS criteria (From Scher et al., 2001).

THE IMPACT OF MIGRAINE

Migraine symptom profiles and degrees of disability vary substantially, both within and among different individuals. The disability of migraine can be severe and has a substantial impact on society, as well as the individual, his/her family, and society. The societal impact of migraine is usually measured through direct costs such as healthcare utilization figures or indirect costs such as work loss (i.e., absenteeism) and reduced productivity while at work due to migraine. The individual impact is often measured by examining attack frequency and severity, as well as the global impact of repeated attacks. Studies of the family members of migraine sufferers provide insight into how the disease affects those around them.

Societal Impact

Direct Costs

Direct costs include all of the costs of diagnosing and treating a particular disorder. In the case of migraine, this includes healthcare utilization figures such as rates of outpatient visits, hospitalization, the use of emergency department services, and costs of prescriptions.

Both Clouse and Edmeads have reported that patients with migraine have higher direct medical costs than the general population, primarily due to greater frequency of physician and emergency department visits [26, 27]. To assess healthcare resource use associated with migraine, Clouse and Osterhaus conducted a study among 1,336 migraine sufferers enrolled in a United Healthcare affiliated plan. Subjects were eligible for enrollment if they had been enrolled in the plan for at least one year, had a medical claim for migraine, and a pharmacy claim for a medication potentially used for migraine treatment. During an 18-month follow-up period, the consultation rates of migraine sufferers (n=1,336) were compared with non-migraine sufferers (n=1,336) matched on the basis of age, sex, duration of enrollment, and subscriber/dependent status. Migraine sufferers made 2,616 visits for migraine, and 19,971 visits for reasons other than migraine. In contrast, non-migraine sufferers made a total of 13,072 visits during the same period. Interestingly, a small proportion of migraine sufferers accounted for the majority of physician visits. While most migraine sufferers reported one to four physician visits per year, only a small proportion (7.6%) reported more than 12 visits. An important limitation of this study is the selected study population: only migraine sufferers who sought treatment were included.

In a recent population-based study, Edmeads and Mackell [27] matched individuals with migraine with a migraine-free control group on the basis of age, sex, employment status, and several comorbidities such as heart attack, angina, stroke, cancer, diabetes, and asthma. Both the frequency and quantity of healthcare utilization was greater for the migraine group than the control group. Migraine sufferers were significantly ($p<0.001$) more likely to report having visited a general practitioner, psychiatrist, or other medical specialist. In addition, while 24% of migraine sufferers reported an emergency department visit during the previous 6 months, only 15% of the comparison group reported a visit ($p<0.001$). Migraine sufferers also reported significantly more frequent physician visits (3.5 vs 2.8, $p<0.001$) and emergency department visits (0.4 vs. 0.2, $p<0.001$) than the control population.

This study has two important limitations. First, it included only self-reported migraine sufferers, although 60% reported that they had been diagnosed by a physician. Secondly, because of the study methodology, it was not possible to distinguish between migraine related visits and those related to comorbid conditions. However, matching the migraine sufferers with a control population should have minimized the extent to which comorbidities confound the results.

According to population-based studies conducted in 1989 and 1999, physician consultation among migraine sufferers increased over the last decade. A recent study of the epidemiology and patterns of health care use for migraine in the United States found that 48 percent of migraine sufferers had seen a doctor for headache within the last year, 21 percent were lapsed consulters (had not consulted for at least one year), while 31 percent had never consulted a doctor for headache [28]. In comparison with the American Migraine Study conducted in 1989, [29] the self-reported rates of current consultation have tripled.

The American Migraine Study also reported that certain demographic features and headache characteristics are associated with physician consultation [29]. For example, consultation is more common among females than males and with increasing age. In addition, more severe attacks, reflected by higher pain intensity, the number of migraine symptoms, attack duration, and disability are all associated with an increased likelihood of physician consultation.

Two population-based studies have translated healthcare use into direct costs [27,30]. Hu et al. [30] reported the direct costs of migraine based on a US population-based sample. In this study, the annual treatment costs of migraine were estimated to be over $1 billion, about

$100 per migraine sufferer per year. Physician visits (60%) and prescription drugs (30%) accounted for the majority of treatment related costs. Emergency department visits accounted for a small proportion of total costs (1%).

Edmeads and Mackell [27] estimated direct medical costs among self-identified migraine sufferers compared with a matched control group. Over a 6 month period, total direct medical costs, including physician visits, emergency department visits, and hospitalization were significantly higher (p=0.039) in the migraine group ($522) than the control population ($415). The costs of physician and emergency department visits were strong drivers behind the significant difference in total direct medical costs. The cost of outpatient physician visits was $221 for the migraine group, and $177 for the comparison group (p<0.001). Emergency department visits were also significantly higher (p<0.001) in the migraine group ($33) versus the control population ($18). The direct costs in this study are underestimated because they do not include the cost of prescription medications.

Headache severity is related to the direct costs. In one study [31], a four- point grading system that scaled pain and disability was used to classify subjects. According to the results of this scale, Grade 1 patients are defined by relatively low or moderate pain intensity without activity limitations. Grade 2 patients are defined by high pain intensity without activity limitations. Grade 3 patients are defined by moderate activity limitations. Grade 4 patients are defined by severe activity limitations. Using data collected in a self-administered questionnaire, the investigators classified members of the managed care organization, Group Health of Puget Sound, into the grading system and then followed the patients for two years. Claims data for these patients indicated that as headache severity grade increased, so did headache treatment costs. Among Grade 1 patients, treatment costs were $200 per patient per year. In contrast, Grade 4 patients had headache treatment costs that were $800 per patient per year.

Edmeads compared the direct medical costs among a population-based sample of self-identified moderate and severe migraine sufferers [27]. The average numbers of physician and emergency department visits were significantly higher for the severe group compared to the moderate group (p<0.004). Total medical costs were higher in the severe group ($605.38) than the moderate group ($471.96). The difference was not statistically significant.

Indirect Costs

While the direct costs of migraine are substantial, the indirect costs are even greater. Indirect costs include the aggregate effects of migraine on productivity at work, at home and in other roles. Many migraine sufferers miss work because of their headaches, and reduced productivity as a result of working during a migraine is common. Since it is important to measure absenteeism as well as work loss due to reduced productivity, many studies examine actual days of missed work, time at work with headache and percent effectiveness while at work with a headache. The components are sometimes combined in an index termed lost work day equivalents (LWDE) which equals actual days of missed work plus days at work with headache times one minus percent effectiveness while at work with headache [31].

Several studies have been conducted in population-based samples of migraine sufferers, and two used daily disability diaries to minimize recall bias. Von Korff et al. [3230] estimated the number of lost work days and LWDEs in a population-based sample of employed migraine sufferers who completed a daily diary for three months. A daily diary was used to improve the accuracy of the work loss data. During the three-month period, migraine sufferers missed an average of 1.1 days due to headache. Subjects who continued to work during a headache attack reported work effectiveness that was reduced by 41 percent. Migraine sufferers reported an average of 3 LWDEs.

Michel et al. [33] conducted a three-month prospective daily diary study examining work loss data among 231 migraine sufferers and 188 non-headache prone subjects. Participants used a daily diary to record the presence or absence of headache and the work situation that day (unemployment, holiday, weekend, medical reason, nonmedical reason). Absenteeism was classified into two groups: sickness related absenteeism (i.e., number of workdays missed or interrupted for medical reasons) and headache related absenteeism (i.e., number of workdays missed or interrupted on days with headache). In this study, migraine sufferers reported an average of 1.45 missed days due to medical reasons, 0.25 of which were due to headache. Sickness related absenteeism was statistically higher in migraine sufferers than non-headache prone subjects. The control population, on the other hand, reported 0.96 sickness related days, 0.7 of which were due to headache. The difference was due to higher absenteeism related to comorbid medical conditions, not headache reasons.

While most studies have reported time lost from work due to a migraine, few studies have recorded the number of days missed from household activities. Edmeads and Mackell [27], however, calculated the number of days missed from both employment and household activities over a 6-month period. Among full and part-time workers, the migraine sufferers missed 5 days of work, while the control group missed only 3 days (p<0.001). The migraine sufferers who were not employed missed more days of household duties (n=18 days) than their counterparts (n=14 days). However, the difference was not statistically significant (p=0.177).

Since migraine sufferers avoid sick leave for headache, it is important to measure time lost due to reduced productivity while working with a headache; however, Michel et al. [33] did not report LWDE data. The amount of lost work time due to LWDEs is significant. For example, as Von Korff et al. [32] reported, migraine sufferers lost only 1.1 days due to headache over a three-month period, but lost 3 days due to headache related reduced productivity. Not including reduced productivity time is one weakness of the Michel et al. [33] and Edmeads [27] studies. Additionally, some of the variation in work loss data may be due to cultural differences in the acceptability of medically-related absences.

While several studies have estimated lost workdays and reduced effectiveness at work, only a few studies have estimated the costs associated with lost productivity. Some of these studies had significant methodological weaknesses because they included biased populations [23,31]. Other studies, including more representative populations have also been published.

Hu et al. [30] estimated the indirect costs of migraine in a population-based sample of migraine sufferers. In this study, prevalence estimates were derived from two existing population-based databases: the American Migraine Study and the Baltimore County survey. The American Migraine Study was a national probability sample of over 20,000 individuals, while the Baltimore County survey was comprised of over 13,000 participants. The authors estimate that migraine costs American employers over $13 billion per year due to absenteeism and reduced effectiveness at work. Assuming that the percentage of people working for pay among migraine sufferers is the same as the general population (i.e., 73% of males and 57% of females), lost productivity costs per year are $690 for males and $1,127 for females.

Michel et al. [33] reported the indirect costs of migraine in a population-based sample, but they reported much lower cost estimates. The total indirect costs as reported in the Michel et al. study were $240 per migraine sufferer per year. The Michel et al. estimate is lower because the number of lost workdays reported by this population was on the low end, and the investigators did not account for LWDEs that would have further increased the estimate. Furthermore, the scale upon which the wages were calculated was not specified. However, since this was a French study, the wages may be different than that used for the studies conducted in the United States.

Edmeads and Mackell [27] calculated the cost of lost workdays and household days among a population-based sample of migraine sufferers and a control population. The cost of time missed from paid employment was significantly higher (p=0.018) in the migraine group ($477.47) than the control group ($309.90). Among migraine sufferers who were not employed, the average lost productivity cost was $1214.44. In the control population, however, the average lost productivity cost was lower ($912.48). This difference was not statistically significant (p=0.174).

In a recent publication, Stewart et al. [34] used data from the American Productivity Audit to estimate the pain related lost productive time and the associated costs due to headache and other conditions in the US workforce. Overall, 5.4% of the workforce reported lost productive time due to headache (pain in the past 2 weeks). The mean lost productive time for headache was 3.5 hours per week. Lost productive time due to headache was much more common than absenteeism. The cost of lost productive time due to headache is substantial: the total cost of lost productive time due to headache in the US workforce is $19.6 billion; $4.2 billion because of absenteeism and $8.7 billion because of impaired work due to pain.

Individual Impact

Attack Characteristics

The individual impact of migraine can be measured in many ways. It is important to assess the pattern of symptoms as well as the frequency and severity of attacks. Factors such as the level of pain intensity, the presence and severity of associated symptoms (nausea, vomiting, photophobia, phonophobia), and attack duration are important determinants of the severity of an individual attack. However, migraine also has a cumulative impact over time. Quality of life studies help quantify the impact of individual attacks as well as quality of life between episodes. Several studies indicate that most migraine sufferers report severe pain and the presence of associated symptoms with their migraine attacks.

In a US population-based study of migraine sufferers [22], 80 percent reported pain that is severe or very severe. The remainder of subjects reported mild to moderate pain. In addition to pain, associated symptoms were common. More than half of the subjects reported photophobia (81.9%) and phonophobia (77.9%). Approximately 60 percent reported nausea that accompanies their migraine headache more than half of the time. Vomiting was uncommon.

The overall impact of the illness is determined not just by attack characteristics, but also by attack frequency. On average, migraine sufferers report one to two migraine attacks per month. The duration of an untreated attack varies by gender. Among females, approximately 71 percent of attacks last longer than 24 hours. In contrast, 48 percent of males reported attacks that last longer than 24 hours. These findings are similar to those reported in other studies [35-37].

Health-Related Quality of Life

HRQoL studies are generally considered a more qualitative assessment of the burden of migraine. They measure the individual impact of a disease in the following domains: physical, psychological, social, spiritual and role-functioning, and general well being. Both generic and disease specific measures have been used to evaluate quality of life among migraine sufferers. While generic quality of life instruments are designed to measure the impact of a range of illnesses using a common scale, disease specific measures contain questions that address the quality of life impact of a specific illness.

Several population-based studies in the United States and Europe have evaluated HRQoL among migraine sufferers and a control population [38-41]. Each of these studies used a generic quality of life measure: the Medical Outcomes Study (MOS) instrument developed by the RAND corporation. Terwindt et al [38] used the SF-36, while Steiner et al [40] and Lipton et al [41] used the SF-12.

All of these studies included a contemporaneous nonmigraine control population. HRQoL scores in the migraine population were significantly lower than those in the control population. These studies also described the relationships between HRQoL, migraine frequency, disability, and depression. As migraine frequency and disability increased, HRQoL decreased [38,39]. The study reported by Lipton et al [41] confirmed that migraine and depression are comorbid. Furthermore, they found that migraine status was associated with decreased HRQoL scores, even after controlling for depression.

Another group of researchers is developing a novel approach to study the quality of life of migraine sufferers by designing a scale to evaluate the severity of the disease [42]. Based on expert consensus and surveys among migraine sufferers, El Hasnaoui et al. found seven items that reflected severity: intensity of pain, tolerability, disability in daily activities, presence of nausea or vomiting, resistance to treatment, and frequency of attacks. In addition, there was very good correlation between the severity items and the migraine sufferers quality of life.

Perspectives on Treatment Options and Cost Effective Intervention

Both pharmacological and non-pharmacological methods are used to treat headaches. Pharmacological treatment may be acute (abortive) or preventive (prophylactic). Acute treatments are given at the time of the attack to relieve pain and other symptoms. Prophylactic treatments are taken on a daily basis whether or not headache is present to prevent migraine attacks and reduce their severity.

Acute treatments may be specific or nonspecific. Nonspecific treatments may be used to treat many pain states from backache to migraine, while specific treatments are used exclusively to treat migraine attacks. Nonspecific treatments are generally used for mild to moderate migraine and include both over-the-counter (OTC) and prescription drugs. OTC treatments include aspirin, acetaminophen, ibuprofen, and the combination of aspirin, acetaminophen, and caffeine.

Nonspecific prescription drugs include ibuprofen, naproxen sodium, indomethacin, or the combination of acetaminophen, isometheptene, and dichloralphenazone. Antiemetics such as domperidone or metoclopramide are also prescribed to combat nausea. The following section summarizes the characteristics of some of the available prescription migraine-specific drugs.

Migraine specific drugs such as the 'triptans' (e.g., sumatriptan, naratriptan, rizatriptan, zolmitriptan, almotriptan, etc.) are available only by prescription in the United States and are available in various dosage forms including injections, intranasal sprays, tablets, and quick-dissolving tablets. The triptans are believed to be 5-HT1 agonists, a class of drugs that have similar chemical structures and mechanisms of action. All seven triptans are effective in relieving the pain and associated symptoms of migraine including nausea, photophobia, phonophobia, and functional disability. As a class, the triptans are contraindicated in patients with cardiovascular risk factors. Serious cardiac events, including death, have been reported in association with the triptans. However, these events are rare and most occurred in patients with risk factors predictive of coronary artery disease. Common side effects associated with these drugs are paresthesia, warm/cold sensations, chest pain/tightness/pressure and/or heaviness, neck/throat/jaw - pain/tightness/pressure, vertigo, and malaise/fatigue [43].

Dihydroergotamine (DHE), a derivative of ergotamine, is an alternative to the triptans. It is available as an injection or intranasal spray. Similarly to the triptans, it is contraindicated in patients with cardiac risk factors. Side effects that are commonly associated with DHE nasal spray include dizziness, parasthesias, abdominal cramps, and chest tightness [43].

Opiates are useful under special circumstances, such as in patients who cannot take ergotamine or triptans, or when nonnarcotic drugs fail [44]. They should only be used when headaches are infrequent. Narcotic drugs used to treat migraine include the combination of codeine and a simple analgesic, butorphanol, meperidine, morphine, and hydromorphone.

Prophylactic treatment of migraine falls into three categories: pre-emptive, short-term, or chronic [44]. Pre-emptive treatment is used when there is a known headache trigger such as exercise or sexual activity. In this case, the treatment is administered, often as a single dose, prior to the exposure. Short-term prophylactic treatment is administered over several days, during exposure to a trigger such as menstruation. In chronic prophylaxis, the drug is administered everyday. Examples of prophylactic treatments include beta-adrenergic blocker, antidepressants, calcium channel antagonists, serotonin agonists, anticonvulsants, and nonsteroidal anti-inflammatory drugs (NSAIDs).

Non-pharmacological treatments such as relaxation and biofeedback are helpful for some headache sufferers. Behavioral interventions such as maintaining a regular schedule, getting adequate sleep and exercise, and giving up tobacco may also be beneficial [44].

The acute migraine treatment options have varying costs and efficacy profiles. In general, the triptans are highly efficacious in most patients, but they are costly in comparison with some of the older treatments such as ergotamine. In clinical trials of oral sumatriptan, 54 percent to 61 percent of participants reported pain relief two hours after a 50 mg dose with a mean response rate of 60 percent [43,45]. By four hours, 68 percent to 78 percent of patients reported relief. Ergotamine, on the other hand, is slightly less efficacious, however, it has a longer duration of action and is less expensive. In order to examine the tradeoffs between cost and efficacy, several studies have examined the cost-effectiveness of acute migraine treatments.

Zhang et al. [46] compared the cost-effectiveness of rizatriptan 10mg, sumatriptan 50mg, and ergotamine tartrate plus caffeine in the treatment of acute migraine attacks over a one-year period. Both rizatriptan and sumatriptan were more cost-effective than ergotamine. The net annual savings were $622.98 and $620.90 per patient for rizatriptan and sumatriptan, respectively.

In another study, Willaims and Reeder [47] examined the cost-effectiveness of almotriptan 12.5 mg and rizatriptan 10 mg in the treatment of a single acute migraine attack. These investigators calculated cost-effectiveness ratios (CERs) based on an effectiveness measure that was defined as the proportion of patients who achieved sustained freedom from pain with no adverse events (SNAE). In the base case analysis, the mean CERs for almotriptan 12.5 mg and rizatriptan 10mg were $91.12 and $131.26, respectively; that is, in this study, almotriptan was more cost-effective than rizatriptan in the treatment of acute migraine.

CONCLUSION

Migraine has a significant impact on the sufferer and on society. It affects approximately 11 percent of the population in Western countries, and is more prevalent among women than men. Migraine prevalence peaks during the late 30s to early 40s, typically the most productive years of life. As a result, the condition is estimated to cost American employers over $13 billion per year due to absenteeism and reduced effectiveness as work [30]. There are many cost-effective, efficacious treatments available: physicians should prescribe treatments based on the attack characteristics of each individual patient.

REFERENCES

[1]   Scher AI, Stewart WF, Lipton RB. Migraine and headache: a meta-analytic approach. In: *Crombie IK, ed. Epidemiology of Pain.* Seattle, WA: IASP Press; 1999:159-170.

[2]   Headache Classification Subcommittee of the International Headache Society. *Classification of Headache Disorders*, 2nd ed. Cephalalgia. 2004;24 (suppl 1):1-150.

[3]   Lipton R, Bigal M, Steiner T, Silberstein S, Olesen J. Classification of primary headaches. *Neurology.* 2004;Aug 10;63(3):427-435.

[4]   Jensen K, Tfelt-Hansen P, Lauritzen M, Olesen J. Classic migraine, a prospective recording of sympotms. *Acta Neurol Scand.* 1986;73:359-362.

[5]   Manzoni G, Farina S, Lanfranchi M, et al. Classic migraine: clinical findings in 164 patients. *Eur Neurol.* 1985;24:163-169.

[6]   Bigal ME, Rapoport AM, Tepper SJ, Sheftell FD, Lipton RB. The classification of chronic daily headache in adolescents - a comparison between the second edition of the international classification of headache disorders and alternative diagnostic criteria. *Headache*. 2005, 45:582-589.

[7]   Silberstein SD, Lipton RB, Sliwinski M. Classification of daily and near-daily headaches: field trial of revised IHS criteria. *Neurology*. 1996; 47:871-875.

[8]   Breslau N, Chilcoat H, Andreski P. Further evidence on the link between migraine and neuroticism. *Neurology*. 1996;47:663-667.

[9]   Stewart W, Linet M, Celentano D, Van Natta M, Ziegler D. Age- and sex-specific incidence rates of migraine with and without visual aura. *Am J Epidemiol*. 1991;134:1111-1120.

[10] Stang P, Yanagihara T, Swanson J, Beard C, O'Fallon W, Guess H, Melton L. Incidence of migraine headache: a population-based study in Olmstead County, Minnesota. *Neurology*. 1992;42:1657-1662.

[11] Lyngberg A, Jensen R, Rasmussen B, Jorgensen T. Incidence of migraine in a Danish population-based follow-up study [abstract]. *Cephalalgia*. 2003;23:596.

[12] Stewart W, Lipton R, Celentano D, Reed M. Prevalence of migraine headache in the United States: relation to age, income, race, and other sociodemographic factors. *JAMA*. 1992;267:64-69.

[13] Lipton R, Stewart W, Diamond S, Diamond M, Reed M. Prevalence and burden of migraine in the United States: data from the American Migraine Study II. *Headache*. 2001;41:646-657.

[14] Lipton RB, Diamond D, Freitag F, Bigal ME, et al. Migraine prevention patterns in a community sample. Results from the American Migraine Prevalence and Prevention (AMPP) study. *Headache* 2005;45: 792.

[15] Lipton R, Scher A, Kolodner K, Liberman J, Steiner TJ, Stewart WF. Migraine in the United States: epidemiology and patterns of health care use. *Neurology*. 2002;58:885-894.

[16] Bigal M, Lipton R, Krymchantowski A. The medical management of migraine. *Am J Ther*. 2004;11:130-140.

[17] Lipton R, Stewart W. Migraine in the United States: a review of epidemiology and health care use. *Neurology* 1993;43(suppl 3):S6-S10.

[18] Abu-Arefeh I, Russell G. Prevalence of headache and migraine in schoolchildren. *BMJ* 1994;309:765-769.

[19] Bille B. Migraine in children: prevalence, clinical features, and a 30-year follow up. In: Ferrari M, Lataste X, eds. *Migraine and Other Headaches*. New Jersey: Parthenon, 1989;29-38.

[20] Mortimer J, Kay, J, Jaron A. Epidemiology of headache and childhood migraine in an urban general practice using ad hoc, Valquist and IHS criteria. *Dev Med Child Neurol*. 1992;34:1095-1101.

[21] Raieli V, Raimondo D, Cammalleri R, Camarda R. Migraine headache in adolescents: a student population-based study in Monreale. *Cephalalgia*. 1995;15:5-12.

[22] Stewart W, Lipton R, Liberman J. Variation in migraine prevalence by race. *Neurology*. 1996;16:231-238.

[23] Stang P, Osterhaus J. Impact of migraine in the United States: data from the National Health Interview Survey. *Headache*. 1993;33:29-35.

[24] Launer L, Terwindt G, Ferrari M. The prevalence and characteristics of migraine in a population-based cohort: the GEM study. *Neurology*. 1999;53:537-542.

[25] Steiner T, Scher A, Stewart W, Kolodner K, Liberman J, Lipton R. The prevalence and disability burden of adult migraine in England and their relationships to age, gender, and ethnicity. *Cephalalgia*. 2003;23:519-527.

[26] Clouse J, Osterhaus J. Healthcare resource use and costs associated with migraine in a managed healthcare setting. *Annals of Pharmacotherapy*. 1994;28:659-664.

[27] Edmeads J, Mackell J. The economic impact of migraine: an analysis of direct and indirect costs. *Headache*. 2002;42:501-509.

[28] Lipton R, Stewart W, Kolodner K, Liberman J. Epidemiology and patterns of healthcare use for migraine in the United States. *Headache* 1999;39:363-364.

[29] Lipton R, Stewart W, Simon D. Medical consultation for migraine: results of the American migraine study. *Headache*. 1998;38:87-90.

[30] Hu X, Markson L, Lipton R, Stewart W, Berger M. Burden of migraine in the United States: disability and economic costs. *Arch Intern Med*. 1999;159:813-818.

[31] Osterhaus J, Gutterman D, Plachetka J. Healthcare resource and lost labour costs of migraine headache in the US. *Pharmacoeconomics*. 1992;1:67-76.

[32] VonKorff M, Stewart W, Simon D, Lipton R. Migraine and reduced work performance: a population-based diary study. *Neurology*. 1998;50:1741-1745.

[33] Michel P, Dartigues J, Duru G, Moreau J, Salamon R, Henry P. Incremental absenteeism due to headache in migraine: results from the Mig-Access French national cohort. *Cephalalgia*. 1999;19:503-510.

[34] Stewart WF, Ricci J, Chee E, Morganstein M, Lipton R. Lost productive time and cost due to common pain conditions in the US workforce. *JAMA*. 2003;290:2443-2454.

[35] Stewart W, Lipton R, Celentano D, Reed M. Prevalence of migraine headache in the United States: relation to age, income, race, and other sociodemographic factors. *JAMA*. 1992;276:64-69.

[36] Gobel H, Petersen-Braun M, Soyka D. The epidemiology of headache in Germany: a nationwide survey of a representative sample on the basis of the headache classification of the International Headache Society. *Cephalalgia*. 1994;14:97-106.

[37] Tekl Haimanot R, Seraw B, Forsgren nL, Ekbom K, Ekstedt J. Migraine, chronic tension-type headache, and cluster headache in an Ethiopian rural community. *Cephalalgia*. 1995;15:482-488.

[38] Terwindt G, Launer L, Ferrari M. The impact of migraine on quality of life in the general population: The GEM study. *Neurology*. 1998;50(suppl 4):A434.

[39] Lipton R, Liberman J, Kolodner K, Dowson A, Sawyer J, Stewart W. Migraine headache disability and quality-of-life: a population-based case-control study. *Headache*. 1999;39:365.

[40] Steiner TJ, Lipton RB, Liberman JN, Kolodner KB, Stewart WF. Work and family impact of migraine: a population-based case-control study. *Neurology*. 1999;52 (Suppl 2):A470-A471.

[41] Lipton R, Hamelsky S, Kolodner K, Stewart W. Migraine, quality of life, and depression: a population-based case-control study. *Neurology*. 2000;55:629-635.

[42] El Hasnaoui A, Vray M, Richard A, Nachit-Ouinekh F, Boureau F. Assessing the severity of migraine: development of the MIGSEV scale. *Headache*. 2003;43:628-635.

[43] Silberstein S, Lipton R, Goadsby P. *Headache in Clinical Practice*. Oxford: Isis Medical Media Ltd., 1998.

[44] *Physicians'Desk Reference*. 53rd ed. Montvale, NJ: Medical Economics Company, 2005.

[45] Ferrari MD, Goadsby PJ, Roon KI, Lipton RB. Triptans (seotonin, 5-HT1B/1D agonists) in migraine: detailed results and methods of a meta-analysis of 53 trials. *Cephalalgia*. 2002; 22:633-658.

[46] Zhang L, Hay J. Cost-effectiveness analysis of rizatriptan and sumatriptan versus Cafergot in the acute treatment of migraine. *CNS Drugs*. 2005;19(7):635-642.

[47] Williams P, Reeder C. Cost-effectiveness of almotriptan and rizatriptan in the treatment of acute migraine. Clinical Therapeutics. 2003;25(11):2903-2919.

RECOMMENDED FURTHER READING

1. Scher AI, Stewart WF, Lipton RB. Migraine and headache: a meta-analytic approach. In: Crombie IK, ed. *Epidemiology of Pain*. Seattle, WA: IASP Press; 1999:159-170.

2. Headache Classification Subcommittee of the International Headache Society. Classification of Headache Disorders, 2nd ed. *Cephalalgia*. 2004;24 (suppl 1):1-150.

3. Hu X, Markson L, Lipton R, Stewart W, Berger M. Burden of migraine in the United States: disability and economic costs. *Arch Intern Med*. 1999;159:813-818.

4. Stewart WF, Ricci J, Chee E, Morganstein M, Lipton R. Lost productive time and cost due to common pain conditions in the US workforce. *JAMA*. 2003;290:2443-2454.

In: Handbook of Clinical Neuroepidemiology
Editors: V. L. Feigin and D. A. Bennett, pp. 123-165

ISBN 978-1-60021-511-7
© 2007 Nova Science Publishers, Inc.

Chapter 4

EPILEPSY

Ettore Beghi

Epilepsy Center & Neurophysiology Unit, University of Milano-Bicocca, Monza, Italy;
Laboratory of Neurological Disorders, Institute for Pharmacological Research Mario
Negri, Milano, Italy.

ABSTRACT

Epilepsy is a chronic neurological disorder characterized by repeated unprovoked seizures, with worldwide distribution. The incidence of epilepsy ranges from 23 to 190 per 100,000 population per year and is higher in developing countries than in industrialized countries and in lower socio-economic classes. The incidence of acute symptomatic seizures is 29-39 per 100,000 per year and the incidence of isolated seizures is 61 per 100,000 per year. The incidence of epilepsy is moderately higher in men than in women and is higher in the two extremes of the age spectrum. By age 80, there is a 1.3 to 4% risk of epilepsy, a 8% risk of epilepsy and single seizures, and a 10% risk when including acute symptomatic seizures. A documented etiology of epilepsy has been reported to vary from 14 to 52% of cases in incidence studies, with cerebrovascular disease, congenital neurological disorders, trauma, neoplasms, degenerative disorders and infections in decreasing order. Complex partial seizures are the predominating seizure pattern, followed by generalized tonic-clonic seizures, simple partial seizures, absence seizures, and myoclonic seizures. The incidence varies significantly according to the epilepsy syndrome. The overall prevalence of epilepsy is 2.7-41 per 1,000 (mostly 4-8 per 1,000). The prevalence is lower in industrialized than in developing countries and is higher in patients with lower socio-economic background. The prevalence tends to prevail in men and in blacks and varies with age, with differing rates in children, adults, and the elderly. Documented etiology in prevalent cases varies from 17 to 56%. The overall prognosis of epilepsy is favorable, with 55-68% of newly diagnosed cases achieving seizure remission. The average recurrence risk of a first unprovoked seizure is 51%, about 50% of recurrences occurring within 6 months. Factors influencing the prognosis of epilepsy include etiology, EEG abnormalities, generalized tonic-clonic seizures, the number of seizures experienced after the onset of treatment, and the syndromic pattern. Antiepileptic drugs suppress seizures but do not alter the long-term prognosis of epilepsy. About 50% of patients are successfully controlled by the first drug. The average risk of relapse after treatment discontinuation in seizure-free patients is 25% at one year and 29% at two years. The mortality of epilepsy is mostly 1-2 per 100,000 per year, with a standardized mortality ratio (SMR) of 1.6-5.3. Mortality is higher in developing countries. Status epilepticus, generalized tonic-clonic seizures and myoclonic seizures are associated with an increased mortality. Seizure etiology is one of the strongest risk factors for mortality in epilepsy. Accidents and suicide are among the commonest causes of death. The SMR is inversely correlated to age and disease duration. The incidence of sudden unexplained death (SUDEP) is 1-3.5 per 1,000.

INTRODUCTION

Epilepsy is a chronic clinical disorder affecting both sexes and all ages with worldwide distribution. Epilepsy is a symptom complex arising from a number of disordered brain functions, which may be secondary to a variety of pathologic phenomena. The cardinal manifestations of epilepsy are the *epileptic seizures*, which are recurrent paroxysmal episodes of brain dysfunction characterized by stereotyped alterations in behavior and reflecting the neural mechanisms involved by the epileptic process. In most cases, the disease can be diagnosed through a careful history or by the chance observation of a seizure. The ascertainment of the disease relies on the attentiveness of the patient and his/her family, on the emotional and social impact of the seizures, and on the capabilities of the available health care facilities. The interictal electroencephalogram (EEG) is of limited help in making the diagnosis, as its sensitivity is only about 60% [1]. Although a causative agent can be identified in some instances, in the majority of cases no cause can be found and the diagnosis is only descriptive. The differential diagnosis of epilepsy encompasses a number of clinical conditions characterized by transient alteration of consciousness and/or behavior, which may explain the possibility of false-positive and false-negative diagnoses. These limitations may be a possible explanation of the heterogeneity of the frequency, course and consequences of the disease in the world.

DEFINITIONS OF SEIZURES AND EPILEPSY

While all people with epilepsy experience seizures, not all individuals with seizures have epilepsy. Epileptic seizures may occur in the context of a brain insult (systemic, toxic or metabolic). These events (provoked or acute symptomatic seizures) are presumed to be an acute manifestation of the insult and may not recur when the underlying cause has been removed or the acute phase has elapsed. In contrast, epilepsy is the occurrence of two or more unprovoked seizures [2]. An unprovoked seizure is a seizure or a flurry of seizures occurring within 24 hours in a person over one month of age, occurring in the absence of precipitating factors. Unprovoked seizures include events occurring in the absence of a recognized etiological or risk factor (idiopathic and cryptogenic seizures), in patients with antecedent stable (non-progressing) central nervous system (CNS) insults (remote symptomatic seizures), or in those with progressive CNS abnormalities such as brain tumors, genetic, metabolic or degenerative conditions (progressive symptomatic seizures). Unprovoked seizures may be single or recurrent. Although all patients with single unprovoked seizures may have "potential" epilepsy, seizure recurrence can be observed only in about one-half of cases [3]. The difference between provoked and unprovoked seizures and between isolated and recurrent seizures is relevant to the interpretation of the main epidemiological indexes. Although epilepsy is, by definition, a chronic clinical condition, about two-thirds of patients achieve seizure remission, most of whom immediately after treatment initiation [4]. *Epilepsy in remission with treatment* is defined by the absence of seizures for at least five years in patients still receiving antiepileptic drugs (AEDs) [2]. *Epilepsy in remission without treatment (terminal remission)* is seizure remission for at least five years in patients off medications at time of ascertainment [2]. These cases add up to the so-called *inactive epilepsy*. By contrast, *active epilepsy* is defined as having at least one seizure in the preceding 5 years regardless of treatment with AEDs [2] *Intractable epilepsy* still requires a standard definition. In a prospective U.S. cohort of childhood-onset epilepsy [5], intractability was intended as failure on two or more antiepileptic drugs *and* one or more seizures a month over 18 months or longer.

INCIDENCE AND PREVALENCE OF EPILEPSY

Methodological Issues

Quality of Epidemiological Reports

The results of the published epidemiological studies must be interpreted in the light of methodological differences and the quality of the reports. The major problems with descriptive epidemiology of epilepsy are diagnostic accuracy and completeness of case ascertainment. Check-lists have been developed to assess the methodological quality of observational studies included in meta-analyses [6]. These include the definition of epilepsy and epileptic seizures, the type of study design (retrospective or prospective, review of medical records and/or direct examination of cases, etc.), the study population (with demography), the description of the selection criteria, and the individual study estimates (main epidemiological indexes).

Differentiation between Epilepsy, single Seizures and acute Symptomatic Seizures

A correct differentiation between epilepsy, single seizures and acute symptomatic seizures is uncommon, mostly in studies done in developing countries.

Type of Study

The prospective design is the ideal method to guarantee completeness of case ascertainment and to identify the eligible cases in the light of standard definitions and inclusion criteria and to provide correct incidence rates. However, prospective studies, which are costly and time-consuming, cannot be undertaken in countries with scarce or limited resources. For this reasons, most epidemiological surveys of epilepsy have been conducted using a cross-sectional or retrospective design. Medical records were the main (and in some cases the only) source of cases. Only in some reports were eligible cases re-examined to confirm the diagnosis. Door-to-door surveys have been conducted in few instances.

Population

The patients with epilepsy enrolled in the epidemiological studies should be representative of the general epilepsy population. Multiple sources of cases should be thus explored to maximize case ascertainment. However, this was not the case in the majority of the published studies. The large majority of population-based surveys have been conducted on all patients with epilepsy or in patients in different age groups (children, adults, elderly). Several studies, especially those from the developing countries, were performed only in patients seeking medical advice. Other studies were limited to selected seizure types or epilepsy syndromes. The large majority of the surveys have been from small urban or rural areas, with no nationally-based reports and no international comparisons [7]. The socio-cultural background of the populations at risk (which has been found to significantly affect the frequency and characteristics of the disease) may be a strong confounder when different populations are compared.

Reference figures from the entire national population have been made available only for some studies. This represents a serious limitation as age- and sex-specific incidence or prevalence rates are missing and standardization (a procedure required by the need to adjust the local findings to the entire country) cannot be performed.

Selection Criteria

A correct identification of the population at risk is needed as evidence of the completeness of case ascertainment and to consent proper comparisons with other studies. Patients with mild or infrequent seizures may not receive medical care. Patients may also deny a history of epilepsy in view of the stigma connected to the disease. In community surveys it may be difficult to exclude pseudoseizures and other non-epileptic seizures, which may be present in up to 28% of patients presenting to general practitioners [8]. Although community-based studies including all epilepsy varieties provide a better insight of the whole spectrum of the disease, studies done in patients with selected epileptogenic conditions, although reductive, may help defining the risk of epilepsy attributable to the given conditions.

Epidemiological Surveys in Developing Countries

Methodological constraints and inconsistencies are mostly prevalent in reports from developing countries, which face several problems in terms of case ascertainment and study conduct [9]. The quality and completeness of data collection is impaired by the use of standard screening instruments across populations with diverse social and cultural backgrounds, the lack of specialized personnel, the almost complete absence of diagnostic equipment, and the use of different terminologies to define seizures and epilepsy.

Epidemiological Indexes

The incidence rates provide a better outlook of the clinical spectrum of a disease and of the distribution of the risk factors. However, given the economic and practical constraints (see above), studies on the incidence of epilepsy represent a small fraction of the epidemiological surveys. Most surveys report, in fact, prevalence rates. In contrast to incidence studies, prevalence studies are biased by the inclusion of survivors and by the exclusion of patients with inactive epilepsy. Prevalence studies are thus less reliable than incidence studies, as the variability of the indexes tends to reflect the structure of the population at risk, the incidence of the disease, the chance of remission, and the mortality. This is even more important for the developing countries were lethal epileptogenic conditions may be more common and few or no patients receive treatment of epilepsy.

INCIDENCE OF EPILEPSY AND UNPROVOKED SEIZURES

The incidence of unprovoked seizures is 33-198 per 100,000 and the incidence of epilepsy is 23-190 per 100,000 [10]. The overall incidence of epilepsy in Europe and North America ranges from 24 and 53 per 100,000 per year (Table 1) [10-13]. The incidence in children is eventually higher and even more variable, ranging from 25 to 840 per 100,000 per year, most of the differences being explained by the differing populations at risk and by the study design. In developing countries the incidence of the disease is higher than that of industrialized countries (Table 2) [10,14-16] and is up to 190 per 100,000. Although one might expect a higher exposure to perinatal risk factors, infections and traumas in these countries, the higher incidence of epilepsy may be also explained by the different structure of the populations at risk, which is characterized by a predominant distribution of young individuals and a short life expectancy.

Incidence by Age

In industrialized countries epilepsy tends to affect mostly the individuals at the two extremes of the age spectrum (Figure 1). The size and characteristics of the population at risk and the methods of case ascertainment mostly explain the differences across studies. In the Rochester, Minnesota population, where all medical contacts for seizures were traced over a 50-year period, the incidence of the disease was 86 per 100,000 population per year in the first year of age, then it tended to decrease to about 23-31 per 100,000 in individuals aged 30 to 59 years, and increased thereafter, up to 180 per 100,000 in the 85+ year age class [13]. The peak in the elderly is not detected in developing countries, where the disease peaks in the 10 to 20-year age class. This may depend on the age structure of the population and on a relative under-ascertainment of the disease in older individuals.

Table 1. Incidence (per 100,000 per year) of epilepsy in industrialized countries[†]

Country	Population	Incidence	Design and methods	Reference(s), year
Canada	Children	41.0	MR review	Camfield et al., 1996[(*)]
Denmark	Elderly	87.0	MR review	Luhdorf et al., 1986[(*)]
Denmark	All ages	43.0	MR review	Joensen, 1986[(*)]
Estonia	Children	45.0	Prospective	Beilmann et al., 1999[(*)]
Estonia	Adults	35.0	MR review	Oun et al., 2003[(*)]
Finland	Children	130.0/25.0	MR review	Rantala and Ingalsno, 1999/ ')Sillanpaa, 1973[(*)]
Finland	Adults and elderly	24.0	MR review and examination	Keranen et al., 1989[(*)]
France	All ages	44.0	Screening	Loiseau et al., 1990[11]
Germany	Children	72.4/52.1	Prospective/MR review	Doerfer et al., 1987[(*)]/Doose and Sitepu, 1983[(*)]
Iceland	All ages	46.5	MR review and examination	Olafsson et al., 1996[(*)]
Italy	Children	82.0	MR review	Cavazzuti, 1980[(*)]
Italy	All ages	33.1	MR review and examination	Granieri et al., 1983
Japan	Children	430.0/145.0	MR review	Tsuboi, 1988[(*)]; Ishida, 1985[(*)]
Norway	All ages	32.8	MR review	De Graaf, 1974[(*)]
Serbia	Children	650.0	MR review	Pavlovic et al., 1998[(*)]
Sweden	Children	82.3/53.0/50.0	MR review/MR review/ MR review and examination	Braathen and Theorell, 1995/[(*] Blom et al., 1978/[(*)] Bronson and Wranne, 1987[(*)]
Switzerland	All ages	46.0	MR review	Jallon et al., 1997[(*)]
U.K.	Children	840.0/430.0	Prospective/MR review	Verity et al., 1992/[(Kurtz et al., 1998[(*)]
U.K.	All ages	46.0	Prospective	MacDonald et al., 2000[12]
U.S.	All ages	44.0/35.0	MR review	Hauser et al., 1993/[Annegers et al., 1999[(*)]

MR = Medical record
[(*)] Reference listed in original source.
[†]Modified from [10]

Incidence by Gender

With few exceptions [17-19], the incidence of epilepsy and unprovoked seizures has been reported to be higher in men than in women both in industrialized and in developing countries, although this finding does not attain statistical significance in the large majority of the reports. The different distribution of epilepsy in men and women can be mostly explained by the differing genetic background, the different prevalence of the commonest risk factors in the two sexes, and by the concealment of the disease in women for socio-cultural reasons. However, the inconsistent findings may be also explained by the play of chance.

Table 2. Incidence (per 100,000 per year) of epilepsy in developing countries†

Country	Population	Incidence	Design and methods	Reference(s), year
Burkina-Faso	All ages ?	83.0	Retrospective	Debouverie et al., 1993[14]
Chile	All ages	113.0	MR review	Lavados et al., 1992[*]
China	All ages	25.0	Door-to-door survey	Li et al., 1985[*]
Ecuador	All ages	190.0	Door-to-door survey	Placencia et al., 1992[*]
Ethiopia	All ages	64.0	Door-to-door survey	Tekle-Haimanot et al., 1997[*]
India	All ages	49.3	Door-to-door survey	Mani et al., 1998[*]
Tanzania	All ages	73.3	Door-to-door survey	Rwiza et al., 1992[*]
Togo	All ages?	119.0	Retrospective	Grunitzky et al., 1991[15]
Uganda	All ages?	156.0	Repeated cross-sectional	Kaiser et al., 1998[16]

(*) Reference listed in original source.
†Modified from [10]

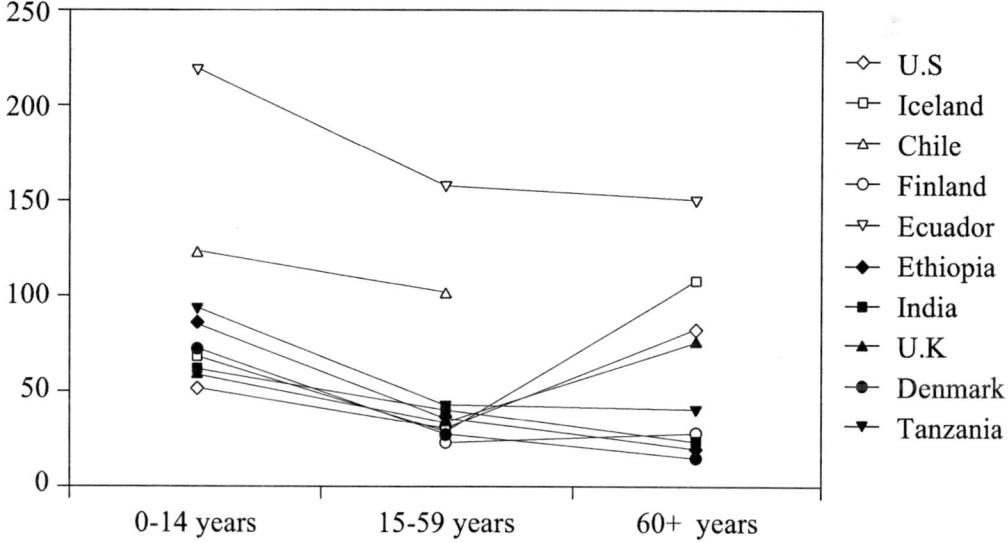

Figure 1. Age-specific incidence rates of epilepsy in selected industrialized and developing countries (Modified from [10]).

Incidence by Etiology

Despite better diagnostic ascertainment in more recent years, the majority of the epilepsies have still an unrecognized etiology. In incidence studies, the proportion of cases with documented etiology has been reported to vary from 13.7% in Ethiopia to 51.6% in Poland [20]. The differences are mostly explained by the structure of the population at risk, the prevalence of the etiological factors in the local environment, the study design, and the extent of the diagnostic ascertainment. In the Rochester, Minnesota study, epilepsy was idiopathic/cryptogenic in about two-thirds of patients [13]. In this population, cerebrovascular disease was the commonest etiology (10.9%), followed by congenital neurological disorders (8.0%), trauma (5.5%), neoplasm (4.1%), degenerative disorders (3.5%), and infection (2.5%). Etiological factors varied significantly with age, congenital disorders being most common in children aged less than 14 years and cerebrovascular disorders in the elderly (Figure 2).

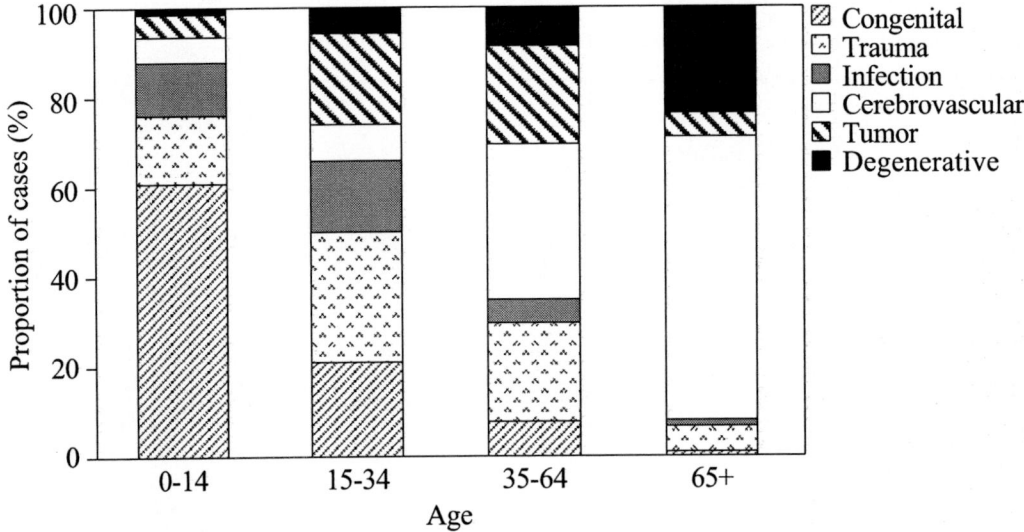

Figure 2. Proportion of cases of newly diagnosed epilepsy assigned to specific etiologic categories within age groups among those with assigned etiologies (From [13] with permission).

Temporal Trends

There are only few observations on the temporal trends of epilepsy. In the Rochester, Minnesota population, where the local population had been actively followed during the period 1935-84, no overall trends were observed [13]. However, age-specific incidence rates of epilepsy tended to decrease in the youngest age groups and to increase in the elderly. In contrast to the U.S. study, reports from Italy [21] and Sweden [22,23] showed a decrease with time of the incidence of the disease, mostly in children. The decreased incidence in the youngest individuals can be explained by the improvement in perinatal care while the increased incidence in the elderly can be attributed to the increased life expectancy (followed by an increasing occurrence of age-related epileptogenic conditions, like stroke and degenerative CNS disorders) and to an increased ascertainment of the disease in this age group.

Incidence by Seizure Type

In the last 20 years, the epidemiological studies have used the ILAE classification of the epileptic seizures [24]. In population-based studies partial seizures are the predominant pattern both in children and in adults. Comparing studies from industrialized and developing countries, Kotsopoulos and co-workers (2002) [10] found a median seizure-specific incidence rate of 30.4 per 100,000 per year (range 10.6-60.8) for partial seizures vs. 19.6 per 100,000 per year for generalized seizures (range 5.6-72.1). In the Rochester, Minnesota study [13], the proportion of all incidence cases by seizure type was the following: complex partial (36%), generalized tonic-clonic (23%), simple partial (14%), other generalized (8%), partial unknown (7%), absence (6%), myoclonic (3%), and unclassified (3%). In contrast to industrialized countries, in most developing countries the predominant seizure pattern is represented by (primarily or secondarily generalized) tonic-clonic seizures [4]. This tends to reflect a relative under-ascertainment of the other seizure types because of their minor impact on the quality of life of the affected individuals.

Incidence of status epilepticus has been found to vary from 6.8 to 41 per 100,000 per year [25]. As with epilepsy and acute symptomatic seizures, status epilepticus incidence is U-shaped, peaking under one year and over 60 years of age. Status epilepticus is more common in men than in women.

Incidence by Race

Virtually all incidence studies have been performed in white or homogeneous populations. The effects of race on the incidence of epilepsy have been mostly explored by studies done in children. No significant differences were found when comparing Japanese and U.S. children in studies using similar definitions and methods [13,26]. A study done in New Haven, Connecticut and comparing different races in children up to age 15 from the same geographic area noted a 1.7 increase in the incidence of epilepsy in blacks compared to whites [27].

Incidence of Epileptic Syndromes

There are only few reports on the incidence of epileptic syndromes. These are mainly studies focusing on selected syndromic patterns. The incidence of the epileptic syndromes in the general population has been calculated in Rochester, Minnesota, and reported in broad categories [28]. In this study, cryptogenic partial epilepsies were the commonest epilepsy syndrome (17.5 cases per 100,000 per year), followed by symptomatic partial epilepsies (17.2), undetermined epilepsies (9.7), symptomatic/cryptogenic epilepsies (4.0), idiopathic generalized epilepsies (3.7), and idiopathic partial epilepsies (0.2). In Bordeaux, France, the incidence of the commonest syndromes was generally lower. The rate was 15.3 per 100,000 for localization-related epilepsies (idiopathic 1.7; symptomatic 13.6), 6.7 per 100,000 for generalized epilepsies (idiopathic 5.6; symptomatic 1.1), and 1.9 per 100,000 for undetermined epilepsies [11]. Some of the differences between the U.S. and the French study can be mostly explained by accuracy in case ascertainment, selection bias, and inclusion (in the French study) of patients with a single seizure. However, the most remarkable difference was found for undetermined epilepsies, which reflects a more or less stringent application of the ILAE syndromic classification [29] and the limitations of this classification for epidemiological purposes. In a referral study of childhood-onset seizures [30], the commonest epilepsy syndromes were, in decreasing order, symptomatic localization-related epilepsies (31.8%), idiopathic generalized epilepsies (20.6%), and idiopathic localization-related epilepsies (10.0%). In an incidence study done in an adult population, 72% of cases had localization-related epilepsies, 16% had generalized epilepsies, and 12% had undetermined epilepsies [31]. There are numerous reports of the incidence of specific syndromes [4,32]. In children aged less than 15 years, idiopathic partial epilepsy with centro-temporal spikes is the commonest syndrome (14%), with an incidence of 10.7 per 100,000 per year [23]. The incidence of absence epilepsy was 7 per 100,000 [33]. The incidence of infantile spasms (West syndrome) is 2-7 per 10,000 live births and the incidence of juvenile myoclonic epilepsy is 1-6 per 100,000 population [32].

Cumulative Incidence

The overall risk of epilepsy by age 80 ranges from 1.3 to 4% in different study populations [4,32]. The differences can be largely interpreted on the basis of the differing accuracy in case ascertainment, especially in the elderly.

Incidence by Socio-economic Status

It is common opinion that the incidence of epilepsy is higher in the lower socio-economic classes. The assumption is supported by the comparison of industrialized and developing countries and by the comparison, within the same population, of people of different ethnic origin. In the New Haven, Connecticut study, the incidence of epilepsy was significantly higher in lower socioeconomic classes even after controlling for race [27].

Incidence and Etiology of Acute Symptomatic and Isolated Seizures

The incidence of acute symptomatic seizures is 29-39 per 100,000 per year [11,34]. Acute symptomatic seizures represent about 40% of all cases of afebrile seizures. Men seem at higher risk than women depending on the differing distribution of the underlying epileptogenic conditions in the two sexes. Acute symptomatic seizures predominate in the youngest age class (less than one year of age) and, to a lesser extent, in the elderly. Traumatic brain injury, cerebrovascular disease, drug withdrawal, infection, and metabolic insults represent the commonest causes.

The incidence of isolated unprovoked seizures can be only estimated from studies with prolonged (virtually lifetime) follow-up. In one of these studies [13], which explored a 50-year period, the age-adjusted incidence of a first unprovoked seizure was 61 per 100,000 person-years, which was approximately 33% higher than the incidence of epilepsy in the same community.

In the Rochester, Minnesota population, the cumulative incidence of single and recurrent epileptic seizures by the age of 80 years was approximately 8% [35]. The incidence was close to 10% when acute symptomatic seizures were also included.

Table 3. Prevalence (per 1,000) of active epilepsy in industrialized countries†

Country	Population	Prevalence	Design and methods	Reference(s), year
Australia	All ages	7.5	MR review	Beran et al., 1985[*]
Denmark	All ages	7.6	MR review	Joensen, 1986[*]
Estonia	Children	3.6	Prospective	Beilmann et al., 1999[36]
Estonia	Adults	5.3	MR review and examination	Oun et al., 2003[*]
Finland	Adults	6.3	MR review and examination	Keranen et al., 1989[*]
Finland	Children	3.9	Retrospective	Eriksson and Koivikko, 1997[*]
				Sillanpaa, 1973[*][*]
		3.2	MR review and examination	
Iceland	All ages	4.8	MR review	Olafsson and Hauser, 1999[*]
Italy	All ages	6.2	MR review and examination	Granieri et al., 1989[*]
			MR review	
		5.1	MR review and examination	Maremmani et al., 1991[*]
		3.9	AED consumption	Beghi et al., 1991[*]
			Door-to-door survey	
		5.2		Giuliani et al., 1992[*]
		3.3		Rocca et al., 2001[*]
Italy	Children	4.5 [+]	MR review	Cavazzuti, 1986[*]
Japan	All ages?	1.5	?	Sato, 1964[*]
Lithuania	Children	4.3	MR review	Endziniene et al., 1997[37]
Norway	Children	5.3	MR review and examination	Waaler et al., 2000[*]
Norway	All ages?	2.3	MR review and GP contacts	Krohn, 1961[*]
Poland	All ages	7.8	MR review	Zielinski, 1974[*]
Spain	Children	3.7[Ø]	Postal/domiciliary questionnaire	Ochoa Sangrador and Luaces, 1991[*]
Spain	Children >10 years and adults	4.1	Two-phase across sectional	Luengo et al., 2001[*]
Sweden	Adults	5.5	Multisource medical register review	Forsgren, 1992[*]
Sweden	Children	4.2	Questionnaire and GP and P inquiry	Sidenvall et al., 1996[*]
		3.5	MR review?	Bronson, 1970[*]
The Netherlands	Adults and elderly	7.7	Door-to-door survey	de la Court et al., 1996[*]
U.K.	All ages	6.2	GP files	Pond et al., 1960[*]
U.K.	Children 4-20 years	4.3	MR review	Tidman et al., 2003[*]
U.S.	All ages	6.8	Screening questionnaire and examination; MR review	Haerer et al., 1986[*]
		6.8		Hauser et al., 1991[*]
U.S.	Children	5.7	Questionnaire and CM inquiry/ MR review	Baumann et al., 1978[*]
		4.7[Δ]		Cowan et al., 1989[*]

[+] = 5-14 years; [Δ] = 6-16 years; + = 5-14 years;

[Δ] = 6-16 years;

[Ø] = 6-14 years.

MR = Medical record; GP = General practitioners; P = Pediatricians; CM = Community members

(*) Reference listed in original source.

†Modified from [4] and [7]

PREVALENCE OF EPILEPSY

There are numerous studies on the prevalence of epilepsy both in industrialized and in developing countries, with differing reports [4,32]. The overall prevalence ranges from 2.7 to 41 per 1,000 population, although in the majority of the published reports, the rate of active epilepsy varies from 4 to 8 per 1,000. The prevalence of active epilepsy is generally lower in industrialized countries (Table 3) [4,7,36-38] than in developing countries (Table 4) [4,19,39,40], which may reflect a lower prevalence of selected risk factors (mostly infections and traumas), a more stringent case verification, and the exclusion of provoked and unprovoked isolated seizures.

Table 4. Prevalence (per 1,000) of active epilepsy in developing countries†

Country	Population	Prevalence	Design and methods	Reference(s), year
Bolivia	All ages	11.2	Door-to-door survey	Nicoletti et al., 1999[(*)]
Chile	All ages	17.7	MR review	Lavados et al., 1992[(*)]
Ecuador	All ages	6.7-8.0$^\Delta$	Door-to-door survey	Placencia et al., 1992[18]
Ethiopia	All ages	5.2	?	Tekle-Haimanot et al., 1990[(*)]
India	All ages	5.3	Descriptive review	Sridharan and Murthy, 1999[(*)]
		4.6	Door-to-door survey	Mani et al., 1998[(*)]
		4.9	Door-to-door survey/	Radhakrishnan et al., 2000[(*)]
		3.6	Door-to-door survey	Bharucha et al., 1988[(*)(*)]
Nigeria	All ages	5.0	Door-to-door survey	Osuntokun et al., 1987[39]
Pakistan	All ages	10.0	Door-to-door survey	Aziz et al., 1994[40]
Panama	All ages?	57.0	Door-to-door survey	Gracia et al., 1990[(*)]
South Africa	Children 2-9 years	6.7	Door-to-door survey	Christianson et al., 2000[(*)]
Tanzania	All ages	10.2	Door-to-door survey	Rwiza et al., 1992[19]
Tunisia	All ages	4.0	Door-to-door survey	Attia-Romdhane et al., 1993[(*)]

$^\Delta$ Including single seizures and afebrile provoked seizures.

(*) Reference listed in original source.

†Modified from [4]

Prevalence by Age

In industrialized countries, the prevalence of epilepsy is lower in infancy and tends to increase thereafter, with the highest rate occurring in the elderly [32,35] (Figure 3). Where available, age-specific prevalence rates of lifetime and active epilepsy from developing countries tend to be higher in the second (254 vs. 148 per 1,000) and third decade of life (94 vs. 145 per 1,000) [41]. The differences between industrialized and developing countries may be mostly explained by the differing distribution of the risk factors and by the shorter life expectancy in the latter.

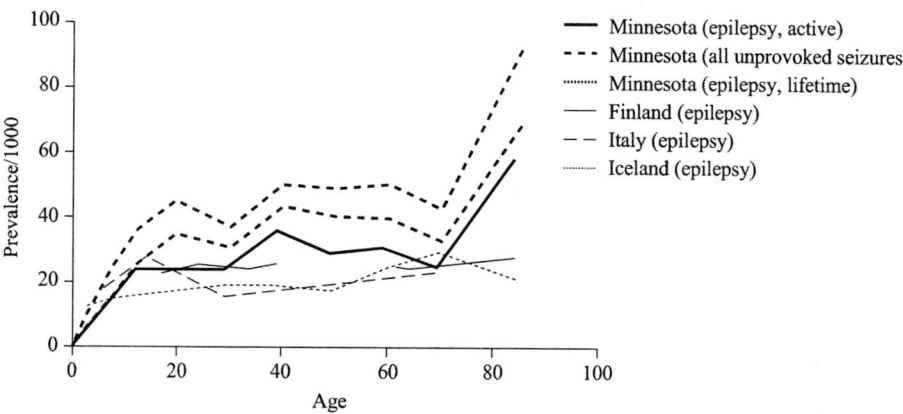

Figure 3. Age-specific prevalence of epilepsy and unprovoked scizures in selected sudies in industrialized countries (Modified from [32]).

Prevalence by Gender

As with incidence, prevalence of epilepsy tends to prevail in men. However, this finding is not consistent across studies and, with few exceptions, is not statistically significant. In individual studies, the dominance in females and males has been found to shift between age groups.

Prevalence by Etiology

The percentage of cases with documented etiology in prevalence studies has been shown to vary from 17 to 56% [20]. The main etiological factors are virtually the same as those reported in incidence studies (see above).

Prevalence by Race

When assessed in multiracial populations, the prevalence of epilepsy was found to prevail in blacks than in whites or Hispanics [32]. Differing risk factors and socio-cultural environments may explain the hererogeneity of the figures.

Prevalence by Seizure Type

Partial seizures are commoner than generalized seizures both in children and adults. As shown by Forsgren [4], in prevalence studies done in adults from industrialized countries, partial seizures were reported in 55-60% of cases, generalized seizures in 26-32%, and unclassifiable seizures in 8-17%. The corresponding numbers in children were 36-66%, 30-62%, and 2-4%. The differing proportions of partial and generalized seizures may be largely explained by the different distribution of the epilepsy syndromes in children and adults. Different figures are present for developing countries (11-55%, 26-86%, and 0-19% respectively), to be mostly interpreted as a consequence of a less accurate diagnostic ascertainment (as many tonic-clonic seizures are thought to be secondarily generalized).

Prevalence of Epileptic Syndromes

As opposed to incidence, the prevalence of epilepsy syndromes has been calculated in several recent reports, all from the Scandinavian and Baltic countries. In a study done in children in Estonia [36], the prevalence of idiopathic epilepsies was 1.2 per 1,000, and that of cryptogenic epilepsies was 1.0 per 1,000. In another study of childhood epilepsies in Lithuania [37], localization-related epilepsies were the commonest syndromic category (1.5 per 1,000) followed by generalized epilepsies (1.3 per 1,000) and undetermined epilepsies (0.6 per 1,000). Localization-related epilepsies were the predominant syndromic category in 41-54% of cases from Sweden, Finland and Norway, followed by generalized syndromes (37-48%) and unclassified syndromes (5-10%) [23,42,43]. The prevalence of specific syndromes in these countries was as follows: idiopathic partial epilepsy with centro-temporal spikes 5-17%, absence epilepsy 6-8%, juvenile myoclonic epilepsy 1-5%, West syndrome 0.5-8%, and Lennox-Gastaut syndrome 2-6%.

Prevalence by Socio-economic Class

Socio-economic background has been found to affect the frequency of epilepsy reports both in industrialized and in developing countries. The different rates found in multiracial populations may have such an explanation. In a study done in Wales, U.K., a strong independent correlation was detected between the prevalence of epilepsy and social deprivation, defined by unemployment, no car in the household, overcrowded households, and households not occupied by the owner [44]. In developing countries prevalence rates have been shown to be greater in the rural compared to the urban context [18,40,45] or in the lower compared to the higher socioeconomic classes [46]. However, opposite figures were reported in a meta-analysis of epidemiological studies from India [47], which confirms that rural and urban environments should not be invariably intended as proxies of lower vs. higher socioeconomic conditions.

ETIOLOGY OF EPILEPSY

Methodological Issues

Factors having a clear association with the development of epilepsy must be identified before accepting the concept of a causal association between a brain insult and the occurrence of epileptic seizures [48]. First, the timing of the seizure(s) must be identified, to separate acute symptomatic from unprovoked seizures. Second, the frequency and spectrum of epilepsy and putative etiological factors in the general population must be assessed to define the fraction of epilepsies associated to a given risk factor and the risk of epilepsy attributable to that factor. Third, the accuracy and validity of the diagnostic work-up must be considered. Fourth, evidence of a causal relationship should be produced to exclude the possibility of a chance association even at the presence of a well-established etiological factor.

Timing of the Seizure(s)

Every brain insult involving the cerebral cortex may be accompanied by immediate or early seizures (acute symptomatic seizures). Acute symptomatic seizures may occur as part of the brain insult and are associated with an increased risk of remote symptomatic seizures and epilepsy, but they should not be considered epilepsy *per se* because they might not relapse when the brain insult has been adequately treated or the acute phase has elapsed.

Incidence and Prevalence of Acute and Remote Symptomatic Seizures and Epilepsy

As previously indicated, the knowledge of the incidence of acute and remote symptomatic seizures and epilepsy in well-defined populations is needed to calculate the fraction of seizures and epilepsy attributable to known etiologic factors, the frequency of well-established risk factors for acute symptomatic and unprovoked seizures, and the fraction of known etiology attributable to each given factor (attributable risk). The etiology of epilepsy in populations may thus reflect the differing distribution of the etiologic factors, which may in turn explain a different proportion of cases with acute and remote symptomatic seizures and a different attributable risk. This is particularly important in developing countries where exposure to epileptogenic risk factors differs from industrialized countries [49].

Accuracy and Validity of the Diagnostic Assessment

Etiology of seizures is documented based on the quality, completeness and validity of diagnostic assessment, which includes history, biochemical and neuroimaging tests. The completeness of the diagnostic ascertainment depends on the availability of the diagnostic tests, the validity and reliability of each test, and the practical use, which depends upon the clinical judgment of the caring physician.

Genetic Epidemiology of Epilepsy

At least in part, the risk of epilepsy is accounted for by genetic factors. The role of the genetic components has been mostly explored by studies of familial aggregation of epilepsy, studies on maternal transmission, and twin studies [50]. As indicated by studies of familial aggregation of epilepsy, siblings and offspring of patients with epilepsy have a two- to threefold increased risk to develop epilepsy [51]. In offspring of patients with epilepsy, the cumulative incidence of unprovoked seizures to age 25 is about 6%, as opposed to 1-2% of the general population [52]. The risk of seizures among offspring of mothers with epilepsy exceeds that of offspring of fathers with epilepsy. If a proband has an early age at onset of seizures, there is an increased risk of seizures among siblings and offspring. The risk of unprovoked seizures is highest among siblings of probands with generalized epilepsy, in whom the risk is related to seizure type (mostly tonic-clonic or absence) and EEG abnormalities (mostly generalized spike and slow wave patterns). Twin studies show a higher concordance for epilepsy in monozygotic compared to dizygotic twin pairs. For a more comprehensive review of the genetics of epilepsy, see Hauser & Hesdorffer, 1990 and Privitera, 2001 [50,53].

Mechanisms of Inheritance in Epilepsy

As indicated by Johnson and Sander [54], there are four different patterns of inheritance in epilepsy: 1.Epileptic seizures occurring in the context of multi-organ hereditary disorders; 2. Idiopathic epilepsies with simple mendelian inheritance; 3. Epilepsies with complex inheritance (involving multiple contributing factors); 4. Idiopathic epilepsies associated with cytogenetic (chromosomal) abnormalities. Genetic disorders associated with epilepsy [20] include epilepsy secondary to multi-organ hereditary disorders (chromosome disorders, metabolic disorders, neurocutaneous disorders, genetic disorders of brain development), idiopathic epilepsies with simple mendelian inheritance (generalized epilepsy with febrile seizures plus, familial adult myoclonic epilepsy, familial autosomal recessive idiopathic myoclonic epilepsy of infancy, X-linked infantile spasms, benign familial neonatal convulsions, benign familial infantile convulsions, autosomal dominant nocturnal frontal lobe epilepsy, familial temporal lobe epilepsy, autosomal dominant rolandic epilepsy with speech dyspraxia, autosomal recessive rolandic epilepsy with paroxysmal exercise-induced dystonia and writer's cramp, familial partial epilepsy with variable foci). Genetic or chromosomal syndromes associated with epilepsy account for 2-3% of all epilepsies, while syndromes characterized by simple mendelian inheritance or cytogenetic abnormalities account for about 1%. Epilepsies with complex inheritance include the majority of the epileptic syndromes and are the result of complex and as yet unknown mechanisms reflecting a gene-environment interaction [55]. Epilepsies with complex, non-mendelian, genetic transmission include idiopathic generalized and partial epilepsies. These disorders may have more than one genetic etiology and phenotypes can be caused by mutations at different genetic loci. In this context, the concept of epilepsy syndromes as discrete entities is contrasted by the concept of a neurobiologic continuum, with idiopathic epilepsies that are *largely* genetic at one end, and symptomatic epilepsies that are *predominantly* acquired at the other [56]. Thus, the interaction between genes and environment affects the risk of disease in susceptible individuals and defines the phenotype.

The genetically-determined idiopathic generalized epilepsies account for about 40-60% of all epilepsies, most having complex inheritance patterns. These include infantile absence epilepsy, juvenile absence epilepsy, juvenile myoclonic epilepsy, and epilepsy with generalized tonic-clonic seizures only, the latter accounting for 25-31% of all epilepsies. The corresponding numbers for infantile absence epilepsy, juvenile absence epilepsy, and juvenile myoclonic epilepsy are 4-11%, 8-9%, and 3-7%, respectively. In families with multiple affected individuals the majority have idiopathic generalized epilepsies or febrile seizures, but the specific syndrome often differs from that of the proband. Within the same family, two individuals are more likely to have similar syndromes if they have a close genetic relationship. Studies in twins have shown that affected monozygotic pairs have the same syndrome, but dizygotic pairs, like ordinary siblings, tend to have different syndromes.

Acquired Causes of Epilepsy

Prenatal and Perinatal Risk Factors

Included are toxemia and eclampsia during pregnancy, low birth weight, asphyxia and other neonatal abnormalities, and other less defined conditions [50]. Although the role of these factors in the etiology of epilepsy seems established, most of the studies provide inconsistent findings and indicate, at best, a moderate association. These results may be explained by the use of differing definitions of pre- and perinatal factors, the study populations, the methods of ascertainment of the cause-effect relationship, and the sample size.

Cerebral Palsy and Mental Retardation

Mental retardation and cerebral palsy are markers of brain dysfunction, which explains their significant association with epilepsy. Epilepsy occurred in 34% of children with cerebral palsy and cerebral palsy was present in 19% of children developing epilepsy in the U.S. National Collaborative Perinatal Project, a study following newborns prospectively up to age 7 [57]. In this cohort, the risk of mental retardation was 5.5 times higher among children developing epilepsy following a febrile seizure than in children with a febrile seizure alone [58]. In a prospective cohort of children with mental retardation from Aberdeen, U.K. the risk of epilepsy was 15% by age 22 years (38% when cerebral palsy was concurrently present) [59]. Epilepsy is more common in individuals with severe or profound mental retardation compared to mild to moderate mental retardation [60].

CNS Infections

In industrialized countries, the lifetime cumulative risk of CNS infections for women and men is almost 1.5 and 2.5% respectively [61] and may be even higher in developing countries. CNS infections are a worldwide risk factor for epilepsy involving all ages. In the Rochester, Minnesota population, survivors of a CNS infection had a threefold increased risk of epilepsy [62]. The risk was highest during the first five years after infection and tends to decrease thereafter, but it remains elevated up to 15 years. The risk varied according to the infection type, being highest with encephalitis (16.2), followed by bacterial meningitis (4.2) and aseptic meningitis (2.3, non-significant). The presence of acute symptomatic seizures greatly influences the risk of subsequent unprovoked seizures and epilepsy. As encephalitis and bacterial meningitis are more prevalent in infants, children and young adults, most post-infectious epilepsies tend to occur in these individuals. Partial seizures are the commonest pattern. The most epileptogenic infectious agents include herpes simplex virus, cytomegalovirus, Epstein-Barr virus, HIV and arboviruses [63]. Toxoplasma can produce seizures in patients with AIDS. There is no clear epidemiological evidence for immunizations to be considered risk factors for epilepsy.

In developing countries, where infectious diseases are commoner than in industrialized countries, infectious causes of epilepsy have higher prevalence in rural compared to urban areas. In these countries, mostly in South America, neurocysticercosis is a major cause of epilepsy [64], followed by cerebral malaria, tuberculosis and toxoplasmosis.

Dementia

Dementing disorders have an overall prevalence of 6% in persons 65 years and older [65] and increase exponentially as a function of age [66]. Alzheimer's disease is the most common cause of dementia in industrialized countries, followed by vascular dementia. A relative risk of 10 (95% CI 4.3-19.7) was found for recurrent seizures in patients with autopsy-proven Alzheimer's disease residing in a nursing home [67]. Compared to non-demented individuals matched for age and sex, patients with Alzheimer's disease have a sixfold risk of unprovoked seizures [68] and people with other types of dementia have an eightfold risk. Seizures may occur at different times during the course of dementia. Partial seizures are the prevailing type in Alzheimer's disease and generalized seizures tend to predominate in other dementing disorders. Myoclonus is another common finding occurring as a late manifestation in about 10% of cases [67].

Cerebrovascular Disease

Stroke is one of the leading causes of disability in the industrialized countries, with an incidence of 100-300 per 100,000 per year [69], and is the most common cause of epilepsy in the elderly [13]. Silent stroke may be also the cause of some cryptogenic epilepsies in aged individuals [70]. The prevalence of seizures and epilepsy after stroke has been reported to vary widely depending on the study population and design and on the inclusion of acute symptomatic seizures and single unprovoked seizures. In patients with ischemic stroke, the cumulative incidence is 2-33% for acute symptomatic seizures, 3-67% for unprovoked seizures, and 2-4% for epilepsy [71]. Cortical site, severity and size of the lesion were independent predictors of acute symptomatic seizures in ischemic stroke. A history of stroke has been found to be associated with an increased lifetime occurrence of epilepsy in the Rotterdam study (OR 3.3; 95% CI 1.3-8.5) [72]. In the Oxfordshire Community Stroke Project, one or more seizures were present in the first 5 years in 11.5% of stroke survivors (95% CI 4.8-18.2) [73]. Compared to the general population, the risk of seizures was 35.2 in the first year and 19.0 in the second year. Acute symptomatic seizures (onset seizures) occurred in 2.1% of cases during the first 24 hours. In a U.S. population-based study of seizure disorders after cerebral infarction, acute symptomatic seizures occurred in 6% of patients [74]. In patients with acute symptomatic seizures, cerebral infarcts were more likely located in the anterior hemisphere (OR 4.0; 95% CI 1.2-13.7). The SIR for epilepsy was 5.9 (95% CI 3.5-9.4). The SIR for an unprovoked seizure was 6.4 (95% CI 4.2-9.3). About two thirds of patients with an unprovoked seizure developed epilepsy within 5 years. The risk was highest during the first year and tended to decrease during the ensuing three years. There was an inverse correlation between age and risk of seizures with a peak in patients aged less than 55 years. The risks were higher after recurrent stroke. Acute symptomatic seizures and recurrent strokes were the only independent predictors of unprovoked seizures and epilepsy.

Compared to ischemic stroke, hemorrhagic stroke (subarachnoid hemorrhage and, to a lesser extent, primary intracerebral hemorrhage) is followed by a higher risk of seizures [73]. The cumulative probability of seizures after a first stroke was about 6% at one year and rised to 11% at 5 years, with significant differences across stroke subtypes (cerebral infarction 4 and 10%; primary cerebral hemorrhage 20 and 26%; subarachnoid hemorrhage 22 and 34%). The risk of epilepsy among survivors of subarachnoid hemorrhage caused by ruptured cerebral aneurysm is highest in patients with acute symptomatic seizures (RR 7.0; 95% CI 2.3; 21.6) or severe neurological sequelae (RR 2.5; 95% CI 0.9-6.3) [75].

Among the other vascular determinants, a history of hypertension was associated with the occurrence of unprovoked seizures (OR 1.6; 95% CI 1.0-2.4) [76]. The risk of unprovoked seizures rises to 4.1 (95% CI 1.5-11.0) at the presence of stroke and hypertension.

Vascular Malformations

Arterovenous malformations cause epilepsy in 17 to 40% of cases. Risk factors include the size and depth of the malformation, age at diagnosis, presentation with hemorrhage, and surgical intervention [77].

Demyelinating Disorders

Individuals with multiple sclerosis appear to be at increased risk of seizures. In a small population-based study, patients with multiple sclerosis had a threefold increase (SIR 3.0; 95% CI 0.6-8.8) in the risk of epilepsy compared to the general population [78]. The cumulative risk of epilepsy after multiple sclerosis was 1.1% at 5 years, 1.8% by 10 years, and 3.1% by 15 years. The mean interval from the onset of multiple sclerosis and epilepsy was about seven years. In a Scandinavian study, a 10 times higher than expected risk of epilepsy was found in patients with multiple sclerosis [79].

Head Trauma

Traumatic brain injury is a fairly common clinical event. Population-based studies in the U.S. suggest an annual incidence of 180-250 per 100,000 [80]. Even higher incidence rates are expected in developing countries. The occurrence of epilepsy after head injury depends on the severity of the trauma [81]. The kinetic energy imparted to the brain tissue produces pressure waves, which disrupt tissue and lead to epileptogenic histopathological changes. In addition, iron liberated from hemoglobin generates free radicals that are considered epileptogenic as they disrupt cell membranes [82].

In the civilian population, traumatic events provoking concussion defined by either loss of consciousness or posttraumatic amnesia but no evidence of tissue disruption, usually are not followed by epilepsy [83]. In a large U.S. population-based study, five years after concussion, the cumulative probability of post-traumatic epilepsy was 0.7% after mild injuries, 1.2% after moderate injuries, and 10% after severe injuries. The risk was highest during the first year and diminished during the ensuing years. After 10 years, only severe injuries still exhibited an increased risk of seizures. The 30-year cumulative incidence of seizures was 2.1% for mild injuries, 4.2% for moderate injuries, and 16.7% for severe injuries. As shown by military series, the highest risk of post-traumatic epilepsy occurs following missile wounds with brain volume loss [81]. Unprovoked seizures were reported in up to 41% of the veterans involved in the Vietnam Head Injury Study [84]. Additional risk factors include focal neurological signs, hematoma, the presence of metal fragments, and the location of the lesion [85]. Significant risk factors for the occurrence of acute symptomatic seizures include acute intracerebral hematoma (especially subdural hematoma), younger age, increased severity of brain injury, and chronic alcoholism [81]. Significant risk factors for the occurrence of unprovoked seizures include acute symptomatic seizures, brain contusion, intracerebral hematoma (especially subdural hematoma), increased severity of brain injury, and age 65 years or older.

Brain Tumors

Although brain tumors account for a substantial proportion of elderly patients included in epilepsy referral series, there are no quantitative data from population-based studies [51]. Seizures are more often the presenting symptoms in low-grade tumors than in rapidly invasive tumors. The epileptogenicity of tumors is related to their location. In large neurosurgical series epilepsy was present in approximately 50% of patients with supratentorial tumors [86]. In a U.K. referral study 28% of patients undergoing surgery for malignant brain tumors had seizures prior to surgery [86]. In contrast, unsuspected brain tumors have been detected in patients undergoing surgery for drug resistant epilepsy [87,88]. Individuals with tumors in the centro-temporo-parietal region have the highest incidence of epilepsy. Epilepsy is more frequent in patients with superficial and cortical tumors than those with deep and noncortical tumors. Although most seizures caused by brain tumors are partial and associated with abnormal clinical and electrophysiological changes [88], sensitivity and specificity of seizure type, neurological examination and EEG are no higher in brain tumors than in other causes of epilepsy. Despite the potential carcinogenicity of antiepileptic drugs (AEDs) [89], at present there is no evidence of an increased risk of brain tumors attributable to antiepileptic medication [90].

Neurosurgery

Surgery on the brain *per se* may be a risk factor for seizures. Based on information derived from clinical series, in patients with no prior seizures, a 17% cumulative incidence of post-operative seizures was observed over 5 years [91]. The risk of unprovoked seizures is greater in patients with younger age, early postoperative seizures, severe neurological deficit, and repeated surgical interventions. It also varies with the underlying pathology.

Effect of Treatment in the Primary Prevention of Seizures and Epilepsy

Based on the results of randomized clinical trials and meta-analyses, AED prophylaxis seems to control provoked seizures in patients with head trauma [92] and craniotomy [93] but it does not seem to prevent the subsequent development of post-traumatic epilepsy and it can be poorly tolerated and even detrimental to cognitive and behavioral functions. The results of these studies are confirmed by a meta-analysis of published randomized clinical trials on seizure prevention [94]. In that review, several AEDs were found to be effective for the control of acute symptomatic seizures: phenobarbital for febrile seizures (relative risk, RR 0.51; 95% confidence interval, 95%CI 0.32-0.82) and cerebral malaria (RR 0.36; 95% CI

0.23-0.56); diazepam for contrast media (RR 0.10; 95% CI 0.01-0.79); phenytoin for craniotomy (RR 0.42; 95% CI 0.25-0.71) or head trauma (RR 0.33; 95% CI 0.19-0.59); carbamazepine for head trauma (RR 0.39; 95% CI 0.17-0.92); and lorazepam for alcohol-related seizures (RR 0.12; 95% CI 0.04-0.40). By contrast, no drug (among those examined) has been shown to be effective for the prevention of subsequent unprovoked seizures. In addition, phenobarbital compared to placebo or no treatment in patients with cerebral malaria was followed by an increased mortality (RR 2.0; 95% CI 1.2-3.3). There is no evidence that AED prophylaxis is effective in seizure prevention in patients with brain tumors [95]. Surprisingly, no studies are available which tested the efficacy of AEDs for the primary prevention of seizures and epilepsy in patients with CNS infections (other than cerebral malaria), stroke and other common neurological conditions.

Incidence and Common Causes of Acute Symptomatic Seizures

In a study done in the Rochester, Minnesota population, the age-adjusted incidence rate of acute symptomatic seizures was 40 per 100,000 person-years [34]. The rate was higher in men than in women (52 vs. 29) and in the first year of life. The rate decreased in childhood and early adulthood, with a nadir at 25-34 years and then it tended to increase, with a second peak at age 75 and older. The most common precipitating causes were, in decreasing order, head trauma, cerebrovascular disease (16% each), infection (15%), alcohol or drug withdrawal (14%), and metabolic disturbances (9%). The distribution of these causes varied with age (infectious and metabolic disorders being most common in children and cerebrovascular diseases in the elderly [34].

Although a wide range of substances, including drugs and illicit compounds, increase the risk of acute symptomatic and unprovoked seizures [20], the cause-effect relationship between drug exposure and seizure occurrence is virtually unknown. Seizures were recorded in less than 1% of 32,812 consecutive patients undergoing prospective monitoring of drug toxicity [96]. A variety of agents may be associated with an increase in seizure occurrence. These mostly include antidepressant drugs (maprotiline, bupropion, amitriptyline, imipramine, nortriptyline, desipramine, doxepin, protriptyline), antipsychotic drugs (clozapine and phenothiazines), analgesics and anesthetics (mostly meperidine and propofol), iodine contrast media, antibacterial agents (penicillins, isoniazid, mefloquine), antiviral agents (zidovuline), antineoplastic and immunosuppressant agents (cyclosporin, iphosphamide, chlorambucil, busulphan), respiratory agents (teophylline, phenylpropanolamine), alcohol, cocaine, amphetamines, phencyclidine, and withdrawal of meprobamate, barbiturates and benzodiazepines [20,97,98].

PROGNOSIS OF EPILEPSY AND EFFICACY OF TREATMENT

As epilepsy is a treatable clinical condition, the prognosis of the disease is generally intended as the probability of attaining seizure freedom after treatment start, during treatment, and after drug withdrawal. There are only few reports, mostly done in developing countries, on the prognosis of untreated epilepsy.

Methodological Issues

As with every chronic clinical condition, the prognosis of epilepsy reflects the characteristics of the population at risk, the choice of the inception point, the spectrum of the disease, the duration of follow-up, and the definition of the prognostic predictors, including treatment. More specifically, the design of an ideal study on the prognosis of epilepsy should have the following pre-requisites: 1. Well-defined criteria for the inclusion of patients; 2. Standard (homogeneous) definitions of the prognostic predictors and outcome measures; 3. Adequate duration of follow-up and proper statistical methods to adjust for drop-outs and limited periods of observation. Ideally, patients should be enrolled at a similar point in the course of the disease (for example, the time of diagnosis) and be representative of the underlying epileptic population. As in many studies on the prognosis of epilepsy, patients are referred from specialized services and a high proportion of them does not seek medical advise prior to having one or more seizure relapses, selection bias is most likely to affect the prognosis of epilepsy. Homogeneous (preferably standard) definitions for the commonest prognostic indicators are encouraged. For example, there are inconsistent reports that family history of epilepsy increases the risk of seizure recurrence. This may be explained by the fact that family history is difficult to ascertain or is unreliable. Details should be also given of *all* the putative prognostic predictors, to provide a comprehensive overview of the prognosis of the disease in question and give the best explanation of the results after controlling for the known prognostic indicators. Prolonged follow-up is required with an attempt to obtain information on the outcome in *all* patients. Outcome measures should be clearly defined and, if possible, reliable indicators should be used. Proper statistical methods (including multivariable analysis models) should be employed to assess the independent role of each prognostic predictor.

Most of the differences among studies on the prognosis of epilepsy can be explained by the different methodology, with particular reference to the study design (retrospective or prospective; community-based or clinic-based), the target population (children and/or adults), the timing of enrolment (interval between seizure and admission), the type of seizure (generalized tonic and/or clonic, partial and other), the length of follow-up, and the use of antiepileptic drugs.

Table 5. Population-based studies on the prognosis of epilepsy

Country	Population	% (duration) remission	Source	F-up (yrs)	Notes
USA	All ages	55% (10-yr) at 20 years	Records linkage	33	Included isolated seizures
UK	All ages	69% (5-yr) at 9 years	General practitioners	9	Included isolated seizures
Sweden	Adults	58% (5-yr) at 11 years	Multiple	10	Included isolated seizures
France	All ages	62% (complete) at 5 years	Neurologists	5	Included isolated seizures
Switzerland	All ages	68% (complete) at 10 years	Neurologists	10	Included isolated seizures
Ecuador	All ages	21% (complete) at 4 years	Hospitals	4	Only two or more seizures
Holland	Children	62% (2-yr) at 5 years	Hospitals	5	Included isolated seizures
Canada	Children	55% (complete) at 7 years (average)	Child neurologists	>20	Included isolated seizures
Finland	Children	68% (5-yr) at 30 years	Multiple	>30	Only two or more seizures

Source: [100]

Overall Prognosis of Epilepsy

The overall prognosis of epilepsy is favorable in the majority of patients. There are several pieces of evidence in support to this assumption. First of all, reports from several developing countries (where patients with epilepsy are largely untreated) give prevalence rates that tend to overlap to those of industrialized countries (see Tables 3 and 4). As in most developing countries the incidence of epilepsy is higher than that of industrialized countries (see Tables 1 and 2) and increased mortality may explain only in part the difference between incidence and prevalence, spontaneous remission is the most likely explanation in several cases. Second, contrary to the old reports [99], studies done in newly diagnosed patients have consistently shown that 55-69% of cases tend to achieve prolonged seizure remission (Table 5) [100].

Early Prognosis of Unprovoked Seizures and Epilepsy

Prognosis after the first Unprovoked Seizure

The risk of relapse of a first unprovoked seizure has been reported to range from 23 to 71% [101] and from 14 to 68% when actuarial methods are used. The rates at two and five years are 21-69% and 34-≥71%. Population-based studies [102,103] provided more homogeneous relapse rates at one (36-37%) and two years (43-45%). In a systematic review of 16 reports [3], the average recurrence risk was 51% (95% CI 49-53%). By two years, the recurrence risk was 36 and 47% in prospective and retrospective studies. After a first unprovoked seizure, the probability of a relapse decreases with time. About 50% of recurrences occur within 6 months of the initial seizure and 76-96% within 2 years [3].

Risk Factors for Relapse of a first Unprovoked Seizure

The two most consistent predictors of recurrence are a documented etiology of the seizure and an abnormal (epileptiform and/or slow) EEG pattern [3]. The pooled recurrence risk in patients with an idiopathic or cryptogenic first seizure is 32% (95% CI 28-35%) as compared to 57% (95% CI 51-63%) with a remote symptomatic seizure. The recurrence risk ranges from 27% (95% CI 21-33%) with a normal EEG tracing to 58% (95% CI 49-66%) with an EEG showing epileptiform abnormalities. Epileptiform abnormalities tend to be associated with a higher risk of seizure recurrence than nonepileptiform abnormalities. The pooled two-year recurrence risk is lowest for an idiopathic or cryptogenic first seizure with a normal EEG (24%; 95% CI 19-29%), intermediate for a remote symptomatic seizure (48%; 95% CI 34-62%) with normal EEG *or* an idiopathic/cryptogenic seizure with an abnormal EEG (48%; 95% CI 40-55%), and highest with a remote symptomatic seizure with an abnormal EEG (65%; 95% CI 55-76%). Seizures occurring during sleep tend to be associated with a higher risk of recurrence both in children and in adults [104-106]. Partial seizures, which are mostly associated with a documented brain injury, are also correlated with a higher risk of recurrent seizures, even after controlling for etiology and EEG abnormalities [102,107]. A positive correlation between seizure relapse and family history of seizures was confirmed in patients with idiopathic or cryptogenic first seizures in only one study [108]. History of prior acute symptomatic seizures has been occasionally found to increase the risk of relapse, while evidence is inconclusive or lacking for sex, age, and status epilepticus [3].

Treatment, Risk of Recurrence and Long-term Prognosis of a first Seizure

There are at least five published randomized studies assessing the effects of treatment of the first unprovoked seizure [109-115]. The results of these studies consistently show that treatment of the first seizure seems to reduce the risk of short-term relapse but is apparently ineffective on the chance of long-term seizure remission. In the Italian First Seizure Trial Group (FIRST) trial [114], the cumulative time-dependent risk of recurrence in treated patients was 17% at 12 months and 25% at 24 months (untreated, 41 and 51%), but the differences tended to disappear when the end-point was the chance of initiating a 2-yr remission. The cumulative probability of long-term remission tended to overlap in the two treatment groups by the second-year of follow-up up to 15 years after randomization [116]. In the MESS study, the largest of these trials [113], at the two-year follow-up, 32% with a single seizure had had a recurrence with immediate treatment as opposed to 39% of those with deferred treatment. The results of these trials tend to confirm several observational reports that the long-term prognosis of the first seizure is substantially unaffected by immediate treatment. However, the comparative effects of the treatment of the first seizure and the treatment of the relapse on the chance of long-term *permanent* remission (ie, off drugs) have not yet been assessed.

Prognosis of Untreated Epilepsy

With one exception [117], the prognosis of untreated epilepsy has been assessed only in developing countries where epilepsy is largely untreated (treatment gap ranging from 70 to 94%). In a population-based study done in Ecuador [18] the cumulative annual incidence rate was 190 per 100,000 and the prevalence rate of active epilepsy was 7 per 1,000, which implies a remission rate of at least 50%. Similar prevalence rates of active epilepsy (5 per 1,000) were found in Nigeria [39], where only 4% of patients were treated at the time of the survey, and in Ethiopia [118]. In a smaller study done in Malawi [119] duration of active epilepsy was similar to that of industrialized countries. All these findings lend support to the hypothesis that spontaneous remission of epilepsy is a common event.

Prognosis of newly Diagnosed Epilepsy

Treatment of epilepsy is generally started at the time of diagnosis, which is made when at least two unprovoked seizures have occurred. In fact, after a second unprovoked seizure, the risk of a third seizure has been estimated as 73% and the risk of a fourth seizure as 76% [120]. Population-based studies on the long-term prognosis of treated epilepsy report a 58-65% cumulative 5-year remission rate at 10 years [121,122] (see also Table 5). This number rises to about 70% by 20 years following seizure onset [121]. The 5-year remission rate at 10 years is 61% in adults [123] and the 3 to 5-year remission rate at 12-30 years in children is 74-78% [4]. In the Finnish cohort of patients with childhood-onset epilepsy, 64% of cases were in 5-year terminal remission off medications [124].

Principal Prognostic Predictors

Etiology of epilepsy is by far the strongest prognostic predictor for seizure recurrence. In general, idiopathic epilepsy has a better chance of seizure remission than symptomatic or cryptogenic epilepsy. In the population-based study from Rochester, Minnesota, symptomatic epilepsies have been found to achieve a significantly lower chance of 5-year remission compared to idiopathic epilepsies (30 vs. 42% at 15 years) [121]. Within this group, patients with neurological dysfunction present at birth had the lowest chance of remission (46% and 30% off-drugs at 20 years). Lower, albeit less significant, remission rates in patients with symptomatic epilepsies were also found in the UK, Sweden (adults) and Finland (children) [100]. A documented etiology of epilepsy was also found to be a significant predictor of seizure intractability in childhood-onset epilepsy [125]. In the Connecticut childhood-onset epilepsy, early predictors of intractability included etiology, high initial seizure frequency, and focal EEG slowing [5]. Other indicators of 5-year remission in the Rochester, Minnesota population, included absence of EEG epileptiform abnormalities and absence of generalized tonic-clonic seizures [126]. In the National General Practice Study of Epilepsy (NGPSE), the only independent predictor of 1-year and 2-year remission was the number of seizures experienced by the patient after the first seizure [12,122]. When other prognostic predictors are excluded, there is no evidence that age at onset of seizures affects seizure outcome. With the exception of rare inherited sex-linked disorders, sex has not been indicated as a significant prognostic predictor.

Prognosis of Epilepsy Syndromes

An epileptic syndrome is a symptom-complex that, taken together, is characterized by a fairly uniform clinical, laboratory, and instrumental manifestation. The features defining an epileptic syndrome include family history, age at onset, putative etiology, EEG and neuroimaging findings [29]. To some extent, the epileptic syndromes, particularly in children, have a differing outcome and response to treatment. As proposed by Sander [127], epilepsy syndromes can be classified into four different prognostic groups: 1. Excellent prognosis (about 20-30% of the total) with high probability of spontaneous remission; these include neonatal seizures, benign partial epilepsies, benign myoclonic epilepsy in infancy, and epilepsies provoked by specific modes of activation; 2. Good prognosis (about 30-40%) with easy pharmacological control and possibility of spontaneous remission; these include infantile absence epilepsy, epilepsies with GTC seizures secondary to specific conditions, and some partial epilepsies; 3. Uncertain prognosis (about 10-20%), which may respond to drugs, but tend to relapse after treatment withdrawal; these include juvenile myoclonic epilepsy, and most partial epilepsies (symptomatic or cryptogenic); 4. Bad prognosis (about 20%) in which seizures tend to recur despite intensive treatment; these include epilepsies associated with congenital neurological defects, progressive neurological disorders, and some symptomatic or cryptogenic partial epilepsies. The prognosis of specific epilepsy syndromes may be significantly different and reflects, at least in children, the inherent severity of epilepsy more than the quality of the therapeutic approach [128].

Antiepileptic Drugs and Seizure Outcome

AEDs are successful in suppressing seizures, but they do not seem to alter the long-term prognosis of epilepsy. In addition, in the FIRST and MESS studies [110,113] there was evidence of less than optimal outcome of seizures in about 20% of patients with newly diagnosed epilepsy.

There are virtually no reports on the comparative efficacy of old and new AEDs on the long-term outcome of epilepsy and there is no evidence to suggest that the newer medications are more efficacious [129]. Although individuals seem to present differing responses to the available drugs, all first-line AEDs seem to be equally effective at a community level. In a single-center hospital-based study of 470 patients diagnosed, treated and followed for a mean period of 5.6 years, 47% of cases became seizure-free with the first prescribed drug [130]. There was no significant difference in the proportion of cases with inadequate seizure control among those treated with carbamazepine, valproate, or lamotrigine. The majority of seizure-free patients required only a moderate daily AED dose.

Prognosis of Epilepsy after Treatment Withdrawal

A long-term population-based study has shown that 5-year terminal remission (i.e. off-drugs) of epilepsy is 61% [121]. Discontinuation of drug treatment is thus a valuable option in patients with epilepsy who are seizure-free for two years or longer. In a critical review of 28 studies accounting for 4615 cases (2802 children and 1020 adults), most of which with at least two years of seizure remission, the proportion of patients with relapses during or after treatment withdrawal ranged from 12 to 66% [131]. Using life-table analysis, the cumulative probability of remaining seizure-free in children was 66-96% at one year and 61-91% at two years. The corresponding values in adults were 39-74%, and 35-57% respectively. The relapse rate was highest in the first 12 months (especially in the first 6 months) and tended to decrease thereafter. In a meta-analysis of 25 studies, the pooled relapse risk was 25% (95% CI, 21-30%) at one year and 29% (95% CI, 24-34%) at two years [132].

In the only randomized trial on the effects of AED withdrawal on seizure relapse [133], patients randomized to continued treatment showed a 22% relapse at two years, while patients randomized to slow drug withdrawal had 41% relapse. This differential risk of relapse was maximal between 1 and 2 years and declined thereafter. After 2 years, the risk of subsequent relapse was the same for both treatment groups. The risk of recurrence was also similar in patients who relapsed after withdrawal of AEDs and in those who relapsed while remaining on treatment [134].

Factors Predicting Seizure Relapse after Treatment Withdrawal

A number of factors have been associated with favourable or unfavourable seizure outcome after treatment discontinuation. Factors consistently indicating a higher-than-average risk of seizure relapse included adolescent-onset epilepsy, partial seizures, presence of an underlying neurological condition, and abnormal EEG findings (children). Factors associated with a lower-than-average risk were childhood epilepsy, idiopathic generalized epilepsy, and – for children – normal EEG. Selected epilepsy syndromes (eg, benign epilepsy with centro-temporal spikes and juvenile myoclonic epilepsy) may be associated with significantly different outcomes after treatment withdrawal [131]. In the MRC AED withdrawal study, independent predictors of relapse included history of partial seizures (primarily or secondarily), generalized tonic-clonic seizures, or myoclonic seizures, use of more than one AED, seizures after treatment start, and a shorter seizure-free period at randomization [133]. In a meta-analysis of 25 studies, adolescent age at onset of seizures had a 1.34 risk of relapse (95% CI 1.00-1.81) compared to adult age at onset [132]. Patients with remote symptomatic seizures had a 1.55 risk of relapse (95% CI 1.21-1.98). An abnormal EEG prior to drug discontinuation was associated with a 1.45 risk of relapse (95% CI 1.18-1.79). In the same review, prognosis following drug withdrawal was similar whether a 2-year or a 4-year seizure-free interval was considered. As well, a randomized trial comparing a 6-week taper with a 9-month taper after 2-year seizure remission in patients with pediatric epilepsy showed no difference in recurrence risk at 2 years [135].

Psychosocial Outcome

The prevalence of unemployed individuals in people with epilepsy is consistently higher than that of the general population, with rates ranging from 24 to 36% [136]. In a population-based study of childhood-onset epilepsy, independent predictors of low socio-economic status included poor fine-motor performance (OR 14.8), poor short-term outcome after treatment (OR 9.8), and presence of psychoneurotic symptoms (OR 3.2) [137]. In that study, 15% required little assistance in daily living activities and about 50% were socially disabled, with up to 30% having moderate to severe handicap.

School achievement in children and adolescents with epilepsy is lower than that of the general population. This may be present even when epilepsy is not associated to other neurological sources of impairment [123]. The lower intellectual level is the most likely explanation for the school under-achievement. Learning disabilities and cognitive dysfunction are commonly reported in children with epilepsy [138]. Factors associated with school under-achievement include epilepsy, AEDs and psychosocial factors. The strongest independent predictors of school under-achievement include early onset of seizures and cumulative number of seizures [139]. Alteration of cognition might reflect a chronic adverse effect of AEDs but the negative effects of the drugs are only one of several factors that may influence cognition. In addition, subjective complaints about cognitive deficits (e.g. memory problems or attention) may also reflect other aspects of adverse effects than those concerning specific cognitive functions (e.g. mood and anxiety) [140]. Although intuitive, the correlation between school under-achievement and psychosocial factors is not supported by studies with robust methodological implant.

Lower rates of marriage and fertility (even after adjustment for marriage) have been also reported in people with epilepsy when compared to the general population [141]. Several socio-cultural limitations may explain the lower likelihood of marriage at the presence of epilepsy. Although adverse treatment effects may be implicated, the cause of decreased fertility remains unclear.

In the absence of seizures (with or without treatment), the risk of accidents and injuries is clearly decreased in people with epilepsy and tends to be close to that of the general population [142,143]. The proportion of road accidents attributable to active epileptic seizures is extremely low, ranging from 0.02% to 0.2% [144,145].

In a multicenter cohort study done in six western European countries (Italy, Germany, England, Holland, Spain, and Portugal) and three eastern European countries (Russia, Estonia, and Slovenia), 951 children and adults with early idiopathic, cryptogenic or remote symptomatic epilepsy and 909 matched controls were followed prospectively for 17,484 and 17,206 person-months [143,146]. Two hundred and 70 accidents were reported by 199 patients (21%) compared to 149 accidents reported by 124 controls (13%). About one fourth of accidents in patients with epilepsy were seizure-related. The most common accidents in patients with epilepsy were, in decreasing order, contusions, wounds, fractures, abrasions, and brain concussions. Contusions, followed by wounds and sprains or strains predominated in the controls. About one-third of brain concussions, contusions and fractures were seizure-related compared to one-fifth of burns and to less than one-sixth of wounds. Most accidents occurred at home, followed by traffic, sports and other leisure activities, work, and school. About one half of domestic accidents were seizure-related. About one third of school accidents and one fourth of traffic accidents were seizure-related. Except for brain concussion, accidents occurring in patients with epilepsy and non-epileptic controls were mostly trivial.

MORTALITY OF EPILEPSY

Methodological Issues

The epidemiological approach to epilepsy mortality depends on the accuracy of the information on the causes of death and the survey methods [147]. For a more precise calculation of the mortality attributable to epilepsy, studies should be population-based and large and involve incident patients. Significant differences in mortality rates are expected when comparing incidence-based and prevalence-based studies. Patients with epilepsy should be assessed separately from patients with a first unprovoked seizure. As well, children and adults and persons with acute symptomatic seizures and with unprovoked seizures should be examined separately. The mortality in the general population should be made available for comparison. In that case, mortality can be expressed as the standardized mortality ratio (SMR), which is the ratio between the deaths observed in the epileptic cohort and the deaths expected in the reference population with a similar age distribution. Another measure is the proportionate mortality ratio (PMR), which is the percentage of deaths in patients with epilepsy attributed to a given cause. However, in the absence of the distribution of the causes of death in a referent non-epileptic population, PMR in epilepsy is difficult to assess from most of the available reports. A third measure is the case-fatality ratio (CFR), which is the number of deaths divided by the number of patients with epilepsy in the study population. The CFR is affected by the distribution of prognostic factors and by differences in medical care. The source of deaths (death certificates, registries, etc.) may also explain the variability of the available reports.

Mortality Rate of Epilepsy

The mortality rate of epilepsy ranges from 1 to 8 per 100,000 population per year, but international vital statistics give annual mortality rates of 1-2 per 100,000 [148]. In a population-based cohort of patients with childhood-onset epilepsy followed up to 35 years, a mortality rate of 6.23 per 1,000 person-years was reported [124]. In this cohort, the probability of survival at 10, 20 and 40 years after seizure onset was 0.94 (95% CI 0.91-0.97), 0.88 (95% CI 0.84-0.92), and 0.75 (95% CI 0.74-0.86).

Overall Mortality in Epilepsy

Based on a meta-analysis of studies investigating mortality in the past 100 years, the SMR for epilepsy was found to range from 1.3 to 9.3 (0.3-3.1 in community-based studies and 1.9-5.1 in institutionalized populations) [149]. In prospective and retrospective incidence cohorts, the SMR for epilepsy ranges from 1.6 to 5.3 in children and adults [148] (Table 6) [151-157]. These rates were not significantly different from those of selected populations followed for differing periods. The higher SMRs reported by the French and Swiss studies may be partly explained by the inclusion of provoked seizures.

Table 6. Community-based studies of mortality in epilepsy

Country	Population	SMR	95% CI	Design and methods	Person-years	Reference, year
Canada	Children	8.8	4.1-13.4	Retrospective incident cohort	NA	Camfield et al., 2002[151]
Finland	Children	6.2 per1000 p-y (*)	5.7-6.7	Prospective incident cohort	NA	Sillanpaa et al., 1998 [124]
France	Mixed	4.1	2.5-6.2	Prospective incident cohort	804	Loiseau et al., 1999[152]
Iceland	Mixed ?	1.6	1.2-2.2	Prospective incident cohort	6,308	Olafsson et al., 1998[153]
Poland	Mixed	1.8	NA	Retrospective prevalent cohort	~20,000	Zielinski, 1974[154]
Sweden	Adults	2.5	1.6-3.8	Prospective incident cohort	850	Lindsten et al., 2000[155]
U.K.	Mixed	2.1	1.8-2.4	Prospective incident cohort	11,400	Lhathoo et al., 2001[156]
U.S.	Mixed	2.3	1.9-2.6	Retrospective incident cohort	8,233	Hauser et al., 1980[157]

(*) Mortality rate; p-y = person-years

NA = not available

Mortality of Epilepsy in Selected Clinical Conditions

Mortality after a First Seizure

There are few reports on the mortality in patients with a first epileptic seizure. In a population-based study reporting one-year mortality in a sample of children and adults with a first epileptic seizure in Gironde, France, the SMR was 9.3 (95% CI 7.9-10.9) [152]. The SMR was 4.1 (95% CI 2.5-6.2) for unprovoked seizures, 6.5 (95% CI 3.8-10.5) for remote symptomatic seizures, 10.1 (95% CI 8.1-12.4) for acute symptomatic seizures, and 19.8 (95% CI 14.0-27.3) for seizures secondary to progressive neurological conditions. There were no deaths in patients with idiopathic seizures and mortality was not increased in patients with cryptogenic seizures (SMR 1.6; 95% CI 0.4-4.1). In an adult Swedish population-based cohort, the SMR in patients with a newly diagnosed unprovoked seizure was 2.5 (95% CI 1.2-3.2), with a peak (SMR 7.3; 95% CI 4.4-12.1) during the first two years after diagnosis and a second peak (SMR 5.4; 95% CI 2.7-11.2) at years 9-11 [155]. These figures were comparable with those from other population-based studies, reporting SMRs ranging from 2.3 to 3.3 [157,158]. Mortality risk was higher with remote symptomatic etiology and age younger than 60.

In a retrospective U.S population-based cohort study, the 30-day mortality of a first episode of status epilepticus was 19% [159], 89% of deaths occurring with nonfebrile acute symptomatic seizures. In the same population, 40% of patients surviving the first 30 days after the seizure died within the ensuing 10 years [160]. The SMR was 2.8 (95% CI 2.1-3.5) and was significantly elevated in symptomatic status epilepticus. By contrast, patients with idiopathic/cryptogenic status epilepticus had no increased risk of death compared to the general population. Age, duration of status epilepticus, seizure type, and etiology were independent predictors of mortality.

Seizure etiology is the single most important risk factor for the increased mortality in patients with a first epileptic seizure. The highest mortality risk in the youngest age groups can be interpreted in part in the light of the underlying epileptogenic conditions and of the lower number of competing causes of death.

Predictors of Mortality in Epilepsy

Etiology of epilepsy is one of the strongest predictors of mortality in epilepsy. Patients with symptomatic epilepsy have a two- to sixfold mortality risk than the general population. Patients with a CNS lesion presumed to be present at birth present the highest mortality, with an SMR between 7 and 50 [4]. Severe functional neurological deficit was the only independent determinant of mortality in children in the Nova Scotia population-based cohort study [151]. However, remote symptomatic seizures and refractory epilepsy mostly account for the increased mortality in childhood-onset epilepsy [128]. Mortality is greater in men than in women, as shown in the majority of the population-based studies. Most studies have also detected an inverse correlation between SMR and age. In neurologically normal children with idiopathic or cryptogenic epilepsy in remission, mortality does not appear to be substantially higher than that of the general population. The highest mortality in children may be thus explained by the rate expected in the general population, which is lowest in children, and by the higher proportion of neurodeficits in this age group. In the Finnish cohort of patients with childhood epilepsy followed into adulthood [124], patients not in remission had a 9.3 RR of death (95% CI 3.8-22.7) compared with patients in 5-year remission. There is also an inverse correlation between SMR and duration of epilepsy during the first 10 to 14 years of disease. Generalized tonic-clonic seizures have been associated with an increased mortality in several studies from the U.S. and Europe. Myoclonic seizures, but not absence seizures, have been associated with an increased SMR in the US (4.1) [157]. By contrast, data regarding the mortality in patients with partial seizures are inconsistent. Status epilepticus is associated with a significant mortality. In prospective population-based studies, the CFR reached 22% [161] and 39% [162]. Although the idiosyncratic reactions and the oncogenic potential of AEDs is well-known, drug-related deaths cannot be estimated, as comparative estimates of the rate of occurrence of such deaths per treatment-years are not available.

Mortality in Epilepsy Associated to Selected Clinical Conditions

Differing mortality rates have been found with different epileptogenic conditions. Accident-related deaths range between 1 and 6% of all deaths, with SMR ranging between 2.4 and 5.6 [163]. Patients with epilepsy are reported to be at higher risk of suicide than the general population. However, the PMRs range from 0 to 20% and the SMRs from 1 and 5.8. The wide difference in rates may be mostly explained by the small size of the studied populations and the different methods of analysis. Patients with severe epilepsy have a fivefold and patients with temporal lobe epilepsy a 25-fold increased risk of suicide [164]. Suicide rates may be even higher (SMR 87.5; 95% CI 35-180) in patients with temporal lobe epilepsy undergoing surgical treatment [165]. Antipsychotic drug intake was associated with a 4-fold increase in the risk of suicide in a Swedish case-control study [166], after adjusting for psychiatric illness and alcohol abuse. Psychiatric comorbidity, psychosocial stressors and iatrogenic factors may thus explain the increased risk of suicide in patients with epilepsy.

While seizure-related mortality is rare in new onset epilepsy, in patients with chronic epilepsy the majority of deaths appear to be seizure-related [167]. In these populations, sudden unexpected death (SUDEP) accounts for 24-67% of all deaths [168]. SUDEP is defined as a non-traumatic, unwitnessed death occurring in a previously healthy patient with epilepsy in whom no cause of death is detected even after post-mortem examination. The incidence of SUDEP ranges from 1 per 1,000 in prevalence studies [169] to 3.5 per 1,000 in incidence studies [170]. The patient at risk for SUDEP is a young or middle-aged person with chronic refractory epilepsy, generalized tonic-clonic seizures, and a complicated and unstable treatment [150]. SUDEP is rare in community-based series of childhood epilepsy [171,172]. In most cases, SUDEP is triggered by a seizure, and seizure-induced cardio-respiratory alterations are a plausible hypothesis [173].

In patients undergoing epilepsy surgery, the SMR was found to range from from 4.5 to 32 [150]. In a population-based study comparing SMR and SUDEP in surgical patients, the SMR (all causes) was 4.9 (95% CI 2.7-8.3) vs. 7.9 (95% CI 2.6-18.4) in non-surgical patients and the incidence of SUDEP was 2.5 vs. 6.3 per 1,000 [174].

There is some indication that carbamazepine could increase the risk of SUDEP by causing arrhythmia or by altering the cardiac autonomic function. However, this evidence is tenuous and most studies have found no association between carbamazepine or any other AED and SUDEP [175].

Mortality in Developing Countries

In a prospective hospital-based incidence cohort in Ecuador, the SMR was 6.3 [176]. In this study, definite or probable SUDEP were the leading causes. There is common belief that mortality in patients with epilepsy is significantly higher in developing countries than in industrialized countries. However, this assumption cannot be confirmed by sound epidemiological data. In follow-up studies of cohorts of patients with epilepsy from Tanzania, Kenya, Ethiopia and Mali, several deaths were reported, mostly seizure-related [177-180]. However, most of these patients were untreated. Mortality was significantly lower in communities of patients with treated epilepsy in Kenya and Ecuador [181,182].

CONCLUSIONS

Although seizures are the cardinal manifestations of epilepsy, not all individuals with seizures have epilepsy. Seizures may occur in fact in the context of an acute brain injury and are risk factors for epilepsy, but they are not intended as epilepsy *per se*. In addition, about 50% of cases have isolated unprovoked seizures during their life. For these reasons, epilepsy is defined as a clinical condition characterized by repeated unprovoked seizures. Epilepsy is a heterogeneous symptom complex with differing etiology and variable distribution according to sex, age, time and geographic area. The changing temporal patterns of the disease (which has been shown to decrease with time in children and increase in adults) may be explained at least in part by better medical care (at least in industrialized countries) and a better case ascertainment. The frequency of the disease is influenced by a complex interaction between genetic and environmental factors. The exposure to different etiological agents and the lower socio-economic background may explain the higher incidence, prevalence and mortality of the disease in developing countries. Although the prognosis of epilepsy is largely influenced by the syndromic patterns, community surveys and prospective studies on referral patients done in the last 30 years have reported that up to 90% of newly diagnosed patients with epilepsy tend to achieve prolonged seizure remission, and about 40–60% of these enter remission as soon as treatment is initiated. This reflects a radical change in the views on the prognosis of epilepsy and enforces the concept of a permanent remission of the disease. Despite a fairly low mortality rate, patients with epilepsy are at higher risk of death than the general population. The higher mortality among the youngest individuals may be explained by the low expected mortality and the low risk of competing causes in these patients.

REFERENCES

[1] Goodin, D.S., Aminoff, M.J. (1984) 'Does the interictal EEG have a role in the diagnosis of epilepsy?' *Lancet 1*, 837-838.

[2] Commission on Epidemiology and Prognosis, International League Against Epilepsy. (1993) 'Guidelines for epidemiologic studies on epilepsy' *Epilepsia 34*, 592-596.

[3] Berg, A.T., Shinnar, S. (1991) 'The risk of seizure recurrence following a first unprovoked seizure: a quantitative review' *Neurology 41*, 965-972.

[4] Forsgren, L. (2004) 'Epidemiology and prognosis of epilepsy and its treatment' In: Shorvon, S., Perucca, E., Fish D., Dodson, E. (eds.) *The Treatment of Epilepsy* (2nd edition). Malden, MA: Blackwell Science. 21-42.

[5] Berg, A.T., Shinnar, S., Levy, S.R., et al (2001) 'Early development of intractable epilepsy in children: a prospective study' *Neurology 56*, 1445-1452.

[6] Stroup, D.F., Berlin J.A., Morton, S.C., et al. (2000) 'Meta-analysis of observational studies in epidemiology: a proposal for reporting. Meta-analysis Of Observational Studies in Epidemiology (MOOSE) group' *Journal of the American Medical Association 283*, 2008-2012.

[7] Forsgren, L., Beghi, E., Oun, A., Sillanpaa, M. (2005) 'The epidemiology of epilepsy in Europe – a systematic review' *European Journal of Neurology 12*, 245-253.

[8] Sander, J., Hart, Y., Johnson, A., Shorvon, S. (1990) 'National general practice study of epilepsy: newly diagnosed epileptic seizures in a general population' *Lancet 336*, 1257-1271.

[9] Preux, P.-M., Druet-Cabanac, M. (2005) 'Epidemiology and aetiology of epilepsy in sub-Saharan Africa' *Lancet Neurology 4*, 21-31.

[10] Kotsopoulos, I.A.W., van Merode, T., Kessels, F.G.H., et al. (2002) 'Systematic review and meta-analysis of incidence studies of epilepsy and unprovoked seizures' *Epilepsia 43*, 1402-1409.

[11] Loiseau, J., Loiseau, P., Guyot, M., et al. (1990). 'Survey of seizure disorders in the French southwest. I. Incidence of epileptic syndromes' *Epilepsia 31*, 391-396.

[12] MacDonald, B.K., Johnson, A.L., Goodridge, D.M., et al. (2000) 'Factors predicting prognosis of epilepsy after presentation with seizures' *Annals of Neurology 48*, 833-841.

[13] Hauser, W.A., Annegers, J.F., Kurland, L.T. (1993) 'The incidence of epilepsy and unprovoked seizures in Rochester, Minnesota, 1935-1984' *Epilepsia 34*, 453-468.

[14] Debouverie, M., Kaboré, J., Dumas, M., et al. (1993) 'Epidémiologie de l'epilepsie au Burkina-Faso' In : Dumas, M., Giordano, C., Gentilini, M., Chieze, F. (eds.) *Neurologie Tropicale.* Paris; John Libbey Eurotext. 57-61.

[15] Grunitzky, E.K., Dumas, M., Mbella, E.M., et al. (1991) 'Les épilepsies au Togo' *Epilepsies 3*, 295-303.

[16] Kaiser, C., Asaba, G., Leichsenring, M., Kabagambe, G. (1998) 'High incidence of epilepsy related to onchocerciasis in West Uganda' *Epilepsy Research 30*, 247-251.

[17] Cockerell, O.C., Eckle, I., Goodridge, D.M., et al. (1995) 'Epilepsy in a population of 6000 re-examined: secular trends in first attendance rates, prevalence, and prognosis' *Journal of Neurology Neurosurgery and Psychiatry 58*, 570-576.

[18] Placencia, M., Shorvon, S.D., Paredes, V., et al. (1992) 'Epileptic seizures in an Andean region of Ecuador. Incidence and prevalence and regional variation' *Brain 115*, 771-782.

[19] Rwiza, H.T., Kilonzo, G.P., Haule, J., et al. (1992) 'Prevalence and incidence of epilepsy in Ulanga, a rural Tanzanian district: a community-based study' *Epilepsia 33*, 1051-1056.

[20] Beghi, E. (2004) 'Aetiology of epilepsy' In: Shorvon, S.D., Perucca, E., Fish D., Dodson, E. (Eds) *The Treatment of Epilepsy* (2nd edition). Malden, MA: Blackwell Science. 50-63.

[21] Granieri, E., Rosati, G., Tola, R., et al. (1983) 'A descriptive study of epilepsy in the district of Copparo, Italy, 1964-1978' *Epilepsia 24*, 502-514.

[22] Blom, S., Heijbel, J., Bergfors, P.G. (1978) Incidence of epilepsy in children: a follow-up study three years after the first seizure' *Epilepsia 19*, 343-350.

[23] Sidenvall, R., Forsgren, L., Blomquist H.K., Heijbel J. (1993) 'A community-based prospective incidence study of epileptic seizures in children' *Acta Paediatrica 82*, 60-65.

[24] Commission on Classification and Terminology of the International League Against Epilepsy (1981) 'Proposal for revised clinical and electroencephalographic classification of epileptic seizures' *Epilepsia 22*, 489-501.

[25] Chin, R.F., Neville, B.G., Scott, R.C. (2004) 'A systematic review of the epidemiology of status epilepticus' *European Journal of Neurology 11*, 800-810.

[26] Tsuboi, T. (1988). 'Prevalence and incidence of epilepsy in Tokyo' *Epilepsia 29*, 103-110.

[27] Shamansky, S.L., Glaser, G.H. (1979). 'Socioeconomic characteristics of childhood seizure disorders in the New Haven area: an epidemiologic study' *Epilepsia 20*, 457-474.

[28] Zarrelli, M.M., Beghi, E., Rocca, W.A., Hauser, W.A. (1999) 'Incidence of epileptic syndromes in Rochester, Minnesota: 1980-1984' *Epilepsia 40*, 1708-1714.

[29] Commission on Classification and Terminology of the International League Against Epilepsy. (1989) 'Proposal for revised classification of epilepsies and epileptic syndromes' *Epilepsia 30*, 389-399.

[30] Berg, A.T., Shinnar, S., Levy, S.R., Testa, F.M. (1999) 'Newly diagnosed epilepsy in children: presentation at diagnosis' *Epilepsia 40*, 445-452.

[31] Forsgren, L., Bucht, G., Eriksson, S., Bergmark, L. (1996) 'Incidence and clinical characterization of unprovoked seizures in adults: a prospective population-based study' *Epilepsia 37*, 224-229.

[32] Hauser, W.A. (1997) 'Incidence and prevalence' In: Engel Jr, J., Pedley, T.A. (eds.) *Epilepsy: A Comprehensive Textbook*. Philadelphia: Lippincott-Raven. 47-57.

[33] Olsson, I. (1988) 'Epidemiology of absence epilepsy. I. Concept and incidence' *Acta Paediatrica Scandinavica 77*, 860-866.

[34] Annegers, J.F., Hauser, W.A., Lee, J.R., et al. (1995). 'Incidence of acute symptomatic seizures in Rochester, Minnesota: 1935-1984' *Epilepsia 36*, 327-333.

[35] Hauser, W.A., Annegers, J.F., Rocca, W.A.(1996) 'Descriptive epidemiology of epilepsy; contributions of population-based studies from Rochester, Minnesota' *Mayo Clinic Proceedings 71*, 576-586.

[36] Beilmann, A., Napa, A., Soot, A., et al. (1999) 'Prevalence of childhood epilepsy in Estonia' *Epilepsia 40*, 1011-1019.

[37] Endziniene, M., Pauza, V., Miseviciene, I. (1997) Prevalence of childhood epilepsy in Kaunas, Lithuania' *Brain Development 19*, 379-387.

[38] Sidenvall, R., Forsgren, L., Heijbel, J. (1996) 'Prevalence and characteristics of epilepsy in children in Northern Sweden' *Seizure 5*, 139-146.

[39] Osuntokun, B.O., Adeuja, A.O.G., Nottidge, V.A., et al. (1987) 'Prevalence of the epilepsies in Nigerian Africans: a community-based study' *Epilepsia 28*, 272-279.

[40] Aziz, H., Ali, S.M., Frances, P., et al. (1994). 'Epilepsy in Pakistan: a population-based epidemiologic study' *Epilepsia 35*, 950-958.

[41] Bharucha, N.E., Shorvon, S.D. (1997) 'Epidemiology in developing countries' In: Engel Jr, J., Pedley, T.A. (eds.) *Epilepsy: A Comprehensive Textbook*. Philadelphia: Lippincott-Raven. 105-118.

[42] Eriksson, K,J., Koivikko, M.J. (1997) 'Prevalence, classification, and severity of epilepsy and epileptic syndromes in children' *Epilepsia 38*, 1275-1282.

[43] Waaler, P.E., Blom, B.H., Skeidsvoll, H., Mykletun, A. (2000) 'Prevalence, classification, and severity of epilepsy in children in western Norway' *Epilepsia 41*, 802-810.

[44] Morgan, C.L., Ahmed, Z., Kerr, M.P. (2000) 'Social deprivation and prevalence of epilepsy and associated health usage' *Journal of Neurology Neurosurgery and Psychiatry 69*, 13-17.

[45] Aziz, H., Guvener, A., Akhtar, S.W., Hasan, K.Z. (1997) 'Comparative epidemiology of epilepsy in Pakistan and Turkey: population-based studies using identical protocols' *Epilepsia 38*, 716-722.

[46] Placencia, M., Sander, J.W., Roman, M., et al. (1994) 'The characteristics of epilepsy in a largely untreated population in rural Ecuador' *Journal of Neurology Neurosurgery and Psychiatry 57*, 320-325.

[47] Sridharan, R, Murthy, B.N. (1999) 'Prevalence and pattern of epilepsy in India' *Epilepsia 40*, 631-636.

[48] Schlesselman, J.J. (1982) 'Case-control studies. Design, conduct, analysis' New York, Oxford: Oxford University Press.

[49] Shorvon, S.D., Farmer, P.J. (1988) 'Epilepsy in developing countries: a review of epidemiological, sociocultural and treatment aspects' *Epilepsia 29 (suppl 1)*, S36-S54.

[50] Hauser, W.A., Hesdorffer, D.C. (eds.) (1990) 'Genetics' In: *Epilepsy: Frequency, Causes and Consequences*. New York: Demos Publications. 93-118.

[51] Hauser, W.A. (1994) 'Epidemiology of epilepsy' In: Gorelick, P.B., Alter, M. (eds.) *Handbook of Neuroepidemiology*. New York: Marcel Dekker. 315-353.

[52] Ottman, R., Annegers, J.F., Hauser, W.A., et al. (1988) 'Higher risk of seizures in offspring of mothers than of fathers with epilepsy' *American Journal of Human Genetics 43*, 257-264.

[53] Privitera, M.D. (editor). (2001) 'Epilepsy Genetics: The 21st Century' *Epilepsia 42* (suppl. 5), 1.

[54] Johnson, M.R., Sander, J.W.A.S. (2001) 'The clinical impact of epilepsy genetics' *Journal of Neurology Neurosurgery and Psychiatry 70*, 428-430.

[55] Serratosa, J.M. (1999) 'Idiopathic epilepsies with a complex mode of inheritance' *Epilepsia 40 (Suppl 3)*, 12-16.

[56] Berkovic, S.F., Andermann, F., Andermann, E., Gloor, P. (1987) 'Concepts of absence epilepsies: discrete syndromes or biological continuum?' *Neurology 37*, 993-1000.

[57] Nelson, K.B., Ellenberg, J.H. (1986) 'Antecedents of seizure disorders in early childhood' *American Journal of Diseases in Childhood 140*, 1053-1061.

[58] Nelson, K.B., Ellenberg, J.H. (1978) 'Prognosis in children with febrile seizures' *Pediatrics 61*, 720-727.

[59] Goulden, K.J., Shinnar, S., Koller, H., et al. (1991) 'Epilepsy in children with mental retardation: a cohort study' *Epilepsia 32*, 690-697.

[60] Forsgren, L., Edvinsson, S.O., Blomquist, H.K., et al. (1990) 'Epilepsy in a population of mentally retarded children and adults' *Epilepsy Research 6*, 234-248.

[61] Nicolosi, A., Hauser, W.A., Beghi, E, Kurland, L.T. (1986) 'Epidemiology of central nervous system infections in Olmsted County, Minnesota, 1950-1981' *Journal of Infectious Diseases 154*, 399-408.

[62] Annegers, J.F., Hauser, W.A., Beghi, E., et al. (1988) 'The risk of unprovoked seizures after encephalitis and meningitis' *Neurology 38*, 1407-1410.

[63] Labar, D.R., Harden, C. (1997) 'Infection and inflammatory diseases' In: Engel Jr, J., Pedley, T.A. (eds.) *Epilepsy: A Comprehensive Textbook*. Philadelphia: Lippincott-Raven. 2587-2596.

[64] Carpio, A., Escobar, A., Hauser, W.A. (1998) 'Cysticercosis and epilepsy: a critical review' *Epilepsia 39*, 1025-1040.

[65] Lobo, A., Launer, L.J., Fratiglioni, L., et al. (2000) 'Prevalence of dementia and major subtypes in Europe: a collaborative study of population-based cohorts. Neurologic Diseases in the Elderly Research Group' *Neurology 54 (Suppl 5)*, S4-S9.

[66] Fratiglioni, L., Launer, L.J., Andersen, K., et al. (2000) 'Incidence of dementia and major subtypes in Europe: a collaborative study of population-based cohorts' *Neurology 54 (Suppl 5)*, S10-S15.

[67] Hauser, W.A., Morris, M.L., Heston, L.L., Anderson, V.E. (1986) 'Seizures and myoclonus in patients with Alzheimer's disease' *Neurology 36*, 1226-1230.

[68] Hesdorffer, D.C., Hauser, W.A., Annegers, J.F., et al. (1996) 'Dementia and adult-onset unprovoked seizures' *Neurology 46*, 727-730.

[69] Feigin, V.L., Lawes, C.M.M., Bennett, D.A., Anderson, C.S. (2003) 'Stroke epidemiology: a review of population-based studies of incidence, prevalence, and case-fatality in the late 20th century' *Lancet Neurology 2*, 43-53.

[70] Roberts, R.C., Shorvon, S.D., Cox, T.C., Gilliatt, R.W. (1988) 'Clinically unsuspected cerebral infarction revealed by computed tomography scanning in late onset epilepsy' *Epilepsia 29*, 190-194.

[71] Camilo, O., Goldstein, L.B. (2004) 'Seizures and epilepsy after ischemic stroke' *Stroke 35*, 1769-1775.

[72] Li, X., Breteler, M.M., de Bruyne, M.C., et al. (1997) 'Vascular determinants of epilepsy: the Rotterdam study' *Epilepsia 38*, 1216-1220.

[73] Burn, J., Dennis, M., Bamford, J., et al. (1997) 'Epileptic seizures after a first stroke: the Oxfordshire community stroke project' *British Medical Journal 315*, 1582-1587.

[74] So, E.L., Annegers, J.F., Hauser, W.A., et al. (1996) 'Population-based study of seizure disorders after cerebral infarction' *Neurology 46*, 350-355.

[75] Olafsson, E., Gudmundsson, G., Hauser, W.A. (2000) 'Risk of epilepsy in long-term survivors of surgery for aneurysmal subarachnoid hemorrhage: a population-based study in Iceland' *Epilepsia 41*, 1201-1205.

[76] Ng, S.K., Hauser, W.A., Brust, J.C., Susser, M. (1993) 'Hypertension and the risk of new-onset unprovoked seizures' *Neurology 43*, 425-428.

[77] Crawford, P.M., West, C.R., Shaw, M.D., Chadwick, D.W. (1986) 'Cerebral arterovenous malformations and epilepsy: factors in the development of epilepsy' *Epilepsia 27*, 270-275.

[78] Olafsson, E., Benedikz, J., Hauser, W.A. (1999) 'Risk of epilepsy in patients with multiple sclerosis: a population-based study in Iceland' *Epilepsia 40*, 745-747.

[79] Kinnunen, E., Wikstrom, J. (1986) 'Prevalence and prognosis of epilepsy in patients with multiple sclerosis' *Epilepsia 27*, 729-733.

[80] Bruns J., Jr, Hauser W.A. (2003) 'The epidemiology of traumatic brain injury: a review' *Epilepsia 44 (suppl 10)*, 2-10.

[81] Frey, L.C. (2003) 'Epidemiology of posttraumatic epilepsy: a critical review' *Epilepsia 44 (suppl 10)*, 11-17.

[82] Willmore, L.J. (1990) 'Post-traumatic epilepsy: cellular mechanisms and implications for treatment' *Epilepsia 31 (Suppl 3)*, S67-S73.

[83] Annegers, J.F., Hauser, W.A., Coan, S.P., Rocca, W.A. (1998) 'A population-based study of seizures after traumatic brain injuries' *The New England Journal of Medicine 338*, 20-24.

[84] Caveness, W.F., Meirowsky, A.M., Rish, B.L., et al. (1979) 'The nature of post traumatic epilepsy' *Journal of Neurosurgery 50*, 545-553.

[85] Salazar, A.M., Jabbari, B., Vance, S.C., et al. (1985) 'Epilepsy after penetrating head injury. I. Clinical correlates: a report of the Vietnam Head Injury Study' *Neurology 35*, 1406-1414.

[86] Le Blanc, F., Rasmussen, T. (1974) 'Cerebral seizures and brain tumors' In: Vinken, P.J., Bruyn, G.W. (eds.) *Handbook of Clinical Neurology.* Amsterdam: North-Holland. 295-301.

[87] Spencer, D.D., Spencer, S.S., Mattson, R.H. (1984) 'Intracerebral masses in patients with intractable partial epilepsy' *Neurology 34*, 432-436.

[88] Blume, W.T., Girvin, J.P., Kaufmann, J.C. (1982) 'Childhood brain tumors presenting as chronic uncontrolled focal seizure disorders' *Annals of Neurology 12*, 538-541.

[89] Singh, G., Driever, P.H., Sander, J.W. (2005) 'Cancer risk in people with epilepsy: the role of antiepileptic drugs' *Brain 128*, 7-17.

[90] Shirts, S.B., Annegers, J.F., Hauser, W.A., et al. (1986) 'Cancer incidence in a cohort of patients with seizure disorders' *Journal of the National Cancer Institute 77*, 83-87.

[91] Foy, P.M., Copeland, G.P., Shaw, M.D. (1981) 'The natural history of postoperative seizures' *Acta Neurochirurgica 57*, 15-22.

[92] Schierhout, G, Roberts, I. (1998) 'Prophylactic antiepileptic agents after head injury: a systematic review' *Journal of Neurology Neurosurgery and Psychiatry 64*, 108-112.

[93] Kuijlen, J.M., Teernstra, O.P., Kessels, A.G., et al. (1996) 'Effectiveness of antiepileptic prophylaxis used with supratentorial craniotomies: a meta-analysis' *Seizure 5*, 291-298.

[94] Temkin, N.R. (2001) 'Antiepileptogenesis and seizure prevention trials with antiepileptic drugs: meta-analysis of controlled trials' *Epilepsia 42*, 515-524.

[95] Glantz, M.J., Cole, B.F., Forsyth, P.A., et al. (2000) 'Practice parameter: anticonvulsant prophylaxis in patients with newly diagnosed brain tumors. Report of the Quality Standards Subcommittee of the American Academy of Neurology' *Neurology 54*, 1886-1893.

[96] Porter, J., Jick, H. (1977) 'Drug-induced anaphylaxis, convulsions, deafness, and extrapyramidal symptoms' *Lancet 1*, 587-588.

[97] Garcia, P.A., Alldredge, B.K. (1994) 'Drug-induced seizures' *Neurologic Clinics 12*, 85-99.

[98] Franson, K.L., Hay, D.P., Neppe, V., et al. (1995) 'Drug-induced seizures in the elderly. Causative agents and optimal management' *Drugs and Aging 7*, 38-48.

[99] Rodin, E.A. (1968) 'The prognosis of patients with epilepsy' Springfield, IL: Charles C Thomas.

[100] Jallon, P. (2003) 'Prognosis of Epilepsies' Montrouge: John Libbey Eurotext.

[101] Beghi, E. (2003) 'Prognosis of first seizure' In: Jallon, P. (ed.) *Prognosis of Epilepsies.* Montrouge: John Libbey Eurotext. 21-28.

[102] Annegers, J.F., Shirts, S.B., Hauser, W.A., Kurland, L.T. (1986) 'Risk of recurrence after an initial unprovoked seizure' *Epilepsia 27*: 43-50.

[103] Hart, Y.M., Sander, J.W., Johnson, A.L., Shorvon, S.D., for the NGPSE. (1990) 'National General Practice Study of Epilepsy: recurrence after a first seizure' *Lancet 336*, 1271-1274.

[104] Hopkins, A., Garman, A., Clarke, C. (1988) 'The first seizure in adult life. Value of clinical features, electroencephalography, and computerised tomographic scanning in prediction of seizure recurrence' *Lancet 1*, 721-726.

[105] van Donselaar, C.A., Geerts, A.T., Schimsheimer, R.J. (1991) 'Idiopathic first seizure in adult life: who should be treated?' *British Medical Journal 302*, 620-623.

[106] Shinnar, S., Berg, A.T., Moshe, S.L., et al. (1996) 'The risk of seizure recurrence after a first unprovoked afebrile seizure in childhood: an extended follow-up' *Pediatrics 98*, 216-225.

[107] Camfield, P.R., Camfield, C.S., Dooley, J.M., et al. (1985) 'Epilepsy after a first unprovoked seizure in childhood' *Neurology 35*, 1657-1660.

[108] Hauser, W.A., Rich, S.S., Annegers, J.F., Anderson, V.E. (1990) 'Seizure recurrence after a 1st unprovoked seizure: an extended follow-up' *Neurology 40*, 1163-1170.

[109] Gilad, R., Lampl, Y, Gabbay, U, et al. (1996) 'Early treatment of a single generalized tonic-clonic seizure to prevent recurrence' *Archives of Neurology 53*, 1149-1152.

[110] Musicco, M., Beghi, E., Solari, A., et al. (1997) 'Treatment of first tonic-clonic seizure does not improve the prognosis of epilepsy' *Neurology 49*, 991-998.

[111] Das, C.P., Sawhney, I.M., Lal, V., Prabhakar, S. (2000) 'Risk of recurrence of seizures following single unprovoked idiopathic seizure' *Neurology India 48*, 357-360.

[112] Camfield, P., Camfield, C., Smith, S., et al. (2002) 'Long-term outcome is unchanged by antiepileptic drug treatment after the first seizure: a 15-year follow-up from a randomized trial in childhood' *Epilepsia 43*, 662-663.

[113] Marson, A., Jacoby, A., Johnson, A., et al. (2005) 'Immediate versus deferred antiepileptic drug treatment for early epilepsy and single seizures: a randomised controlled trial' *Lancet 365*, 2007-2013.

[114] First Seizure Trial Group. (1993) 'Randomized clinical trial on the efficacy of antiepileptic drugs in reducing the risk of relapse after a first unprovoked tonic-clonic seizure' *Neurology 43*, 478-483.

[115] Chandra, B. (1992) 'First seizure in adults: to treat or not to treat' *Clinical Neurology and Neurosurgery 94 Suppl,* S61-S63.

[116] Leone, M., Solari, A., Beghi, E., FIRST Group. (2006) 'Treatment of the first tonic-clonic seizure does not affect long-term remission of epilepsy' *Neurology 67,* 2227-2229.

[117] Keranen, T., Riekkinen, P.J. (1993) 'Remission of seizures in untreated epilepsy' *British Medical Journal 307*, 483.

[118] Tekle-Haimanot, R., Forsgren, L., Abebe, M., et al. (1990) 'Clinical and electroencephalographic characteristics of epilepsy in rural Ethiopia: a community-based study' *Epilepsy Research 7*, 230-239.

[119] Watts, A.E. (1992) The natural history of untreated epilepsy in a rural community in Africa' *Epilepsia 33*, 464-468.

[120] Hauser, W.A., Rich, S.S., Lee, J.R.-J, et al. (1998) 'Risk of recurrent seizures after two unprovoked seizures' *The New England Journal of Medicine 338*, 429-434.

[121] Annegers, J.F., Hauser, W.A., Elveback, L.R. (1979) 'Remission of seizures and relapse in patients with epilepsy' *Epilepsia 20*, 729-737.

[122] Cockerell, O.C., Johnson, A.L., Sander, J.W.A.S., et al. (1997) 'Prognosis of epilepsy: a review and further analysis of the first nine years of the British National General Practice Study of Epilepsy, a prospective population-based study' *Epilepsia 38*, 31-46.

[123] Lindsen, H., Stenlund, H., Forsegren, L. (2001) 'Remission of seizures in a population-based adult cohort with a newly diagnosed unprovoked epileptic seizure' *Epilepsia 42*, 1025-1030.

[124] Sillanpaa, M., Jalava, M., Kaleva, O., Shinnar, S. (1998) 'Long-term prognosis of seizures with onset in childhood' *The New England Journal of Medicine 338*, 1715-1722.

[125] Sillanpaa, M. (1993) 'Remission of seizures and predictors of intractability in long-term follow-up' *Epilepsia 34*, 930-936.

[126] Shafer, S.Q., Hauser, W.A., Annegers, J.F., Klass, D.W. (1988) 'EEG and other early predictors of epilepsy remission: a community study' *Epilepsia 29*, 590-600.

[127] Sander, J.W. (1993) 'Some aspects of prognosis in the epilepsies: a review' *Epilepsia 34*, 1007-1016.

[128] Shinnar, S., Pellock, J.M. (2002) 'Update on the epidemiology and prognosis of pediatric epilepsy' *Journal of Child Neurology 17*, S4-S17.

[129] LaRoche, S.M., Helmers, S.L. (2004) 'The new antiepileptic drugs: scientific review' *Journal of the American Medical Association 291*, 605-614.

[130] Kwan, P., Brodie, M.J. (2001) 'Effectiveness of first antiepileptic drug' *Epilepsia 42*, 1255-1260.

[131] Specchio, L.M., Beghi, E. (2004) 'Should antiepileptic drugs be withdrawn in seizure-free patients?' *CNS Drugs 18*, 201-212.

[132] Berg, A.T., Shinnar, S. (1994) 'Relapse following discontinuation of antiepileptic drugs: a meta-analysis' *Neurology 44*, 601-608.

[133] MRC Antiepileptic Drug Withdrawal Study Group. (1991) 'Randomised study of antiepileptic drug withdrawal in patients in remission' *Lancet 337*, 1175-1180.

[134] Chadwick, D., Taylor, J., Johnson, T. (1996) 'Outcomes after seizure recurrence in people with well-controlled epilepsy and the factors that influence it' *Epilepsia 37*, 1043-1050.

[135] Tennison, M., Greenwood, R., Lewis, D., Thorn, M. (1994) 'Discontinuing antiepileptic drugs in children with epilepsy: a comparison of a six-week and a nine-month taper period' *The New England Journal of Medicine 330*, 1407-1410.

[136] Sander, J.W.A.S., Sillanpaa, M. (1997) 'Natural history and prognosis' In: Engel Jr, J., Pedley, T.A. (eds.) *Epilepsy: A Comprehensive Textbook*. Philadelphia: Lippincott-Raven. 69-86.

[137] Sillanpaa, M. (1990) 'Children with epilepsy as adults: outcome after 30 years of follow-up' *Acta Paediatrica Scandinavica 368 (Suppl)*, 1-78.

[138] Bourgeois, B.F.D. (1998) 'Antiepileptic drugs, learning, and behavior in childhood epilepsy' *Epilepsia 39*, 913-921.

[139] Seidenberg, M, Beck, N, Geisser, M, et al. (1986) 'Academic achievement of children with epilepsy' *Epilepsia 27*, 753-759.

[140] Brunbech, L., Sabers, A. (2002) 'Effect of antiepileptic drugs on cognitive function in individuals with epilepsy: a comparative review of newer versus older agents' *Drugs 62*, 593-604.

[141] Schupf, N, Ottman, R. (1994) 'Likelihood of pregnancy in individuals with idiopathic/cryptogenic epilepsy: social and biologic influences' *Epilepsia 35*, 750-755.

[142] Krauss, G.L., Krumholz, A., Carter, R.C., et al. (1999) 'Risk factors for seizure-related motor vehicle crashes in patients with epilepsy' *Neurology 52*, 1324-1329.

[143] van den Broek, M., Beghi, E., for the RESt-1 Group. (2004) 'Accidents in patients with epilepsy: types, circumstances and complications: a European cohort study' *Epilepsia 45*, 667-672.

[144] Black, A.B., Lai, N.Y. (1997) 'Epilepsy and driving in South Australia - an assessment of compulsory notification' *Medicine and Law 16*, 253-267.

[145] Sheth, S.G., Krauss, G., Krumholz, A., Li, G. (2004) 'Mortality in epilepsy: driving fatalities vs other causes of death in patients with epilepsy' *Neurology 63*, 1002-1007.

[146] Beghi, E, Cornaggia, C., and the RESt-1 Group (2002) 'Morbidity and accidents in patients with epilepsy: results of a European cohort study' *Epilepsia 43*, 1076-1083.

[147] Tomson, T. (2003) 'Mortality studies in epilepsy' In: Jallon, P., Berg, A., Dulac, O., Hauser, A. (eds.) *Prognosis of Epilepsies*. Paris: John Libbey. 12-21.

[148] Massey, E.W., Schoenberg, B.S. (1985) 'Mortality from epilepsy. International patterns and changes over time' *Neuroepidemiology 4*, 65-70.

[149] Shackleton, D.P., Westerndorp, R.G.J., Kastelejin-Nolst Trenite, D.G.A., et al. (2002) 'Survival of patients with epilepsy: an estimate of the mortality risk' *Epilepsia 43*, 445-450.

[150] Jallon, P. (2004) 'Mortality in patients with epilepsy' *Current Opinion in Neurology 17*, 141-146.

[151] Camfield, C.S., Camfield, P.R., Veugelers, P.J. (2002) 'Death in children with epilepsy: a population-based study' *Lancet 359*, 1891-1895.

[152] Loiseau, J., Picot, M.C., Loiseau, P. (1999) 'Short-term mortality after a first epileptic seizure: a population-based study' *Epilepsia 40*, 1388-1392.

[153] Olafsson, E., Hauser, W.A., Gudmundsson, G. (1998) ,Long-term survival of people with unprovoked seizures: a population-based study' *Epilepsia 39*, 89-92.

[154] Zielinski, J.J. (1974) 'Epilepsy and mortality rate and cause of death' *Epilepsia 15*, 191-201.

[155] Lindsten, H., Nystrom, L., Forsgren, L. (2000) 'Mortality risk in an adult cohort with a newly diagnosed unprovoked epileptic seizure: a population-based study' *Epilepsia 41*, 1469-1473.

[156] Lhatoo, S.D., Sander, J.W.A.S., Shorvon, S.D. (2001) 'The dynamics of drug treatment in epilepsy: an observational study in an unselected population based cohort with newly diagnosed epilepsy followed up prospectively over 11-14 years' *Journal of Neurology Neurosurgery and Psychiatry 71*, 632-637.

[157] Hauser, W.A., Annegers, J.F., Elveback, L.R. (1980) 'Mortality in patients with epilepsy' *Epilepsia 21*, 399-412.

[158] Cockerell, O.C., Johnson, A.L., Sander, J.W.A.S., et al. (1994) 'Mortality from epilepsy: results from a prospective population-based study' *Lancet 344*, 918-921.

[159] Logroscino, G., Hesdorffer, D.C., Cascino, G., et al. (1997) 'Short-term mortality after a first episode of status epilepticus' *Epilepsia 38*, 1344-1349.

[160] Logroscino, G., Hesdorffer, D.C., Cascino, G.D., et al. (2002) 'Long-term mortality after a first episode of status epilepticus' *Neurology 58,* 537-541.

[161] DeLorenzo, R.J., Hauser, W.A., Towne, A.R., et al. (1996) 'A prospective, population-based epidemiologic study of status epilepticus in Richmond, Virginia' *Neurology 46*, 1029-1035.

[162] Vignatelli, L., Tonon, C., D'Alessandro, R, on behalf of the Bologna Group for the Study of Status Epilepticus. (2003) 'Incidence and short-term prognosis of status epilepticus in adults in Bologna, Italy' *Epilepsia 44*, 964-968.

[163] Gaitatzis, A., Sander, J.W. (2004) 'The mortality of epilepsy revisited' *Epileptic Disorders 6*, 3-13.

[164] Barraclough, B.M. (1987) 'The suicide rate of epilepsy' *Acta Psychiatrica Scandinavica 76*, 339-345.

[165] Harris, E.C., Barraclough, B. (1997) 'Suicide as an outcome for mental disorders. A meta-analysis' *British Journal of Psychiatry 170*, 205-228.

[166] Nilsson, L., Ahlbom, A., Farahmand, B.Y., et al. (2002) 'Risk factors for suicide in epilepsy: a case control study' *Epilepsia 43*, 644-651.

[167] Tomson, T., Beghi, E., Sundqvist, A., Johannessen, S.I. (2004) 'Medical risks in epilepsy: a review with focus on physical injuries, mortality, traffic accidents and their prevention' *Epilepsy Research 60*, 1-16.

[168] Pedley, T.A., Hauser, W.A. (2002) 'Sudden death in epilepsy: a wake-up call for management' *Lancet 359*, 1790-1791.

[169] O'Donoghue, M.F., Sander, J.W. (1997) 'The mortality associated with epilepsy, with particular reference to sudden unexpected death: a review' *Epilepsia 38 (suppl 11),* S15-S19.

[170] Nashef, L., Fish, D.R., Garner, S., et al. (1995) 'Sudden death in epilepsy: a study of incidence in a young cohort with epilepsy and learning difficulty' *Epilepsia 36*, 1187-1194.

[171] Callenbach, P.M., Westendorp, R.G., Geertz, A.T., et al. (2001) 'Mortality risk in children with epilepsy: the Dutch study of epilepsy in childhood' *Pediatrics 107*, 1259-1263.

[172] Donner, E.J., Smith, C.R., Snead, O.C. 3rd (2001) 'Sudden unexplained death in children with epilepsy' *Neurology 57*, 430-434.

[173] Nashef, L., Walker, F., Allen, P., et al. (1996) 'Apnoea and bradycardia during epileptic seizures: relation to sudden death in epilepsy' *Journal of Neurology Neurosurgery and Psychiatry 60*, 297-300.

[174] Nilsson, L., Ahlbom, A., Farahmand, B.Y., Tomson, T. (2003) 'Mortality in a population-based cohort of epilepsy surgery patients' *Epilepsia 44*, 575-581.

[175] Walczak, T. (2003) 'Do antiepileptic drugs play a role in sudden unexpected death in epilepsy?' *Drug Safety 26*, 675-683.

[176] Carpio, A. (2003) 'The Ecuadorial study of prognosis of epilepsy' In: Jallon, P., Berg, A., Dulac, O., Hauser, A. (eds.) *Prognosis of Epilepsies*. Paris: John Libbey, 85-101.

[177] Jilek-Aall, L., Rwiza, H.T. (1992) 'Prognosis of epilepsy in a rural African community: a 30-year follow-up of 164 patients in an outpatient clinic in rural Tanzania' *Epilepsia 33*, 645-650.

[178] Snow, R.W., Williams, R.E., Rogers, J.E., et al. (1994) 'The prevalence of epilepsy among a rural Kenyan population. Its association with premature mortality' *Tropical and Geographic Medicine 46*, 175-179.

[179] Tekle-Haimanot, R., Forsgren, L., Ekstedt, J. (1997) 'Incidence of epilepsy in rural central Ethiopia' *Epilepsia 38*, 541-546.

[180] Carpio, A., Bharucha, N.E., Jallon, P., et al. (2005) 'Mortality of epilepsy in developing countries' *Epilepsia 46 (suppl 11)*, 28-32.

[181] Feksi, A.T, Kaamugisha, J., Sander, J.W.A.S. (1991) 'Comprehensive primary health care antiepileptic drug treatment programme in rural and semi-urban Kenya' *Lancet 337*, 406-409.

[182] Placencia, M, Sander, J.W., Shorvon, S.D., et al. (1993) 'Antiepileptic drug treatment in a community health care setting in northern Ecuador: a prospective 12-month assessment' *Epilepsy Research 14*, 237-244.

RECOMMENDED FURTHER READING

1. Beghi, E. (2004) 'Aetiology of epilepsy' In: Shorvon, S., Perucca, E., Fish D., Dodson, E. (eds.) *The Treatment of Epilepsy* (2nd edition). Oxford: Blackwell Science. 50-63.

2. Forsgren, L. (2004) 'Epidemiology and prognosis of epilepsy and its treatment' In: Shorvon, S., Perucca, E., Fish D., Dodson, E. (eds.) *The Treatment of Epilepsy* (2nd edition). Oxford: Blackwell Science. 21-42.

3. Hauser, W.A., Hesdorffer, D.C. (1990) *Epilepsy. Frequency, causes and consequences.* New York: Demos Publications.

4. Hauser, W.A. (1997) 'Incidence and prevalence' In: Engel Jr, J., Pedley, T.A. (Eds) *Epilepsy: A Comprehensive Textbook.* Philadelphia: Lippincott-Raven. 47-57.

5. Jallon, P. (2003) *Prognosis of epilepsies.* Montrouge (France): John Libbey Eurotext.

6. Kotsopoulos, I.A.W., van Merode, T., Kessels, F.G.H., et al. (2002) 'Systematic review and meta-analysis of incidence studies of epilepsy and unprovoked seizures' *Epilepsia 43*, 1402-1409.

7. Tomson, T., Beghi, E., Sundqvist, A., Johannessen, S.I. (2004) 'Medical risks in epilepsy: a review with focus on physical injuries, mortality, traffic accidents and their prevention' *Epilepsy Research 60*, 1-16.

In: Handbook of Clinical Neuroepidemiology   ISBN 978-1-60021-511-7
Editors: V. L. Feigin and D. A. Bennett, pp. 167-177   © 2007 Nova Science Publishers, Inc.

Chapter 5

LOW BACK PAIN

Kern Singh and Gunnar B. J. Andersson

Department of Orthopaedic Surgery, Rush University Medical Center, Chicago,
Illinois, USA

ABSTRACT

Epidemiologic research on back pain is difficult in large part because of the lack of
agreement on a diagnostic classification. This creates an imposing problem when making
comparisons between studies and precludes the development of a general database. The
goals and expectations of the patient should be addressed when making decisions about
treatment. More clinical work is needed to help address the pathologic basis for low back
pain and to help to improve how we treat these patients.

INTRODUCTION

In the United States, back pain is the most common cause of activity limitation in people
younger than 45 years [1]. It is the third most common cause of surgical procedures and
results in 2% of the American work force being compensated for back injuries each year [2].
The economic impact of back pain is witnessed in other western countries as well. Low back
pain is the largest single reason for absence from work in the United Kingdom resulting in
12.5% of all sick days [3]. Similar findings were also reported in Swedish populations in
1987, where a diagnosis of back pain was found in 8% of the insured population [4].
Epidemiologic research on back pain is difficult in large part because of the lack of
agreement on a diagnostic classification. This creates an imposing problem when making
comparisons between studies and precludes the development of a general database.

DEFINITION

Low back pain is usually defined as pain, muscle tension, or stiffness localized below the costal margin and above the inferior gluteal folds, with or without leg pain (sciatica) [5]. Approximately 90% of cases of back pain have no identifiable cause and are designated as nonspecific [6]. Currently, no reliable and valid classification system exists. Although acute episodes that last up to 3 months are the most common presentations of low back pain, chronic back pain ultimately is more disabling because of the physical impediment it causes and its psychological effects. Many doctors order elaborate studies when nonspecific back pain is presented, including radiographs and magnetic resonance imaging. The result is little guidance with regards to treatment decisions.

INCIDENCE AND PREVALENCE OF LOW BACK PAIN

Information on the prevalence and incidence of back pain is available from several sources including national registries, insurance and hospital data, and selective prospective and retrospective clinical studies [7]. Assessing or comparing prevalence studies of back pain can be hampered by the lack of agreement on a clear definition of low back pain. Furthermore, period prevalence studies may be biased by poor recall and incomplete responses. Given these caveats, recently published data continue to confirm that low back pain is a common disorder in Western and developing nations [7-10].

In the US population, the third National Health and Nutrition Examination Survey (NHANES III, 1988-94) estimated that the 12-month period prevalence of back pain episodes lasting for at least 1 month was 17.8% [11]. In the adult Greek population, the 1-month prevalence of back pain has been estimated at 32% [12]. This figure is somewhat higher than reported in other population surveys and may reflect the relatively high proportion of the Greek population engaged in manual work such as agriculture. A direct comparison of back pain between the United Kingdom and Germany not only showed differences in prevalence between the two countries (22% compared with 44.9% in women) but also demonstrated marked differences in the prevalence of current back pain within each country or region [13]. West Germans carry a risk of back pain 2.5 to 3.5 times higher than the British, even after adjusting for potential confounders. The authors hypothesize that intercultural differences between the British and Germans in pain perception or pain reporting may be a plausible explanation for the variation where none was expected to occur.

In developing countries with large work forces, prevalence data on back disorders, and particularly back pain, have been recently reported. In a nationwide study of 1-year prevalence of musculoskeletal disorders among workers in Taiwan, pain in the lower back and waist was among the most frequently cited symptom, occurring in 18% of male workers and 20% of female workers. Workers between the ages of 45 and 64 years had the highest prevalence of back pain in both sexes [8]. The overall prevalence of low back pain lasting more than 1 day among Chinese workers was relatively high reaching 50% [9]. The prevalence declined considerably as the period of recall shortened from 61% (lifetime) to

20% in the past week. The most frequent occurrence of low back pain was among garment workers, who showed a four-fold increase in comparison with teachers.

Murphy and Volinn reported a decline in frequency of occupational low back pain reported over a 9-year period [14]. Data from a workers' compensation provider, Liberty Mutual Insurance Company (1987-1995), the Washington State Department of Labor and Industry (1991-1995), and the Bureau of Labor Statistics (1992-1995) were reviewed for frequency of low back claims from industrial settings. The US estimates of annual low back pain claims decreased by 34% between 1987 and 1995. More important, annual costs decreased during this time period by 58%. However, because the rate of filing remained 1.8 per 100 workers, the estimated cost of low back pain claims for 1995 was 8.8 billion USD. In an attempt to determine the proportion of costs of components of back care, Williams et al. reported data derived from the National Council on Compensation Insurance on health care use and indemnity costs within the natural history of work-related low back pain disability [15]. Health care costs were disproportionately distributed along the disability curve, with 20% of claimants with back pain for four months or more accounting for 60% of health care costs. These data confirm reports by Federspiel et al. emphasizing that a small proportion of individuals with chronic disability account for a disproportionate amount of resources [16].

NATURAL HISTORY

The outcome of low back pain is closely linked to natural history. True natural history may be difficult to establish because we are all affected by our surroundings and the effect that this has on our strategies for managing the situation. We receive recommendations from family, friends and health care providers. All this may influence the course of the episode because different strategies may result in different outcomes. How the health professionals regard the condition, what kind of education is given, and what groups are studied may give us different answers [17-21]. To establish a true natural history may therefore be a difficult task.

Data on the natural history of low back pain are conflicting, but most patients are likely to recover from their acute, presenting episode of back pain. Rates of recovery within 2-3 weeks vary from 30-70%, and 90% are back at work within two months [7]. However, 5-10% develop chronic back pain lasting more than 3 months. The median time to recover is about 7 weeks, but relapses are common. Of the 15% who seek medical help, about 35-80% are still in pain a year later, although perhaps only 10-15% will be highly disabled [22-24].

RISK FACTORS

Inconsistencies remain in the literature over the relative contributions of physical and psychological risk factors to the occurrence of back disorders and back pain. More recently, genetic and biomechanical models have contributed to the understanding of the development of back disorders that present as back pain.

Individual Risk Factors

The presence and severity of low back pain is associated with several socio-demographic factors, among them sex, age, education level, smoking and occupation [12,13,25]. Although the prevalence of back pain increases with age, the dose-response relation between age and low back pain is not linear [8]. Growing evidence suggests that low back pain starts early in life, between the ages of 8-10 years [26-28]. One study of young adolescents (12-22) demonstrated an overall prevalence of back pain of 7% (pain > 30 days during the past year) [29]. The same investigators showed a statistically significant association between high birth weight and risk of developing low back pain in male patients but not in female patients, suggesting that factors that predispose to low back pain could operate in the prenatal environment [30].

Psychosocial Risk Factors

Predictors of new-onset chronic back pain using prospective data in the general household population identified general health and psychosocial factors in both men and women [31]. Psychological variables associated with low back include stress, distress, mood and emotions, cognitive functioning, pain behavior, and depressive disorder [32]. Studies show a strong association between back pain and depressive disorders, but a cross-sectional analysis cannot establish cause and effect [33]. In a prospective study, however, lifetime depressive disorder has been shown to be an independent risk factor for a first-ever report of back pain during a 13-year follow-up period in comparison with those who did not have depressive disorder at baseline [34]. The combination of chronic back pain and major depression is associated with greater disability than either condition alone [33].

Occupational Risk Factors

Studies on the association between occupational risk factors and low back pain are hampered by the difficulties of measuring specific exposures. The relative timing of the onset of low back pain and work exposure is also often uncertain. Workplace factors, including physical and psychosocial factors and their interaction, are strong determinants of back pain [35]. Psychosocial risk factors at work (perceived high pressure on time and workload, low job control, job dissatisfaction, monotonous work, and low support from coworkers and management) appear to independently increase the risk of hospitalization for back disorders, with a 3.2-fold increase in a low-control job compared with a high-control job [36]. Other factors such as heavy physical work, night shifts, lifting, bending, twisting, pulling and pushing have often been associated with low back pain [37].

MANAGEMENT STRATEGIES

Treatments for non-specific low back pain cover a multitude of different modalities. Many of these modalities have been tested in randomized control trials, but it has been difficult to establish the efficacies of different modalities, reflecting the inconclusiveness of systematic reviews.

In a prospective cohort study in six countries concerning the effect on pain, back function, and return to work of received treatments for chronic low back pain, the results indicated that "almost none of the frequently practiced medical interventions for patients who are sick-listed because of low back pain had any positive effects of either the recorded health measures or work resumption" [38].

Manipulation has been an established tradition in the treatment of low back pain and has been studied quite extensively in several randomized control trials. However, its effect has been difficult to establish despite several clinical studies. Systematic reviews have come to varying conclusions suggesting that even if manipulation has some effect it does not seem to be highly effective [39-41]. A recent meta-analysis by Assendelft et al. concluded that there is no evidence that spinal manipulative therapy is superior to other standard treatments for patients with acute or chronic low back pain [42].

Varying forms of exercises have been the primary modality of treatment for both acute and chronic low back pain. The prevailing theory being that strong abdominal and back muscles help provide a solid foundation for support of the spine and may therefore help alleviate pain. The popularity of this treatment modality and the myriad of different exercises may give an impression of effectiveness. Despite numerous clinical trials, the efficacy of physical therapy has been difficult to establish. A recent Cochrane review on physical therapy concluded that there is no proven benefit in the treatment of acute low back pain [43]. Normal activity seems to be as effective as specific exercises. However, vigorous exercises for chronic back pain have been shown to have some positive effect. From a clinical perspective, the important conclusion made regarding exercise is that it is important to get patients with low back pain active regardless of strategy.

Multidisciplinary rehabilitation treatments of different intensities have been developed in accordance with the biopsychosocial model for the development of chronic low back pain. These treatments emphasize fitness, specific exercises, work hardening complemented with cognitive-behavioral therapy [44]. The results have varied, but the current literature suggests that it has an effect on back function and on low back pain [45]. The effect on return to work is still undefined.

Fear-avoidance behavior has been proposed as an important factor in patients not being able to resume normal activity or return to work [23]. In this model, patients' disability is not only a function of their pain, but also of their response to pain. The model maintains that there are two extreme responses to pain, either a confronting response or an avoidance response. Since the relationship between pain and disability has been shown to be low, it is proposed that fear is more linked to fear of injury or re-injury than to pain. Although being an important factor, fear does not seem to explain the main mechanism for the development of chronic low back pain. Cognitive-behavioral treatments designed to reduce pain-related fear seem to be effective, but it is still unknown what type of patient is most likely to benefit from this kind of behavioral treatment.

The inability for target interventions to show a substantial effect strongly suggests that the modalities applied in the cure for unspecific low back pain have unspecific-pain-modulating effects. This may be important for patients during the time the condition heals itself and may have an effect on return to work. The trend in treatment of low back pain seems to be focused on giving the patient support through physical examination and education to resume activity, in other words to focus on treating the disability rather than the pain itself [46].

The role of opioid analgesics for chronic low back pain patients engenders considerable differences of opinion. Apprehensions exist concerning efficacy, adverse effects, tolerance, and addiction associated with the use of narcotics. Jamison et al. reported on a pharmaceutical-sponsored study of 36 patients with back pain who were randomly assigned to naproxen alone, fixed-dose oxycodone, or titrated dose of oxycodone and sustained-release morphine sulfate [47]. At the 1-month post-treatment period, the authors monitored pain, activity, mood, medication, hours awake, and adverse effects associated with abuse. The titrated-dose group had less pain and emotional distress than the other groups. Only one patient had complete pain relief. Patients were able to taper off the narcotic, but experienced no long-lasting effect on function.

The role for surgical treatment of persistent disabling low back pain remains controversial [48]. The most common surgical treatment for persistent low back pain with degenerative changes is spinal fusion. A small, randomized trial (64 patients) compared spinal fusion with an aggressive rehabilitation program [49]. The rehabilitation program used a cognitive behavioral approach among patients. The study demonstrated no differences between groups at one year in back pain, function, use of medication, work status, or general satisfaction. The likelihood that spinal fusion surgery will be beneficial for common degenerative changes may be improved by selecting patients without coexisting psychosocial disorders (including serious psychological distress or disputed compensation issues) and those with severe degenerative changes [50].

MEDICAL AND SOCIOECONOMIC OUTCOMES

The literature regarding the long-term course of low back pain is confusing because of variations in definitions of low back pain as well as a lack of distinction between outcome parameters. A recent review to investigate the long-term course of incident and prevalent cases of low back pain showed that the reported proportion of patients who still experienced pain after 12 months was 62% (range, 42-75%), dispelling the popular notion that up to 90% of low back pain episodes resolve spontaneously within 1 month [51].

Psychological distress (in the form of depressive symptoms) emerged as the strongest single baseline predictor of 4-year outcome and greatly exceeded the influence of pain intensity [52]. Fear-avoidance beliefs and heightened somatic concern are also determinants of recurrence in the longer term. Their influence goes beyond the accepted relation with short-term pain and disability outcomes. In patients over the age of 70, duration and severity of pain are significantly associated with function/disability and underscore the need to optimize pain treatment in independent older adults and delay dependent living status [53].

When work-related back pain is considered, type of treatment, response to therapy, severity of injury, and type of job are factors influencing the duration of disability [54]. Economic, social, and legal factors also influence recovery. Longer duration of work disability as measured by workers' compensation is a powerful predictor of recurrence of low back pain; therefore, early return to work contributes to better outcomes.

An important component of the biopsychosocial model of low back pain management is exercise. Exercise is thought to reduce fear-avoidance behavior and facilitate functional improvements despite ongoing pain, and results are largely maintained at follow-up [55,56]. Graded behavioral interventions reinforce the concept that "hurt does not mean harm" [57]. Early mobilization programs can reduce duration of sick leave over 3 years and result in economic gains for society [58]. Cognitive intervention and exercise program may be just as effective in improving disability in patients with chronic back pain and disc degeneration compared with patients undergoing lumbar fusion surgery [58].

Other important determinants of the outcome of low back pain beyond activity modification include attitudes and perceptions of the patients [59]. Patients are affected by their surroundings and receive recommendations from family, friends, and health care providers. For example, as many as 50-60% of the Norwegian population believe in the importance and benefit of radiographs and other imaging tests and consequently have expectations for such services. Population beliefs have an important impact on how the health professionals regard the condition and determine the kind of education given to patients [37].

CONCLUSION

Guidelines are playing an increasingly important role in the evidence-based practice for low back pain in an effort to improve outcomes. Unfortunately, good guidelines alone do not guarantee that they will be used in daily practice, and their implementation may need to be reinforced. The natural history of low back pain seems to be favorable, but the consequences of long-term or permanent disability is of concern. Cognitive intervention, designed to remove fear and uncertainty and to give the patient confidence appear to have promising results. The goals and expectations of the patient should be addressed when making decisions about treatment. More clinical work is needed to help address the pathologic basis for low back pain and to help to improve how we treat these patients.

REFRENCES

[1]   Taylor, V.M., et al., Low back pain hospitalization. Recent United States trends and regional variations. *Spine*, 1994. 19(11): p. 1207-12; discussion 13.

[2]   Hart, L.G., R.A. Deyo, and D.C. Cherkin, Physician office visits for low back pain. Frequency, clinical evaluation, and treatment patterns from a U.S. national survey. *Spine*, 1995. 20(1): p. 11-9.

[3]   Frank, A., Low back pain. *Bmj*, 1993. 306(6882): p. 901-9.

[4]   Nachemson, A., Back Pain. Causes, diagnosis and treatment. The Swedish Council of Technology Assessment in Health Care., 1991.

[5]   Indahl, A., Low back pain: diagnosis, treatment, and prognosis. *Scand J Rheumatol*, 2004. 33(4): p. 199-209.

[6]   van den Bosch, M.A., et al., Evidence against the use of lumbar spine radiography for low back pain. *Clin Radiol*, 2004. 59(1): p. 69-76.

[7]   Andersson, G.B., Epidemiological features of chronic low-back pain. *Lancet*, 1999. 354(9178): p. 581-5.

[8]   Guo, H.R., et al., Prevalence of musculoskeletal disorder among workers in Taiwan: a nationwide study. *J Occup Health*, 2004. 46(1): p. 26-36.

[9]   Jin, K., G.S. Sorock, and T.K. Courtney, Prevalence of low back pain in three occupational groups in Shanghai, People's Republic of China. *J Safety Res*, 2004. 35(1): p. 23-8.

[10] Latza, U., et al., Can health care utilization explain the association between socioeconomic status and back pain? *Spine*, 2004. 29(14): p. 1561-6.

[11] Dillon, C., et al., Skeletal muscle relaxant use in the United States: data from the Third National Health and Nutrition Examination Survey (NHANES III). *Spine*, 2004. 29(8): p. 892-6.

[12] Stranjalis, G., et al., Low back pain in a representative sample of Greek population: analysis according to personal and socioeconomic characteristics. *Spine*, 2004. 29(12): p. 1355-60; discussion 1361.

[13] Raspe, H., et al., Variation in back pain between countries: the example of Britain and Germany. *Spine*, 2004. 29(9): p. 1017-21; discussion 1021.

[14] Murphy, P.L. and E. Volinn, Is occupational low back pain on the rise? *Spine*, 1999. 24(7): p. 691-7.

[15] Williams, D.A., et al., Health care and indemnity costs across the natural history of disability in occupational low back pain. *Spine*, 1998. 23(21): p. 2329-36.

[16] Federspiel, C.F., et al., Expenditures for nonspecific back injuries in the workplace. *J Occup Med*, 1989. 31(11): p. 919-24.

[17] Haldorsen, E.M., et al., Musculoskeletal pain: concepts of disease, illness, and sickness certification in health professionals in Norway. *Scand J Rheumatol*, 1996. 25(4): p. 224-32.

[18] Kvien, T.K., H. Nilsen, and P. Vik, Education and self-care of patients with low back pain. *Scand J Rheumatol*, 1981. 10(4): p. 318-20.

[19] Lapossy, E., et al., The frequency of transition of chronic low back pain to fibromyalgia. *Scand J Rheumatol*, 1995. 24(1): p. 29-33.

[20] Leino, P.I., M.A. Berg, and P. Puska, Is back pain increasing? Results from national surveys in Finland during 1978/9-1992. *Scand J Rheumatol*, 1994. 23(5): p. 269-76.

[21] Smedbraten, B.K., et al., Self-reported bodily pain in schoolchildren. *Scand J Rheumatol*, 1998. 27(4): p. 273-6.

[22] Burton, A.K. and K.M. Tillotson, Prediction of the clinical course of low-back trouble using multivariable models. *Spine*, 1991. 16(1): p. 7-14.

[23] Burton, A.K., et al., Psychosocial predictors of outcome in acute and subchronic low back trouble. *Spine*, 1995. 20(6): p. 722-8.

[24] Deyo, R.A. and Y.J. Tsui-Wu, Functional disability due to back pain. A population-based study indicating the importance of socioeconomic factors. *Arthritis Rheum*, 1987. 30(11): p. 1247-53.

[25] Leino-Arjas, P., et al., Occupational exposures and inpatient hospital care for lumbar intervertebral disc disorders among Finns. *Am J Ind Med*, 2004. 46(5): p. 513-20.

[26] Leboeuf-Yde, C., et al., Back pain reporting in children and adolescents: the impact of parents' educational level. *J Manipulative Physiol Ther*, 2002. 25(4): p. 216-20.

[27] Wedderkopp, N., et al., Back pain reporting pattern in a Danish population-based sample of children and adolescents. *Spine*, 2001. 26(17): p. 1879-83.

[28] Wedderkopp, N., et al., Back pain in children: no association with objectively measured level of physical activity. *Spine*, 2003. 28(17): p. 2019-24; discussion 2024.

[29] Hestbaek, L., et al., Comorbidity with low back pain: a cross-sectional population-based survey of 12- to 22-year-olds. *Spine*, 2004. 29(13): p. 1483-91; discussion 1492.

[30] Hestbaek, L., et al., Heredity of low back pain in a young population: a classical twin study. *Twin Res*, 2004. 7(1): p. 16-26.

[31] Kopec, J.A., E.C. Sayre, and J.M. Esdaile, Predictors of back pain in a general population cohort. *Spine*, 2004. 29(1): p. 70-7; discussion 77-8.

[32] Turk, D.C., Understanding pain sufferers: the role of cognitive processes. *Spine J*, 2004. 4(1): p. 1-7.

[33] Currie, S.R. and J. Wang, Chronic back pain and major depression in the general Canadian population. *Pain*, 2004. 107(1-2): p. 54-60.

[34] Larson, S.L., M.R. Clark, and W.W. Eaton, Depressive disorder as a long-term antecedent risk factor for incident back pain: a 13-year follow-up study from the Baltimore Epidemiological Catchment Area sample. *Psychol Med*, 2004. 34(2): p. 211-9.

[35] Ferguson, S.A., W.S. Marras, and D.L. Burr, The influence of individual low back health status on workplace trunk kinematics and risk of low back disorder. *Ergonomics*, 2004. 47(11): p. 1226-37.

[36] Eriksen, W., D. Bruusgaard, and S. Knardahl, Work factors as predictors of intense or disabling low back pain; a prospective study of nurses' aides. *Occup Environ Med*, 2004. 61(5): p. 398-404.

[37] Houben, R.M., et al., Health care providers' orientations towards common low back pain predict perceived harmfulness of physical activities and recommendations regarding return to normal activity. *Eur J Pain*, 2005. 9(2): p. 173-83.

[38] Hansson, T.H. and E.K. Hansson, The effects of common medical interventions on pain, back function, and work resumption in patients with chronic low back pain: A prospective 2-year cohort study in six countries. *Spine*, 2000. 25(23): p. 3055-64.

[39] Bronfort, G., Spinal manipulation: current state of research and its indications. *Neurol Clin*, 1999. 17(1): p. 91-111.

[40] Koes, B.W., et al., Spinal manipulation for low back pain. An updated systematic review of randomized clinical trials. *Spine*, 1996. 21(24): p. 2860-71; discussion 2872-3.

[41] Shekelle, P.G., et al., Spinal manipulation for low-back pain. *Ann Intern Med*, 1992. 117(7): p. 590-8.

[42] Assendelft, W.J., et al., Spinal manipulative therapy for low back pain. A meta-analysis of effectiveness relative to other therapies. *Ann Intern Med*, 2003. 138(11): p. 871-81.

[43] Manniche, C., et al., Clinical trial of intensive muscle training for chronic low back pain. *Lancet*, 1988. 2(8626-8627): p. 1473-6.

[44] Haldorsen, E.M., et al., Multimodal cognitive behavioral treatment of patients sicklisted for musculoskeletal pain: a randomized controlled study. *Scand J Rheumatol*, 1998. 27(1): p. 16-25.

[45] Guzman, J., et al., Multidisciplinary bio-psycho-social rehabilitation for chronic low back pain. *Cochrane Database Syst Rev*, 2002(1): p. CD000963.

[46] Loisel, P., et al., Training the next generation of researchers in work disability prevention: the Canadian Work Disability Prevention CIHR Strategic Training Program. *J Occup Rehabil*, 2005. 15(3): p. 273-84.

[47] Jamison, R.N., et al., Opioid therapy for chronic noncancer back pain. A randomized prospective study. *Spine*, 1998. 23(23): p. 2591-600.

[48] Errico, T.J., Authors' reply to drs. Deyo, mirza, and nachemson. *Spine J*, 2005. 5(6): p. 699-700.

[49] Brox, J.I., et al., Randomized clinical trial of lumbar instrumented fusion and cognitive intervention and exercises in patients with chronic low back pain and disc degeneration. *Spine*, 2003. 28(17): p. 1913-21.

[50] Carragee, E.J., S.J. Paragioudakis, and S. Khurana, 2000 Volvo Award winner in clinical studies: Lumbar high-intensity zone and discography in subjects without low back problems. *Spine*, 2000. 25(23): p. 2987-92.

[51] Hestbaek, L., C. Leboeuf-Yde, and C. Manniche, Low back pain: what is the long-term course? A review of studies of general patient populations. *Eur Spine J*, 2003. 12(2): p. 149-65.

[52] Burton, A.K., et al., Long-term follow-up of patients with low back pain attending for manipulative care: outcomes and predictors. *Man Ther*, 2004. 9(1): p. 30-5.

[53] Weiner, D.K., et al., How does low back pain impact physical function in independent, well-functioning older adults? Evidence from the Health ABC Cohort and implications for the future. *Pain Med*, 2003. 4(4): p. 311-20.

[54] Wasiak, R., et al., Risk factors for recurrent episodes of care and work disability: case of low back pain. *J Occup Environ Med*, 2004. 46(1): p. 68-76.

[55] Liddle, S.D., G.D. Baxter, and J.H. Gracey, Exercise and chronic low back pain: what works? *Pain*, 2004. 107(1-2): p. 176-90.

[56] Patrick, L.E., E.M. Altmaier, and E.M. Found, Long-term outcomes in multidisciplinary treatment of chronic low back pain: results of a 13-year follow-up. *Spine*, 2004. 29(8): p. 850-5.

[57] Staal, J.B., et al., Graded activity for low back pain in occupational health care: a randomized, controlled trial. *Ann Intern Med*, 2004. 140(2): p. 77-84.

[58] Karjalainen, K., et al., Mini-intervention for subacute low back pain: a randomized controlled trial. *Spine*, 2003. 28(6): p. 533-40; discussion 540-1.

[59] Ihlebaek, C. and H.R. Eriksen, The "myths" of low back pain: status quo in norwegian general practitioners and physiotherapists. *Spine,* 2004. 29(16): p. 1818-22

RECOMMENDED FURTHER READING

1. Andersson GB. (1999) Epidemiological features of chronic low-back pain. *Lancet 354*:581-5.

2. Brox JI, Sorensen R, Friis A, et al. (2003) Randomized clinical trial of lumbar instrumented fusion and cognitive intervention and exercises in patients with chronic low back pain and disc degeneration. *Spine 28*:1913-21.

3. Ihlebaek C, Eriksen HR. (2004) The "myths" of low back pain: status quo in norwegian general practitioners and physiotherapists. *Spine 29*:1818-22.

4. Kopec JA, Sayre EC, Esdaile JM. (2004) Predictors of back pain in a general population cohort. *Spine 29*:70-7; discussion 7-8.

In: Handbook of Clinical Neuroepidemiology　　　　　ISBN 978-1-60021-511-7
Editors: V. L. Feigin and D. A. Bennett, pp. 179-195　© 2007 Nova Science Publishers, Inc.

Chapter 6

DEMENTIA

Amos D. Korczyn, Veronika Vakhapova and Simon Korn

Department of Neurology, Sackler School of Medicine,
Tel-Aviv University Ramat-Aviv 69978, Israel.

ABSTRACT

Because of the aging of the population, dementia – already the third most expensive disease in developed countries – will become even more common in the next few decades, reaching pandemic proportions. Understanding of this problem, with its huge clinical, social and economic implications, necessitates action. Like in other epidemics, prevention is easier than cure. Due to epidemiologic research, several common risk factors for dementia have been identified which can be treated.

In the present paper, we shall discuss the nosology of old age dementia, and particularly Alzheimer's disease and vascular dementia, and the effect of the definitions of these disorders on our understanding of the epidemiology of dementia and of measures which can be taken to reduce its prevalence. Because it is impossible to discuss at length all risk factors, we shall focus on the relationship between smoking with dementia and the role of brain trauma in triggering dementia.

INTRODUCTION

Data on the epidemiology of dementia are largely limited to old-age dementia in developed countries [1,2,3], although attention has lately been directed towards the developing world [3,4]. The evidence from several studies gives a clear picture. The frequency is rather high and increases steeply with age. The most striking fact about the epidemiology of Alzheimer's disease (AD) is the exponential increase in incidence with age (see Figure 1). The Baltimore longitudinal study of aging examined the incidence rates of AD among 1236 participants over 3 years [5]. Incidence rates of AD increased from 0.08% per year (95% CI 0.00 to 0.43) in the 60 to 65 age group to 6.48% per year (95% CI 5.01 to 8.38) in the 85+ age group for men and women combined. The doubling time of incidence rates was estimated to be approximately 4.4 years. Data from the Cache county study [6] and other epidemiological data also seem to demonstrate that incidence doubles every 4-5 years. Data are also available about the relative frequency in men and women and the importance of various risk factors. Female gender and fewer years of education are associated with higher incidence rates [5]. Nevertheless, much remains to be clarified. An interesting but yet unresolved issue is whether the incidence of AD continues to rise in the same rate in the tenth decade and beyond. The underlying mechanisms predict that the incidence would continue to rise [6], but data are lacking to substantiate this suggestion. The issue is of course very important because of the aging of the population and the number of centenarians.

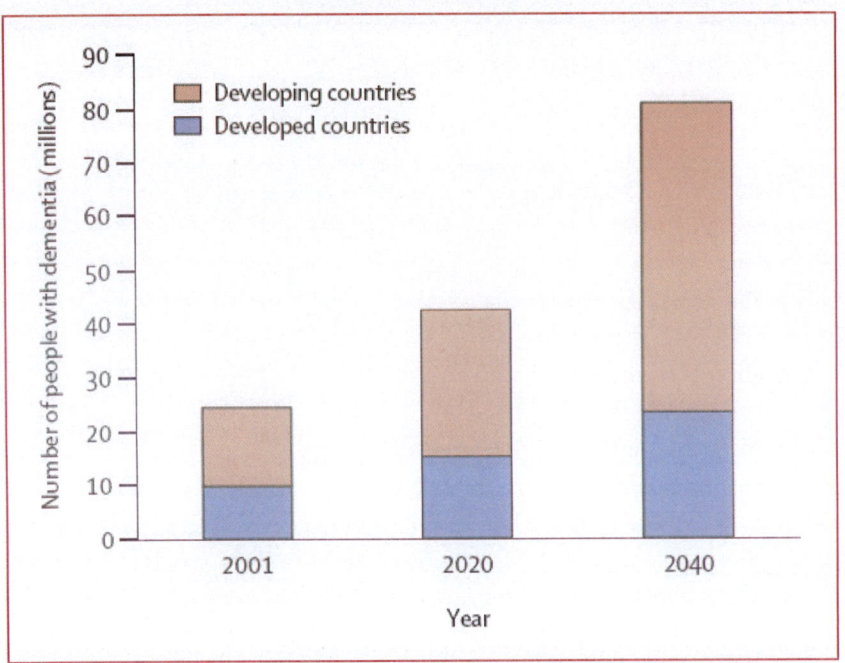

Figure 1. Number of people with dementia in developed and developing countries. (From: Ferri CP Global prevalence of dementia: a Delphi consensus study. The Lancet 2005, 366, 2112-2117)

DEFINITIONS

Diagnostic criteria for dementing disorders are still not quite acceptable. The main difficulty is that the definition of dementia is largely based on the concept of AD as a progressive disorder starting with memory impairment. However, the disease may begin with aphasia, behavioral disturbances or a dysexecutive syndrome [7]. Such patients may have, at least initially, relatively preserved memory and thus may not fulfill the formal diagnostic criteria, such as those of the DSM [8].

The transition from normal cognition to dementia is rarely abrupt. Most cases develop insidiously, and the decision when they become demented is arbitrary. The concepts of age associated memory impairment (AAMI), mild cognitive impairment (MCI) and cognitively impaired not demented (CIND), which are popular in the last 20 years, illustrate this point. The transition from any of these to frank dementia may reflect not only biological processes but also environmental influences.

The borders between normal aging and MCI on the one hand, and between MCI and dementia on the other, are arbitrary and quantitative rather than biological or qualitative. The disease states underlying dementia cannot be accurately identified in vivo, lacking validated biological markers, particularly such which can be used in large scale epidemiological studies. This makes data on prevalence of MCI, AD or vascular dementia (VaD) inaccurate.

VASCULAR CONTRIBUTION TO DEMENTIA

A lot of attention has been focused on the subtypes of dementia and their risk factors. One important point of interest is the recognition that VaD and AD are usually not separate entities, since they overlap in risk factors, clinical manifestations and pathology (and even treatment) [9]. These entities are considered to be the most common forms of dementia, and several attempts have been made to define each [8,10-13] and to distinguish between them. However, the clinical distinction between these two nosological entities is impossible, particularly in epidemiologic studies [9,14,15]. Because AD as well as atherosclerosis are age-dependent disorders, and because they are both so common, they inevitably occur together very frequently. The onset of dementia is typically insidious in AD, but even when vascular damage underlies the cognitive decline or contributes to it, this does not necessarily take a "step-like" onset or course [16]. In cases of insidious cognitive decline it may be impossible to decide about the underlying pathology, which in cases lacking clear clinical evidence of strokes, is traditionally attributed to AD [17], although in reality many of these cases have unsuspected vascular lesions in the brain [18].

Vascular lesions to the brain are frequently asymptomatic, and the distinction between a primary neurodegenerative process such as AD and vascular brain damage cannot always be made even by pathologists. (There are several reasons why pathologists cannot accurately diagnose either VaD or AD [19]).

The suggestion that many cases diagnosed as VaD are actually due to mixed (degenerative-vascular) etiology [9] is supported by three lines of evidence. Undoubtedly AD is a generalized brain disorder. In the cortex, widespread neuronal loss occurs accompanied (or preceded) by loss of synapses, leading to shrinking of the brain and increased sulcal width. This generalized process, however, is primarily observed in the parietal and temporal lobes. The main histopathologic changes, depositions of amyloid and accumulation of neurofibrillary tangles, are similarly pronounced in these regions, although not following an identical pattern. While these changes are the hallmark of the pathological diagnosis of AD such as the Khachaturian or CERAD criteria (see Tables 1, 2) [20-22], these are by themselves insufficient. There is no biological dividing line between the identical changes that are the inevitable consequences of aging, and any separation is arbitrary. In fact, it is well known that many elderly may harbor identical changes without showing cognitive changes [23]. While these ubiquituous changes are seen as pathognomonic for AD (and they are, by definition of the disorder), the fact that they can occur in non-demented elderly people poses an important question. If these changes are necessary but insufficient to cause dementia of the Alzheimer type, what are the added pathological changes that are required to produce dementia? The answer, in many cases, is that vascular ischemic changes to the brain may tip the balance towards the development of cognitive decline. One possible hint was provided by the famous "Nun study" [24]. In this study, many elderly nuns who came to autopsy had the brain changes required for a pathological diagnosis of AD, but only about half of those have been diagnosed as demented when examined before death. The two subgroups, those with and those without dementia, did not differ significantly by the amount of deposited amyloid or the load of neurofibrillary tangles, but rather by the co-occurrence of vascular lesions to their brains, sometimes quite discrete. It is possible that the small vascular lesions identified were actually just an indicator of a more widespread vascular damage to the brain interfering with cerebral blood supply and metabolism. This damage could be generalized or more restricted, e.g. limited to the medial temporal lobes and basal forebrain. Thus, vascular lesions to the brain must be an important factor causing dementia, frequently on the background of Alzheimer changes.

Table 1. *Khachaturian autopsy criteria for the diagnosis of AD

• In any patient *less than 50 years of age*, the number of senile or neuritic plaques and of neurofibrillary tangles anywhere in the neocortex should exceed two to five per field (1 sq mm microscopic magnification x 200 field).
• In any patient *between the ages of 50 and 65 years*, there may be some neurofibrillary tangles, but the number of senile plaques must be eight or more per field.
• For any *patient between 66 and 75 years of age*, some neurofibrillary tangles may again be present, but the number of senile plaques must be greater than ten per field.
• In any patient *greater than 75 years old*, neurofibrillary tangles may sometimes not be found in the neocortex, but the number of senile plaques should exceed 15 per microscopic field.

*Khachaturian [20].

The classical view of VaD as being associated with step-like deteriorations obviously does not cover the full spectrum of the disease. Clinically evident strokes typically cause identifiable motor or sensory deficits (and sometimes "cognitive" changes such as aphasia or apraxia); however their association with insidious cognitive decline is more complex. In many cases the cognitive changes are only identified, and possibly develop, slowly over weeks or months after the occurrence of a stroke [25]. However, another type of vascular cognitive syndrome, first described by Binswanger [26], is related to progressive white matter lesions due to very small ischemic changes, such as on the basis of diabetes mellitus [27] and lipohyalinosis. Although Binswanger suggested that such white matter changes are sufficient, by themselves, to impair cognition, similar lesions can frequently be seen on CT or MRI imaging in cognitively intact individuals, particularly in old age or on the background of hypertension or diabetes mellitus [28]. The cognitive features seen in some subjects who underwent strokes can only partially be explained by the size or location of the ischemic lesions; additional factors must contribute, which are largely elusive.

Table 2. CERAD neuropathology diagnostic criteria for Alzheimer's disease

Normal (with respect to AD or other dementing processes)	No histologic evidence of Alzheimer's disease (age-related plaque score is allowed), with or without history of dementia.
Definite	(age-related plaque score is allowed), with or without history of dementia.
Probable	An age-related plaque score (histologic findings SUGGEST the diagnosis of Alzheimer's disease) *and* clinical history of dementia, *and* presence or absence of other neuropathologic disorders likely to cause dementia.
Possible	An age-related plaque score that indicates or suggests the diagnosis of Alzheimer's disease and presence or absence of clinical manifestations of dementia.

The central role of the hippocampus in memory processes has led to particular examination of changes to this structure in demented individuals. Indeed, medial temporal (or hippocampal) atrophic changes are the earliest pathological changes in AD [29], and are constantly seen in AD patients on imaging. Unfortunately these imaging changes too are not specific to AD but seen very frequently in cases fulfilling VaD diagnostic criteria [30].

A third cardinal manifestation of AD is the loss of neurons in the nucleus basalis of Meynert [31]. These cholinergic cells in the basal forebrain are the origin of much of the cholinergic innervation of the cerebral cortex and their degeneration leads to cholinergic deficiency, which presumably is responsible for, or at least contributes to, the cognitive deficits. This deficiency forms the basis of the therapy of AD with cholinesterase inhibitors. However, similar changes can be seen frequently in patients fulfilling diagnostic criteria for VaD [32,33]. Therefore it is likely that those Alzheimer changes are also important contributing factors in VaD.

Neuroimaging plays a central role in the diagnosis of dementia subtypes. Its primary role is to identify lesions that could cause cognitive impairment (tumor, subdural hematomas or hydrocephalus). Brain neuroimaging is also sensitive in diagnosing vascular lesions, but has many of the same limitations as pathological examinations, namely inability to determine the time at which the changes have appeared and particularly unable to determine the relationship to the cognitive decline - causative, contributory or coincidental. The frequent identification of white matter lesions in patients otherwise diagnosed as suffering from AD [34,35] is of special relevance to the present discussion, since the lesions are predominantly due to vascular causes, suggesting that vascular factors are involved in classical AD [36]. In addition to coexistent atherosclerosis, these may either be due to perivascular amyloid deposits.

One central problem of the neuroimaging studies in dementia in general, and VaD in particular, is that specific lesions that can account for cognitive decline are rarely demonstrated. The general approach in diagnostic guidelines such as the DSM or the National Institute of Neurological Disorders and Stroke and Association Internationale pour la Recherche et l'Enseignement en Neurosciences (NINDS-AIREN) criteria is that VaD should be diagnosed if stroke-related changes are seen on neuroimaging. These changes should, *in the judgment of the clinician*, be responsible for the cognitive changes. Unfortunately no directive is provided to assist in the evaluation of the presumed relationship.

In conclusion, most patients diagnosed as VaD actually have evidence of hippocampal atrophy and cortical cholinergic deficiency, both typically regarded as markers of AD. Demented patients with vascular brain disease frequently have some degree of amyloid deposits and neurofibrillary changes which, even if insufficient to fulfill the arbitrary criteria set for the diagnosis of AD, may nevertheless contribute to the cognitive changes. Like the AD changes, the vascular damage may develop slowly and impair neuronal metabolism and function, eventually causing cell death. Similarly, cases with full-blown AD frequently have coexistent lacunes or white matter changes.

The frequency of mixed dementia may be under-estimated because of the lack of criteria for this disorder. The common diagnostic criteria for AD and VaD, like those in the DSM IV and the ICD-10, are mutually exclusive, while the NINDS-AIREN criteria [12] specifically forbid the use of the term mixed dementia. Nevertheless, the term continues to be used and in fact its use seemingly increases.

If the differential diagnosis between VaD and AD is questionable, no widely accepted tools are available to separate out fronto-temporal dementia (FTD). FTD is considered by some to be the second most common cause of dementia [37,38], but even if the true frequency is lower, it is still significant. Most if not all epidemiological studies looking for risk factors for AD have included FTD cases, thus reducing the power of these studies.

Another consideration relates to infective dementias. Syphilis, once a common cause of dementia, has largely disappeared whereas HIV-related dementia becomes a common disorder in some communities. The dementias accompanying other neurodegenerative diseases, such as Parkinson's disease and multiple sclerosis also receive more attention lately [39,40].

RISK FACTORS

The study of risk factors for dementia suffers from the lack of diagnostic instruments, but in addition is limited because of unreliable data regarding the onset time. Many researchers believe that AD starts several years prior to the appearance of even the earliest clinical signs. This means that when performing studies on risk factors for AD in incidence studies, the "normal" control group is likely to include a substantial number of preclinical AD cases. Depending on the age of the study population, this may significantly jeopardize any conclusion reached; particularly negative results should be viewed with suspicion.

Retrospective data collection is associated with reporter bias, and this may be considerable, especially since the reporter is cognitively impaired and the control not.

Several epidemiological studies have attempted to identify risk factors for AD. In younger people, this was very rewarding by identifying several genetic mutations that can cause the disease, in the amyloid precursor protein (APP) gene on chromosome 21, on the presenilin 1 (PS1) gene on chromosome 14, and on the presenilin 2 gene on chromosome 1. Together these mutations account for approximately half of the familial early-onset AD cases [41]. Their identification had huge importance on the understanding of the biochemical pathways leading to AD, and also on therapeutic attempts.

In elderly people, dementia is more commonly sporadic. However, information on familiality is limited because data on illness among parents is frequently inaccessible or inaccurate. Nevertheless it is usually agreed that there is a genetic background although its effect is smaller than in early onset AD. Among the genetic factors responsible for dementia in old age, only one has been definitely identified so far, apolipoprotein E ε4 (APOE4) [42]. Remarkable, APOE4 is a factor also in other neurodegenerative diseases [43]. While APOE4 is usually considered a risk factor for AD, a more correct interpretation of the data is that it advances the age of onset of the disease. People with AD who carry the APOE4 haplotype have an earlier onset age than those who do not carry APOE4 (this of course translates to higher prevalence of dementia among APOE4 carriers in any given age). However, other factors must operate to cause cognitive decline on the genetic background of each person.

A long list of factors have been identified which have a higher prevalence among AD cases than in controls, and many have been confirmed as risk factors also in prospective studies. The most remarkable finding is that several of these are cardiovascular risk factors as well (see Table 3). The commonality of risk factors for dementia (including cases diagnosed clinically as either "pure AD" or as VaD), for vascular disease in general and for stroke in particular is of great interest, since this has not been anticipated. Data are still not available regarding some vascular risk factors and how they relate to dementia, including sleep apnea and migraine.

Table 3. Established risk factors for dementia

- Age
- Female sex
- Head trauma
- Low level of education
- Smoking
- Diabetes mellitus
- Hypertension
- Apolipoprotein E status
- Coronary artery disease
- High dietary saturated fat and cholesterol
- Midlife cholesterol
- Hyperhomocysteinemia
- History of depression

Of the so-called risk factors identified for dementia, differentiation has to be made between real risk factors, risk indicators, and disease manifestations. Several genetic markers for the disease have been identified [41], but yet these cannot be changed. Others, like mid-life hypertension and hyperlipidemia [44], behave as risk factors. They can of course be treated but although it is possible to assume that normalization of these values will reduce the incidence of dementia, the evidence in this direction is incomplete. Coronary artery disease [44-46] is likely to behave as a risk indicator rather than a risk factor, while falls in the elderly may be a manifestation of the disease process itself [47].

The relationship of smoking to AD has been controversial for many years. Several large epidemiological studies initially came up with results supporting an inverse relationship between smoking and the *prevalence* of AD, concluding that smoking protects against dementia. Other studies, however, suggested that the AD *incidence* is actually <u>higher</u> among smokers [48]. There is no clear theoretical reason to assume the existence of either a positive or negative relationship between smoking and AD, and these results were interpreted in different ways. For example, data are available from autopsy studies showing a decrease of brain nicotinic receptors in AD [31,49], and attempts are being made to treat AD patients with nicotinic agonists. Smoking is a known risk factor for vascular disease in general, frequently affecting the brain, as well as for coronary artery disease, which itself is associated with AD [50].

One possible explanation for the difference between prevalence studies (showing a lower AD frequency among smokers) and incidence studies (suggesting that smoking is a risk factor for AD) is reduced survival of AD patients who are also smokers. This issue is yet not completely resolved.

TRAUMATIC BRAIN INJURY AS A RISK FACTOR FOR ALZHEIMER'S DISEASE

Dementia developing late following head trauma is described in the medical literature for at least 50 years both on a histological autopsy level and on a clinical level [51]. The first case-control studies to demonstrate an association between traumatic brain injury (TBI) and AD were by Heyman, Mortimer and their colleagues [52,53] respectively. The well-recognized condition in boxers, *dementia pugilistica*, has prompted research activity to determine whether and by what mechanisms TBI and AD may be linked.

If, in fact, TBI can lead to AD (usually after a long period of apparent complete or partial recovery from the trauma), this may be of significant theoretical and practical interest. The main question is: what pathophysiologic processes or cascades are triggered by brain injury which then continue to operate and cause further insidiously progressive brain damage? If these processes are identified this could open up avenues for pharmacologic intervention (for example anti-inflammatory, anti-glutamatergic or anti-apoptotic therapy), which could be generalized also to prevent dementia not related to trauma.

Mechanisms which may act synergistically or consequentially following brain trauma include: (1) damage to cholinergic pathways, (2) an inflammatory process, (3) amyloid beta (Aβ) deposition, (4) tau pathology, (5) APOE4 genotype, and (6) lipid peroxidation.

There are many methodological problems and sources of bias in studies examining the role of TBI as a risk factor for AD, including recall and reporter bias, a lack of consistent scoring systems for TBI, and diagnostic criteria for AD.

Firstly, retrospective studies rely on recall of head injury events that may have occurred decades earlier, while for individuals with more severe cognitive impairment a proxy history needs to be taken.

A lack of consistent scoring systems for assessing the severity of head injury and unreliable information on duration of loss of consciousness limit the ability to ascertain a dose-response relationship, although some studies have in fact demonstrated such a relationship [54,55]. Importantly, it should be noted that the severity or "dose" of TBI is measured by the duration of unconsciousness. Thus, it is the *effect* of the trauma, in particular on the brain-stem, rather than the trauma itself, which is being scored. The cognitive changes, however, may be the result of involvement of cortical or subcortical hemispheric damage (such as the cholinergic pathways), rather than the brain-stress.

Prospective follow-up cohort studies eliminate some of the biases above but many of these studies lack the necessary statistical power to detect the association of head injury with AD [53]. Many case-control studies show an association between TBI and AD. Heyman et al [52] performed a case-control study on 40 patients with onset of AD (diagnosed according to rigorous clinical criteria) prior to age 70 and from 80 community control subjects. A history of TBI was obtained significantly more often among the patients (15%) than among the controls (3.8%). The odds ratio (OR), calculated by logistic regression, was 5.31. With the exception of thyroid disease among female patients or a family history of dementia no other associations were found. Similar results were obtained by Mortimer et al. [53], Rasmusson et al. [56] and Salib and Hillier [57] (only amongst the male subjects), while other case-control studies, however, demonstrated no association [58-62].

Mortimer et al. [63] performed a meta-analysis of clinical trials demonstrating a pooled relative risk for head trauma of 1.82 (95%, CI: 1.26 to 2.67).

Prospective studies have the advantage of eliminating some of the biases associated with retrospective or cross-sectional studies. However, they too have limitations. In particular, if registry data are used, the data are not collected for the purpose of the study and there may well be missing information. Nevertheless, some prospective studies have shown a positive association between head injury and AD, for example [64] (more than threefold) and [55] (hazard ratio [HR] nearly 5). Other prospective studies have found no evidence to support the hypothesis that head injury is a risk factor for AD or dementia [65-69].

Breteler et al. [67] performed a 9 year follow-up study comparing a patient group of people aged 50-75 with a history of Parkinson's disease (PD), epilepsy or severe TBI (patients with no explicit mention of loss of consciousness or intracranial injury were excluded) to a control group based on the linked databases of three Dutch nationwide morbidity registers. Although a significant relative risk was found for epilepsy and PD, severe TBI was not associated with an increased risk of dementia (RR = 1.0, 95% CI 0.9-1.1). This study examined dementia incidence in general (not specifically AD).

Nemetz et al. [69] did not demonstrate a higher incidence overall in subjects post TBI versus controls. 1,283 traumatic brain injury cases were followed over 40 years. 31 developed AD, giving a standardized incidence ratio of 1.2, 95% confidence interval 0.8-1.7. However, the observed time from traumatic brain injury to AD was less than the expected time to onset of AD (median = 10 years, expected = 18 years, p = 0.015).

Mayeux et al [70] suggested a synergistic relationship between TBI and APOE4 on the risk of developing AD. Head injury in subjects not possessing an APOE4 allele was not associated with an increased risk of AD. With APOE4 alone there was a 2-fold increase in risk but there was a 10-fold increase in the risk of AD in people carrying two APOE4 alleles and a history of TBI. Some authors have demonstrated a worse clinical outcome and poorer recovery after TBI associated with the APOE4 genotype [71-73].

NEUROPSYCHOLOGICAL CONSEQUENCES OF TBI

Many studies have shown different measures of memory and attention impairments following TBI. These include impairments in strategic planning and prospective memory [74], sustained attention [75] and 'pre-attentive' deficits [76]. These neuropsychological deficits result in functional and psychosocial problems that may be just as significant following moderate head injury as severe head injury [77]. Many sports result in repetitive mild TBI and the condition *dementia pugilistica* demonstrates a relationship between concussion and neuropsychological decline in professional boxers [78]. This relationship has later been demonstrated in American football players [79] and professional soccer players [80].

POST-MORTEM AND HISTOLOGICAL STUDIES

In a post-mortem series of 152 patients who died between 4 hours to 2.5 years after a severe TBI, approximately 30% showed intracerebral deposition of β-amyloid ($A\beta$) in one or more cortical areas. Increasing age seemed to accentuate the extent of $A\beta$ deposition [81]. The presence of large numbers of 'diffuse' non-congophilic $A\beta$ plaques with little or no neuritic component observed in post-traumatic dementia is similar to that observed in the brains of boxers with *dementia pugilistica* [82]. This supports the hypothesis of TBI having an etiologic role in AD (at least in early onset post-traumatic AD).

Ikonomovic et al. [83] used immunohistochemical techniques to determine the extent of AD-related changes in temporal cortex resected from 18 subjects (ages 18-64 years) who were treated surgically for severe TBI. Diffuse cortical $A\beta$ deposits were observed in one third of subjects (aged 35 - 62 years) as early as 2 hours after injury, with only one (35-year old) individual exhibiting "mature", dense-cored plaques. In plaque-positive cases, the only statistically significant change in cellular immunostaining was increased neuronal APP. There was no significant correlation between the distribution of $A\beta$ plaques and markers of neuronal degeneration (tau, ubiquitin and synuclein). Tau-positive, NFT-like changes were detected in only two subjects, both of more advanced age and who were without $A\beta$ deposits.

A battery of antisera that specifically stained the tangles in AD brains also stained the tangles in cases of *dementia pugilistica* [84] thus suggesting a common pathogenesis. However, Hof et al. [85] found that in dementia pugilistica cases, NFT were concentrated in the superficial layers in the neocortex, whereas in AD they predominated in the deep layers. Thus an inverse NFT distribution as compared to AD in the association cortex of brains from dementia pugilistica patients was demonstrated. Some studies have shown that the hippocampus is sensitive to mild head injury [86,87].

Although clinically and experimentally most work has been focused on acute severe head injury there is now increasing interest in repetitive mild TBI (rmTBI). Although no acute deterioration in cognitive test performance was found in participants in a 7-day amateur boxing tournament, with the exception of 7 out of 82 participants whose contest was stopped by the referee [88], it is possible that the effects of rmTBI are cumulative over a longer period of time as in dementia pugilistica.

Thus there is convincing evidence of similarities in the neuropathological processes that follow brain trauma with those seen in AD. It is still not quite clear how this processes are triggered by the trauma, but the similarity suggests the possibility that interventions against the neurodegeneration following head trauma may also be applicable in spontaneous neurodegeneration.

CONCLUSIONS

Dementia is a multifactional syndrome, most common in the elderly. In this age-group, most patients have a mixed pathogenesis. While the risk factors of the neurodegenerative processes are largely unknown, a large amount of data has been accumulated during the past two decades to indicate an important contribution of vascular risk factors for the cognitive deterioration. These work, presumably, through vascular damage to the brain that enhances the effects of the neurodegenerative processes. While there is not much that can be done, at present, to slow the neurodegenerative process, there is a lot of data indicating how the vascular components can be manipulated. Such methods have proved successful in reduction of cardiovascular mortality. Assuming that a similar effect can delay the onset of dementia by five years, the age-specific prevalence rates will be reduced by one half or more.

Better understanding of the mechanisms underlying progressive brain degeneration and cognitive decline following head trauma is important since it may well indicate processes which also operate in similar degenerative changes not triggered by trauma.

REFERENCES

[1] Rocca WA, Amaducci LA, Schoenberg BS. Epidemiology of clinically diagnosed Alzheimer's disease. *Ann Neurol* 1986; 19:415-424.

[2] Rocca WA, Hofman A, Brayne C, et al. The prevalence of vascular dementia in Europe: facts and fragments from 1980-1990 studies. *Ann Neurol* 1991; 30:817-824.

[3] Ferri CP, Prince M, Brayne C, et al. Global prevalence of dementia: a Delphi consensus study. *Lancet* 2005; 366:2112-2117.

[4] Kalaria RN. Dementia comes of age in the developing world. *Lancet* 2003; 361:888-889.

[5] Kawas C, Gray S, Brookmeyer R, Fozard J, Zonderman S. Age-specific incidence rates of Alzheimer's disease: the Baltimore Longitudinal Study of Ageing. *Neurology* 2000; 54:2072-2077.

[6] Miech RA, Breitner JC, Zandi PP, Khachaturian AS, Anthony JC, Mayer L. Incidence of AD may decline in the early 90s for men, later for women: The Cache County study. *Neurology* 2002; 58:209-218.

[7] Petersen RC. Clinical subtypes of Alzheimer's disease. *Dement Geriatr Cogn Disord* 1998; 9:16-24.

[8] American Psychiatric Association. *Diagnostic and Statistical Manual of Mental Disorders* (DSM-IV). Washington, D.C. 1994.

[9] Korczyn AD. Mixed dementia - the most common cause of dementia. *Ann NY Acad Sci* 2002; 977:129-134.

[10] McKahnn G, Drachman D, Folstein M, Katzman R, Price D. Clinical diagnosis of Alzheimer's disease: Report of NINCDS-ADRDA Work Group under the auspices of the Department of Health and Human Services Task Force on Alzheimer's disease. *Neurology* 1984; 34:939-944.

[11] Chui HC, Victoroff JI, Margolin D, Jagust W. Criteria for the diagnosis of ischemic vascular dementia proposed by the State of California Alzheimer's disease diagnostic and treatment centers. *Neurology* 1992; 42:473-480.

[12] Roman GC, Tatemichi TK, Erkinjuntti T, et al. Vascular dementia: Diagnostic criteria for research studies. *Neurology* 1993; 43:250-260.

[13] Rockwood K, Stadnyk K. The prevalence of dementia in the elderly: a review. *Can J Psychiatry* 1994; 39:253-257.

[14] Wallin A. The overlap between Alzheimer's disease and vascular dementia: the role of white matter changes. *Dement Geriatr Cogn Disord* 1998; 1:30-35.

[15] Kalaria RN, Ballard C. Overlap between pathology of Alzheimer's disease and vascular dementia. *Alzheimer Dis Assoc Disord* 1999;13:S115-123.

[16] Aharon-Peretz J, Daskovski E, Mashiach T, Tomer R. Natural history of dementia associated with lacunar infarctions. *J Neurol Sci*. 2002; 203-204:53-5.

[17] Nussbaum M, Treves TA, Korczyn AD. DSM-III-R criteria for primary degenerative dementia and multi-infact dementia. *Alzheimer Dis Assoc Disord* 1992; 6:111-118.

[18] Jellinger K, Danielczyk W, Fischer P, Gabriel E. Clinicopathological analysis of dementia disorders in the elderly. *J Neurol Sci* 1990; 95:239-258.

[19] Korczyn AD. The complex nosological concept of vascular dementia. *J Neurol Sci* 2002; 203-204:3-6.

[20] Khachaturian ZS. Diagnosis of Alzheimer's disease. *Arch Neurol* 1985; 42:1097-1105.

[21] Mirra SS, Heyman A, McKeel D, et al. The consortium to establish a registry for Alzheimer's disease (CERAD). Part II. Standardization of the neuropathologic assessment of Alzheimer's disease. *Neurology* 1991; 41:479-486.

[22] Mirra SS, Gearing M, Hughes J, et al. Interlaboratory comparison of neuropathology assessments in Alzheimer's disease: A study of the Consortium to Establish a Registry for Alzheimer's Disease (CERAD). *J Neuropath Exp Neurol* 1994; 53:303-315.

[23] Knopman DS, Parisi JE, Salviati A, et al. Neuropathology of cognitively normal elderly. *J Neuropathol Exp Neurol* 2003; 62:1087-1095.

[24] Snowdon DA, Greiner LH, Mortimer JA, Riley KP, Greiner PA, Markesbery WR. Brain infarction and the clinical expression of Alzheimer's disease. The Nun Study. *JAMA* 1997; 277:813-817.

[25] Treves TA, Aronovich BD, Bornstein NM, Korczyn AD. Risk of dementia after a first-ever ischemic stroke: A 3 year longitudinal study. *Cerebrovasc Dis* 1997; 7:48-52.

[26] Roman GC. Senile dementia of the Binswanger type. A vascular form of dementia in the elderly. *JAMA* 1987; 258:1782-1788.

[27] Biessels GJ, Stackenborg S, Brunner E, Brayne C, Scheltens P. Risk of dementia in diabetes mellitus: a systematic review. *Lancet Neurol* 2006; 5:64-74.

[28] Hachinski VC, Potter P, Merskey H. Leucoaraiosis. *Arch Neurol* 1987; 44:21-23

[29] Braak H, Braak E. Neuropathological stageing of Alzheimer-related changes. *Acta Neuropathol* 1991; 82:239-259.

[30] Barber R, Gholkar A, Scheltens P, Ballard C, McKeith IG, O'Brien JT. Medial temporal lobe atrophy on MRI in dementia with Lewy bodies. *Neurology* 1999; 52:1153-1158.

[31] Whitehouse P. Clinical and neurochemical consequences of neuronal loss in the nucleus basalis of Meynert in Parkinson's disease and Alzheimer's disease. *Adv Neurol* 1987; 45:393-397.

[32] Perry EK, Perry RH, Smith CJ, et al. Nicotinic receptor abnormalities in Alzheimer's and Parkinson's disease. *J Neurol Neurosurg Psychiatry* 1987; 50:806-809.

[33] Gottfries CG, Blennow K, Karlsson I, Wallin A. The neurochemistry of vascular dementia. *Dementia* 1994; 5:163-167.

[34] Brun A, Englund E. A white matter disorder in dementia of the Alzheimer type: a pathoanatomical study. *Ann Neurol* 1986; 19:253-262.

[35] Rezek DL, Morris JC, Fulling KH, Gado MH. Periventricular white matter lucencies in senile dementia of the Alzheimer type and in normal aging. *Neurology* 1987; 37:1365-1368.

[36] de la Torre JC. Alzheimer disease as a vascular disorder: Nosological evidence. *Stroke* 2002; 33:1-3.

[37] Neary D, Snowden J, Man D. Frontotemporal dementia. *Lancet* 2005; 4:771-780.

[38] Ikeda M, Ishikawa T, Tanabe H. Epidemiology of frontotemporal lobar degeneration. *Dement Geriatr Cogn Disord* 2005; 17:265-268.

[39] Korczyn AD. Dementia in Parkinson's disease. *J Neurol* 2001; 248 (Suppl 3):III/1-III/4.

[40] Calabrese P. Neuropsychology of multiple sclerosis--an overview. *J Neurol* 2006; 253:110-115.

[41] Cacabelos R. Diagnosis of Alzheimer's disese: defining genetic profiles (genotype vs phenotype). *Acta Neurol Scand* 1996; 165:72-84.

[42] Roses AD, Saunders AM. APOE is a major susceptibility gene for Alzheimer's disease. *Curr Opin Biotechnol* 1994; 5:663-667.

[43] Chapman J, Korczyn AD, Karussis DM, Michaelson DM. The effects of APOE genotype on age at onset and progression of neurodegenerative diseases. *Neurology* 2001; 57:1482.

[44] Kivipelto M, Halkala EL, Laakso MP, Hanninen T, Hallikainen M, Alhainen K, Soininen H, Tuomilehto J, Nissinen A. Midlife vascular risk factors and Alzheimer's disease in later life: longitudinal, population based study. *BMJ* 2001; 322:1447-1451.

[45] Kalaria RN. Vascular factors in Alzheimer's disease. *International Psychogeriatrics* 2003; 15:47-52.

[46] Newman AB, Fitzpatrick AL, Lopez O, Jackson S, Lyketsos C, Jagust W, Ives D, Dekosky ST, Kuller LH. Dementia and Alzheimer's disease incidence in relationship to cardiovascular disease in the Cardiovascular Health Study cohort. *J Am Geriatr Soc* 2005; 53:1101-1107.

[47] Giladi N Mordechovich M, Gruendlinger L, Shabtai H, Merims D, Naor S, Baltadzhieva R, Hausdorff JM, Gur AY, Bornstein NM. "Brain Screen": A self-referral, screening program for strokes, fall and dementia risk factors. *J Neurol* 2006; 253:307-315.

[48] Letenneur L, Larrieu S, Barberger-Gateau P. Alcohol and tobacco consumption as risk factors of dementia: a review of epidemiological studies. *Biomed Pharmacother.* 2004; 58:95-99.

[49] Whitehouse PJ, Au KS. Cholinergic receptors in aging and Alzheimer's disease. *Prog Neuropsychopharmacol Biol Psychiatry* 1986; 10:665-676.

[50] Breteler MM, Bots ML, Ott A, Hofman A. Risk factors for vascular disease and dementia. *Haemostasis* 1998; 28:167-173.

[51] Corsellis JA, Brierley JB. Observations on the pathology of insidious dementia following head injury. *J Ment Sci* 1959; 105:714-720.

[52] Heyman A, Wilkinson WE, Stafford JA, et al. Alzheimer's disease: a study of epidemiological aspects. *Ann Neurol* 1984; 15:335-341.

[53] Mortimer JA, French LR, Hutton JT, et al. Head injury as a risk factor for Alzheimer's disease. *Neurology* 1985; 35:264-267.

[54] Guo Z, Cupples LA, Kurz A, Auerbach SH, Volicer L, Chui H, Green RC, Sadovnick AD, Duara R, DeCarli C, Johnson KA, Go RC, Crowdon JH, Haines JL, Kukull WA, Farrer LA. Head injury and the risk of AD in the MIRAGE study. *Neurology* 2000; 54:1316-1323.

[55] Plassman BL, Havlik RJ, Steffens DC, et al. Documented head injury in early adulthood and risk of Alzheimer's disease and other dementias. *Neurology* 2000; 55:1158-1166.

[56] Rasmusson DX, Brandt J, Martin DB, Folsdtein MF. Head injury as a risk factor in Alzheimer's disease. *Brain Inj* 1995; 9:213-219.

[57] Salib E, Hillier V. Head injury and the risk of Alzheimer's disease: a case control study. *Int J Geriatr Psychiatry* 1997; 12:363-368.

[58] Chandra V, Kokmen E, Schoenberg BS, Beard CM, Head trauma with loss of consciousness as a risk factor for Alzheimer's disease. *Neurology* 1989; 39:1575-1578.

[59] Aronson MK, Ooi WL, Morgenstern H, et al. Women, myocardial infarction, and dementia in the very old. *Neurology* 1990; 40:1102-1106.

[60] Fratiglioni L, Ahlbom A, Viitanen M, Winblad B, Risk factors for late-onset Alzheimer's disease: a population-based, case-control study. *Ann Neurol* 1993; 33:258-266.

[61] Li G, Shen YC, Li YT, Chen CH, Zhau YW, Silverman JM. A case-control study of Alzheimer's disease in China. *Neurology* 1992; 42:1481-1488.

[62] Mendez MF, Underwood KL, Zander BA, Mastri AR, Sung JH, Frey WH. Risk factors in Alzheimer's disease; a clinicopathologic study. *Neurology* 1992; 42:770-775.

[63] Mortimer JA, van Duijn CM, Chandra V, et al. Head trauma as a risk factor for Alzheimer's disease: a collaborative re-analysis of case-control studies. *Int J Epidemiol* 1991; 20:S28-S35.

[64] Schofield PW, Tang MX, Marder K, Bell K, Dooneief G, Chun M, Sano M, Stern Y, Mayeux R. Alzheimer's disease after remote head injury: an incidence study. *J Neurol Neurosurg Psychiatry* 1997; 62:119-124.

[65] Katzman R, Aronson M, Fuld P, et al. Development of dementing illnesses in an 80-year-old volunteer cohort. *Ann Neurol* 1989; 25:317-324.

[66] Williams DB, Annegers JK, Kokmen E, O'Brien PC, Kurland LT. Brain injury and neurologic sequelae: a cohort study of dementia, parkinsonism, and amyotrophic lateral sclerosis. *Neurology* 1991; 41:1554-1557.

[67] Breteler MMB, de Groot RR, van Romunde LK, Hofman A. Risk of dementia in patients with Parkinson's disease, epilepsy, and severe head trauma: a register-based follow-up study. *Am J Epidemiol* 1995; 142:1300-1305.

[68] Mehta KM, et al. Head trauma and risk of dementia and Alzheimer's disease: The Rotterdam Study. *Neurology* 1999; 53:1959-1959.

[69] Nemetz PN, Leibson C, Naessens JM, Beard M, Kokmen E, Annegers JF, Kurland LT. Traumatic brain injury and time to onset of Alzheimer's disease: a population-based study. *Am J Epidemiol* 1999; 149:32-40.

[70] Mayeux R, Ottman R, Maestre G, et al. Synergistic effects of traumatic head injury and apolipoprotein-epsilon 4 in patients with Alzheimer's disease. *Neurology* 1995; 45:555-557.

[71] Teasdale GM, Nicoll JA, Murray G, Fiddes M. Association of apolipoprotein E polymorphism with outcome after head injury. *Lancet* 1997; 350:1069-1071.

[72] Friedman LR, Froom P, Sazbon L, et al. Apolipoprotein E-epsilon4 genotype predicts a poor outcome in survivors of traumatic brain injury. *Neurology* 1999; 52:244-248.

[73] Lichtman SW, Seliger G, Tycko B, et al. Apolipoprotein E and functional recovery from brain injury following postacute rehabilitation. *Neurology* 2000; 55:1536-1539.

[74] Fortin S, Godbout L, Braun CM. Cognitive strurcture of executive deficits in frontally lesioned head trauma patients performing activities of daily living. *Cortex* 2003; 39:273-291.

[75] Robertson IH, Manly T, Andrade J, Baddeley BT, Yiend J. 'Oops!': performance correlates of everyday attentional failures in traumatic brain injured and normal subjects. *Neuropsychologia* 1997; 35:747-758.

[76] Polo MD, Newton P, Rogers D, Escera C, Butler S. ERPs and behavioural indices of long-term preattentive and attentive deficits after closed head injury. *Neuropsychologia* 2002; 40:2350-2359.

[77] Hellawell DJ, Taylor RT, Pentland B. Cognitive and psychosocial outcome following moderate or severe traumatic brain injury. *Brain Inj* 1999; 13:489-504.

[78] Corsellis JA. Boxing and the brain. *BMJ* 1989; 298:105-109.

[79] Collins MW, Grindel SH, Lovell MR, Dede DE, Moser DJ, Phalin BR, et al. Relationship between concussion and neuropsychological performance in college football players. *J Am Med Assoc* 1999; 282:964-970.

[80] Matser JT, Kessels AG, Lezak MD, Troost J. A dose-response relation of headers and concussions with cognitive impairment in professional soccer players. *J Clin Exp Neuropsychol* 2001; 23:770-774.

[81] Roberts GW, Gentleman SM, Lynch A, Murray L, Landon M, Graham DI. Beta amyloid protein deposition in the brain after severe head injury: implications for the pathogenesis of Alzheimer's disease. *J Neurol Neurosurg Psychiatry* 1994; 57:419-425.

[82] Clinton J, Ambler MW, Roberts GW. Post-traumatic Alzheimer's disease: preponderance of a single plaque type. *Neurpathol Appl Neurobiol* 1991; 17:69-74.

[83] Ikonomovic MD, Uryu K, Abrahamson EE, Ciallella JR, Trojanowski JQ, Lee VM, Clark RS, Marion DW, Wisniewski SR, Dekosky ST. Alzheimer's pathology in human temporal cortex surgically excised after severe brain injury. *Exp Neurol* 2004; 190:192-203.

[84] Roberts GW. Immunocytochemistry of neurofibrillary tangles in dementia pugilistica and Alzheimer's disease: evidence for common genesis. *Lancet* 1988; 2:8626-8627.

[85] Hof PR, Bouras C, Buee L, Delacourte A, Perl DP, Morrison JH. Differential distribution of neurofibrillary tangles in the cerebral cortex of dementia pagulistica and Alzheimer's disease cases. *Acta Neuropathol* 1992; 85:23-30.

[86] Lowenstein DH, Thomas MJ, Smith DH, McIntosh TK. Selective vulnerability of dentate hilar neurons following traumatic brain injury: a potential mechanistic link between head trauma and disorders of the hippocampus. *J Neurosci* 1992; 12:4846-4853.

[87] Lyeth BG, Jenkins LW, Hamm RJ, Dixon CE, Phillips LL, Clifton GL, et al. Prolonged memory impairment in the absenxce of hippocampal cell death following traumatic brain injury in the rat. *Brain* 1990; 526:249-258.

[88] Moriarity J, Collie A, Olson D, et al. A prospective controlled study of cognitive function during an amateur boxing tournament. *Neurology* 2004; 62:1497-1502.

RECOMMENDED FURTHER READING

1. Lichtenberg PA, Murman DL, Mellow AM (Editors). *Handbook of Dementia: Psychological, Neurological, and Psychiatric Perspectives.* Wiley, 2003.

2. Levesque L, Bird M, Meulemans, and Herrman F. *The Clinical Management of Early Alzheimer's Disease: A Handbook.* LEA, Inc., 2003.

3. Sink KM. Holden KF. Yaffe K. Pharmacological treatment of neuropsychiatric symptoms of dementia: a review of the evidence. JAMA. 293(5):596-608, 2005

4. Langa KM. Foster NL. Larson EB. Mixed dementia: emerging concepts and therapeutic implications. JAMA. 292(23):2901-8, 2004

5. Ritchie K. Lovestone S. The dementias. Lancet. 360(9347):1759-66, 2002

In: Handbook of Clinical Neuroepidemiology
Editors: V. L. Feigin and D. A. Bennett, pp. 197-232

ISBN 978-1-60021-511-7
© 2007 Nova Science Publishers, Inc.

Chapter 7

TRAUMATIC BRAIN INJURY

Hans von Holst

Department of Clinical Neuroscience, Section of Neurosurgery, Karolinska Institutet
Stockholm, Sweden;
School of Technology and Health, Royal Institute of Technology, Stockholm, Sweden.

ABSTRACT

The present chapter gives the non-specialist clinician an overview of traumatic brain injury, which is one of the most challenging problems to face worldwide as it remains a burden to patients, relatives and the society as a whole. The epidemiological pattern of traumatic brain injuries is described including an overview of the clinical pathophysiology after a mechanical impact. An outline of evidenced based practice is presented about recommendations of management at the scene of accident and on admission to the emergency hospital. Further, the neurosurgical and rehabilitation management of mild, moderate and severe traumatic brain injury is reviewed before prognosis and preventative strategies are discussed.

INTRODUCTION

Traumatic brain injury is a frequently occurring disease worldwide. The overall incidence pattern is not possible to define completely since many countries do not have access to an injury surveillance system. For the same reason, it is difficult to define the prevalence pattern of traumatic brain injury. A rough estimation can be performed in most industrialized countries. It is, however, not realistic to extrapolate these figures to the emerging and developing countries due to regional differences. In contrast to many other diseases, the etiology to traumatic brain injury is well known. The causes are to be found mainly in accidents due to traffic, falls, violence, and at leisure. Although there is an increased awareness from the society, the number of victims is still unacceptably high.

Further, with an increased aging population during the next decades, we can foresee a further increased number of falls resulting in traumatic brain injury. It is therefore important to collect data aiming at prevention of the disease together with finding the best evidence based medical treatment of choice. With an improved social standard and awareness of the disease, primary prevention will be the ultimate choice of activity in order to reduce the number.

In general traumatic brain injury is defined as mild, moderate and severe although there is a considerable overlap in the use of such terminology. About 80 % is defined as mild, 10 % to moderate and another 10 % to severe injuries. In contrast of most other diseases, it has a sudden onset with a substantial impact also on the patients close relatives. Except for the medical consequences, it should be looked upon as complicated from a psychological perspective since in many cases a personality change is shown and therefore difficult to handle for the relatives in its onset.

Although improvements in outcome have been presented during the last decades, there are significant differences in the medical treatment. The recommended treatment is predominately based on clinical practice and personal experience. With an increased interest in evidence-based medicine, we will face an even more comprehensive and generally accepted treatment of traumatic brain injuries resulting in an improved outcome. The present chapter gives a brief overview of what is known about traumatic brain injury and recommended treatment of choice.

EPIDEMIOLOGY

Incidence and Mortality Rates

Injury is the leading cause of death in youth and early middle age. It has become a substantial burden not only for the victim but also to the relatives and the society as a whole. The vast majority of these injuries are to be found in traffic, fall, violence, sport and recreational activities in combination with a large number of different risk factors. For instance, traffic related injuries are an increasing problem throughout the world, affecting both old industrial and new industrialized countries. A study from Harvard University, World Bank and World Health Organisation showed that traffic related injuries will be ranked third in terms of global burden of disease in coming decades, unless promotion and control of safety are given greater priority. The global burden is unequally distributed not only between continents but also between countries and within their different regions and communities. Certainly, the different epidemiological scenarios are, to some extent, caused by insufficient statistical data evaluation. The same disproportionate pattern holds true also among age and gender as well as economically and socially marginal groups. It has been estimated that in 2002 there were about 5 million deaths from injuries worldwide constituting about 9 % of all deaths [1]. Further, for every death due to injuries, there are hundreds of individuals who suffer non-fatal physical and mental disabilities, often for the rest of their lives. This means that the disability adjusted life years lost account for a significantly higher percentage than the estimated death rate [2]. Not to be forgotten is the interpersonal violence with a global statistics, however underestimated due to incomplete reporting systems, of more than half a million victims of homicide in 2000 [3].

Injuries can be divided into different anatomical structures. Although not knowing the pattern completely, traumatic brain injuries are responsible for a substantial percentage of all injuries presented. Traumatic brain injury accounts for up to half of all deaths from trauma [4]. More than 50% of all multiple injured patients suffer from traumatic brain injury. About 20 % of the combined injuries are found on the head and extremities. Since the definition of traumatic brain injury differs between regions, it is not possible to fully compare statistical data for epidemiological purposes. For instance, some data of traumatic brain injury may include trauma to the face while others exclude such injuries. In 1992 the World health Organisation published the revised International Classification Diseases 10 [5]. The ICD system is well accepted by hospitals in most countries. It will certainly improve the epidemiological statistics thereby giving a clearer pattern of traumatic brain injuries among injuries as a whole.

Although there is a value in comparing the statistics across countries, precaution must be stressed. The traumatic brain injury incidence varies due to several important reasons that limit comparison such as different statistical data available, differences between developing and developed regions, age, gender and socio-economic level, number of traumatic brain injured cases admitted to a hospital etc. Despite these limitations, however, from existing publications it is possible to estimate the mortality rate of head injuries to about 15 per 100 000 inhabitants while the incidence rate is estimated to about 200 per 100 000 inhabitants [6].

In parallel with an increased awareness of the physical, mental and economic burden for the society, many countries over the continents are presenting their respective statistical data on incidence of traumatic brain injuries. This gives an opportunity to compare not only the epidemiological pattern of traumatic brain injury worldwide but also the effect of primary prevention strategies for the future.

In Europe there is a large variation between countries and regions [7]. Traumatic brain injury in the United Kingdom with a population of 62 million is estimated to at least 1 million patients admitted to hospital annually [8]. This gives an incidence ratio of 1600 per 100 000 inhabitants per year. Mild traumatic brain injury was defined to about 90 % while the other 10 % were equally divided on moderate and severe traumatic brain injury. In Germany 280 000 patients were admitted to hospital due to a traumatic brain injury in 1996. Based on a population of 82 million this gives an annual incidence rate of about 350 per 100 000. The mortality rate was defined to 11.5 per 100 000 per year [9]. In Sweden with a population of 9 million, statistical data from the National Board for Health and Welfare showed that during 1987-2001 there was an annual frequency of about 22 000 traumatic brain injury seeking hospital care. This gives an incidence rate of 220 per 100 000 per year. Mild traumatic brain injury was found in 85 % while 15 % were divided on moderate and severe traumatic brain injuries [10].

In Asia there are some reports presented on traumatic brain injury during the last years. Thus, from a hospital based epidemiological study in Bangalore, India, the incidence rate was defined to 160 per 100 000 per year while the mortality rate was 20 per 100 000 per year. However, the report stresses on the lack of large-scale population or hospital based epidemiological studies and which results in difficulties in analysing the present situation for the country as a whole [11]. In Japan there is a trend of gradual reduction of traumatic brain injuries. So far the statistics are available from only traffic accidents. Based on a population of about 126 million the overall traumatic brain injury pattern was 106 469 divided on 90 427 mild traumatic brain injury, 11 198 severe traumatic brain injury and 4844 deaths. Thus, the statistical data gives an incidence and mortality rate of 85 and 5 per 100 000 per year, respectively, as a consequence of road traffic accidents [12]. In the Peoples' Republic of China with a population of 1.3 billion, an epidemiological investigation of traumatic brain injury was performed 1983 and 1985 in six large cities and in 21 rural areas. In the cities the incidence rate was 55.4 per 100 000 inhabitants per year and 64.1 in rural areas. The mortality rate was defined to 6.2 and 9.7 in the cities and rural areas, respectively. In Taiwan the incidence and mortality rates are given from two different regions and based on hospital admissions and deaths. The Hualien Province study from 1991 presents an incidence and mortality rate of 333 and 89, respectively, per 100 000 per year [13]. In Taipei City, Taiwan, the incidence and mortality rates were defined to 180 and 23, respectively, per 100 000 per year [14].

In Australia the incidence of hospital-treated traumatic brain injury in a community was reported to approximately 100 per 100 000 per year [15]. Another epidemiological study from South Australia indicated an incidence rate of 322 per 100 000 per year.

In South Africa the epidemiological pattern of traumatic brain injury has been evaluated in Johannesburg. The incidence rate was defined to 316 per 100 000 per year while the mortality rate ranged between 45 for Coloured, 54 for White and 88 for Africans per 100 000 per year [16].

In the United States with a population of 180 million, there are several regional studies performed on the incidence and mortality rates. Several important differences limit comparison between these publications. However, based on a conservative estimation, the incidence rate is defined to 200 per 100 000 per year [17]. A review of the traumatic brain injury death between 1986-1989 defined the mortality rate to 16.9 per 100 000 per year.

Population based studies on the incidence and mortality rate including causes of traumatic brain injury in developing countries has been reported during the last 10 to 15 years. However, it is somewhat difficult to compare these data with those from developed countries since the definition and methodology differ a lot due to lack of standardized guidelines. Also, data from different regions in one country may differ quite a lot due to a number of different factors. It is therefore not meaningful to extrapolate data from developed countries to developing countries.

Causation

A review of the literature shows that the causes of traumatic brain injury are similar in the industrial world. In the majority of published data, traffic accidents are responsible for about 50 % of all traumatic brain injuries followed by falls with 20 to 25 %. Violence, sport and recreation is responsible for another 15 to 25 %. While traffic accidents are most frequently found in the younger population, falls are most frequently to be seen among the elderly population. It should be stressed that falls are the most common cause of injury among children aged 0 to 15 years. Also, it is notified that of more severe injuries, the head is the most commonly injured region in this age group. Sport and recreation accounts for a significant number of traumatic brain injuries depending on type of activity [18]. The incidence of traumatic brain injury due to sport and recreation is expected to increase due to more freedom in life style combined with the leisure based industrial expand. Not to be forgotten is the interpersonal violence.

Exposure Risk Characteristics

Studies of occurrence of traumatic brain injury worldwide show that high rates are found in individuals under the age of 10 and between 15 to 24 years of age. After 24 the incidence rate declines in the middle years before the rates increase again around 60 to 65 years of age. All incidence studies so far have reported that traumatic brain injury is two to three times more common in males compared to females. Socio-economic status, as measured by a number of indicators, shows that traumatic brain injuries are more common in families with the lowest income levels [19].

There is a general agreement between governmental and nongovernmental authorities that blood alcohol concentration may have a profound risk of injury. Although there is significant variation in individual tolerance, alcohol has a negative effect on neuronal physiology. For instance, alcohol was found to be positively associated with physician-diagnosed neurological impairment together with clinical complications and length of hospital stay. Not only alcohol but also other substances, which may influence the human behaviour, have a substantial impact on traumatic brain injury incidence. Thus, a recent study showed that as much as 80 % of patients with traumatic brain injury due to violence had a history of substance abuse [20].

Classification of Severity

In order to classify an injury optimally a number of different scoring systems have been developed during the last decades. The purpose has been to better coordinate the primary assessment by the trauma team, to predict the likelihood of outcome, that is, triage, to collect statistical data for comparative studies and to define strategies for primary prevention. It has to bear in mind that all of the scoring systems used today have their respective limitations for optimal judgement of an injured patient. The most common score systems presently used are the Abbreviated Injury Scale (AIS), the Injury Severity Score (ISS), the Glasgow Coma Scale (GCS), and the Revised Trauma Score (RTS). The AIS is solely based on the anatomy by using a numerical method of ranking injury by body region from 1 (minor) to six (major). The ISS calculates the sum of the squares of the highest AIS score in three different body regions thereby providing a range from 1 (mild) to 75 (most severe). The GCS is used for observation of neurological condition, severity grading and prognosis. It is a numerical method analysing eye opening, verbal and motor responses ranging from 3 (most severe) to 15 (normal neurological condition). The RTS evaluates the clinical condition of the patient by including the respiratory rate, systolic blood pressure and the GCS.

There is no single system of classifying traumatic brain injury that is fully accepted worldwide due to limitations of all systems available. Nevertheless, the GCS is the most internationally accepted score to be used in quantifying the neurological condition and the most common evaluation to traditionally classify the severity of traumatic brain injury as mild, moderate and severe [21]. Thus, traumatic brain injury is defined as mild with a GCS of

13 to 15. About 80% of all traumatic brain injuries admitted to the hospital are mild. Moderate traumatic brain injuries are defined with a GCS of 9 to 12 and accounts for 10 %. Severe traumatic brain injuries are those with a GCS of 3 to 8 and accounts also for 10 % of the traumatic brain injured patients.

The social ramifications are important and mild traumatic brain injury can have a substantial impact on both the patients´ and their families´ well being. Most mild traumatic brain injury patients recover promptly and without complications. Despite being classified as mildly injured, however, some patients deteriorate shortly after the accident, or present with long-term disability symptoms. A recent best evidence synthesis has evaluated the dimension of mild traumatic brain injury from the large number of scientific literature and defined the incidence rate of about 100 to 300 per 100 000 per year. This number is probably well underestimated since a large number of mild traumatic brain injuries are not admitted to the hospital [22].

Mechanisms of Head Injury

According to the definition, the term trauma refers to an external source of kinetic energy causing a physical injury to the scalp, skull bone, vessels or brain tissue. Individual mechanisms of impact result in different types of traumatic brain injury. Therefore, several factors must be considered in accurately determining the type and severity of injury following an accident. Generally, traumatic brain injury is the result from acceleration of the head in response to the impact. Radial and tangential impacts result in linear and rotational or angular accelerations, respectively. The angular acceleration of the head is much more deleterious compared to linear acceleration. However, the most common head impact is a combination of both radial and tangential directions and defined as the oblique impact. The severity of the traumatic brain injury is not only sensitive to the force and direction of the impact. It is also time dependent since a high level of acceleration acting for a short time on the head may be less injurious compared to a lower level of acceleration acting over a longer time.

While the mechanical impact to the head can be calculated in milliseconds, the chemical consequences starts momentary and last from seconds, minutes, hours and days to weeks. Thus, may be the most comprehensive way to review what is known at present, is to define the knowledge into neuromechanical and neurochemical aspects.

Neuromechanical Aspects

The mechanical impact to the head is caused either by a stationary or a dynamic force. The stationary force is a rare event and originates from a slow moving force to the head resulting in fractures, intracranial hematomas and contusions of various degrees while axonal injury is absent. Instead, by far the most common impact is the dynamic force, which causes an injury due to contact with the head, acceleration / deceleration or both. The dynamic force then results in a chock wave influencing the tissue by pressure, strain and shear thereby injuring the bone, vascular system and nervous tissue.

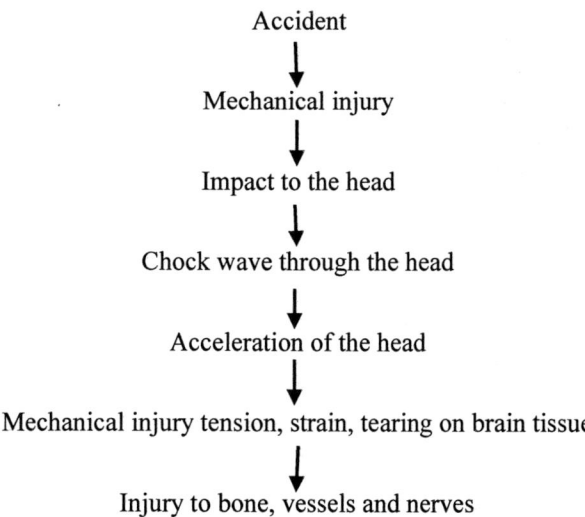

Neuromechanical cascade

Accident

↓

Mechanical injury

↓

Impact to the head

↓

Chock wave through the head

↓

Acceleration of the head

↓

Mechanical injury tension, strain, tearing on brain tissue

↓

Injury to bone, vessels and nerves

Neurochemical Aspects

Neurochemical cascade

Mechanical injury

↓

Reduced cerebral blood flow

↓

Disturbance in electrolyte homeostasis

↓

Reduced cerebral metabolism

↓

Release of degradating proteins

↓

Reduced cell function

↓

Cerebral infarction

In line with the neuromechanical events, the neurochemical pattern after traumatic brain injury has become better understood especially during the last two decades. However, in contrast to the neuromechanical event lasting in milliseconds after the impact, the neuochemical cascade may last from seconds to hours, days and weeks. Briefly, the neurochemical reaction initiates an ischemia thus altering the blood supply with oxygene reduction together with depletion of energy production on the cellular level. As a consequence, the ion homeostasis is altered thereby giving raise to membrane depolarisation simultaneously with the release of neurotransmitters into the extracellular space. An increased concentration of intracellular $Ca2+$ ions then activates phospholipases, which causes the destruction of membrane lipids and the cellular metabolism ceases in a negative spiral.

Cerebral ischemia has introduced the concept of a *penumbra zone* and identified by the use of Positron Emission Tomography. This area is anatomically localised outside the infarction area but inside the normal cerebral tissue and with a cerebral blood flow of 15 ml / 100 mg / min. In the penumbra zone the neural tissue is said to be vital, however non-functional and thereby potentially salvageable from further extension of the infarction area.

Imaging and Clinical Neuropathology

Imaging techniques are the modality of choice in the evaluation of acute traumatic brain injuries admitted to the hospital after a mechanical impact but also for the subsequent follow up of treatment and outcome of especially moderate and severe traumatic brain injuries. Computed tomography (CT) and magnetic resonance (MR) have, due to their respective specialties, replaced skull radiography parallel with the installation of modern technique worldwide during the last two decades. CT is the technique of choice since it is rapidly performed to a low cost giving the clinician the first information of the neuropathology pattern of both the skull bone and significant lesions in the cerebral tissue on the admission to the hospital. Also, CT is frequently used in the subacute stage to identify patient at high risk of deterioration. Although MR is more sensitive than CT, it is not used in the acute stage since it takes longer to perform, is usually placed in some distance from the emergency room and is more expensive. Instead, MR is used more for the evaluation of non-hemorrhagic diffuse axonal injuries and hemorrhagic and non-hemorrhagic cortical contusions and should be used as a complementary technique to CT. MR is of special support for the clinician in the assessment of rehabilitation and prognosis after moderate to severe traumatic brain injury. Hence, both CT and MR are of great value in analysing primary and secondary head injuries.

The functional impairment of the neurological condition as measured by the Glasgow Coma Scale (GCS) does not consider the underlying pathological structure of the central nervous tissue. It is common to find different lesions in size and anatomical location in patients having similar GCS score. The difference is a consequence of several factors influencing the external and internal structures of the head disproportionately. The best way to clinically define the pathophysiology pattern following a mechanical impact is to classify the traumatic brain injuries into primary and secondary events.

PRIMARY HEAD INJURIES

Primary traumatic brain injuries are the direct result of the mechanical forces on the head at the moment of impact. These injuries are further divided into focal and diffuse injuries (Panel 1).

The focal injuries consist of macroscopic damages more or less located to a well-defined area and visible with imaging technique such as CT scan. They include external injuries such as scalp wounds and skull fractures, and internal injuries such as vascular injury leading to different types of hemorrhage depending on their locations within the skull, contusions and lacerations. Approximately two thirds of the traumatic brain injury deaths are attributable to focal injuries with subdural hematomas and diffuse axonal injuries as the two most important causes.

Panel 1. Primary head injury

Focal injuries	Diffuse injuries
• Scalp wound	• Concussion
• Skull fracture	• Axonal injury
• Intracranial hemorrhage	

- Epidural hematoma (EDH)
  - Subdural hematoma (SDH)
  - Intracerebral hematoma (ICH)
  - Subarchnoid hemorrhage (SAH)
  - Intraventricular hemorrhage (IVH)	

• Contusion	
• Laceration	

Focal Injuries

Scalp wounds are frequently seen following a traumatic brain injury. They range from small to very large in size. As the blood supply to the scalp is luxary, the blood loss can be severe although hypotension should not be attributable to bleeding from such a wound. The localisation of a scalp wound may lead the clinician to define an intracranial lesion.

Skull fractures are the result of significant mechanical impact to the skull. They may be classified as anatomically located to the cranial vault or the skull base, simple or compound and linear, comminute or depressed. Configuration of the different skull fractures depends much on the mechanical force with linear fractures occurring with less force compared to the mechanical force to perform a comminute or depressed skull fractures. Linear fractures are found in more than half of severe traumatic brain injured patients. The incidence of depressed fractures are about 20 per 100 000 per year while the incidence of fractures in the skull base are present only in about 4%. A rare complication is the growing skull fracture detected in less than 1% of linear fractures among children mostly before the age of 3 years. The mortality rate of different skull fractures is not possible to define since the death of traumatic brain injured patients with skull fractures often have a concomitant injury which in fact is responsible for the poor outcome.

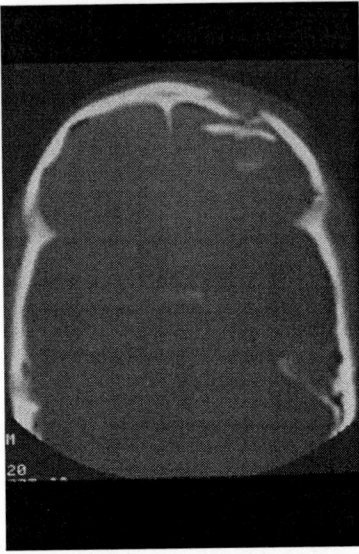

Figure 1. CT scan showing a depressed fracture in the right frontal skull bone (seen from below).

Intracranial Hemorrhage

The etiology of hematomas after traumatic brain injuries is the rupture of arteries, veines, sinuses or diploe at the time of injury. According to the anatomical localisation the hemorrhage is defined as epidural hematomas (EDH), subdural hematomas (SDH), subarachnoid (SAH), intracerebral (ICH) and intraventricular hemorrhage (IVH). Intracranial hematomas are the most common causes to neurological deterioration and death among patients presenting a lucid interval after the trauma event. Also, hemorrhage in the brain is usually combined with other injuries with SDH in 28% and with EDH in 10%.

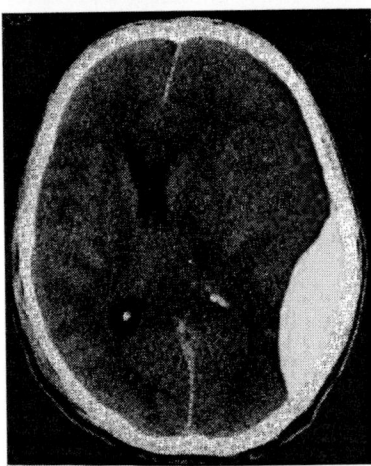

Figure 2. CT scan showing an epidural hematoma in the left temporo-paritel lobe with a significant midline shift to the right (seen from below).

An *EDH* is located between the inner surface of the skull bone and the dura. The most important risk factor is an associated fracture. Usually the EDH originates from a teared artery such as the middle cerebral artery as a result of skull fracture. The vast majority of EDH is found in the temporo-parietal region due to a fracture damaging the meningeal artery although approximately 10% are found in the frontal or the posterior fossa. The incidence of EDH occurs in about 2 to 4 % of all head injuries. Although EDH is seen at all ages, they are very rare in young children and primarily found in males under the age of 40 years. From a clinical aspect the patient may experience a lucid interval without unconsciousness in about 20% before a neurological deterioration is seen. However, patients with EDH may be presented as briefly unconscious or comatose since the traumatic brain injury occurred. In about 30 % of EDH other significant intracranial injuries are also present.

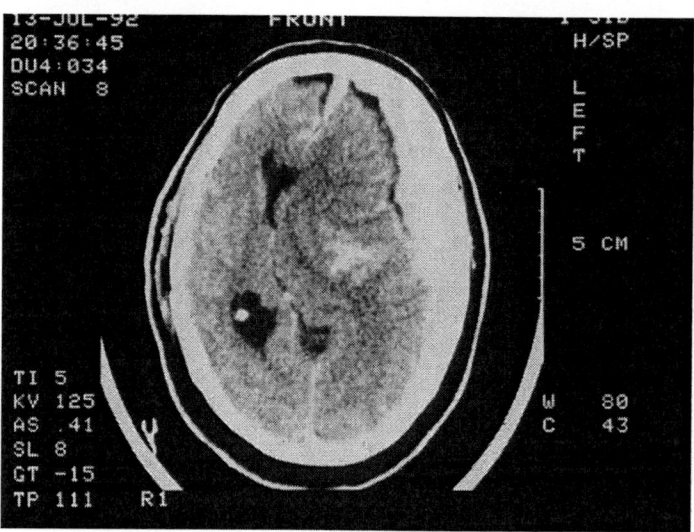

Figure 3. CT scan of an acute subdural hematoma and contusion on the left hemisphere with a significant midline shift to the right (seen from below).

A *SDH* is located between the dura and the arachnoid. SDH are usually divided into acute (ASDH) and chronic (CSDH) hematomas. ASDH is found in connection with the relative movement and displacement of the brain following a strong mechanical force and the result of either a ruptured artery or rupture of bridging veins on the cerebral surface. The incidence of ASDH is seen in about 20% of severe traumatic brain injured patients and is the most common and severe type of intracranial hematomas after trauma. Also, it results in the worst clinical outcome of these patients and the mortality rate ranges from 30 to 90% depending on the clinical treatment. Another major reason to the poor outcome is the presence of ischemic cerebral tissue damage due to an increased intracranal pressure caused by the movement of the brain and the hematoma itself.

CSDH, on the other hand, evolves over a period of weeks after the trauma. The mechanism is tearing of veins bridging the space between cortex and venous sinuses. However, in many patients there is no history of any trauma at all. The incidence rate is about 1 to 2 per 100 000 per year. Important predispositions are older age, chronic alcoholism and cerebral atrophy.

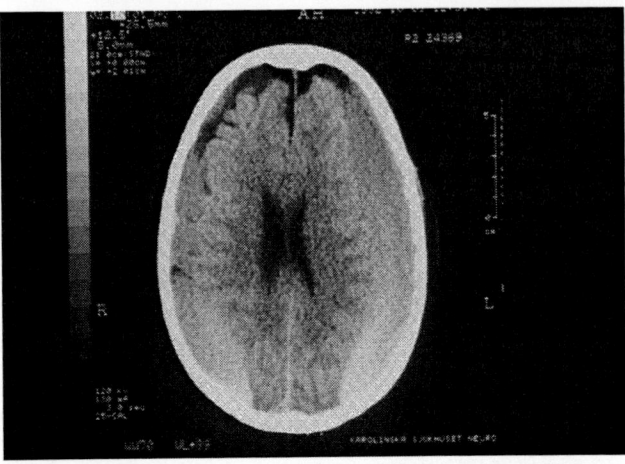

Figure 4. A CT scan showing chronic subdural hematoma between the skull bone and brain on both.

SAH is usually found on the CT scan after traumatic brain injury. Normally the amount of blood is minimal and, hence, of minor clinical significance. When this type of hemorrhage is significant, it may be associated with contusion or laceration.

ICH is located in the brain parenchyma. With CT scan ICH is found in as much as 30% of more severe traumatic brain injuries. Primary ICH is caused by rupture of cerebral arteries while secondary ICH is a consequence of contusion or laceration usually located in the frontal and temporal lobes.

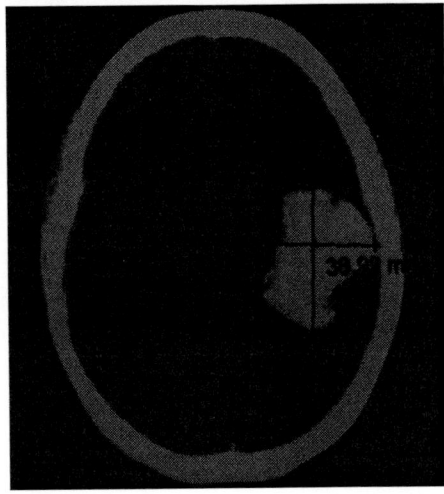

Figure 5. A CT scan showing an intracerebral hematoma on the left temporo-parietal lobe (seen from below)

IVH is usually found in small amounts in an incidence of 1 to 10% depending on the severity of the traumatic brain injury. In 1 out of three patients IVH is secondary to intracerebral hematomas disrupting the ventricular wall. Further, in about half of the patients presenting diffuse axonal injury on CT scan, there is an IVH [23].

Acute posttraumatic posterior fossa hematomas have an incidence rate of 1-2%. When the hematoma supersides 15 to 30 ml in the subtentorial space, it may result in severe neurological dysfunction since they may interfere negatively with the brain stem or result in the obstruction of CSF fluid.

A **Contusion** is the focal damage of cerebral tissue caused by a mechanical force due to contact between the surface of the cerebral tissue and the irregular bone at the frontal and middle fossa thereby located in the inferior of the frontal and temporal lobes. It damages the small vessels and neural parenchyma. There are various types of contusion. Most commonly used are the coup and contre coup lesions. A coup contusion is located in the vicinity of the contact injury while a contre coup contusion is located opposite to the impact site. The mortality rate varies from 25 to 60%.

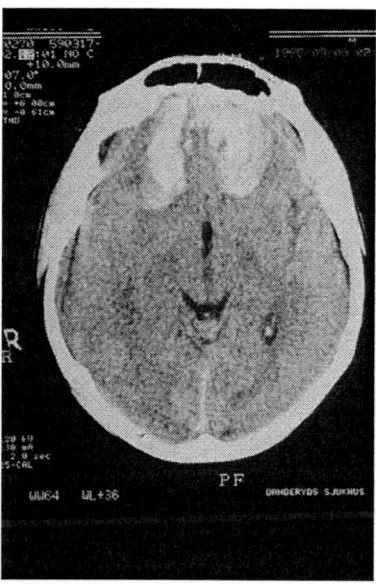

Figure 6. A CT scan showing an acute contusion on left and right frontal lobes.

Laceration is defined as a tearing disruption of the neural parenchyma produced at the time of trauma, however not always so easy to differentiate from contusion.

Diffuse Injuries

Concussion is a general term that is usually defined as a temporary disturbance in neurological function. The impact, which is caused by the mechanical force of rapid acceleration / deceleration, may result in either preserved or brief loss of consciousness. In the mild concussion a variable of symptoms are present and does not necessarily result in unconsciousness. In the more advanced concussion, unconsciousness may be present together with other neurological abnormalities. As the neurological symptoms dissipate in the vast majority of patients within a short time after the trauma, the concussion is usually considered a mild traumatic brain injury. Health care providers generally look upon the word concussion as being synonymous with mild traumatic brain injury defining the GCS within the range of 13 to 15. There are two criteria usually defined with concussion, namely loss of consciousness and posttraumatic amnesia.

Diffuse Axonal Injury (DAI)

Following a severe mechanical impact to the head, it is generally accepted that there is a considerable movement of the whole brain. The consequence will be damage of diffuse pattern in different areas of the cerebral tissue, especially in the white matter. DAI is defined by the disruption of neurones in the cerebral tissue. It originates from substantial tangential mechanical force applied to the skull and similar to that producing SDH. The mechanical impact causes diffuse axonal damage from primary to secondary axonal degeneration leading to neurophysiological failure of communication in targeted areas localised to the hemispheres, corpus callosum and brain stem [24]. The incidence of DAI among severe head injuries is found in about 50% and is the most common cause of severe disability and vegetative state. The mortality rate is 1 in 3 of all deaths after traumatic brain injury.

Secondary Head Injury

Secondary traumatic brain injuries (Panel 2) are the result of the chemical events in the nervous tissue as a direct consequence to the primary focal and diffuse injuries. Of those to be mentioned are cerebral ischemia, cerebral edema and raised intracranial pressure.

Panel 2. Secondary head injury

> - Cerebral ischemia
> - Cerebral swelling
> - Increased intracranial Pressure

Cerebral ischemia is a common finding in severe traumatic brain injuries and in autopsies. The incidence of cerebral ischemia has been found in more than 80% of severe traumatic brain injuries at autopsy. In a broad aspect ischemia is defined as the mismatch between cerebral blood flow and the metabolic need. Normally, the cerebral blood flow is about 55 ml / 100 mg / min and constant with a mean arterial blood pressure ranging between about 6.5 and 20 kPa. When the cerebral blood flow is reduced below 20 ml /100g /min, the ischemic threshold is passed with loss of the neuronal electrical activity. A further decrease to 15 ml / 100 mg / min makes the ischemic pattern becomes evident. A cerebral blood flow below 10 ml / 100 mg /min causes loss of cellular homeostasis and infarction occurs [25]. Ischemia may result from different reasons such as the reduction of cerebral blood flow, space occupying hematomas, brain edema and raised intracranial pressure.

Cerebral swelling is defined as an increased amount of water content in the nervous tissue. The incidence of swelling after severe traumatic brain injury is very high. It seems to be associated with either a single factor or multiple factors although the exact causes are only to some extent clearly explained. The swelling, which may be well localised or general, is either caused by an increased cerebral blood volume, so called congestive brain swelling, or an increased water content defined as cerebral edema. Congestive swelling is present when the cerebral blood flow is increased and caused by either a vasodilatation of arteries and / or an obstruction of the venous system. Cerebral swelling differentiates between cytotoxic, vasogenic, interstitial, hydrostatic and osmotic edema [26]. Of these, cytotoxic and vasogenic edema are those dominating after traumatic brain injury. In cytotoxic edema there is an increase of water content within the cells due to hypoxic and/or ischemic damage resulting in the derangement of normal ion homeostasis. In vasogenic edema there is a disruption of the blood brain barrier resulting in an accumulation of protein rich fluid in the extracellular environment. Due to the oncotic pressure an accumulation of water is found between the cells. It has been shown that cytotoxic edema dominated the cerebral edema after traumatic brain injury while vascular edema is responsible for about 25% [27].

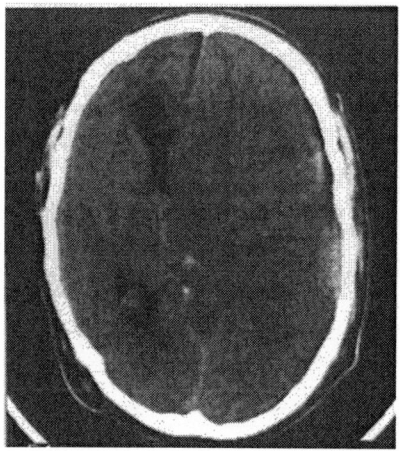

Figure 7. A CT scan showing a large edema in the left hemisphere resulting in a midline shift (seen from below).

Raised *intracranial pressure* (ICP) is found in the majority of severe traumatic brain injuries and may be deleterious for the patient unless treated effectively. The incidence of raised ICP following autopsy of severe traumatic brain injuries were found to be as high as 75% mainly caused by intracranial hematomas and brain swelling [28]. Also, a raised ICP can in itself set in motion various processes which strengthern a raised ICP. Under normal physiological condition ICP is defined as up to 2.7 kPa. This is present as long as the three intracranial components of central nervous tissue, cerebral blood volume and cerebrospinal fluid compensate in relation to each other. However, following a mechanical impact leading to an intracranial hematoma or brain swelling of larger size, the compensation mechanisms are ruled out. In such scenarios even a small increase of the intracranial volume causes a large increase in ICP. A raised ICP above 2.7 kPa is found in more than half of severe traumatic brain injured patients and may, untreated, lead to ischemic damage and even herniation of the cerebral tissue. Post-mortem studies have shown that herniation of the medial part of the temporal lobe through the tentorium was very much correlated with a raised ICP ranging between 2.7 kPa and 5.3 kPa in life. Thus, strong evidence has been presented that a raised ICP following traumatic brain injury is associated with a poor outcome.

PREHOSPITAL MANAGEMENT

A modern infrastructure includes the use of ground as well as airborne transportation facilities together with the introduction of effective trauma teams prepared for the acute management of the victim at the emergency room in the hospital. The organisation of using advanced equipped ambulance cars nearby and the addition of ambulance helicopter for those accidents more distant from the hospitals, have greatly shortened the transportation from the scene of accident to the hospital. Such a modern infrastructure of aftercare following an accident with traumatic brain injury is of most importance since early neurosurgical care may improve the outcome [29].

The general view of a trauma team (Panel 3) consists of the staff dealing with the post care handling of an accident. Although not involved as a member of the trauma team, by-passers are indeed the first to start the rescuing the patient immediately after the accident. Among the first to show up are professionals from the police department and responsible for the primary investigation together with the primary prevention of further injury at the site of accident. The staff from the fire department is equally important since they are often those arriving first to, for instance, a motor vehicle accident among professionals and responsible for the first care of the patient.

Panel 3. The trauma team

Prehospital care members	Hospital care members
• By-passers	• Physicians representing the general surgery, anesthesiology, orthopedic surgery, ENT and neurosurgery
• Police department	• Emergency room staff
• Fire department	
• Paramedics	

Perhaps it is time to change the pattern of the trauma team. Since many people with different competence and knowledge in one or another way are involved in the society as a whole, the optimal trauma team should also include pre-crash competence such as epidemiologists, statisticians and those dealing with primary prevention. Moreover, not to be forgotten are those people and institutions responsible for the long-term care taking such as family members and societies. All named personnel should participate in the design of an effective trauma system including primary prevention of injuries. Such a holistic view would certainly expand the field of competence and knowledge.

Prehospital care of the trauma patient (Panel 4) is the most essential phase for a successful long-term outcome. Several studies have indicated that this is the part of care during which a significant number of deaths can be prevented. The application of effective protocols and priorities of resuscitation should be stressed. Thus, the management of a traumatic brain injured patient, as well as in all accidents, should start already at the scene of accident according to the generally adopted basic principles defined as *ABC*, which relates to Airway care, Breathing and Circulation. An individual passing by and witnessing the accident may very well start such fundamental and lifesaving first aid until paramedics arrive. A prerequisit to this view is that by-passers are familiar with such a management system. The first *assessment* performed by the paramedics is brief and incomplete in order to get a comprehensive picture of the patient's condition. Of significant importance is to reach an optimal *respiratory status* for normal breathing and oxygenation. In maxillofacial injuries the mouth may be filled by debris, which has to be removed. Simultaneously, the tongue should be pulled in a frontal position. Next to be prioritised is the *circulation*. Control of external bleeding is vitally important in order to prevent significant blood volume loss. Internal bleeding common among multitrauma patients should also be considered although this cannot be performed sufficiently at the scene of accident. Traumatic brain injured patients with fractures of the long bones and abdominal trauma are particularly vulnerable to rapid neurological deterioration since the blood loss may be substantial.

Panel 4. Management at the scene of accident

- Assessment
- Airway
- Breathing
- Circulation
- Stabilization
- Transportation

The incidence of concomitant spinal injuries among traumatic brain injuries ranges between 5 to 10% [30]. Thus, as cervical fractures may be present, however not discovered immediately, or the patient may suffer from sensory and motor disturbances due to instability of the neck, the paramedics must stabilize the cervical spine with a rigid collar prior to transportation.

After the acute care including ABC management and stabilization of potential fractures, the paramedics should keep the time spent at the scene as short as possible. Parallel with the introduction of high skilled paramedics, trauma teams and level 1 trauma centres, the patients are more frequently transported directly to such a hospital instead of passing through a primary hospital.

General and Neurological Examination on Admission

On arrival at the hospital the responsibility of the patient is handed over to a senior officer of the medical staff. Usually the trauma surgeon or the anaesthesiologist is initially in command of the team and should be in complete charge throughout the acute care in order to establish priorities. The members of the trauma team are forced to obey orders from the leader and proceed to manage the severed injured patient in an organised and coordinated pattern. The senior officer in leader takes the responsibility for a more thoroughful general examination of the patient (Panel 5) while the members of the trauma team is taking active support in whatever is needed. This means that none of the physicians is allowed to leave the emergency room until excused by the leader.

Panel 5. Management at the emergency room

Part I. General assessment
1. History of event from paramedics
2. Detailed physical examination
3. Multitrauma or not?
4. Radiological investigation
5. Acute treatment of choice
6. Observation or Intensive care unit

As soon as the ambulance has handed over the patient to the trauma team, the senior officer receives a *general overview* of the accident from the paramedics simultaneously with the conduction of a rapid and *detailed physical assessment* of the patient starting with the respiratory and circulation system. When airways, breathing and circulation is secured, *trauma on other organs* has to be excluded. Then, depending on type of injury, it has to be decided what kind of further investigation has to be performed. Based on the clinical examination and what has been found on other investigations, the treatment of choice is very much dependent on the patients clinical condition. Whenever in a good condition, the patient is transported to a ward for further observation. However, when severely injured, the patient is transferred to the intensive care unit.

When the trauma team leader has completed necessary priorities and depending on type of injury, he or she is in the position to command a physician from one of the other surgical subspecialties to take over the responsibility of the patient before discharged from the resuscitation procedure. Prior to that all physicians have to complete a record documenting what has been found and how this has been treated.

When the patient has been diagnosed with a traumatic brain injury, the neurosurgeon in the trauma team will be responsible for the next step of treatment. To define the exact way for management of the traumatic brain injured patient is a challenge due to its complexity of concomitant injuries together with the unpredictable course of intracranial processes found on the initial CT scan.

Neurological Examination

First of all the neurological examination starts to evaluate the severity of the traumatic brain injury with regard to GCS (Panel 6). The GCS score separates those with mild, moderate and severe traumatic brain injury. According to the GCS, patients with mild traumatic brain injury having a score of 13-15 can open the eyes either spontaneous or to speech, obeys commands or localize pain and are oriented or confused in the conversation. Patients with moderate traumatic brain injury are scored between 9-12. As the vast majority of the severe traumatic brain injuries are comatose, they cannot respond properly to the criteria of the GCS and thus scored 3-8.

Panel 6. Part II Neurological assessment

Associated systemic injuries
• Maxillofacial injuries
• Thoracic injuries
• Abdominal injuries
• Orthopedic injuries
• Spine injuries
Radiological investigations
Conservative versus surgical treatment
Neurosurgical intensive care

Associated Systemic Injuries

Since the incidence of associated systemic injuries among severe traumatic brain injured patients is as much as 50%, it is of most importance to exclude such injuries already at the emergency room. Some of these are mentioned here since they may cause neurological deficits of various degrees.

Maxillofacial injuries are common in patients with trauma in general. The incidence of maxillofacial trauma in traumatic brain injured patients is about 5 % 31. Of special importance are those injuries having the potential risk to negatively influence the normal breathing and those fractures influencing frontal skull base.

Thoracic injuries may be caused by hemothorax, hemopneumothorax or pneumothorax due to rib fractures. This may result in decreased vital capacity. Further, injury to the vascular tree in the thoracic region may result in hypotension, embolism or vascular occlusion. These associated injuries can cause neurological deterioration with harbouring of an already existing brain damage.

Abdominal injuries may be very difficult to evaluate since no or little external evidence of such an injury may be present. Shock in a traumatic brain injured patient may be caused by abdominal injury. If a traumatic brain injury patient has associated trauma to the chest, pelvis or has signs of hypotension, there is an increased risk of also having an injury to the abdomen.

Orthopedic injuries may be either obvious or difficult to find at the first sight. A fracture of the long bones may contain a substantial amount of blood due to vascular injury of femur. Some of the fractures may alter the traumatic brain injured patients neurological condition in the sense of substantial blood loss resulting in hypotension.

Spinal injuries are, as mentioned above, frequently associated with traumatic brain injuries. In contrast to conscious patients, a spinal injury may be very difficult to discover in comatose patients. Thus, a spinal injury should always be suspected until proven otherwise.

Radiological Investigations

As stated out earlier, CT scan is the primary choice of imaging technology at the emergency room. The presence of a CT scan obviates indications for skull x-ray as CT scan can determine whether a skull fracture is present or not. A CT scan is indicated in all traumatic brain injured patients with a depressed consciousness. It should be stressed that even when there is no sign of any pathological finding on the initial CT scan, it does not exclude a worsening of the patient in a later stage. Some of the patient with a good neurological condition on admission may deteriorate within a few hours to days. The incidence of such a phenomenon defined as "talk and deteriorate", is seen in about 25 % of severe traumatic brain injuries. These patients were lucid and talked at some point after the accident and before coma ensued [32]. Hence, the combination of repeated neurological examination including GCS scoring and repeated CT scan is of most importance in order to discover an early deterioration after moderate and severe traumatic brain injuries. This holds true also in mild traumatic brain injured patients based on their initial level of consciousness.

Conservative Versus Surgical Treatment

The neurosurgeon in charge of the trauma team has to decide whether a traumatic brain injured patient should be sent home, observed during the next few days or surgically treated. This is much dependent on the patients' neurological condition and what has been found on a CT scan. Of natural reasons traumatic brain injuries having a GCS scored 3-13 should always be observed at the hospital. Of the mild traumatic brain injuries having a GCS scored 13-15, it much depends on whether there has been any signs of neurological dysfunction or not.

Indications for surgical treatment or not depends on the presence of associated injuries, the patients neurological condition and what has been found on a CT scan. A patient with neurological deterioration harbouring any mass lesion, which causes a significant mass effect, should be treated surgically as soon as possible in order to prevent secondary complications.

Neurosurgical Intensive Care

The final decision for the neurosurgeon in charge of the trauma team has to take is whether the patient is in the need for neurosurgical intensive care or not. Traumatic brain injured patients defined with a GCS score of 3-8 and unconscious should always be treated at the neurointensive care unit. Further, traumatic brain injured patients with a GCS score of 8-13 and with intracranial lesions on CT scan may have the potential risk to deteriorate rapidly and should therefore be observed at the neurointensive care unit. If not possible, these patients should be under continuous observation outside the neurointensive care unit.

Neurosurgical Treatment

The guidelines for neurosurgical treatment of extra- and intracranial damage originate from the best evidence synthesis of practice at neurosurgical departments worldwide. Timing of neurosurgical treatment depends on a variety of factors such as severity of neurological condition on admission and type of traumatic brain injury presented by the CT scan.

Scalp Wounds

All uncomplicated soft tissue injuries on the scalp and in the face should be closed either at the emergency room or at best opportunity. Wounds are cleaned and sutured primarily after careful evaluation of foreign bodies, which have to be removed and for any visible skull fracture.

Fractures

Simple linear fractures do not need any surgical treatment. Simple depressed fracture may be surgically elevated due to cosmetic aspects. Compound depressed and comminute fractures are generally in the need for surgical treatment. After careful cleaning of the wound including removal of foreign bodies and debridement of devitalised scalp tissue, the inspection should look for any leakage of cerebrospinal fluid or lacerated brain tissue due to dural rift. If this holds true a careful inspection of the dura should be performed in order to exclude underlying intracranial hematoma, contusion or laceration, which has to be treated surgically. The dural rift is then closed with primary suturing. Large dural defects, however, may need duraplasty with material from pericranium, fascia lata or xenograft.

Fractures in the face should be treated second to neurosurgical procedures and, whenever possible, within the next 24 to 48 hours and together with physicians from other surgical subspecialites. Depressed fractures in the frontal region interfering with the frontal sinus are repaired as soon as possible in order to avoid infections due to fistulas between the nasal part of the face and the anterior skull base, pneumocephalus, meningitis and abscesses. The surgical procedure uses a bi-coronal scalp flap in combination with a low bilateral frontal bone flap. The posterior wall of the frontal sinus is removed together with the mucosa in the sinus, which is finally plugged with either muscle or fat tissue. The dura is then inspected with regard to rift or laceration and treated in routine fashions as is the closure of the bone and scalp flap, respectively. The fracture system is aimed at getting rigidly fixed. This can be achieved with different fixation systems such as titanium plates and screws.

Of special importance are those traumatic brain injuries presenting cerebrospinal fluid (CSF) rhinorrhea or otorrhea due to CSF fistulas. The incidence of such CSF fistulas may be as high as 9% after traumatic brain injury. They have the potential risk of initiating infections such as meningitis with an incidence of 20 to 40%. However, about 80% of the CSF fistulas are closed successfully with bed rest alone or in combination with CSF drainage.

Intracranial Hematomas

The outcome of patients presenting an intracranial hematoma is mainly dependent on the neurological condition at the time of evaluation, the time elapse from traumatic brain injury to neurosurgical treatment but also what is found on the CT scan.

Epidural hematomas (EDH) with a thickness of more than 0.5-1 cm verified on CT scan and a midline shift verified on CT scan in the comatose patient should be surgically removed urgently. Instead of only burr holes, a complete craniotomy is the ultimate choice. This technique makes it possible for the surgeon to evacuate the whole clot. Also, the acute bleeding is controlled by coagulation of arteries located on the dura, plugging of the meningeal artery in the middle temporal fossa and waxing any bleeding from the diploe.

Acute subdural hematomas (ASDH) in moderate and severe traumatic brain injuries must be promptly removed when the mass effect of the haematoma results in midline shift of more than 0.5 –1 cm, the ventricular system or the basal cisterns are compromised. The technical procedure is similar to that for EDH.

Chronic subdural hematomas (CSDH) are treated either conservatively or surgically. The most common treatment is evacuation of the liquefied haematoma via an enlarged burr hole under local anaesthesia and sedatives.

Intracerebral hematomas have, in contrast to EDH and ASDH, resulted in controversy in best neurosurgical practice. There are studies recommending a conservative view as well aggressive view 33 in the care taking of ICH. However, traumatic brain injured patients with ICH, even though large, which do not produce elevated ICP or any midline shift should be treated conservatively. This guideline holds true also in multiple ICH as well as deeply located ICH. The only ICH to be evacuated are those located superficially and large enough to produce midline shift and / or elevated ICP. Nevertheless, clinical experience in neurosurgery may eliminate a surgical procedure in about 60% of ICH [34].

Intraventricular hemorrhage (IVH) is best treated with the insertion of a catheter in either one or both lateral ventricles to prevent obstructive hydrocephalus.

Acute posttraumatic posterior fossa hematomas should be evacuated as soon as possible mainly due to the potential life-threatening risk by their negative influence to the brain stem. The surgical procedure consists of a unilateral or bilateral craniotomy with subsequent opening of the dura before the haematoma can be fully removed. It is mandatory to identify any vascular injury, which should be coagulated. As some of these patients may have blood also in the ventricular system a ventricular catheter is liberally indicated.

Contusions and lacerations may be treated either conservatively or surgically. The conservative approach includes severe traumatic brain injured patients with a stable neurological condition with lesions confined to the deep white matter. However, lesions over 2 cm in size should be surgically evacuated if there is a mass effect, a midline shift over 0.5 cm or raised ICP difficult to control. The surgical procedure is to perform a craniotomy large enough for the resection of contused or lacerated brain tissue, which usually are surrounded by edema.

Axonal injury is treated conservatively as there is no indication at present to surgically improve such a condition. The same view holds true for all diffuse injuries, which are not lifethreatening. The exception is diffuse cerebral edema, which may result in severe swollen with a significant midline shift. In these patients a frontal or temporal lobe resection is indicated.

Concussion is conservatively treated in the vast majority of patients. The estimated prevalence of intracranial CT scan abnormalities is 5 % in patients presenting to hospital with a GCS score of 15 and 30 % or higher in patients with a GCS score of 13. Also, there is evidence that skull fracture is a risk factor for intracranial lesion among these patients. The incidence of having a neurological deterioration due to mass lesion in the need for surgical treatment is about 1%. A systematic search has been performed and found 41 guidelines published for recommended treatment of mild traumatic brain injury. Following appraisal only 3 of the guidelines were categorized as evidence-based and rigorously designed [35]. Another systematic search of the literature for non-surgical intervention found 45 publications of which 16 (32%) articles were accepted for best-evidence synthesis. There was no evidence for routine administration of intensive assessment and intervention to reduce post-concussion symptoms. The evidence supports education about long-term sequelae of persisting complaints and the time course for recovery.

Neurointensive Care Management

The combined increased activities of primary prevention prehospital care and neurosurgical intervention has certainly improved the outcome following traumatic brain injury. The introduction of neurointensive care units during the last decade has further improved the treatment and outcome. In contrast to the care at the scene of accident and at the emergency room, the neurointensive care may continue over days and weeks. During this period it is of vital importance that clinicians from several subspecialties share their respective knowledge and competence in a comprehensive view aiming at reaching the best outcome for the individual traumatic brain injured patient.

As mentioned earlier approximately 50% of multitrauma involves the central nervous system with intracranial complications in the need for intensive care from a general as well as from a neurological aspect. The aim is to minimize already existing injury by maintaining an optimised airway breathing and circulation but also to prevent further deterioration due to secondary complications thereby reducing morbidity and mortality rates.

Whether a traumatic brain injured patient has to be treated at the neurointensive care unit or not, is a decision for the neurosurgeon in charge at the emergency room. It is custom that multitrauma patients always are admitted directly to the intensive care unit after acute treatment. Parallel with general intensive treatment of the system as a whole, focus is simultaneously directed toward the head since both are closely linked together. For instance, disturbance in the airway will soon reduce the oxygen concentration with negative influence on the brain metabolism as a consequence. Likewise, secondary insults such as systemic hypotension due to reduced blood circulation undoubtedly reduces the chances for the brain to maintain a normal cerebral metabolism.

Head Position

It is generally accepted to have the patients' head elevated to about 30 degree. The position improves the oxygenation by increasing the functional residual capacity and the chest wall compliance. Further, in those traumatic brain injured patients not intubated, it reduces the risk for pneumonia due to aspiration.

Neurological condition and repeated CT scan

Of special importance is the continuous observation of the traumatic brain injured patients *neurological condition*. This is best achieved by monitoring the GCS score frequently. The ongoing process of evaluating the patients' GCS score can early predict a neurological deterioration. The neurological condition is dependent also on cerebral pathophysiology after an injury. Since more than half of the patients demonstrate new findings on repeat CT scan, it is of significant value to use serial CT scan evaluation for the optimal treatment.

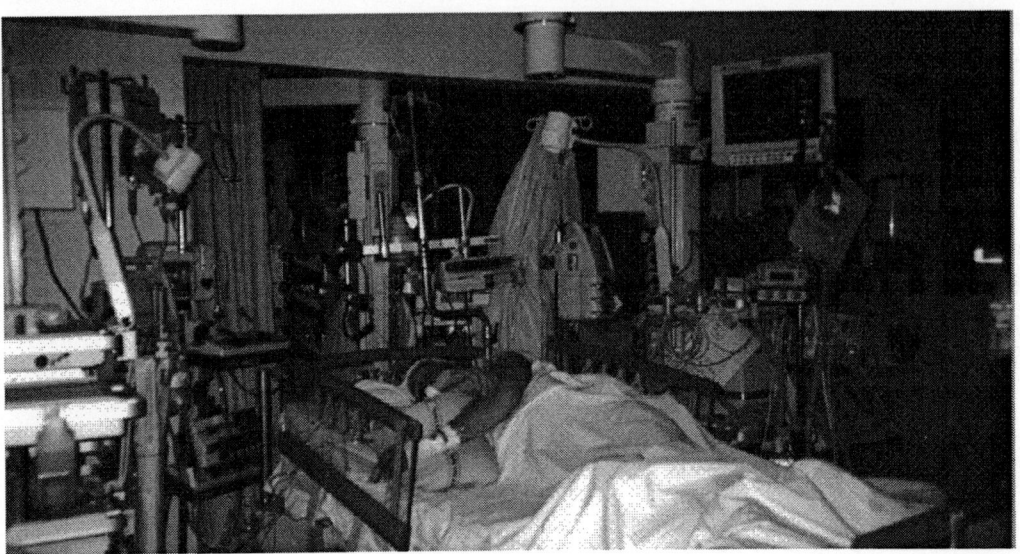

Figure 8. A head injured patient in the neurointensive care unit with all technical equipment needed.

Oxygenation and blood pressure

Earlier studies have shown that the incidence of hypoxemia and hypotension each was found in one third of the severely traumatic brain injured patients in the prehospital environment. This complication will significantly increase the morbidity and mortality rates. By comparison, in non-hypoxemic patients the mortality rate was about 15 % while hypoxemia resulted in a mortality rate of about 50%. Thus, a correct mean arterial blood pressure (MAP) should be maintained above 12 kPa and is reached by continuous infusion of fluids.

Intracranial pressure monitoring

Many of the severe traumatic brain injuries present elevated ICP, which may be detrimental on already existing traumatic brain injuries. Indication for monitoring includes unconscious patients with a GCS score between 3-8 together with a pathological CT scan. The upper normal limit is defined to about 2.5 kPa. By normalising the ICP the mortality rate decreased from 50 % to one third among the severe traumatic brain injuries. Available data support the monitoring with a ventricular catheter connected to an external strain gauge. So far there is no prospective randomised clinical trial showing that ICP monitoring favours a good outcome among these patients.

Cerebral Perfusion Pressure

Cerebral perfusion pressure (CPP) is defined as the MAP – ICP and should be kept over about 9 kPa. A normal CPP is vital for the cerebral metabolism. Maintenance of the CPP is thus reached by simultaneous monitoring of blood pressure and ICP. Earlier aggressive hyperventilation after severe traumatic brain injury is nowadays not accepted since it results in reduced CPP and the potential risk in developing an increased ICP and cerebral ischemia. The mechanism goes via vascular vasoconstriction and the subsequent reduction in an already existing cerebral blood flow among these patients. At present there is no prospective randomised controlled clinical trial published supporting hyperventilation. Instead, several class II clinical studies published during the last decade show that cerebral oxygenation is independent CPP as long as the pressure is above 8 kPa [36].

Mannitol

The primary mechanism of Mannitol is its rheologic effect as it reduces the blood viscosity thereby favorising an increased cerebral blood flow. As a consequence, the cerebral autoregulation decreases the ICP via its vasoconstrictive effect on cerebral arterioles. Some clinical class III studies support the view that Mannitol is effective when ICP is high or when CPP is low. At present there is no prospective randomised clinical trial that shows an improved outcome by the use of Mannitol.

Steroids

At present there is no evidentiary indication that corticosteroids have any significant effect on the outcome of moderate and severe traumatic brain injuries. Instead, steroids may initiate several complications in an already stressed patient with traumatic brain injury. Thus, the routine use of steroids in these patients is not recommended.

Long-term Neurological Complications

Despite full awareness and aggressive prevention of neurological complication after head injury from a clinical perspective, the incidence is significant and depending on type of complication. Educating both the patient and family members about these complications is a necessity for an overall good outcome.

Infection

Infection after traumatic brain injury is less than 10% and mainly found in severe injuries. Late infection after traumatic brain injury is the result of delayed or inadequate treatment and ranging from small scalp wounds to more severe intracranial complications such as meningitis and abscesses. The incidence of bacterial meningitis following traumatic brain injury ranges from 0.2% to as much as 17.8% and where CSF leakage is a major risk factor. The incidence of abscesses following neurosurgery and trauma may be as high as 20% with seizures reported in about 30%. On the other hand, the mortality rate from brain abscesses has been reduced to about 5%.

Seizure

The incidence of posttraumatic seizure is in the acute stage about 2% with focal seizure in the majority of patients. In the late stage the incidence is about 5% varying significantly depending on type of lesion and with the majority of patients presenting a general convulsion seizure with or without focal onset. The risk for developing seizure is higher in patients with coma and those with surgery compared to mild traumatic brain injuries.

Intracranial Hematomas

The incidence of intracranial hematomas due to altered neurological condition and skull fractures is high. It has been shown that the overall risk is 1 in 348 among adults and 1 in 2400 among children younger than 15 years of age. With decreased level of consciousness the risk increases to 1 out of 4 among adults and to 1 in 12 among children younger than 15 years of age [37].

Post-Concussion Syndrome

The most frequent symptoms correlated to post-concussion are headache, cranial symptoms and signs and psychological and somatic complaints including many subtle symptoms. Neither of these symptoms is unique following traumatic brain injury since they are also evident in other types of injury and, not least, in the healthy population. Further, evidence exists that other non-injury related external causes may be attributable to longstanding post-concussion symptoms. A meta-analysis of 17 studies after mild traumatic brain injury showed that financial compensation was a strong risk factor for long-term post-concussion symptoms and that compensation-seeking strongly predicted delayed return to work [38].

Evidence-based Guidelines in Neurotrauma Care

The treatment for the same traumatic brain injury may vary due to different experience in clinical practice. When searching the literature most published experience is based on Level II and Level III evidence with very few Level I studies. The most reliable clinical research is a Level I study, defined as prospective, randomised, controlled, blind clinical trials. In the absence of such trials, a guideline recommendation is usually based on the systematic review of existing relevant literature.

The number of existing guidelines can be long and most of these guidelines are based on expert opinions. In neurosurgery there is a significant number of clinical trials classified as II and III. The introduction of evidence-based guidelines is the only way at present to compare best treatment of choice. Although this is a complex methodology, a systematic review of the literature provides some information how best to manage clinical problems in traumatic brain injured patients.

Three larger evidence based systematic reviews of the literature have been published recently.

One systematic review includes two parts, namely guidelines for the management of severely traumatic brain injured patient and early indicators of prognosis in severe traumatic brain injuries comprising 14 topics ranging from trauma systems and prehospital resuscitation to monitoring and treatment of intensive care. The other part had the purpose to identify those early indicators that may be prognostic for outcome following severe traumatic brain injury [39]. The second systematic review includes common questions after severe traumatic brain and spinal injuries and recommendations about their management [40]. This is of special interest since an evaluation had been performed of the former guidelines in three Class III studies. The result showed a successful outcome of implementation regarding mortality rate,

ICU days and hospital cost per patient. The third systematic review deals with mild traumatic brain injury. This task force undertook a best evidence synthesis of the literature on mild traumatic brain injury addressing epidemiology, prognosis, treatment and economic costs in order to make recommendations to reduce the consequences [41].

REHABILITATION

There is no distinct transition between critical care and rehabilitation. Instead, it should be emphasized that rehabilitation starts at the same moment as the patient is admitted to the emergency room. The variety of long-term disabilities identified among traumatic brain injured patients originates from the primary and secondary injuries. Thus, in order to reach the best prognosis rehabilitation medicine should be a natural feature of an interdisciplinary trauma team already from the very early beginning.

The admission of a new traumatic brain injured patient to the rehabilitation medicine demands a smooth transition from the acute and short-term intensive care toward a more lengthy and extended period of partial or total dependence of others. Although a part of the trauma team, rehabilitation medicine has its own profile of staff members including physician, nurse, physical and occupational therapists, psychologist, speech trainer and almoner. A definition of an action plan for the individual patient implies a complete knowledge of the extent of injury. Although some prediction of outcome can be made at an early posttraumatic stage, there is a considerable variation in rate and extent of recovery following traumatic brain injury. These variations may be caused by the patients´ premorbid condition and site of injury location. Of special importance is the documentation of cognitive disorders influencing perception and communication, language, learning and memory, complex information processing and planning. The deficiencies may be carefully analysed simultaneously with the patients´ state of readiness of rehabilitation is achieved.

Mild traumatic brain injuries may suffer from the post-commotional syndrome including headache, irritability, vertigo and disturbance in memory, concentration and perseverance. Moderate traumatic brain injuries usually present a mixed pattern of neurological symptoms such as disturbance in sensory and motor coordination, reduced alertness memory and concentration together with disturbance in emotional life, behaviour and personality. Among severe traumatic brain injuries problems with consciousness is dominating and frequently accompanied by various cognitive and behavioural changes. Headache and pain is usually seen in the acute and sub-acute stage in all types of traumatic brain injuries. In the long-term run these complications will disappear.

Although frequently seen after traumatic brain injury, posttraumatic amnesia is more pronounced among severe traumatic brain injuries with lack of memory both before as well as after the time of accident. Amnesia may last for minutes and hours or lasts for weeks following consciousness has returned and can be tested with Galvestone Orientation Amnesia Test (GOAT). Of specific importance are those complications expected to be seen after returning home. These include personality changes, cognitive disorders, deficits in activities of daily living, and communication and relationship disturbances with other family members.

The *personality* before the traumatic brain injury is of importance for the outcome. It is therefore essential that each patients´ intellectual capacity is defined. For instance, if the patient has had intellectual problems at school, this may delay the recovery. Also, elderly patients need a longer time for recovery than younger patients as the aging brain has difficulties in readapting toward the earlier situation the patient was familiar with. If the patient has abnormal behaviour paaterns prior to the accident, such as low stress tolerance, depression, drug abuse or hyperactivity, the recovery may be further complicated. The same holds true for those patients´ who have had an earlier neurological deficiency. Moreover, complicated relationships within the family or at the place of work, prior to the accident, may also prolong the recovery.

Cognitive disorders include deficits in learning and memory, thinking and perceptual skills and slowness in information processing and may have a profound effect on a patients´ personality. Sometimes these changes can be related to various forms of organically localized brain areas. The site of injury together with different premorbid factors may significantly influence the process of recovery. Cognitive recovery has been found to be hierarchical beginning with the recovery of attention mechanisms, discrimination, memory association and finally those skills in the need for analysis and synthesis of input and output.

Expected complications after return to home
Personality
Cognitive deficits
Activity of Daily Life deficits
Communication Disturbance
Relations to Family System and Colleagues

Activities of daily living are all influenced by the various intellectual problems present. Usually these problems have a profound effect not only on the patient but also on family members. Deficits of daily living may slightly or profoundly interfere with the patients´ capacity to perform an independent living compared to activities performed before the trauma. To optimise rehabilitation program, the retraining must assess the patients´ personality, profession and employment, leisure interest activities and social role as a whole. The incidence of impaired physical function of self-feeding is significant in the early period. Deficiency such as poor head control, facial paresis, hemiplegia in one of the upper extremities or sensory disturbances is well addressed by the respective staff members. Dressing is another frequently occurring deficiency due to impaired physical skills or perception. Likewise, deficits in hygiene maintenance are often significant. All the examples of deficiency in daily life must be incorporated into the patients´ routine while still at the rehabilitation ward. Except for teaching and learning the traumatic brain injured patient, many of the deficiencies of daily activities may be improved by a variety of technical devices.

Communication disorders are essential to recognize early since these may complicate the dialogue between the patients and the people involved in the recovery process. This may be caused by motor or sensory disturbances. The recovery of communication skills is closely related to the cognitive recovery.

Stages of Family Reactions
Denial
Exhilaration
Distraction
Helplessness

Family members and friends are looking forward to welcoming the patient back home. As these persons usually are expecting a speedy return to normal life, they may be disappointed when they meet the patient again. After realising hard facts many friends will leave the family system alone to deal with the patients' problem. Usually there is a distinction between sorrow following bereavement and sorrow following severe trauma. The sorrow after death of a close relative or friend can be defined as periods of shock, reaction, revision and reorientation lasting for about a year. In contrast, the sorrow after a severe traumatic brain injury with complications for the patient may identify four steps lasting for different times. The first stage is defined as *denying* of the accident. This stage is followed by *exhilaration* when they have met the patient making progress in rehabilitation in the hospital. The third stage is *distraction* when the patient comes home and all the complications are presented to the relatives. Finally, when the relatives realize the prognosis they progress into a state of *helplessness*.

Acute care and rehabilitation is an ongoing process for months and even years after discharge from the hospital. To meet a person who has slightly or significantly changed in personality is very strenuous especially since there is no answer for how long this situation may persist. It is therefore of most importance that also the family is educated in due time about problems to be expected such as poor control of temper, loss of affection, lack of energy, cruelty, memory disturbance and inability to reasoning. Except for emotional and behavioural changes, the financial consequences may be a frequent source of great stress. Thus, it is of value for those involved to fully understand how psychological maladjustments among these families develop in order to prevent them on an early stage. Posttraumatic stress disorder is recognized as a major obstacle to a full recovery after head injury. Of importance to reduce stress among the family members, is their awareness of frequent and continuous follow-up contacts with the rehabilitation team for a long time after discharge. Early assessment and referral to a psychologist will probably improve the long-term outcome and shorten the recovery process significantly. Evidence based best practice will be of great value in designing rehabilitation programmes after traumatic brain injury.

PROGNOSIS AND OUTCOME

The prognostication of traumatic brain injuries is an important factor for designing an individual rehabilitation program and for adequate information to the family. While the GCS is used in the acute stage, the Glasgow Outcome Scale (GOS), is frequently used for the evaluation of outcome and should be looked upon as rough scoring of the individual patient at discharge. GOS is a five degrees scale ranging from 5 to 1 and where five defines a completely recovered situation while scoring one is defined as death. The score 4 is given the patient who has recovered moderately, 3 with significant neurological deficiency and 2 when the patient is in a vegetative stage.

Along with the high incidence and prevalence rates of head injuries due to trauma, considerable progress has been made in defining how to measure the outcome of these patients. The prediction of outcome after traumatic brain injury is of most importance during the acute care of the patient since an aggressive treatment may result in a good outcome. With the publication of a significant number of both retrospective and prospective clinical studies, sometimes evaluated on a best-evidence synthesis methodology, some realistic conclusions of the prognosis following traumatic brain injuries can be stated.

In a best-evidence synthesis on prognosis for *mild traumatic brain injury*, 428 studies related to prognosis and 120 (28%) of theses articles were accepted after critical review [42]. It was found that although cognitive deficits and symptoms were common in the acute stage, the majority of patients with mild traumatic brain injury were recovered after 3 to 12 months.

The outcome following *moderate traumatic brain injury* shows that about 60% made good recovery. The outcome seems dependent on the presence or absence of intracranial complications. For those patients with delayed and progressive intracranial complication verified with CT scan, the long-term outcome was worse compared to those without such complications [43]. The mortality rate ranges between 1 to 2.5% during hospitalisation.

The outcome for *severe traumatic brain injuries* has improved parallel with development of new technology together with an increased experimental and clinical knowledge. Comparing the prediction of outcome with mild and moderate traumatic brain injuries, it is not so easy to define the outcome among severe traumatic brain injured patients although a strong correlation was found between initial GCS score and outcome [44].

The incidence for the overall outcomes after intracranial hemorrhage varies profoundly mainly depending on the extensive of secondary injuries together with associated injuries. The mortality rate in patients with EDH, which does not damage the brain tissue, ranges between 20 to 40% while combinations with secondary brain damage increases the mortality rate to as much as 60%. The prognosis in ASDH is usually poor. The mortality rate ranges from 42 to 90% much depending on the concomitant secondary and associated injuries. The incidence of good outcome following surgical treatment of CSDH is about 75% while the mortality rate is less than 10% in uncomplicated situations. The outcome following ICH is much dependent on the patient's condition right after the mechanical impact together with other associated injuries. The prognosis of acute hematomas in the posterior fossa is best with early surgical procedure with an incidence rate of good outcome as high as over 80%. On the other hand, when these patients are admitted late to hospital with coexisting intracerebral hematomas, the mortality rate is about 80%.

Earlier studies have shown that patients with a low GCS but with the same severity have a mortality rate ranging between 9 to 74% and a good outcome ranging from 6 to 68% according to type of lesion. The mortality rate among patients with ASDH and DAI was as high as 78 % when associated with coma for more than 24 hours. Cerebral edema and contusion are associated with an immediate mortality rate while isolated contusion had the lowest mortality rate. Further, in a retrospective study examining the relationship between CT scan midline shift and outcome, the rate of poor outcome was set to 50 % when midline shift was present and 14% with a midline shift while a normal CT scan had a poor outcome rate of only 5% [45].

Prognostic probabilities are assessed by a number of different criteria. The identification of one, single and strong factor for the evaluation of outcome after traumatic brain injury is at the present moment not realistic, especially since head injuries are mainly divided into mild, moderate and severe traumatic brain injuries. Instead, neurosurgeons dealing with neurotraumatology usually attempt to take a wide range of factors into account. Even this attempt makes it difficult to perform a holistic prognostic pattern of guideline. Also, the definition of prognostic guidelines is, to some extent, controversial since these may be used to allocate resources. Further, the existence of prognostic guidelines may interfere with individual neurosurgical treatment in a negative way due to ethical and cultural differences. Thus, despite a great interest to both epidemiologists and clinicians within the neurological field in defining the optimal guideline for predicting the outcome following mild, moderate and severe traumatic brain injury, the design of such a guideline has not been possible [46]. Nevertheless, it is possible to predict the outcome with about 80 to 90 % accuracy when parameters such as GCS, CT scan features and the GOS are combined.

PREVENTATIVE STRATEGY

The increased awareness of primary prevention is based on our experience in the field. Thus, the implementation of new laws has significantly reduced the number of traumatic brain injuries due to an increased awareness of effective outcome. Individual behaviour is evidently changed when faced with legislative penalties. Thus, the incidence rate of seat belt use has significantly increased as a consequence of the introduction of laws making seatbelt use mandatory. Simultaneously, the number of traffic related injuries fell drastically. Also, in regions where laws enforcing mandatory use of helmets among motorcyclists and cyclists, significant reductions of incidence, prevalence and mortality rates for traumatic brain injuries are presented. Likewise, the same pattern of reduced injuries holds true in regions where alcohol controls in traffic and during various leisure activities is a natural feature. Further reduction of traumatic brain injuries can be foreseen with the introduction of a number of different safety systems in the society as a whole.

Traumatic brain injury education programmes should be directed towards different age groups at school and other important areas. One important step in primary prevention is the designing and presentation of education programmes to persuade individuals to change their risk-taking behaviour in traffic and during leisure activities. For instance, technical innovations are introduced faster than peoples´ adaptation to them. The incorporation of new technical innovations for primary prevention demands changes in peoples´ behaviour may impede the effectiveness.

Of special interest is the introduction of traumatic brain injury surveillance systems on national levels [47]. The construction of a surveillance system gives statistical information about incidence, prevalence and mortality rates of traumatic brain injuries. Where hospital data are present, the system includes age, gender, ICD codes, codes for causes of injury and treatment statistics. When constructed in a similar manner, the statistics can be compared with and implemented by different regions and nations. By analysing the information from such a database, the injury surveillance system can be used for preventative purposes. This system is also available to be used by people coming from different professions.

The enhanced continuous information process between the trauma team responsible for the acute care and life-threatening treatment and rehabilitation medicine responsible for the long-term processes, has improved the quality of secondary and tertiary prevention and treatment. Indeed, primary prevention of traumatic brain injuries is nowadays receiving much attention from governmental and non-governmental authorities. In contrast to many diseases, the etiological factors to traumatic brain injury such as accidents related to traffic, fall and leisure activities, is completely understood. Through communicating knowledge about prevention, acute care and rehabilitation, the incidence, prevalence and mortality rates of traumatic brain injuries can most probably be reduced considerably. The unacceptable epidemiological pattern of traumatic brain injuries worldwide demands the creation of a new paradigm for traumatic brain injury prevention. The old paradigm where the victim alone was responsible for an injury is nowadays transformed into the new one where society per se has a significant responsibility. In technical terms an injury can be defined as defective systems while in medical terms an injury is defined as pathological tissue and emotional complications. In societal terms the injury can be defined as an economic burden.

A step toward a new paradigm is to improve the coordination in ongoing preventative activities by breaking down the barriers between professionals dealing with primary, secondary and tertiary prevention. The introduction of a new paradigm by removing existing barriers may lead us to design and build a more comprehensive team. Such a head trauma team includes technology with competence in engineering and infrastructure, medicine with competence in emergency care, rehabilitation processes and representatives of brain trauma foundations. The society represents both non-governmental as well as governmental authorities. The ongoing activities within this team should include epidemiology, reconstruction accidents, health care programmes, individual rehabilitation processes, economic analyses, research action and quality assurance of all steps.

CONCLUSION

The health consequences of traumatic brain injury in economic terms result in a significant burden for the society. Of all injuries presented to the society in the world, traumatic brain injury is probably the most devastating event since it has such a profound impact not only to the victim him/herself but also to their close relatives as well as society as a whole. Statistical data from a large number of reports continue to demonstrate an unacceptably large number of traumatic brain injured victims worldwide. For every traumatic brain injury fatality, there are many victims in the need for hospital care not to mention the number of patients requiring outpatient treatment. The actual overall global cost of traumatic brain injuries is difficult to even estimate due to the lack of statistical data in many regions of the world. It is, however, certain to conclude that the global demands on an already overstretched health care cost level is enormous. On the other hand, it is much more difficult to consider the cost to society of long term absence from work, child and spousal stress in caring for the patient, and impact on the quality of life for both traumatic brain injured patients as well as their family members.

Of great importance is the awareness of the epidemiological pattern of traumatic brain injuries. Today the overall pattern is insufficient as incidence prevalence and mortality rate studies are suffering from methodological flaws. Also, a traumatic brain injury is not an all or nothing event but an ongoing dynamic process lasting for a long time. Thus, the introduction of standardized injury surveillance systems worldwide is necessary in order to significantly improve evidenced based practice among physicians dealing with traumatic brain injury.

The causes of traumatic brain injuries are, as mentioned, well known for the society. Both governmental and nongovernmental authorities can be of substantial help in organising the strategies to prevention of traumatic brain injuries. Primary prevention should be successful by the construction of local, regional, national and international networks of interdisciplinary knowledge. These networks aim at providing coordination and promote synergy in the response to head injury including the use of available resources and competences. By coordinating the networks under the auspicious of the World Health Organisation, all experience of primary prevention can be disseminated worldwide in the most effective way.

Parallel with an increased knowledge of the mechanisms behind a traumatic brain injury, the medical treatment has made big steps forward resulting in the improvement of outcome. For instance, the mortality rate of severe traumatic brain injury has decreased during the last decades because of an increased effective treatment strategy. Thus, the combination of increased biomechanical knowledge with new imaging and neurointensive care techniques has reduced the mortality rate of traumatic brain injuries with about 30%. The efficiency of the prehospital care taking already at the scene of accident is therefore of most importance for the outcome of the patient. Mathematical modelling, neuroimaging technology and neurointensive care includes the close interdisciplinary collaboration between technology and health care providers. To catch up with the increased technical and medical knowledge and to meet the demand for global goals for the prevention of traumatic brain injuries, a traumatic brain injury trauma team is suggested. The main objective of such a team is to initiate a cascade of activities achieved by the integration of knowledge originating from technology, medicine and society thereby creating a comprehensive picture of the traumatic brain injury pattern. The stress among family members to a traumatic brain injured patient has been underestimated. There is no doubt that the silent suffering is significant and that this should be encountered when defining the overall pattern of traumatic brain injury. Without their substantial support in assisting the patient with their re-integration back into society, the health care costs would have been much more expensive. To look upon prevention of traumatic brain injuries as a public health and family issue, the unacceptable large number of deaths and disabled can be significantly reduced, thereby resulting in reduced health care costs as well as reduced physical and mental impact to the society as a whole.

REFERENCES

[1]   Krug E, Dahlberg, L, Mercy J A et al. World report on violence and health, *World Health Organisation*, Geneva. 2002.

[2]   Injuries in the WHO European Region: burden, challenges and policy response. Background paper for the 55th Session of the WHO Regional Committee (RC55) 2005.

[3]   Waters H, Hyder A, Rajkotia Y et al.: The economic dimensions of interpersonal violence, *World Health Organisation*, Geneva. 2004.

[4]   Kraus J F: Epidemiology of head injury. In: Cooper PR, Ed. *Head Injury*, 3rd ed. Baltimore, MD: William Wilkins. 1993.

[5]   WHO report: International Statistical Classification of Diseases and Related Health Problems, ICD –10, 10th revision, *World Health Organisation*, Geneva.1992.

[6]   Fernside M R, Simpson D A: Epidemiology, 3-23. In *Head Injury – Pathophysiology and management of severe head injury*. Eds: Reilly P and Bullock R. Chapman & Hall, London. 1997.

[7]   Murray G D, Teasdale G M, Braakman R, Cohadon F et al: The European Brain Injury Consortium survey on head injuries. *Acta Neurochir*. 1999;141: 223-230.

[8]   Kay A, Teasdale G M: Head injury in the United Kingdom. *World J Surg*, 2001; 25: 1210-1220.

[9]   Firsching R, Woischneck M D: Present status of neurosurgical trauma in Germany. *World J. Surg.* 2001; 25, 1221-1223.

[10]   Kleiven S, Peloso P, von Holst H: Incidence of Head Injuries in Sweden during 1987 and 2000. *J Injury Control and Safety Promotion*, 2003; Vol 10, No. 1, 173-180).

[11]   Gururaj G: Epidemiology of traumatic brain injuries: Indian scenarios. *Neurol Res.* 2002; 24:24-28.

[12]   Maejima M D, Katayama Y: Neurosurgical trauma in Japan. *World J. Surg.* 2001; 25: 1205-1209.

[13]   Hung C, ChiuW, Tsai C: The epidemiology of head injury in Hualien County, Taiwan, *Journal of the Formosan Medical Association*.1991; 90: 1227-1233.

[14]   Lee L, Shih Y, Chiu W et al.: Epidemiological study of head injuries in Taipei City, Taiwan. *Chinese Medical Journal (Taipei)*. 1992; 50:219-225.

[15]   Tate R L, McDonald S, Lulham J M: incidence of hospital-treated traumatic brain injury in a community. *Brain Inj*. 1997 Sep; 11 (9): 649-59.

[16]   Nell V, Brown S O D: Epidemiology of traumatic brain injury in Johannesburg II: Morbidity, mortality and etiology. *Soc. Sci Med*. 1991; 33:289-292.

[17]   Kraus J F, McArthur D L, Silverman T A, et al.: Epidemiology of brain injury. 13-30. In *Neurotrauma*, (Ed: Narayan R K, et al) McGraw-Hill. 1996.

[18]   Bailes J E, Cantu R C,: Head Injury in Athletes. Neurosurgery. 2001; Vol 48, No 1, 26-46.

[19]   Collins J G: Types of injuries by selected characteristics: United States 1985-1987. *Vital Health Stat.* 1990; 10:17.

[20]   Bogner J A, Corrigan J D, Mysiw W J et al: A comparison of substance abuse and violence in the prediction of long-term rehabilitation outcomes after brain injury. *Arch Phys Med Rehabil*, 2001; 82: 571-7.

[21]   Teasdale G, Jennett B: Assessment and prognosis of coma after head injury. *Acta Neurochir*, 1976; 34:45- 47.

[22]   Cassidy D, Carroll L J, Peloso P M et al: Incidence, risk factors and prevention of mild traumatic brain injury. *J Rehabil Med*, 2004; February Suppl No 43: 28-60.

[23]   Wilberger J E, Rothfus W E, Tabas J et al: Acute tissue tear hemorrhage of the brain: computed tomographyand clinicopathological correlations. *Neurosurgery*, 1990; 27: 208-213.

[24]   Povlishock J T: Traumatically induced axonal injury: pathogenesis and pathobiological implications. *Brain Pathology*, 1992; 2:1-12.

[25]   Siesjö B: Pathopgysiology and treatment of focal cerebral ischemia. Part II: Mechanism of damage and treatment. *J Neurosurg*. 1992; 77:337-354.

[26]   Miller J D: Traumatic brain swelling and edema, in *Head Injury* (Ed. Cooper P J) Williams and Wilkins, Baltimore, MD, 1993; pp351-354.

[27]   Marmarou A, Fatouros P, Bandoh K et al: *The contribution of brain edema to brain swelling, ICP and craniospinal dynamic, in Intracranial Pressure VIII*, (eds. Avezaat C J J et al), Springer Verlag, Berlin, 1993; pp 525-528.

[28]   Graham D I, Lawrence A E, Adams J H et al: Brain damage in non-missile head injury secondary to high intracranial pressure. *Neuropathol Appl Neurobiol*. 1987; 13:209.

[29]   Wilberger J E, Harris M, Diamond D: Acute subdural hematoma: Morbidity and mortalityrelated to timing of operative intervention. *J Trauma* 1990; 30:733-736.

[30]   Pagni C A, Massaro F: Concomitant cranio-cerebral and vertebro-medullary injuries: Analysis of 121 cases. *Acta Neurochir (Wien)*, 1991; 111:1-10.

[31]   Goodisson D, MacFarlane M, Snape L et al (2004): Head injury and associated maxillofacial injuries. *N Z Med J*, Sep 10: 117 (1201):U1042).

[32]   Lobato R D, Rivas J J, Gomez P A et al: Head injured patients who talk and deteriorate into coma: Analysis of 211 cases studied with computerized tomography. *J Neurosurg*, 1991; 75: 256-261.

[33]   Cooper P R: Post-traumatic intracranial mass lesions, 275-329, in Cooper P R (Ed): *Head Injury* (3rd Edition) 1993; Baltimore, Williams&Wilkins

[34]   Kwiakowski S: Contemporary verification of posttraumatic intracerebral hematoma treated conservatively before the CT era. *Neurol Neurochir Pol Suppl 2*, 1994; 229-234.

[35]   Peloso, P M, Carroll L J, Cassidy D et al: Critical evaluation of the existing Guidelines on mild traumatic brain injury, *J Rehabil Med Suppl*, 2004; 43:106-112.

[36]   Hlatky R, Robertson C S: Does raising the cerebral perfusion pressure help head injured patients? In *Neurotrauma* 2005; (Ed: Valadka A B) Thieme pp 75-82.

[37]   Teasdale G, Murray G, Andersson E et al: Risks of acute traumatic intracranial hematoma in children and adults: implications for managing head injuries. *BMJ* 1990; 300: 363-367.

[38]   Paniak C, Reynolds S, Toller Lobe G et al (2002): A longitudinal study of the relationship between financial compensation and symptoms after treated mild traumatic brain injury. *J Clin Exp Neuropsychol*. 2002; 24: 187-193.

[39]   (Ed: Povlishock J T: Management and prognosis of severe traumatic brain injury. *J Neurotrauma*. 2000; Vol 17, 6/7, June/July).

[40] (Ed: Valadka A B): *Neurotrauma, Evidence-based answers to common questions.* 2005; Thieme.

[41] (Ed: Grimby G: Best evidence synthesis on mild traumatic brain injury: Results of the WHO collaborating centre for neurotrauma prevention, management and rehabilitation task force on mild traumatic brain injury. *J Rehabil Med Suppl 43*, 2004.

[42] Carroll L J, Cassidy D, Peloso P M et al: Prognosis for mild traumatic brain injury: Results of the WHO collaborating centre task force on mild traumatic brain injury. *J Rehabil Med Suppl*, 2004; 43: 84-105.

[43] Colohan A R T, Oyesiku N M (1992): Moderate head injury: An overview. *J Neurtotrauma*,1992; 9 (suppl.), S 259-S 264.

[44] Waxman K, Sundine M J, Young R F: Is early prediction of outcome in severe head injury possible? *Arch Surg* 126, 1991: 1237-1241.

[45] Quatrocci K B, Prasad P, Willits N H et al: Quantification of midline shift as a predictor of poor outcome following head injury. *Surgical Neurol* 35, 1991; 183-188.

[46] Choi S C, Barnes T Y: Prediction outcome in the head-injured patient. pp 779-792. In *Neurotrauma*, 1996; (Ed Narayan R K) McGraw-Hill.

[47] Injury surveillance guidelines (Ed Holder Y et al), 2001; *World Health Organisation,* Geneva.

RECOMMENDED FURTHER READING

1. Rosenthal M (Editor). *Rehabilitation of the adult and child with traumatic brain injury.* 3rd Edition. FA Davis Company, Philadelphia, 1999.

2. Narayan RK, Povlishock and Wilberger JE. *Neurotrauma.* McGraw-Hill Companies, 1996.

3. Reilly P and Bullock R. *Head injury. Pathophysiology and management of severe closed injury.* A Hodder Arnold Publication, 1997.

4. *Prehospital trauma care systems.* World Health Organisation, Geneva, 2005.

In: Handbook of Clinical Neuroepidemiology

Editors: V. L. Feigin and D. A. Bennett, pp. 233-300

ISBN 978-1-60021-511-7

© 2007 Nova Science Publishers, Inc.

Chapter 8

PERIPHERAL NEUROPATHY

Nadir E. Bharucha[1,2] and Christopher D. Ward[3]

[1]Bombay Hospital Institute of Medical Sciences, Bombay, India;
[2]Department of Neuroepidemiology, Medical Research Centre, Bombay Hospital, Bombay, India;
[3]University of Nottingham School of Community Health Sciences, UK.

ABSTRACT

This chapter reviews the epidemiology of distal, symmetrical polyneuropathy. There are few reliable data on the epidemiology of peripheral neuropathy in general, and there have been no published attempts to measure the burden of disability in the population. We survey the evidence on a series of groups of conditions: genetic, diabetic, inflammatory, infective, toxic (including drugs), nutritional and paraneoplastic. Again, there are few data on the extent of disability attributable to neuropathies due to individual causes. A recurring theme in the chapter is the need for rigorous diagnostic criteria, since clinical classification of peripheral neuropathy is in many conditions neither specific nor sensitive.

INTRODUCTION

Peripheral neuropathy is a frequent diagnosis in clinical neurology [31,30]. In this section we will review population-based data on peripheral neuropathy with regard to prevention and management at the individual and public health levels. We will discuss evidence relevant to the burden of disability attributable to peripheral neuropathy in populations, although data are scarce. The main focus of the section will be on symmetrical, diffuse polyneuropathy. We will not discuss individual rare neuropathies where population data are not available and we will not cover compressive neuropathies.

DEFINITIONS AND EPIDEMIOLOGY OF POLYNEUROPATHIES

Overviews of the epidemiology of peripheral neuropathy produce widely discrepant statistics. Thus, for example, estimates of the annual incidence of peripheral neuropathy have varied from 1.6 to 99 per 100,000 [187*]. Possible reasons for such variation are (a) that the interpretation of epidemiological data is more dependent on case definition in peripheral neuropathy than in most neurological conditions; (b) electrophysiological abnormalities are much more sensitive than clinical criteria; and (c) clinical criteria themselves vary in specificity: sensory symptoms may be of very questionable significance in the absence of signs, and some signs, such as absent vibration sensation are non-specific. Diagnostic specificity can be greatly enhanced by standardised methods of sensory assessment [124]. Formal operational definitions comprising combinations of features are required in specific conditions, such as diabetic neuropathy and also in specific research contexts, such as house-to-house surveys. Epidemiological generalisations from multiple studies of peripheral neuropathy are of limited value unless due allowance is made for variations in case definition. Conversely, the technical challenges entailed in the diagnosis of neuropathy must be taken into account when interpreting other epidemiological data. An Indian study [151] found that 94 of 125 patients thought to have ill-defined or functional disorders had neuropathy.

Criteria for the etiological classification of neuropathies are also highly variable from one publication to another. For example, investigation of patients with diabetes revealed alternative diagnoses in less than 10% in one carefully conducted study [89], but in another American study 55 (53%) of 103 patients with diabetes had additional causes for distal sensory polyneuropathy, including neurotoxic medications, excessive alcohol intake, B_{12} deficiency and renal disease. Laboratory investigations showed abnormally low levels of vitamin B_6 and of B_1, monoclonal gammopathy and hypertriglyceridaemia [107]. Again, generalizations from multiple studies are difficult because data on the relative prevalence of different types of neuropathy must take into account different investigation protocols. When symmetrical neuropathies are lumped together with compressive neuropathies, heterogeneity is even more of a problem and the possibility of making useful inferences from broad descriptive statistics is further reduced.

Overall Incidence and Prevalence of Peripheral Neuropathy

There is a shortage of prospective data from which incidence figures for peripheral neuropathies as a group can be derived. In a prospective cohort study of diabetic neuropathy, 2% of a control group of older adults had peripheral neuropathy at baseline, and 6% had peripheral neuropathy at 10 years [226].

The prevalence of peripheral neuropathy is best estimated from house-to-house surveys. A study of Parsis in Bombay achieved many of the methodological standards required for reliable population-based data: the participation rate was high, respondents completed a detailed questionnaire, and each individual was examined by an experienced neurologist. In the pilot study of 851 people (89.2% of whom were ≥ 15 years age), the crude prevalence of peripheral neuropathy was 3760 per 100,000 [31]. In the definitive study of 14,010 people (87.7% of whom were ≥ 15 years), peripheral neuropathy was found in 2384 per 100,000 [30]. Table 1 shows the distribution of types of neuropathy in the Bombay study.

In the Bombay study, polyneuropathies constituted about 30% of all peripheral neuropathies and diabetes was the most common cause of polyneuropathy. In a study of patients attending general practitioners in two Italian regions, diabetes was associated with neuropathy in 44% of the cases [142].

Table 1. Estimated prevalences of neuropathies
(Bombay study: Bharucha et al 1991) [30]

	Cases	Crude prevalence per 100,000
Mononeuropathies		
Carpal tunnel syndrome	78	557
Lumbosacral radiculopathy	72	514
Bell's palsy	20	143
Cervical radiculopathy	19	136
Ulnar nerve palsy	14	100
Herpes zoster	12	86
Meralgia paraesthetica	10	71
Compressive neuropathy, cause uncertain	6	43
Trigeminal neuralgia	4	29
Polyneuropathies		
Diabetic neuropathy (all types)	52	371
Idiopathic neuropathy	30	214
Guillain Barre syndrome	4	29
Alcoholic neuropathy	3	21
Iatrogenic neuropathy	3	21
Hereditary motor sensory neuropathy	2	14
Rheumatoid neuropathy	2	14
Ischaemic neuropathy	2	14
Nutritional neuropathy	1	7
TOTAL	334	2384

GENETIC NEUROPATHIES

Genetic polyneuropathies have become an increasingly complex field since the introduction of genetic testing from the 1980s [86*,64*]. From an epidemiological point of view, it would be desirable to be able to collate information on prevalence of genetic polyneuropathies both as a group and as individual syndromes. Ahlstrom et al (1993) [3] reported a total prevalence of 9 per 100,000, but this figure was applicable to southern Sweden. Genetic diseases are subject to large regional variations for a variety of reasons, such as founder effects in dominant conditions and rates of consanguineous unions in recessive conditions. Data on the burden of morbidity and disability would also be valuable, but could rarely be inferred from prevalence data alone, because the clinical severity of genetic neuropathies is extremely variable. Currently available evidence from population-based studies therefore leaves many of the crucial questions unanswered.

Charcot Marie Tooth syndrome (also known as hereditary motor/sensory neuropathies)

Charcot Marie Tooth syndrome (CMT) (also called the hereditary motor/sensory neuropathies - HMSN) causes slowly progressive distal weakness and muscle wasting, largely affecting the legs, typically with pes cavus, areflexia and glove and stocking sensory impairment. It usually begins in the first to third decade. Some subtypes are associated with pyramidal signs. Other important associations of different subtypes include diaphragmatic weakness [171,186], scoliosis [186], laryngeal paralysis [87], hearing loss, and hip dysplasia [193]. The neuropathy of CMT can be painful [48].

Originally defined clinically, in the 1960's the CMT hereditary neuropathies were classified into two groups based on neurophysiological and histological criteria. One group is attributed to slow nerve conduction velocities with hypertrophic demyelinating neuropathy (HMSN type 1 or CMT1). The other group has relatively normal velocities, with axonal and neuronal degeneration rather than demyelination (hereditary motor and sensory neuropathy type 2 or CMT2). With the advent of genetic testing, an ever increasing number of genetic subtypes has been described. In one study, 80% of those with CMT-1 had clinical signs but all had delayed nerve conduction, so that the penetrance was 100% [209].

Among the demyelinating (CMT-1) polyneuropathies the most frequently encountered genotype is CMT-1A. This is due to a 1.4 megabase duplication of chromosome 17 containing the peripheral myelin protein gene. The gene codes for an important protein constituent of nerves, peripheral myelin protein (PMP-22). New mutations were thought to be not uncommon in one study [186], but Mostacciuolo et al (1991) [209] estimated the rate to be 3 to 6 per million gametes. A low mutation rate would be expected, since CMT is unlikely to have a major influence on reproductive fitness. Other CMT-1 genotypes have been identified, including CMT-1B, which is caused by mutations in the myelin protein zero gene on chromosome 1. CMT-1A and 1B are clinically and neurophysiologically indistinguishable. CMT-1 is usually autosomal dominant but can be autosomal recessive.

Axonal (CMT-2) syndromes are also slowly progressive [277]. Some genetic subtypes have somewhat later onset of symptoms. Inheritance can be dominant or recessive. The major cause of autosomal dominant CMT2 is CMT2A secondary to mutations in the mitofusin 2 gene which in recent studies accounts for approximately 20% of autosomal dominant CMT2. The main form of X-linked CMT is caused by mutation in the connexin-32 gene and this form of CMT is the second commonest form after CMT1A.

A large French series of people with CMT-1A genotype, including asymptomatic relatives of probands, showed that functional disabilities, which were usually not severe, were evident in the first decade in 50% of cases and in the second decade in 70% [33]. A more severe disease course was associated with earlier age of onset and with more greatly reduced motor nerve conduction velocity. Neurological deficit and functional disability increased, whereas median nerve conduction velocity (MNCV) and compound muscle action potential (CMAP) amplitude did not change with disease course. Deficits differed widely within as well as between families, with variations in age at onset, clinical severity and MNCV slowing, suggesting that environmental factors may influence clinical manifestations. In support of this suggestion, the clinical features of CMT-1A have been shown to vary between monozygotic twins [101]. Although the study by Birouk et al (1997), [33] was cross-sectional, there was evidence that clinical progression was not related to decreasing motor nerve velocity. In another cross-sectional comparison of neurophysiological and clinical data, disability was correlated with indicators of axonal loss rather than demyelination [162].

Table 2A. CMT prevalence in children

Region	Estimated Prevalence per 100,000		Reference
	Subtypes	All types	
South Sweden	CMT-1 8.0	19.1	Hagberg & Westerberg 1983 [117]
	CMT-2 11.1		
West Sweden	--	13.6	Darin & Tulinius 2000 [77]

Table 2B. CMT prevalence – all ages

Region	Estimated Crude Prevalence per 100,000		Reference
	Subtypes	All CMT	
North Italy	CMT-1 9.4	-	Mostacciuolo e al 1991 [209]
South Wales	CMT-1 10.9	18.1	MacMillan & Harper 1994 [184]
	CMT-2 2.7		
North Sweden	CMT-1 16.2	20.1	Holmberg 1993 [131]
	CMT-2 3.1		
Benghazi Libya	CMT-1 6.4		Radhakrishnan K. et al 1987 [231]
	CMT-2 1.5		
North Spain	CMT-1 15.2	28.2	Combarros O. et al 1987 [65]
	CMT-2 13.0		
West Norway	--	41.0	Skre H. 1974 [262]
Central Italy	CMT-1A 11.2	17.5	Morocutti et al 2002 [208]
West Japan	CMT-1A 3.0	10.8	Kurihara et al 2002 [165]

CMT is one of the most common inherited neurological disorders. Estimates of the population prevalence of CMT have varied from 11 to 41 per 100,000 in different parts of the world (see Table 2). Some of the variation is undoubtedly due to variations in gene frequency in different populations, and some is likely to be due to methodological differences between studies. Case ascertainment usually depends on identifying index cases, often from medical records, and subsequently identifying relatives. Many factors introduce potential error into these procedures.

Estimates of prevalence do not change markedly with age, suggesting that progression is slow. Holmberg (1993) [131] reported a lower age-specific prevalence (12.8 per 100,000) in those aged 5 to 10 years than in subsequent decades, but prevalence rates among children were not markedly different from those in adults in two other studies [117,77].

CMT-1 accounts for 80% of cases of CMT in most studies. The CMT-1A secondary to the chromosome 17 duplication is present in 70% to 80% of unrelated European patients with CMT1 [216,35,210]. Many CMT subtypes have been described in only a few families. Specific ethnic associations are sometimes evident, for example the occurrence of CMT-4D in various communities of Romany origin [241] and recessive inheritance may account for as much as half of the cases in areas where consanguineous marriages are common [286]. In Nigeria, CMT has been reported to be rare, but without formal epidemiological confirmation [4].

Prevalence studies of CMT have invariably found wide variations in clinical severity both between and within families. There are very few data from which to estimate the burden of disability attributable to CMT in populations. Hagberg and Westerberg (1983) [117] estimated the prevalence of severe disability in children to be 1.9 per 100,000. The prevalence of moderate disability was 13.3 per 100,000. Holmberg (1993) [131] found that disability was severe for 15% of people with CMT. One quarter of those aged 20 or more stated that CMT had affected their choice of profession, and 42% of those aged between 30 and 60 were receiving partial or complete disability pensions.

Hereditary Neuropathy with Liability to Pressure Palsies

Hereditary neuropathy with liability to pressure palsies (HNNP) is an autosomal dominant condition, characterized by recurrent mononeuropathies caused by relatively trivial traumas. Recovery is usually good, although in a minority residual disabilities can persist. The condition is caused by a deletion of the same 1.4 megabase part of chromosome17 (containing the PMP-22 gene), which in CMT-1A is duplicated. Meretoja et al [201] found the remarkably high prevalence of 16 per 100,000 in southwest Finland. They pointed out that since CMT-1A and HNNP are considered to be reciprocal deletion/duplication syndromes and since neither disease significantly affects life expectancy, their prevalences would be expected to be similar [201]. The burden of disability is uncertain. Sander et al (2005) [248] failed to find the mutation in a series of patients with carpal tunnel syndrome.

Familial Amyloid Polyneuropathy

Familial amyloid polyneuropathy (FAP) is one form of hereditary generalized amyloidosis, initially showing polyneuropathy and autonomic dysfunction but later involving many visceral organs. This disorder was first clearly described in Portugal in 1952, where the disease is endemic [270], but there are also foci in Sweden [8,269], in the Spanish Balearic islands [212] and in Japan [140]. Smaller clusters have been found elsewhere, for example Ireland [240]. More than 80 mutations, with variable phenotypes, have been identified.

In north Portugal, the crude prevalence rate reported was 90.3 per 100,000, and the frequency of gene carriers was estimated to be 186 per 100,000. About half of these carriers had manifested symptoms [270]. The prevalence in Northern Sweden ranged from 91 to 104 per 100,000 [269]. Holmgren et al (1994) [132] used a monoclonal antibody to screen a random sample of adults, those with evidence of the mutation then having DNA tests. The prevalence of the relevant mutation in the area was 1.5%, ranging from 0.0 to 8.3%. The crude prevalence rate for FAP was 30 per 100,000 compared with a mutation prevalence of 1500 per 100,000 and a similarly low penetrance was found by Reilly et al (1995) [240].

DIABETIC POLYNEUROPATHY

Mono- and polyneuropathies are common complications of diabetes mellitus [39*]. In this review we will focus primarily on polyneuropathy, as well as autonomic neuropathy. There are several reasons why diabetic neuropathy is an important topic for clinical neurologists. Firstly, diabetes is the single most frequent cause of polyneuropathy. Among patients with polyneuropathy of unknown cause investigated in three specialist neuromuscular clinics, 36% had impaired glucose tolerance (pre-diabetes) and 21% had previously undiagnosed diabetes mellitus [274]. Secondly, neuropathic symptoms, such as pain and foot-drop, are important sources of disability in their own right. Thirdly, neuropathy makes a major contribution to two disabling and life-threatening complications, foot ulceration and amputation. Finally, even when not severe in their own right, polyneuropathy and cardiac autonomic neuropathy are markers for the presence of risks of other microvascular conditions as well as macrovascular complications, many of which can be alleviated or prevented with improved blood sugar control. For this reason alone, the presence of painful sensory neuropathy should trigger a full oral glucose tolerance test (OGTT) to exclude pre-diabetes or diabetes [274,261]. Thus, diabetic neuropathy is one of the few conditions in which neurologists have an opportunity for preventive intervention.

The pathogenesis of diabetic neuropathy is not well understood [273*,38*]. Excess glucose is thought to cause oxidative stress and also glycation, a non-enzymatic reaction with proteins and other neural constituents. From a clinical and epidemiological point of view, the key point is that hyperglycemia causes a physiologically reversible reduction in nerve conduction velocity. Structural damage and cell death may result from impaired microcirculation and other factors. Schwann cells are also thought to be affected, leading either to cell death or to demyelination [285].

Interpretation of epidemiological data on diabetic polyneuropathy must generally take into account (1) the population characteristics including geographical and ethnic factors, as well as quality of clinical care; (2) year of publication (in view of time-trends in incidence and prevalence), and (3) criteria for case definition.

Diagnostic Definition of Diabetic Neuropathy

As in other neuropathies, definitional problems greatly complicate the analysis of epidemiological data about diabetic neuropathy. In one study, for example, the majority of adults with established diabetes had decreased reflexes at baseline. Only a minority (4 to 13 %) had definite neuropathy on clinical grounds alone, while around four times as many had abnormal nerve conduction studies [82]. No single clinical or physiological test provides an adequate diagnostic criterion because the pathogenesis of diabetic neuropathy involves both large and small fibres in complex ways. Hence, standardized protocols are required [66,88]. No single protocol will be suitable both for community-based epidemiological studies and for more intensive clinic-based studies.

A further definitional problem arises because a causal relationship between diabetes and neuropathy can never be established with certainty. Other etiologies are likely to be present in populations with presumed diabetic neuropathy, especially since the prevalences of diabetes itself and of both diabetic neuropathy and other neuropathies increase with age (Table 3 a,b). In the study of diabetic distal sensory polyneuropathy already mentioned [107], over half the participants had one additional cause and 25% had more than one. Nine (9%) had three or more demyelinating features on EMG.

Incidence and Prevalence of Diabetic Neuropathy

Incidence

The annual incidence of diabetic polyneuropathy in *the general population* was estimated to be 54 (CI 33, 83) per 100,000 in one U.K study based on general practice records [183].

The incidence of neuropathy has been investigated more thoroughly in populations of *people with diabetes*. From an analysis of the case records of a Rochester, MN cohort with DM2, using clinical criteria, Palumbo et al (1978) reported polyneuropathy to have a point prevalence of 4% at the time of diagnosis, compared with 15% after 20 years of follow-up [225]. Using vibration perception threshold (VPT) as a criterion, Coppini et al (2001) [68] found that 20% of patients developed neuropathy over a 12 year period. The remaining 80% retained a "normal" VPT after a mean diabetes duration of 16 years, despite less than optimal blood sugar control, suggesting that other factors such as genetics may influence the incidence of diabetic polyneuropathy [68]. Partanen et al (1995) [226] found neurophysiological evidence of neuropathy in 8.3% of people newly diagnosed with DM2, compared with 16.7% at five years and 41.9% at 10 years. At baseline, there was no difference between diabetics and controls in the frequency of neuropathic pain or paraesthesiae, but after 10 years, 20% of the diabetic group experienced neuropathic pain and more than 30% had paraesthesiae. Note that 27% of the patients had died by 10 years. After a mean of 7 years follow-up, 17% of patients with DM1 developed cardiac autonomic neuropathy defined by loss of heart rate variability or postural hypotension on standing [303]. In a study of men with DM1, 25% developed erectile dysfunction over 10 years. The incidence increases with age and with increasing duration of diabetes [158]. Thus, the annual incidence of new cases of neuropathy among diabetics appears to range between 1% and 2%.

Prevalence

Two door-to-door surveys in Sicily and in the Parsi population in Bombay, provide comparable data on prevalence *in the general population*. In these studies, diabetes and polyneuropathy were defined clinically, and neither nerve conduction nor autonomic testing were performed. The estimated prevalence of symptomatic diabetic polyneuropathy in the population as a whole was 268 per 100,000 in Sicily and 371 per 100,000 in Bombay. Both studies showed an age-related rise in prevalence, except in the oldest age-groups where sample sizes were small. Findings from the two studies are summarised in Table 3. In Sicily there was a preponderance of females in the older age groups, which was not found in Bombay.

Table 3 (a,b). Age- and sex-specific prevalences of diabetic neuropathy per 100,000 population in two studies[

Age-group	Prevalence per 100,000 (Number of cases/sample size)					
	Males		Females		Total	
	Sicily	Bombay	Sicily	Bombay	Sicily	Bombay
0-39	0.0 (0/4456)	0.0 (0/2931)	0.0 (0/4226)	0.0 (0/3008)	0.0 (0/8062)	0.0 (0/5939)
40-59	375.0 (6/1600)	213.2 (4/1876)	597.0 (10/1675)	227.8 (5/2195)	488.5 (16/3275)	221.1 (9/4071)
60-79	573.6 (6/1046)	766.8 (12/1565)	1150.4 (14/1217)	1422.3 (26/1828)	883.8 (20/2263)	1119.9 (38/3393)
80+	0.0 (0/133)	1374.6 (4/291)	1604.3 (3/187)	316.5 (1/316)	937.5 (3/320)	823.7 (5/607)
All ages	165.9	300.17	369.6	435.55	268.2	371.16

Numbers of cases and sizes of samples in parentheses
(Sicily Study [251]; Bombay Study: unpublished data [30])

The frequency of neuropathy among *people with diabetes* has been studied repeatedly. Using rigorous criteria including abnormalities in either nerve conduction studies or objective autonomic tests, the Rochester Diabetic Neuropathy Study [89] found polyneuropathy in 54% of those with insulin-dependent diabetes mellitus (Type 1, DM1) and in 45% of those with Type 2 (DM2). Figure 1 is based on the results from this study. In all age groups, the majority of neuropathies were asymptomatic. There was no marked effect of age or of type of diabetes.

The 1989 American National Health Interview Survey, which used less rigorous diagnostic criteria, found that 30.2 % of those with DM1 reported symptoms compatible with sensory neuropathy. Thirty-six percent of men with DM2 and 39.8% of women with DM2 were affected, compared with 9.8 and 11.8% of controls [120]. Other estimates of the prevalence of clinically detectable neuropathy have been around 25% for both Type 1 and Type 2 diabetes (DM1, DM2) [175,133,13]. A similar prevalence has been reported in children with DM1 [217]. A community-based study by Daousi et al (2004) [76] found chronic painful neuropathy in 16% of diabetics compared with only 5% of age and sex matched controls [76].

In summary, the prevalence of polyneuropathy appears to be similar in DM1 and DM2. Using the most rigorous criteria, detectable neuropathy affects about half of all patients, with 10% to 20% being symptomatic. The estimates are higher when less rigorous criteria are applied.

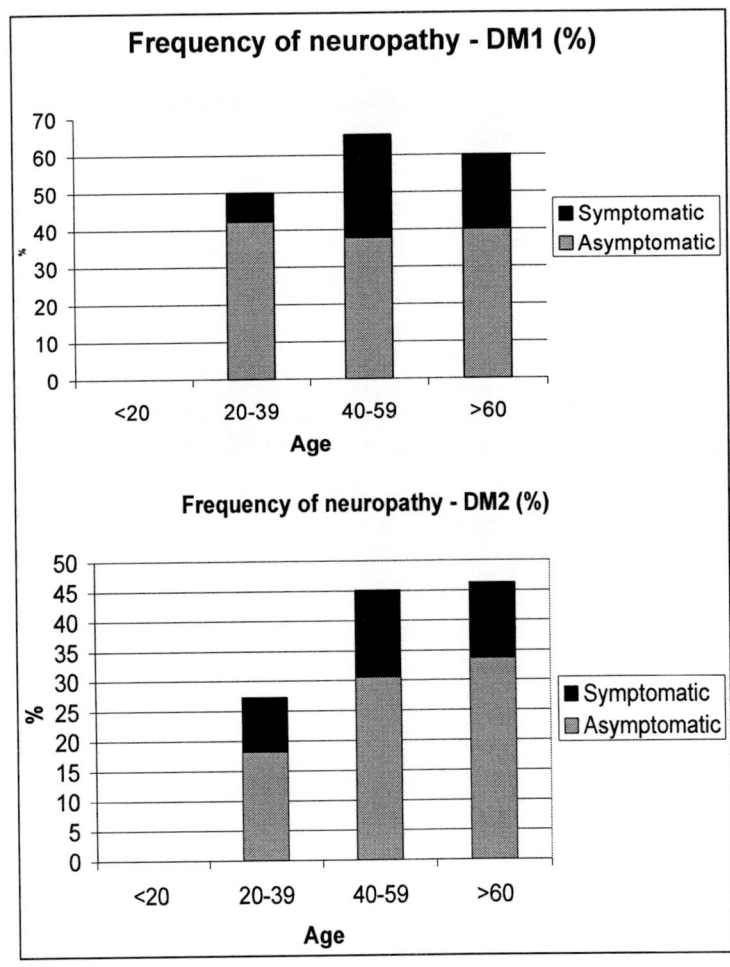

Figure 1. Frequency of neuropathy in diabetes mellitus (based on data from Dyck et al 1993 [89].

Autonomic Neuropathy in Diabetes

Judged from the vasoconstriction index, Freccero et al (2004) [97] found abnormal sympathetic function in 40% of a series of patients with DM1 and in 41% of those with DM2. The expiration/inspiration ratio, indicating parasympathetic dysfunction, was abnormal in 42% with DM1and 65% with DM2 [97]. The prevalence of autonomic neuropathy was 36% in a large European study, with no gender differences. The frequency of orthostatic dizziness was 18%, while only 4% of patients had nocturnal diarrhea and 5% had problems with bladder control [149]. In the Rochester Diabetic Neuropathy Study [89], postural fainting was rare (1% in DM1 and none in DM2). Visceral autonomic neuropathy was found in 5.5%, but nocturnal diarrhea was rare (1% in DM1 and 0.4% in DM2), as was urinary incontinence (1% in DM1, none in DM2). Impotence affected 13% of men with DM1 and 11% of men with DM2. As in the case with diabetic polyneuropathy diabetic autonomic neuropathy is often asymptomatic.

Risk Factors for Diabetic Neuropathy

Diabetic polyneuropathy and autonomic neuropathy are related both to age and to duration of diabetes. Other prominent risk factors include glycemic control (see below), hypertension and smoking [226,71,34,13,149]. Autonomic neuropathy is associated with the presence of cardiovascular disease and with other cardiovascular risk factors in addition to smoking and hypertension, including a lower HDL-cholesterol ratio, a lower total cholesterol/HDL-cholesterol ratio and a higher fasting triglyceride [149]. Diabetic autonomic neuropathy has increased prevalence and severity in Vietnamese diabetic patients, suggesting that genetic factors may be operative [282].

Effect of Glycemic Control

In a randomised comparison of intensive metabolic therapy with conventional therapy in adults with insulin-dependent diabetes mellitus, the reduction in risk of clinical peripheral neuropathy was 71% (CI 34 to 87) in the primary prevention cohort of patients who had had diabetes for between one to five years and who had no retinopathy or albuminuria. The risk reduction was similar (64%, CI 45% to 76%) in the secondary prevention cohort with moderate and non proliferative retinopathy and moderate or no albuminuria [82]. These risk reductions, have been maintained through 7 years of further follow up, even though the difference in mean glycosylated hemoglobin [HbA(1c)] levels of the treatment groups became statistically nonsignificant by 5 years, and rate of progression of complications remained lower in the intensive treatment group after termination of the trial. Thus, the benefits of intensive treatment extend well beyond the period of its most intensive implementation [83]. In keeping with this result, a prospective study from Pittsburgh found an inverse relationship between the development of neuropathy and intensiveness of treatment provided [308]. An association between microvascular complications, including neuropathy, and social deprivation is also likely to reflect poorer glycemic control [32].

Tighter glycemic control may be needed to prevent peripheral neuropathy than to prevent other complications of diabetes mellitus An Australian study of complications in adolescents with DM1 demonstrated a significant decline in retinopathy and in microalbuminuria from 1990 to 2002 despite a highly significant increase in peripheral neuropathy. Autonomic nerve abnormalities remained unchanged. [205].

Disability, Mortality and Health Care Costs Associated with Diabetic Neuropathy

There are few epidemiological data on the burden of disability associated with diabetic neuropathy. In a Norwegian study based on data from patients referred to a tertiary centre [213], the prevalence of diabetic neuropathy with 'significant polyneuropathy symptoms' was estimated to be 23.2 (15.5-30.9) per 100,000. If the overall population prevalence of diabetic neuropathy was similar to that found in Sicily and Bombay, the Norwegian data may give some indication of the proportion of patients (perhaps 10%) in whom the condition was sufficiently significant to merit neurological referral. Pain is an under-recognized cause of morbidity. In a community-based study, Daousi et al (2004) [76] found that 40% of diabetics with chronic painful neuropathy had received no treatment for pain; one third of these had never reported their symptoms to a physician.

Neuropathy is an independent predictor of reduced mobility, although not of reduced activities of daily living [43]. Comorbidity, for example stroke, contributes to this association, but the predominant factors here are foot ulceration and amputation. Foot ulceration is more strongly associated with neuropathy than with microvascular disease, and accounts for the largest proportion of healthcare costs incurred by neuropathy [106]. In patients with DM2 neuropathy, besides being a major cause of morbidity, is among the variables predictive of mortality [71].

There are important ethnic variations in risk of foot ulceration. In the UK, people of South Asian origin have about one-third the risk of those of European origin. Two of the main reasons for the reduced risk are the reduced frequency of neuropathy and of peripheral vascular disease in this population. People of African-Caribbean origin, particularly males, also have less foot ulceration, largely because of a reduced frequency of neuropathy [2,57]. In Africa, neuropathy is thought to underlie diabetic foot complications more often than peripheral vascular disease, which is less common [189]. However, studies in various parts of Africa have produced widely different estimates of the prevalence of both neuropathy and foot ulceration [1].

INFLAMMATORY NEUROPATHIES

Guillan Barre Syndrome (Acute inflammatory demyelinatng polyneuropathy, AIDP)**

Guillain-Barre Syndrome (GBS) is a subacute, progressive, usually symmetrical polyneuropathy characterized by weakness, areflexia and few sensory signs, despite sometimes prominent symptoms. Progression is complete in 90% of cases by 4 weeks and is followed by a plateau and gradual improvement. It is thought to be due to an autoimmune response towards the peripheral nervous system, triggered by an antecedent infection whose agent is believed to share antigens with the gangliosides of peripheral nerves, the 'molecular mimicry' theory. Campylobacter is thought to be the most important antecedent infection. The commonest form of GBS is acute inflammatory demyelinating polyneuropathy, (AIDP). The axonal forms, thought commoner in Asian countries, e.g. China, Japan and Mexico [113,194,307,233], often in an epidemic form, can present as either an acute motor axonal neuropathy (AMAN) or as an acute motor-sensory axonal neuropathy (AMSAN). The least common is the Fisher Syndrome which comprises ophthalmoplegia, ataxia and areflexia. This syndrome is more frequent in Eastern Asia than elsewhere, accounting for 19% of GB cases in Taiwan and 25% of GB cases in Japan [182,207].

The epidemiology and natural history of the condition are difficult to study because the first NINCDS diagnostic criteria were formulated only in 1978 and have evolved subsequently [12]. Not all studies have used these criteria, nor are the criteria themselves clinically definitive, particularly in those with AMAN and antiGM1 antibodies, who may have preserved reflexes and even hyperreflexia during the course of the illness [305,168]. The criteria may need to be supported by electrophysiology and other investigations, including CSF. Investigations are often negative in the early stages of the disease. Mild cases, or those which arrest spontaneously, may not come to neurological attention. Alternatively, in an epidemic situation, patients who have other illnesses may be misdiagnosed as GBS. This was thought to inflate the incidence of GBS during the swine-flu epidemic in the US in 1976. In countries where paralytic poliomyelitis still occurs, distinguishing GBS from acute polio is a problem. To a lesser extent, the same is true of West Nile Fever and paralytic rabies.

Incidence rates from countries in the developed and developing worlds appear to be fairly uniform. Incidence increases with age with two peaks, the first in young adults aged 16-25 years and the second between 45-60 years [139]. There is a slight preponderance in males. A review of studies based on NINCDS criteria found an annual incidence rate of 0.8 to 1.6 per 100,000 people [60]. In southeast England an estimate of 1.2 per 100,000 was adjusted to 1.5 per 100,000 (CI 1.3 to 1.8) following capture-recapture analysis [239]. Two increases in incidence over time have been reported, possibly due to better case recognition. In northern Italy incidence increased, especially in urban areas and amongst the elderly, from 1.09 to 2.73 per 100,000 population between 1981-1984 and 1991-1993 [109]. In Olmsted County, Rochester, USA there was an increase from 1.2 to 2.7 per 100,000 people between 1953 -1956 and 1970-80 [20]. Assuming the higher incidence of 2.7 per 100,000, and a US population of 280,000,000 (http://www.census.gov/population/www/pop-profile/profile2000. html), the predicted annual number of new cases of GBS in Americans would be 7560, which is remarkably close to the 7874 new cases estimated from American hospital discharge data in 1995 [214].

Between half and two-thirds of patients with GBS have an illness preceding onset by a few weeks. For a long time it was thought that infections and vaccines, drugs, toxins, immune disorders, endocrine and metabolic disturbances, neoplasm's and other conditions were associated with GBS, but the necessary case control studies were lacking [254]. In order to establish a biological association, properly conducted case-control studies are essential.

Association with Infection

Epidemics of GBS have been reported in Jordan following an outbreak of diarrhea, thought to be related to Shigella [152], and also in China [129] where AMAN has been reported in summer [129]. Epidemics of the AIDP form have no seasonal variation [129,194].

Two early case-control studies showed associations with gastroenteritis [150] and with respiratory infections [200]. Kennedy et al (1978) [150] used patients with Bell's palsy as controls, but since Bell's palsy may also be a post-viral phenomenon, the association of GBS with viral infection may have been under-estimated due to over-matching.

C.jejuni, which will be discussed in more detail below, has been identified in 14-36% of GBS patients and 1-12% of controls [301,204,238]. CMV was present in 11% to 13% of GBS patients, and 1% to 2% of controls in two studies [301,145]. EBV and M.pneumoniae were infrequently found in cases and controls in the study of Winer et al, 1988, but more frequently found in cases than controls in the study of Jacobs (1997), where 22% of GBS cases could be attributed to C. jejuni, 12% to CMV, 9% to EB virus and 4% to M. pneumoniae. To establish a link with EB virus requires a younger population than that used in Winer's (1988) study [301]. The choice of controls is also important. In Winer's 1988 [301] series, surgical controls were used and although surgery preceded GBS in 8 out of 99 patients, no meaningful comparison could be made.

There is strong evidence of an association between GBS and infection with Campylobacter jejuni. In China, serological evidence of Campylobacter jejuni infection was found in 66% of GBS patients compared with 16% of controls [129]. Anti-glycolipid antibodies, in particular IgG anti-GMI antibodies, were seen in 42% of GBS cases compared with 6% controls [129]. In a Japanese study, C.jejuni was isolated in 30.4% GBS patients but in only 1.2% of healthy controls [167]. The relationship was further studied in a prospective, case-control study in Britain. C.jejuni infection was confirmed by combinations of rigorous criteria (positive stool cultures, positive serology and a history of diarrhea illness) [144]. Preceding C.jejuni infection was demonstrated in 26% of GBS patients compared with 2% of household and 1% of hospital controls. The association with infection was more common in men than women [238], which could account for the preponderance of GBS in young men. In China, the association between GBS and C.jejuni was found to be stronger for AMAN than for AIDP. Some 76% of the AMAN subgroup tested positive for C. jejuni compared with only 42% of the AIDP subgroup [129]. Similar results were was found in the British study [238].

The nine day interval between diarrhea and development of GBS suggests that the effect of C jejuni is immunological rather than infective or toxic. Anti GM1 and anti-GD1a auto antibodies have been discovered in patients with post-C jejuni GBS. Both act against gangliosides in peripheral nervous tissue. In Fisher syndrome GQIb antibodies are present [143]. Molecular mimicry is likely to be mediated by lipo-oligosaccharides structurally resembling the GMI ganglioside of peripheral nerve. Only a few strains of C.jejuni have these lipo-oligosaccharides. Kuroki [167] in Japan identified one of these strains in 10 out of 12 C.jejuni isolates from patients with GBS and preceding enteritis but in only 1.7% of patients with enteritis without GBS. In a similar study, Yuki found the same strain in 52% of GBS patients but in only 5% of the enteritis only group [306]. There is also some evidence for molecular mimicry in GBS patients with preceding CMV infection: 22% had IgM antibodies of the anti-GM2 type, compared with only 2% of GBS patients without preceding CMV [145].

No host factors which would make a person susceptible to GBS have been identified, although such factors must exist, since infection with strains producing the ganglioside-like moiety produces antibodies to ganglioside only in those who develop GBS and not in those who develop diarrhea only [258].

There is also an accidental human "model" of GBS which lends further support to the autoimmune basis for this disease. In 1993, a study in Italy of patients without preceding gastro-intestinal infection, given gangliosides as therapy for a variety of symptoms not considered to be early GBS, later developed symptoms of polyneuropathy, suggesting that ganglioside treatment may actually precipitate GBS [170].

Epidemiology of C.Jejuni

It is important to consider the epidemiology of C jejuni because more effective treatment and prevention of C.jejuni enteritis would be expected to reduce the incidence of GBS. C.jejuni is the commonest zoonotic enteric pathogen in the developed world [214].

It is more common in men than women, usually affecting young adults and children under four [214]. Both these statements also apply to GBS. There is seasonal variation, with more cases in summer in temperate zones. Chicken is the largest potential source of human infection. In Northern Europe, the estimates of incidence range from 60 to 90 per 100,000 population, but these are thought to be gross underestimates. In the USA, the CDC estimated there were 1000 cases per 100,000 population per year [214]. The risk of developing GBS following C jejuni infection could be around 1 in 1000, taking the highest incidence estimate (2.7 per 100,000) and assuming that 30% of these are attributable to C.jejuni.

In developing countries, there are no reliable estimates of incidence, but C jejuni is thought to affect principally young children. C.jejuni enteritis is likely to be more common in developing than in developed countries and this might account for the more frequent occurrence of the axonal form in China and Mexico.

Vaccination

In late 1976 in the USA, the estimated incidence of GBS rose to 8.8 per 100,000 among people vaccinated against influenza A ('swine flu') compared with 1.2 per 100,000 in the unvaccinated population. The reliability of this finding was questioned because of the lack of diagnostic criteria for GBS and because of the potential for ascertainment bias due to heightened awareness amongst patients and physicians [254]. No similar epidemic has been reported in association with Influenza A vaccination elsewhere or in the USA, either before or since 1976 [148,172]. The American influenza vaccine-related GBS epidemic demonstrates very important epidemiological points including the value of a surveillance system to allow calculation of a baseline incidence level, the importance of strict diagnostic criteria and the need to monitor diseases over time, using the same criteria and ascertainment methods. For a rare disease like GBS, this is very expensive and is therefore feasible in practice only in small, not necessarily representative areas such as Olmsted County Minnesota with the Mayo Clinic Record Linkage System.

A variety of other immunizations have been associated with GBS e.g. oral polio vaccine (OPV), anti hepatitis B vaccine, semple type anti rabies vaccine, vaccinia, measles vaccine and tetanus toxoid. Most of these were based on case reports in which onset of GBS was preceded by a particular immunization. A temporal association between the two events does not imply causality. Epidemiologic studies with proper case definition and controls are necessary. Baseline incidence rates of GBS in the community should also be determined. Studies in areas where mass polio, measles and hepatitis B immunization programmes have been carried out, have with the exception of one Finnish study [155], generally not shown an increased incidence of GBS over that expected by chance alone [156,234,72,196].

Treatment

Supportive treatment with attention to respiratory care, prevention of deep venous thrombi and management of autonomic disturbances has reduced the mortality of GBS from 30% to 5% [302]. No trials were necessary to show this dramatic benefit.

Randomised trials however were necessary to show the benefit of plasma exchange. Patients treated with plasma exchange had a significant additional benefit in terms of time to recovery, walking with and without aid, need for and duration of artificial ventilation, full muscle strength recovery and severe sequelae at one year [235]. Subsequently, randomized trials with early use of intravenous immunoglobulin showed it to be as effective as plasma exchange [137]. On the other hand, oral corticosteroids slowed recovery. Intravenous methylprednisolone alone was not useful, but when combined with intravenous immunoglobulin could hasten recovery but without long term benefit [138].

These clinical trials were designed to look at short term outcome. Prospective population based studies, such as the multicentre Italian Study, have not shown treatment with either intravenous immunoglobulin or plasma exchange to have an impact on long term outcome [19]. The two studies from southeast England [301,239], which were conducted 10 years apart, also showed no long term benefit of intravenous immunoglobulin and plasma exchange. Neither of these treatments was in use during the period of the first study and there was no significant difference in mortality and morbidity between the two study periods.

The patients entered into clinical trials may not be representative of the full spectrum of GBS because they include only the more seriously affected patients and exclude patients with coexisting illnesses. In addition, the number of patients enrolled in these trials may be insufficient to show long term benefit. There is also probably a need to develop therapies which will have a greater impact on long term outcome.

Mortality

In their literature review, Chio et al [60] found that mortality at one-month ranged from 3.2 % to 8%, but one study from North Tanzania showed a mortality rate of 15.3%. Factors possibly affecting mortality are older age, dysautonomia leading to cardiac arrest, premorbid lung dysfunction, ventilator dependence, maximum severity of motor deficit, and axonal or mixed EMG pattern rather than a demyelinating one. Death due to cardiac arrest has been largely preventable since the advent of ECG monitoring and improved intensive care. Winer et al [301] found 40% of deaths were due to cardiac arrest as a result of autonomic dysfunction, but there were none in the study of Rees et al in the same area ten years later when ICU monitoring was used. However, in the multicentre Italian study, 5 out of the 7 patients who died due to cardiac arrest from dysautonomia had ICU monitoring. Seven of the 33 who died had shown improvement in their neuropathy.

Morbidity

Recovery after GBS seems to be quite good. From 48 to 88% of patients achieve this by 1-2 years after the illness, as shown in Table 4. Differences in results may be methodological rather than real and due to severity of the illness at entry to the study.

All studies used as an index of good recovery of patients with GBS a Hughes grade of less than or equal to 2, or an equivalent of minimal or no disability

Among the factors that have been related to a poor outcome, the most consistent appears to be age over 40 or 50 [301,239,280,91]. Other negative prognostic factors include lack of history of preceding respiratory infection [60], antecedent gastroenteritis [280], severe disability at time of admission [280], short latency-to-peak deficit [280,301], more severe disability (Hughes Grade $\geq$ 4) at peak deficit [91], longer duration of active disease [280,236,255], clinical features such as need for ventilation [301,255], bulbar palsy [255], quadriplegia at peak of illness [236], and dysautonomia [255]. Neurophysiological markers of poor prognosis include Compound muscle action potential (CMAP) which is 0-20% of the lower limit of normal in the first month of the illness [70], and inexcitable nerves [116].

Table 4. Percentages with good recovery at intervals after GBS

STUDY	3 MONTHS	6 MONTHS	1 YEAR	2 YEARS
Winer et al [301]			80%	
Rees et a l [239]			70%	
Multicentre Italian [280]			70%	82%
Emilia-Romagna [91]		64%		
Sedano [255]	30%	54%		88%
Rafael [236]			48%	68%
Chio [60]				80%

Prognosis of Different Subtypes of GBS

Outcome may also depend on the clinical subtype of GBS. Feasby et al [92] found a poor prognosis in an acute axonal form of GBS. However axonal forms of GBS do not necessarily have a poorer prognosis than demyelinating forms [116]. Ho et al in Northern China also found equally good recovery in 76% of their patients who had AMAN and 19% with AIDP [128]. A neuropathological study of 12 autopsied cases in northern China [113] showed 3 cases to have changes suggestive of AIDP, 3 cases had severe sensory and motor axonal degeneration (AMSAN) and 6 cases had only motor axon involvement (AMAN). Of the 6 cases with AMAN, 3 had severe axonal degeneration similar to the findings in Feasby et al's cases and the other 3 had very mild axonal involvement yet had severe paralysis at the time of death. These findings suggest that there may be mild and severe types of AMAN and these may be difficult to distinguish clinically.

Studies from the Netherlands [146,293,290] have investigated the relationship between clinical subgroups of GBS and outcome. In the mild form, 28% of patients could walk unaided at the peak of the deficit [290]. The investigators believed this mild form was associated with men under 50 years of age. In the same study, the severe form was related to positive serology for CMV, C.jejuni, mycoplasma and EBV. Another study, [146] showed that rapidly progressive, severe, motor neuropathy with a poor prognosis was associated with preceding C.jejuni infection and anti-GM-1 antibodies. The third Dutch study [293] identified a group of patients who had had CMV, who were younger, more often women than men, who had an initially severe course with respiratory insufficiency, cranial nerve involvement and severe sensory loss. This contrasts with the motor involvement in the

C.jejuni-associated form. Both groups suffered delayed recovery compared with those without any history of preceding infection. The mild form was also found in 12% of the patients in Winer's study [301], 23.3% of the patients in the multicentre Italian Study [280], and 24% of patients in the Emilia-Romagna study [91].

Functional and longer Term Outcome

Studies of functional outcome, such as that of Merkies et al [202], have used the International Classification of Impairment, Disabilities and Handicaps (ICIDH) framework (WHO 1980) to distinguish impairments (abnormalities of structure or physiological function) from disability (the inability to perform specific activities) and handicap (perceived disadvantage in fulfilling social roles). They studied 113 clinically stable patients recruited from the Rotterdam Immune-Mediated Polyneuropathy Data Bank and the Dutch GBS Study, 83 of whom had GBS, 22 had CIDP and 8 had monoclonal gammopathy of uncertain significance. Only two thirds of disability could be accounted for by impairment. Psychological and other factors were also implicated. Similarly impairment and disability together accounted for only 80% of the variance in handicap. Other factors contributing to outcome were pain, lack of social support, physical stamina and psychological factors.

Longer term outlook was studied in Denmark [79]. The Danish study, which used controls, looked at outcome 7 years after the illness. Although no disability was found, 48% of patients had a residual neuropathy and all reported lower health status than controls. The Dutch study looked at patients 3-6 years after the onset of GBS and found the psychosocial status changed in 63% of patients, including those who had had a good recovery. This brings us back to the difference between impairment and disability. Psychological factors can contribute to disability, even in the absence of impairment.

Chronic Inflammatory Demyelinating Polyneuropathy (CIDP)

In contrast to GBS, chronic inflammatory demyelinating polyneuropathy (CIDP) produces weakness and sensory disturbance which progresses for two months or more, with liability to subsequent relapses. CSF examination and electrophysiologic evidence of peripheral nerve demyelination help confirm the diagnosis. A sural nerve biopsy finding of demyelination was made mandatory by an AAN adhoc subcommittee, but is no longer considered essential. Indeed, a controlled study did not find biopsy to be of much diagnostic value [36]. Insistence on a greater number of laboratory criteria such as CSF, EMG, NCV, biopsy results in a more specific diagnosis, but many 'true positive' cases of CIDP will be missed.

In clinical practice, CIDP variants are usually distinguished from idiopathic CIDP. These variants include multifocal motor neuropathy with conduction block (MMNCB) a condition in which antiganglioside antibodies are found, multifocal acquired demyelinating sensory and motor neuropathy (MADSAM) or Lewis-Sumner Syndrome and sensorimotor distal acquired demyelinating symmetric neuropathy in which IgM antibodies are often present [160,174,287]. MMNCB may mimic motor neuron disease. It is important to identify MMNCB because it is treatable with intravenous immunoglobulin or cyclophosphamide but not steroids. There are no epidemiologic data other than information on clinical and electrophysiologic outcome and clinical trials of treatment.

CIDP may also be associated with a variety of other conditions including HIV, hepatitis C, connective tissue diseases such as Sjogren's disease, paraproteinemias, malignancies, metabolic disorders (diabetes mellitus and thyrotoxicosis) and even Charcot Marie-Tooth disease.

The associations between diabetes mellitus and CIDP and that between CMTD and CIDP require further investigation. It is important for the clinician to recognize that two conditions may be present in the same patient, worsening the neuropathy. It is therefore imperative that the CIDP component be treated [104,108].

Antecedent infections or immunizations are reported less frequently in CIDP (19 – 32% of cases), than in AIDP [118*]. In case series with children, antecedent events are more commonly found. There were 54% in Nevo et al's series. This difference may be due to the fact that as a subacute onset is common in children, such events are more commonly recalled. Booster immunizations are only rarely related in time with a relapse in a patient with known CIDP or GBS. If the initial attack occurs within 12 weeks following an immunization, particularly with tetanus toxoid, that immunization should never be given again [134].

Genetic factors have also been implicated, but the number of patients studied is too small to be conclusive. Analytic case control studies such as those which have been carried out for AIDP are necessary.

CIDP-Prevalence, Course, Prognosis

A population based study in NSW Australia found a crude prevalence ratio of 1.9 per 100,000 population, an annual incidence rate of 0.15/100,000, onset at age 47.6 years and an age specific prevalence which increased with age to 6.7 per 100,000 population in the 70 – 79 year age group. Fifty one percent had a relapsing and remitting course, the mean duration of illness was 7.1 years and 87% were able to walk without assistance [195]. A similar prevalence (1.24 per 100,000) was found in a population based study in the South east Thames area in England [181], in which 13% of those surveyed needed aid to walk and 54% were on treatment.

In clinical series with a greater proportion of younger patients, there is a predominance of patients who have a relatively good prognosis [121,192]. A series of 92 Australian patients (62% males) a mean age of onset was 35.4 years [192]. In 65% there was a relapsing course and mean age of onset was 26.8 years. In 35% there was a non-relapsing disease with either subacute onset of monophasic disease or clinically progressive disease. Mean age of onset for this group was older, 51.4 years. Follow up at a mean of 10.6 years after disease onset showed 10 patients had died, 5 as a result of their disease and 5 due to unrelated intercurrent illness. Six patients were lost to follow up and 76 patients were still alive. The overall prognosis was good, 73% had disability of grade 2 or less and mortality due to CIDP was 6%. 90% were able to walk without assistance. Patients with relapsing disease had a median disability score of 1 and those with non-relapsing disease a score of 2. This difference was, however, not significantly different.

If patients are older, as in a study from France in which the mean age was 52 years, the proportion of patients with a relapsing course is less (14%). Forty-five percent had a progressive course and the remainder had a progressive onset followed by a relatively stable course [37]. In both the Australian and the French studies, younger patients had a relapsing course; older patients had a monophasic static or progressive course.

Disability data was collected in 83 out of the 100 patients over an average of 6 years [37]. The outcome was as follows:

Good	47
Mild handicap	11
Severe handicap	6
Bedridden	5
Deaths	14
Total	83

Those with axonal loss had greater disability. Also, all those with symptomatic CNS involvement were severely handicapped.

Another study of outcome 5 years after treatment was begun showed that 13% of patients had severe disability and 39% still required immune modulating treatment [168]. A subacute onset and symmetrical symptoms were associated with a better outcome.

CIDP rarely occurs in children. The onset is often subacute, initial response to immune modulating treatment good, progression uncommon after 3 months, relapses and remissions common and there is usually complete remission without necessity for long term treatment within a year [67,121,218,259].

However, even in children, there is a group [218] of severely affected subjects with poor response to initial treatment, progression for more than 3 months, and necessity for prolonged steroids and persistent weakness.

Treatment

Randomized controlled trials have established that intravenous immunoglobulin, plasma exchange and corticosteroids are equally effective in CIDP [291,199,198]. Treatment is determined according to clinical indications and what the patient can afford. Between 60% and 80% of patients respond positively if the treatment is started early, before axonal damage occurs [118].

If this treatment fails, azathioprine, cyclophosphamide and cyclosporine may be tried, although there is no reliable evidence of their efficacy from randomized controlled clinical trials [135]. Other forms and combinations of immuno modulating agents have been reviewed recently [161]. The majority of studies have been open label with small numbers. Even the randomized controlled trials for initial treatment of CIDP have usually been of 6 weeks duration or less, which is rather short for a chronic disease.

NEUROPATHIES RELATED TO INFECTION

Leprosy

Leprosy was known in India in about 1300 BC as "kushtha". It was possibly brought to Europe in about 327 BC by Alexander's army returning from India. Humans constitute the only reservoir apart from armadillos and a few primates. The organism can exist in soil for prolonged periods. Spread of leprosy usually occurs via nasal droplets, but, unlike tuberculosis, infection requires prolonged, close contact. It may also occur via contact with soil, or tattooing. Skin to skin contact is not an important source of infection. After inhalation, the organism enters the bloodstream and spreads via endoneural vessels to peripheral nerves, where it binds to Schwann cells and multiplies. Subsequently, an immune-mediated myelin loss occurs, involving monocytes, macrophages and cytokines. This immune response is particularly important in tuberculoid leprosy [224]. The cooler areas of the skin are also affected by hematogenous spread. The incubation period is estimated to be about 7 years after infection. Resistance to infection may also be determined partly by the presence of a protein, natural resistance-associated macrophage protein 1 (NRAMP 1), which is present in some ethnic groups [224].

The WHO leprosy detection and early treatment programme has resulted in cure of more than 14 million patients globally by multi-drug treatment since 1985 [304]. The aim was to eliminate leprosy by 2005, but leprosy remains a public health problem in six African countries, in India, Nepal and in Brazil. The word "eliminate" as used by WHO, means reducing prevalence to less than 1 case per 10,000 population, so that the primary health care system can subsequently look after leprosy. In 2004, the annual world incidence was 407,791 people but the global registered prevalence was 286,063 at the start of 2005. This incidence-prevalence discrepancy is the result of the WHO considering patients to be 'cases' only while they were on multi-drug treatment and not thereafter. The annual global detection rate is decreasing in India, but increasing in Africa and Brazil. Fifteen percent of new patients are children, suggesting that active transmission is still continuing [178,288]. Even in areas in which there is a decline in detection of new cases, the decline may be artefactual because the method of assessment has been changed from skin smear to clinical detection of a single anesthetic patch which will pick up only 70% of cases, missing the multi-bacillary cases. Prevalence is also artificially reduced by shortening of treatment courses to 12 months for the multi-bacillary form. There are several reasons why total eradication of leprosy and leprosy-related morbidity might not occur even when prevalence is reduced to less than 1 in 10,000. Firstly, the organism is hardy: 5% of the population in endemic areas carry M.leprae DNA in their noses. Secondly, the 5 year relapse rate after a short course of treatment is unknown, but may be significant. Moreover, leprosy is a chronic disease and peripheral nerve damage can occur during the course of treatment due to immunological reactions.

Peripheral nerve involvement is seen in 33 – 56% of patients at diagnosis. In 11-51%, there is no recovery or worsening. Secondary impairment, due to trauma and infection, are already present in 6-27% at diagnosis. Both primary and secondary impairments result in limitation of activities of daily living, or disability. This disability, together with stigma associated with the disease, result in diminished social participation or handicap [289]. The aims of management are:

1. Early diagnosis including techniques to pick up early sensory loss. Nylon Semmes-Weinstein monofilaments are used for this purpose in leprosy programmes and now also in diabetes mellitus programmes [177].
2. Multi-drug treatment.
3. Treatment of nerve damage by steroids or possibly thalidomide, except in women who are, or may become, pregnant.
4. Attempts to prevent nerve damage by the use of steroids. However, a randomized control trial, Tripod I, in Bangladesh and Nepal, found that though damage was prevented at 4 months, improvement was not sustained at 1 year [265].
5. Prevention of disability by taking precaution against injury plus physiotherapy and occupational therapy for those already disabled.
6. Reduction of stigma by education. Patients can also be reassured that they will become non-infectious within 72 hours of commencing multi-drug treatment and will not necessarily develop deformities [177].

Human Immunodeficiency Virus Infection

Worldwide, the WHO estimated that 40.1 million people were living with HIV/AIDS in 2005. The burden fell very largely on low-to-middle income countries, especially in sub-Saharan Africa, and in the WHO South-East Asia region. WHO estimated that 2.6 million people would die from HIV/AIDS during the following 12 months.

Peripheral neuropathy is one of the most important neurological complications related to HIV infection. Since the bulk of people with HIV/AIDS live in developing countries, where access to specific treatment is limited, preventive targeting of at risk groups in the community is obviously imperative. In this section we consider both the neuropathy associated with HIV infection and also the neuropathy induced by anti-HIV treatment.

HIV-related Distal Sensory Polyneuropathy (HIV-DSP): Clinical Features, Risk Factors and Treatment

Distal sensory polyneuropathy (DSP) is a painful neuropathy with preserved proprioception and absent ankle jerks. If proprioception is abnormal and ankle jerks are present, a coexisting myelopathy should be considered. For simultaneous involvement of multiple sites in the nervous system, the term "parallel tracking" is used. Nerve conduction studies are abnormal in most patients with DSP. In a small number, they may be normal because predominantly small fibres have been affected. Skin biopsies with assessment of intra-epidermal nerve fibre density (IENF) are useful in assessing small fibre neuropathies. In the Nerve Growth Factor Trial for DSP [191], reduction in IENF density correlated with increased pain, low CD4 count and elevated HIV-RNA.

'Time locking' is the term used to describe the relationship between the staging of HIV disease and the duration of the illness [41]. It was coined in the pre-HAART era when a longer illness resulted in a correspondingly greater reduction of CD4 count and opportunistic infection, such as CMV polyradiculoneuropathy. With the advent of HAART, the CD4 count remains normal for longer periods and disease manifestation is more closely related to this value (T cell locking) than to the duration of disease.

In early HIV (CD4 ≥ 500) and moderate HIV (CD4 = 200 – 500), peripheral neuropathy is uncommon and although precise figures are unavailable, the incidence of peripheral neuropathy in early and moderately advanced HIV is low. It occurs in approximately 3% of otherwise healthy HIV subjects. The types of peripheral neuropathy found are AIDP-like, CIDP-like or multifocal mononeuropathy.

There is no specific treatment inducing regeneration of diseased peripheral nerve. Controlled clinical trials using lamotrigine [260] and trial of nerve growth factor [191] have shown improvement of pain. Although lamotrigine improved pain in DSP it did not improve pain in ATN. Gabapentin has been shown to improve pain in both DSP and ATN though the study was small and open-label.

Asymptomatic vs. Symptomatic Peripheral Neuropathy

In the pre-HAART era, clinical examination revealed peripheral neuropathy in 55% of 272 HIV positive people with cognitive decline; 20% were asymptomatic, 35% were symptomatic. If all patients had not been examined clinically, much peripheral neuropathy would have been missed [253]. This study suggested that cognitive changes are likely to influence the interpretation of symptoms. In the era before highly active anti-retroviral therapy (HAART) intravenous drug use could be another factor responsible for patients with HIV-DSP not reporting symptoms. In the Manhattan HIV Brain Bank Study (MHBB) [281], 73% of all patients with asymptomatic DSP used intravenous drugs such as opiates, compared with 47% of those with symptomatic neuropathy and 43% of those without any neuropathy. It was concluded that symptomatic opiate users may interpret their symptoms differently from those who did not use opiates, because of altered central pain mechanisms.

Peripheral Neuropathy due to Causes other than HIV

HIV-DSP commonly occurs in groups at high risk for co-morbidity. In a multicenter AIDS cohort study (190), a case-control approach was used to compare peripheral neuropathy in HIV positive, but otherwise healthy, homosexual and heterosexual males with HIV negative homosexual controls. Sensory abnormalities were the commonest finding, but occurred to a similar extent in both groups, 13% in HIV positive and 11% in HIV negative cases. There was no statistical difference between the two. Other factors that need to be considered before diagnosing HIV-DSP are diabetes mellitus, inherited conditions and psychoactive drugs, including alcohol.

Incidence and Prevalence of HIV-induced Polyneuropathy

To the best of our knowledge, there are no door-to-door, population-based incidence studies of HIV neuropathy available. Existing prevalence studies have been conducted on differing populations, using different diagnostic criteria. Comparisons between studies must take into account the staging of the disease, the length of follow-up and the degree of distinction of anti-retroviral toxic neuropathy (ATN) from DSP due to HIV. The prevalence of peripheral neuropathy varied from 13% in HIV positive patients with clinically determined peripheral neuropathy referred to hospital for evaluation [69], to 35% in hospitalized AIDS patients [266], to nearly 100% when autopsy was used [80].

In a study pre-dating HAART, 89% of people with both early and advanced HIV were found to have peripheral neuropathy when they were assessed using a combination of clinical examination, EMG, nerve conduction studies and peripheral nerve biopsy [102]. Following the introduction of HAART, incidence and prevalence of neurological manifestations of HIV began to differ between developed and developing countries [130]. After HAART, there was a decrease in HIV-dementia and opportunistic infections of the nervous system, resulting in peripheral neuropathy becoming the main type of nervous system disease.

In advanced HIV (CD4 < 200), DSP was found in 30% [276], 53% post-HAART [281], and 55% of patients in a pre-HAART group [253]. In the Multi-Centre AIDS Cohort Study 1985-1992 [14], the incidence of peripheral neuropathy rose from 0.49/100 person years if the CD4 count was more than 500, to 7.75/100 person years if the CD4 count was less than 100.

The increased incidence of peripheral neuropathy in advanced AIDS is not solely due to the drop in CD4 count, but also to prolonged survival. Prolonged survival plus HAART, plus the fact that more elderly people are prone to acquire HIV because the CD4 count drops with age in normal older people; mean that the HIV positive AIDS cohort will contain greater number of older people now than in the past.

Risk factors for DSP are increased age, reduced CD4 count, increased HIV-RNA levels in the blood, co-infection with HTLV-2, CMV and VZV and possibly inherited neuropathy. Some studies, such as the MHBB study, have shown no association between DSP with low CD4 count and with increased viral load, but cross-sectional studies could obscure the relationship.

Anti-retroviral Toxic Neuropathy (ATN)

The treatment of HIV-AIDS has been revolutionized by the use of nucleoside analogs. These agents, which function as reverse transcriptase inhibitors, may be considered a new category of acquired mitochondrial toxins [73]. The group includes zalcitabine (ddC, Hivid), didanosine (ddI, Videx), lamivudine (3TC, Epivir), stavudine (d4T, Zerit), fialuridine (FIAU) and zidovudine (AZT). The location of different phosphorylases, whose action is to phosphorylate a particular reverse transcriptase, determines the tissue affected eg. ddC, ddI and 3TC are in peripheral nerve, d4T and FIAU in nerve and muscle and AZT is found in muscle only [73].

Anti-retroviral toxic neuropathy (ATN) is usually a painful, sensory axonal polyneuropathy. It has an incidence of 15-40% and usually develops 4-5 weeks after treatment has started. In one study [24], all patients treated with a high dose of nucleoside ddC developed painful neuropathy within a mean of 7.7 weeks after commencing treatment. The neuropathy progressed for 2-3 weeks even after stopping the toxin i.e. there was coasting. If suspected, anti-retroviral treatment has to be stopped, so that less neurotoxic drugs can be substituted after pain subsides. The co-existence of both HIV neuropathy and toxic neuropathy due to the anti-retroviral drugs is called "layering."

Neuropathy due to AIDS usually occurs later and may be distinguished by the fact that stopping treatment does not result in improvement. If lower doses of the anti-retroviral agent are used, peripheral neuropathy develops less frequently, is less severe and starts later. Overall, in most patients improvement occurs after stopping treatment. In the case of zalcitabine, 10% stop treatment because of side effects. Factors predisposing to peripheral neuropathy include a low CD4 count (<100), polytherapy, a genetic susceptibility and any underlying neuropathy.

TOXIC NEUROPATHIES

This section reviews neuropathies due to drugs and environmental toxins. Peripheral nerves are particularly vulnerable to toxicity because of their high metabolic demands, their limited ability to regenerate and their length and multiple connections. (119)

Neurotoxicology: General Principles

A toxin can affect the entire neuron (neuronopathy), the axon (axonopathy), or the myelin sheath, (myelinopathy). In addition, toxins can affect axonal ion channels (channelopathies) or the neuromuscular junction [119].

Toxic neuronopathies are usually sensory, involving the dorsal root or trigeminal nerve ganglia and producing simultaneous, subacute onset of paraesthesiae in all four limbs and face, with proprioceptive loss, absent reflexes, preserved power and abnormal sensory nerve conduction studies. As the neurons themselves are affected, recovery may be quite slow.

Axonopathies are usually sensory initially, motor later, gradual in onset, affect the largest and longest fibres first and therefore result in distal leg paraesthesiae, numbness, weakness and reflex loss in a glove and stocking distribution, which gradually extends proximally and involves the arms. Recovery is slow. Progression may continue after removal of the toxin ("coasting"). Amplitudes of both sensory and motor action potentials are reduced, but conduction velocities are relatively preserved. CSF examination is usually normal.

In the ion channel syndromes, there may be associated gastrointestinal symptoms. Parasthesiae and numbness commence in the mouth and face, and are followed rapidly by weakness of all four limbs and even respiratory distress.

In the neuromuscular junction syndromes, there is usually early involvement of cranial nerves, with ptosis, diplopia, dysarthria and dysphagia, followed by neck and generalized limb weakness. Tendon reflexes are preserved. There may also be features of cholinergic overexcitation in the case of organophosphate intoxication.

The following criteria suggest that a peripheral neuropathy may have a neurotoxic origin. [126,252].

1. Timing and disease onset are consistent with the time of exposure.
2. Disease severity is related to dosage and duration of exposure. Other factors determining severity are age and pre-existing peripheral neuropathy, differing ability metabolize drugs and multiple factors acting in concert. In sensory neuropathies, symptoms are subjective, which can make quantification of severity difficult.
3. Removal of toxin usually results in improvement of symptoms, although worsening of symptoms, termed "coasting", sometimes occurs [252].
4. The clinical picture is consistent with other known instances of exposure and with the known biological effect of the toxin.
5. The toxin has been identified in the environment or in the patient.
6. There are in vivo and in vitro models of neurotoxicity for the candidate substance.
7. No other sufficient cause of peripheral neuropathy can be found in the patient

The principles of studying neurotoxicology in populations have been systematically stated by Schaumburg in his treatise on neurotoxicology [252].

Studying Neurotoxicology in Populations

Whenever chemical neurotoxicity is suspected, systematic investigation is required in order to obtain unambiguous data. Preliminary survey of a small cohort by a group of unbiased and experienced specialists can direct the attention of a subsequent, larger study to appropriate areas. Definitive, controlled, prospective study of an exposure should have a clearly-defined population, and a pre-determined endpoint. Methodological rigor is especially important. The team of investigators must include experienced clinicians, toxicologists and statisticians. Retrospective studies can document exposures, but causal relationships are difficult to prove. Reassessment at intervals after exposure improves the quality of results by documenting progress and recovery.

The three main situations in which possible toxic exposures occur and require assessment are:

1. Following exposure to a known neurotoxin, people must be surveyed using specific screening methods
2. Following exposure to a chemical not known to be neurotoxic, where people appear to be well, clinical assessment may be needed either to confirm or exclude toxicity.
3. Following development of abnormal neurological symptoms and signs in people exposed to a substance not known to be toxic, those exposed need assessment. Mediation is needed between patients, regulatory agencies and the industry.

Exposure may be limited to workers, as in the case of methyl-n-butyl-ketone, or due to an accident at an industrial plant which results in widespread exposure of the population, as in the gas disaster which occurred in Bhopal, India, in 1984 [28].

With the decline of occupational exposure, the commonest cause of neurotoxicity is likely to be prescribed or recreational drugs.

Neuropathies Due to Therapeutic Agents

Anti-microbial and Anti-parasitic Agents

Drugs for HIV infection, antituberculous agents such as isoniazid, dapsone for leprosy and chloroquine for malaria are among the most widely used potential neurotoxins. HIV and tuberculosis are likely to become more common over the next decades, but the incidence of leprosy is decreasing (see above). Metronidazole, effective against the protozoal diseases which are still widespread in developing countries, and nitrofurantoin, used to treat low grade urinary tract infections for prolonged periods, are also important causes of toxic peripheral neuropathy. Anti-retroviral agents were discussed in the section on HIV-AIDS and will not be covered here.

Metronidazole, if used in high doses over a prolonged period, can produce a sensory neuropathy which persists for years after stopping treatment. Occasionally, even normal doses of 400 mg t.i.d. for periods as short as 9 days can produce neuropathy [246].

Dapsone, if given in doses of more than 300 mg/day for prolonged periods, produces a motor neuropathy, thus distinguishing it from leprosy. It affects the arms more than the legs. In conventional doses of 100 mg/day, peripheral neuropathy is uncommon unless there is a predisposing factor, such as the patient being a slow acetylator.

Isoniazid inhibits the enzyme, pyridoxine kinase, produces a conditioned pyridoxine deficiency and results in a sensory neuropathy after 4-6 months of treatment. In one report, between 2% and 5% of people on 3 to 5mg/kg/day and 17% of those on 6 mg/kg/day sustained peripheral neuropathy [185]. Alcohol intake, poor nutritional status, pregnancy and liver disease are acquired predisposing factors. Slow acetylation is an inherent genetic predisposition. Supplementation of isoniazid with pyridoxine prevents peripheral neuropathy, but does not hasten improvement once neuropathy occurs.

Nitrofurantoin uncommonly produces a sensorimotor axonal neuropathy which is not clearly related to dose or duration of treatment. Occasionally it can produce a GBS-like picture. There is no specific treatment other than stopping the drug. If consumption continues the peripheral neuropathy worsens and ultimate recovery will be incomplete.

Podophyllin, a topical agent used for treatment of condylomata acuminata, affects microtubules and can produce both an axonopathy and a neuronopathy. Causes of poisoning include accidental oral intake and Chinese herbal remedies [52,221]. Ingestion of as little as 350 mg may be lethal.

Chloroquine is not only an antimalarial, but used in the treatment of connective tissue diseases. It is an ampiphyllic drug, damages lysosomes and can affect nerve, muscle and the neuromuscular junction. The neuromyopathy usually develops months to years after treatment with 250 -750 mg/day. Quadriceps weakness is a diagnostic feature. The most serious side effect of chloroquine is a dose-related retinopathy.

Cardiovascular Drugs

Statins: The most commonly prescribed cardiovascular drugs are the statins. It is estimated that there are 25 million people throughout the world on statins. They interfere with membrane function. The early large trials of statins did not find peripheral neuropathy, perhaps because of lower doses and duration of treatment and because peripheral neuropathy was not looked for carefully. Subsequently the UK General Practitioner Data Cohort Study [99] found a relative risk of 2.5 (C1 0.3 – 14.2) for those on statins, compared with controls from the general population and those with untreated hyperlipidemia.

A Danish study [100], used registry data to carry out a case-control study of 166 cases of idiopathic neuropathy, 35 of whom were definite cases. There were 25 age and sex matched controls per definite case. Statin use was associated with an odds ratio (OR) of 14.2 (CI 5.3 to 38) for the definite cases. If treatment duration was 2 years or more, the OR rose to 26.4 (CI 7.8 – 45.4). The effect of confounders such as diabetes and renal insufficiency was minimized, but the possibility of dyslipidaemia per se causing peripheral neuropathy, (136) or of glucose intolerance leading to peripheral neuropathy, (261) could not be excluded. The study also showed that the 'number-needed-to-harm' (an estimate of how many people one would treat before a side-effect or harmful outcome is experienced) in those over 50 years of age was 2,200 (880-7,300). The type of neuropathy found was usually sensorimotor, but rarely a GBS-like illness is produced [230*].

Amiodarone is widely used against cardiac arrhythmias. It produces a subacute or chronic sensorimotor peripheral neuropathy in 5% - 74% of patients [296]. In one study, peripheral neuropathy developed after four months in 6% of patients treated [55]. Neuropathy usually develops when doses of 400 mg/day are given for several months, but can develop even on daily doses of 200 mg/day, even if the duration is just one month. The neuropathy may be severe enough to produce a quadriplegia and the autonomic nervous system may also be affected. As the drug is lipophyllic and tends to enter the lysosome, it can also produce a demyelinating neuropathy. The half-life of amiodarone is long and it tends to accumulate in various organs. Amiodarone concentration was measured in a sural nerve sample from a 65 year old woman who had taken high doses of amiodarone for a prolonged period. It was found to be 80 times higher than in serum [96]. Besides peripheral neuropathy, amiodarone produces a tremor with the characteristics of essential tremor, other movement disorders, gait ataxia, optic neuropathy and myopathy.

Drugs used in Treatment of Cancers

In the doses used and for the duration necessary to treat cancer, anti-neoplastic agents commonly produce peripheral neuropathy. Indeed, with the advent of bone marrow-supporting drugs, peripheral neuropathy is one of the key dose-limiting factors. Factors predisposing to peripheral neuropathy are the type of drug, the dose, any previous exposure to neurotoxic agents, combinations of chemotherapeutic agents such as the taxoids with cisplatin, the presence of diabetes mellitus or alcohol use and hereditary neuropathy [58]. Charcot Marie Tooth disease is a contraindication to the use of vincristine.

Vincristine, used mainly for lymphomas, leukaemias and solid tumours, produces a painful sensory peripheral neuropathy in nearly all patients, usually within 2 months. Vincristine disassembles microtubules. If treatment is continued, there follow motor, autonomic and cranial nerve manifestations, including a painful opthalmoplegia. If single doses are not permitted to exceed 2 mg, the incidence of neuropathy is reduced.

Taxoids, including paclitaxel and docetaxel, which are used to treat solid tumours, induce assembly of disordered microtubules and produce similar types of axonal neuropathy to vincristine. In addition however, they can produce a neuronopathy. In the case of paclitaxel, if doses exceed 250 mg/m^2, 55-100% of patients sustain neuropathy [176,228]. At lower doses, the neuropathy, though frequent, is neither clinically significant nor dose limiting. Docetaxel has a much wider dose range, 50-600 mg/m^2 [10].

Cisplatin and *oxaliplatin,* a second generation platinum compound, are widely used. They almost invariably produce a sensory neuronopathy. In addition, oxaliplatin binds to sodium channels and produces a distinctive neuromyotonia consisting of cold-induced parasthesiae and cramps in the jaw, throat and limbs. Neuromyotonia due to defects in voltage-gated potassium channels, is seen in Isaac's syndrome. Cisplatin produces sensory symptoms with each dose and with cumulative doses beyond 250-500 mg. Some of the neuropathic manifestations may be irreversible. In a review of patients performed 13 years or more after treatment with cisplatin and doxorubicin, 38% had non-symptomatic neuropathy, 28% had symptomatic neuropathy and 6% had disabling neuropathy [272].

Natural History and Treatment of Chemotherapy-Related Neuropathies

Improvement in neuropathy occurs slowly if a drug is discontinued, but may be incomplete, particularly if the sensory ganglia are involved as in the case of thalidomide. The phenomenon of coasting is common. It may be particularly long in the case of suramin, which has a long half-life of 40-50 days. In all cases, paraneoplastic neuropathies need to be excluded by looking for anti-Hu antibodies.

Animal models suggest that chemotherapy-induced peripheral neuropathy can be ameliorated by gene transfer. In one study, HSV vectors containing nerve growth factor (NGF) or neurotrophin-3 (NT-3) were injected subcutaneously 3 days before a 6 week course of cisplatin. The HSV vectors transduced neurons in the dorsal root ganglia to produce NGF or NT-3 [56]. Chemotherapy-induced iatrogenic neuropathies have a known onset and subacute course. Since the patients themselves have life-threatening diseases, the first human gene transfer trials to prevent neuropathy could be carried out in this group.

Besides gene transfer, a number of other agents have been tried experimentally. Examples are alpha lipoic acid to prevent taxoid neuropathy, (103) and FK 506 tacrolimus, to protect against acrylamide neuropathy. Ethosuximide has been shown to reverse paclitaxel-induced mechanical allodynia and paclitaxel-and vincristine-induced cold allodynia [95]. A preliminary, randomized, controlled clinical trial of Vitamin E versus no Vitamin E in cancer patients on chemotherapy (cisplatin ± paclitaxel) found peripheral neuropathy in 25% of those receiving Vitamine E compared with 73% of controls [11].

Other therapeutic Drugs

Thalidomide, which has anti-inflammatory and anti-angiogenic properties, produces a dose-dependent, sensorimotor axonal neuropathy, particularly when the cumulative dose exceeds 20 gms (50). The drug should be used with close clinical and electrophysiological monitoring. As embryopathy can be avoided by contraception, peripheral neuropathy is now the main dose-limiting factor [59].

Suramin is a reverse transcriptase inhibitor with a half life of 40-50 days, which makes it useful in the treatment of protozoal diseases such as onchocerciasis and African trypanosomiasis. It is also used in higher doses for the treatment of refractory neoplasms. It produces neuropathy in 15-40% of those with peak levels of 350μg/ml [267]. The neuropathy is usually dose-dependent, affecting the axon. In one study, 15% of patients developed a GBS-like illness with peak severity by 2-6 weeks [267]. The probability of getting this increased if total dose exceeded 6 gm/m^2. Serial electrophysiological monitoring was found useful for early detection. Plasma exchange has been used for treatment.

Bortezomib, a proteosome inhibitor, produces an axonal and occasionally a GBS-like illness in 36% (147) to 47% (78) of patients.

Misonidazole, which is used as a radiosensitizer and has a chemical structure similar to metronidazole, produces a large fibre neuropathy with secondary demyelination in a third of patients.

Leflunomide, an immunosuppressive pro-drug for rheumatoid arthritis, produces a painful sensorimotor axonal neuropathy about 3 to 6 months after exposure. Treatment should be stopped within a month of onset of symptoms, or else recovery is incomplete. Less commonly it produces an asymmetrical, multifocal, demyelinating neuropathy which begins 2-10 weeks after exposure.

Colchicine, like vincristine, disassembles microtubules in nerve and muscle, producing a neuromyopathy plus a distal axonal neuropathy with proximal weakness and massively raised CPK. The neuromyopathy, which is often missed, occurs commonly with therapeutic doses of colchicine in patients with gout, particularly with chronic use and renal dysfunction causing impaired colchicine excretion. It needs to be distinguished by muscle biopsy from polymyositis, metabolic myopathy due to uremia or hypothyroidism, and from toxic neuromyopathy due to alcohol, amiodarone, chloroquine or vincristine [268,164]. Improvement occurs after the drug is stopped.

Disulfiram or Antabuse is a carbamate used in the treatment of chronic alcoholism. It produces an axonal sensorimotor neuropathy weeks to months after treatment with daily doses higher than 250 mg. Its importance lies in the fact that it needs to be distinguished from alcoholic neuropathy. It produces unusual peripheral nerve morphology. Distended large axons result from neurofilament deposition, which is secondary to a carbon disulfide intermediate.

Self-medication

Pyridoxine (vitamin B$_6$), with chronic use in doses as low as 50 mg/day but usually 200 mg or more per day [25,5], produces a severe sensory neuronopathy. If the drug is stopped in time, recovery is good. There is coasting. If the neuropathy is severe there may be severe residual disability.

Pyridoxine neuropathy may be considered a human model of toxic peripheral neuropathy. Indeed, in one study, healthy volunteers took varying doses of pyridoxine for varying time periods. The study confirmed: 1) a clear relationship between dose, serum level and effect 2) that quantitative sensory testing is a sensitive measure of early peripheral neuropathy and preceded changes in nerve conduction studies 3) that coasting appears unrelated to persistently raised serum pyridoxine levels 4) that large fibres are not necessarily affected selectively by toxins as suggested by animal studies and studies in humans, in which large doses were used for prolonged time periods. When lower doses are used, as in this study, small fibre dysfunction is the earliest predominant abnormality.

Tryptophan:. In 1974 tryptophan became available in the US [197]. It was increasingly used, particularly by women for psychosomatic complaints. In spring 1989, in New Mexico, USA, a large number of patients, mostly women aged 34-44 years, developed a syndrome subsequently termed "eosinophilia-myalgia syndrome," (EMS) consisting of eosinophilia and incapacitating myalgia, with no other underlying illness. The muscle pain and weakness are secondary to peripheral neuropathy, which was found in 6 out of 12 patients studied electrophysiologically. The absence of muscle degeneration on histology, with lack of elevated serum CPK in these patients are against muscle disease. A subsequent review by Swygert [275], found neuropathy in 27% of 1531 cases. The neuropathy is usually axonal but may be demyelinating, suggesting an autoimmune mechanism [98]. The women had taken 1.2 to 2.5 gms tryptophan per day for 3 weeks to 2 years [125]. Initially, it was felt that the tryptophan may have been contaminated, or that the condition was due to abnormal tryptophan metabolism. To determine whether EMS was due to tryptophan itself or to constituents introduced during its manufacture, a case-control study was performed on patients with EMS and healthy people who were tryptophan users [22]. An association was found between intake of a chemical constituent associated with specific tryptophan manufacturing conditions at one company. It was not tryptophan but the contaminant which produced neurotoxicity. Further studies [188], have established that the contaminant responsible was chemically similar to an aniline derivative found in the oil responsible for the Spanish toxic oil syndrome of 1981. There exist also clinical similarities between the two syndromes. Although neither syndrome is currently found, their importance lies in the ease with which toxicity can occur and that similar chemicals can produce toxic effects in such different situations. Hence, the importance of the aware clinician, able to pick up the same syndrome in different circumstances.

Substance Abuse

This section covers the neuropathies which are most commonly associated with abuse although in some cases exposure may sometimes be therapeutic or industrial rather than 'recreational'.

Opiates, sedatives, amphetamines: In a cross-sectional, clinical and electrophysiological study of peripheral neuropathy in 212 HIV-seronegative and HIV-seropositive injection drug users (IDU's), 24% of the HIV-seronegative IDU's had peripheral neuropathy (89% asymptomatic), and 32.1% of the HIV-seropositive IDU's had peripheral neuropathy (71% asymptomatic) [23]. Transient peripheral neuropathy was found in 49% of 198 heroin users in Australia, who were screened by questionnaire [297]. Peripheral neuropathy therefore, is a more common event among IDU's than is generally appreciated. Consequently, these people need close monitoring. Besides the drugs of abuse themselves, other factors requiring consideration are alcohol abuse, malnutrition, B-complex deficiency and compression neuropathy.

Nitrous Oxide (N$_2$O): N$_2$O inactivates the enzyme, methionine synthase, resulting in B$_{12}$ deficiency and symptoms and signs of subacute combined degeneration. This can occur even after one or two anaesthetic doses in patients with subclinical B$_{12}$ deficiency – "anaesthesia paraesthetica" [157]. The drug is also abused by health care professionals and whipped cream dispensers, so called "whippits." There is a dose-response relationship. In one study mild peripheral neuropathy occurred when 100-200 propellant cartridges were used for 3 months and disabling sensory ataxia occurred when the duration extended to 6 months [115]. In a questionnaire study of 30,000 dentists and 30,000 assistants, symptoms of peripheral neuropathy were three times more common in assistants exposed to N_2O and four times more common in exposed dentists than they were in the unexposed group [42].

In Auckland, New Zealand, in a survey by questionnaire of 1782 first year university students, 1360 (76%) responded, 780 (57%) knew about nitrous oxide used as a recreational drug, 158 (12%) used it themselves recreationally, and 39 (3%) inhaled it once a month at least, showing use of the gas to be quite common. Abuse of N_2O should thus be suspected in otherwise healthy young persons with subacute myelopathy [220].

In the process of making the diagnosis, the investigator should look for macrocytic anaemia, although this may be absent. A low serum B_{12} level is not always found, and higher levels of abnormal metabolites such as methyl malonic acid and homocysteine should also be looked for. Treatment is by stopping exposure and administering Vitamin B_{12} supplements. Recovery depends on severity of exposure. Residual defects are common.

Hexacarbons: Gasolene-based solvents contain n-hexane and methyl-butyl-ketone (rarely used today), which are then used in glues, spray paints and coatings in shoemaking, furniture-making, fabric finishes and other industries. Methy-ethyl-ketone, also used in solvents, though non-toxic in its own right, nevertheless potentiates n-hexane neuropathy. 2,5 hexane dione, the toxic intermediary metabolite of n-hexane and methyl-butyl-ketone, produces neurofilament accumulation in axons, resulting in giant axonal swellings, similar to those of acrylamide neuropathy and autosomal recessive giant axonal neuropathy. The main sources of exposure are industrial and recreational abuse (sniffers and huffers). In a study of 93 workers, industrial exposure resulted in sensory neuropathy in 57%, sensorimotor neuropathy in 34%, and amyotrophy in 9%. There was full recovery in 92% after 4 years [263]. In an epidemic in Ohio of methyl-butyl-ketone exposure in a plant making coated fabrics, there were 86 cases of neuropathy among 1157 employees [6]. In 37 patients, neuropathy was identified only electrophysiologically by slowing of nerve conduction. In 38 patients, there was mild neuropathy with sensory signs and 11 patients had moderately severe sensorimotor neuropathy. Elimination of the toxin resulted in improvement in the majority. This study is regarded as a model for epidemiological investigation of an industrial outbreak.

Recreational abuse results in inhalation of higher quantities of the toxin, which produces a picture like Guillain Barre Syndrome or AIDP. Indeed, one should search for a history of toxic exposure in all cases of AIDP [54]. Like acrylamide toxicity, there are sweaty palms and soles, resulting from an autonomic neuropathy. In a study of 18 juveniles with symmetrical, progressive, ascending weakness with wasting and persistent deficit at 8 months, the nerve biopsy suggested glue-sniffers' neuropathy [7]. In this case, methyl-ethyl-ketone potentiated the effect of n-hexane. In glue-sniffing, where high doses are used, recovery is less certain. In industrial exposures, providing exposure is stopped, recovery is the rule after a period of coasting for some months.

Alcoholic Neuropathy

Chronic alcoholism is a world-wide problem. The WHO estimates that there are about 2 billion people worldwide who consume alcoholic beverages and 76.3 million with diagnosable alcohol use disorders (WHO, 2004). Alcohol causes 1.8 million deaths (3.2% of total) and loss of 58.3 million (4% of total) Disability-Adjusted Life Years (DALYs.) (WHO, 2002.). Neuropsychiatric conditions account for 40% of the 58.3 million DALYs. Alcohol produces a peripheral neuropathy, whose incidence varies from 10-50% of alcoholics [206]. If EMG criteria are used, incidence rises. A clinical epidemiological study of 296 alcoholics with polyneuropathy showed 48 subjects (16.2%) had symptoms only, but 144 subjects (48.6%) had polyneuropathy on EMG [294]. Although peripheral neuropathy may not be a prominent feature of the Wernicke-Korsakoff syndrome, it is present in over 80% of people with chronic alcoholism. The neuropathy is usually sensory-motor axonal with painful paraesthesiae [292]. Small fibre involvement accounts for this and for the autonomic component. Rarely, there is an acute GBS-like syndrome [141]. In addition, compressive neuropathies are more common in alcoholics, being radial, brachial plexus, peroneal and ulnar, in order of decreasing frequency.

The aetiology of polyneuropathy in those with chronic alcoholism is probably an interaction between the direct toxic effect of alcohol and B-complex deficiency [292,300]. The precise mechanism of toxicity of alcohol is unknown. Though very difficult to assess, the dose of ethanol required to produce peripheral neuropathy is thought to be 100cc ethanol per day for 3 years [21]. In Vitadini's study, duration of alcohol use was also an important factor. Symptoms of peripheral neuropathy were twice as common after 10 years as they were after 5 years of abuse. The type of alcohol consumed is another factor. Drinking wine is more often associated with neuropathy than drinking beer or spirits. It is possible that lead in wine contributes to alcoholic peripheral neuropathy. Peripheral neuropathy was seen more often in men than women and in older people more than the young [294]. Alcoholism may also be associated with abuse of other toxic substances. The nutritional aspect of alcoholism is multifactorial. Relevant factors are diminished and /or imbalanced food intake, demand for more thiamine due to increased carbohydrate intake, absolute thiamine and/or B-complex deficiency in the diet exacerbated by malabsorption, and all the above compounded by impaired metabolism as a result of alcohol and alcoholic liver disease. Liver disease and macrocytosis are strong correlates of the severity of neuropathy [294].

Analytical case-control studies have attempted to tease out the relative contributions of nutritional deficiency and direct toxicity. Behse and Bucthal (1977), [21] compared 37 patients with alcoholic peripheral neuropathy with 6 patients with post-gastrectomy nutritional neuropathy. Sixty percent of the alcoholic group had no weight loss. The peripheral neuropathy in alcoholics both with and without significant weight loss and in the post-gastrectomy group was clinically identical. Sural nerve biopsy, however, showed more segmental demyelination in the post-gastrectomy group, demonstrating that this peripheral neuropathy was distinct from the ethyl alcohol-related peripheral neuropathy. A study by Koike H. et al (2003) [159] looked at 64 patients with alcoholic peripheral neuropathy, some of whom had B_1 deficiency determined by serum levels and erythrocyte transketolase activity. These were compared with 32 patients with non-alcoholic peripheral neuropathy, but with similarly determined B1 deficiency. The group with high alcohol and normal B_1 had a small fibre sensory neuropathy. The group with B_1 deficiency alone had a large fibre sensorimotor neuropathy and the group with alcoholism and B_1 deficiency showed mixed findings. This study supports a direct toxic effect of alcohol. An electrophysiological study in patients with chronic alcoholism found that parasympathetic dysfunction and reduction in sensory action potential correlated with lifetime dose of alcohol [206]. Controls did not have autonomic neuropathy, although one did have peripheral neuropathy. Autonomic neuropathy and peripheral neuropathy in the alcoholic group correlated with each other and were not related to age or nutrition.

Mild to moderate alcoholic peripheral neuropathy is reversible if intake is stopped [127]. In addition to abstention, treatment is supplemented with B group vitamins, especially B_1. No specific studies have objectively assessed treatment options.

Environmentally Induced Neuropathies

Exposure to toxins in the environment still occurs and is often inadvertent. Exposure to plant and animal toxins must also be considered.

Heavy Metals

Heavy metals (elements with atomic weights between 195 and 207.2, including platinum, gold, mercury, thallium and lead) are potent neurotoxins. Arsenic, with an atomic weight of 74.9, is not a heavy metal, but is grouped with them [299*]. Exposure is either environmental in industry or agriculture, by deliberate ingestion eg. arsenic or thallium, and rarely therapeutic. The general principles of toxicology apply, namely that onset of symptoms is related to exposure and cessation of exposure is related to diminishing of symptoms. As well as the peripheral nervous system, the other systems involved are the gut, the haemopoietic system, bone and the central nervous system. Deposition of heavy metals in bone is of great importance, since after cessation of exposure, the metal is released from bone leading to a recurrence of symptoms.

Lead (Pb): The toxic effects of exposure to lead are now widely appreciated, and direct industrial, occupational and environmental exposures are much less common following precautionary measures or use of alternative materials where possible. At the Mayo Clinic between 1949-89, there were less than 10 cases of lead neuropathy in adults in 3.5 million new patients [299]. Occupational contact with lead can occur in smelting, demolition and battery manufacture. Taking a careful history is mandatory to detect unusual sources of lead poisoning such as pica, lead shot or Asian traditional remedies. Levels of atmospheric lead are rising, as shown by a 400-fold increase in lead in the polar ice cap from prehistory to the present and a 100 fold increase in bone lead from 3000 BC to the present [299].

The neurological features of lead poisoning are encephalopathy in children and peripheral neuropathy in adults. Unlike the other heavy metals and most other toxic neuropathies, it produces a multifocal motor neuropathy, involving the arms more than the legs. Weakness commences in the finger extensors, extends proximally to involve the wrist extensors and also affects the small muscles of the hands, giving the impression of an anterior horn cell disorder. There may also be a mild sensory neuropathy affecting the legs more than the arms. Electrophysiological studies have been widely used to identify neuropathy in asymptomatic workers exposed to lead. Nerve conduction abnormalities, motor plus sensory or motor alone, have been found when blood lead levels exceed 70μgm/dl of whole blood, which is the industrial safe exposure limit [299]. Haematological changes, almost always coexist with lead neuropathy and include microcytic, hypochromic anaemia with basophilic stippling. Other symptoms are abdominal pain and constipation.

In addition to the history of exposure, confirmation of neuropathy and haematological abnormalities, abdominal pain and constipation, the diagnosis is finally made by finding increased lead in tissue. Blood and urine lead levels may be raised, as are urinary delta-aminolevulinic acid and coproporphyrin. Lead in blood and urine reflect recent exposure, as the half-life of lead in the blood is 20 days. The half-life in bone and teeth is 20 years, reflecting chronic exposure. A relationship between lead and ALS [299] has been suspected ever since early clinical neurologists found a history of lead exposure in some patients with ALS and the clinical similarity between the two conditions, except for pyramidal signs in ALS. However, case-control studies and trials of treatment with chelating agents have found either negative, or only slightly positive results.

There are no recent, systematic, clinical trial data as lead neuropathy is rare. Removal from the source of exposure, chelating agents, IV EDTA, oral penicillamine, British Anti Lewisite (BAL) and meso-2,3-Dimercaptosuccinic acid (DMSA) have been used.

Arsenic: Arsenic is one of the most toxic metals derived from the natural environment and can inactivate up to 200 enzymes [237]. The current main source of arsenic exposure is groundwater contamination. In the Indian state of West Bengal, 42.7 million people are exposed to arsenic. In adjoining Bangladesh, the figure is 79.9 million people, as groundwater levels exceed the WHO's maximum permissible limit of 50 μgm/L. In West Bengal, arsenic levels in some tubewells may be as high as 3400 μg/L. Arsenic groundwater levels also exceed permissible levels in parts of some industrial countries as in Millard County, USA.

In West Bengal and Bangladesh, 1331 people with proven arsenic-intoxication were studied. Between 34.2 and 60.3% were found to have arsenic-induced peripheral neuropathy, mainly sensory, with mixed-fibre involvement [211].

Another important source of arsenic ingestion is in traditional Chinese, Korean and Indian medicines. Arsenic contamination has been shown in 14% of products in herbal medicine stores in California [237]. Arsenic in the form of arsenic trioxide (As_2O_3) is used for the treatment of acute promyelocytic leukemia

There are industrial sources of arsenic, but these are much less commonly seen now. Mining, smelting and pesticides used to be major sources. Accidents too are less common now that usage has diminished, with the result that death from arsenic today is usually either murder or suicide.

Acute intoxication produces encephalopathy and abdominal symptoms. Chronic intoxication produces areas of altered pigmentation, particularly in the trunk and abdomen, hyperkeratosis of palms and soles, Mee's lines in the nails and painful, sensory-motor, axonal neuropathy which may affect the trigeminal nerve also. Neuropathy occurs from 10 days to 3 weeks following a single exposure. It may progress for up to 5 weeks [173].

The presence of arsenic is confirmed by finding increased levels of arsenic in the urine, and if chronic toxicity is suspected, by, arsenic-levels of hair and nails. Consumption of seafood within 3 days of testing the urine may result in elevated urinary levels of arsenic, but this form of arsenic is arsenate (As^{5+}) which does not bind to keratin and hence is excreted unchanged.

There have been two trials of BAL (British Anti-Lewisite) [299] and it was not found to be very effective. Recovery is slow. Months to years after initially severe peripheral neuropathy, a permanent deficit may remain.

Prevention in endemic areas requires an alternative source of water. Filtering water may help.

There are individual differences in susceptibility to arsenic poisoning. These may be related to genetic polymorphism, slow or fast methylators, age, sex, nutritional status and role of vitamins, minerals and antioxidants.

Thallium (Tl): Thallium poisoning is currently either accidental or intentional. Its use in pesticides has been banned. Almost always, peripheral neuropathy develops. In addition, there are joint pains, abdominal pain and alopecia, which occurs weeks later, in which there is pathognomic darkening of the hair roots [247]. The patient may die before hair loss occurs [51]. Mee's lines and anaemia without basophilic stippling are also found. The nervous system is affected at several levels. Thallium ions behave like potassium ions, but also combine with sulphydryl groups and produce mitochondrial swelling and axonal damage. The peripheral neuropathy is sensory-motor axonal. There may be cranial nerve involvement with ptosis, respiratory embarrassment, involvement of the autonomic nervous system and, with higher doses, an increasingly prominent encephalopathy. The painful neuropathy can be distinguished from GBS by the preservation of proximal reflexes. Alopecia distinguishes the condition from arsenic poisoning. At the time of thallium ingestion, absorption can be limited by oral administration of Prussian blue (potassium ferric ferrocyanide)

Mercury (Hg) [61]. Mercury exists as elemental liquid mercury, as mercury vapour, as inorganic mercury salts and as organic forms, methyl and ethyl mercury.

Elemental mercury: Dental amalgams containing mercury emit mercury vapour, which is inhaled and absorbed into the circulation. The act of chewing increases blood and urinary levels of mercury. However, no evidence has supported any evidence of mercury amalgams producing peripheral and central nervous conditions, or of removal of oral amalgams producing clinical benefits [299,81]. Indeed, removal of amalgam produces mercury vapour and may be harmful. Liquid mercury, if ingested, is not absorbed and passes out unchanged. Mercury spilt at home produces a vapour close to the ground, which may affect young children. Mercury vapour, in concentrations exceeding $500\mu gm/m^3$, produces peripheral neuropathy, erethism ("mad as a hatter"), intention tremor, gingivitis and proteinuria. The syndrome is now rare.

Methyl mercury is produced by conversion of inorganic mercury in the aquatic food chain. This is the major source of methyl-mercury, which is concentrated as one ascends the chain. Epidemiological studies have demonstrated that eating large fish causes mercury poisoning. In Minamata Bay in Japan birds and cats who ate such fish developed signs of poisoning with mercury, which was detected in their bodies [166]. Mercury toxicity in humans was reported in Iraq, where bread had been made from grain coated with methylmercury, a fungicide [15], and in the USA when people ate pork from a pig that had eaten grain treated with methyl-mercury to prevent fungus [61]. Methyl-mercury produces an encephalopathy, loss of vision and hearing, sensory ataxia, and a painful sensory-neuropathy with simultaneous circumoral and distal extremity paraesthesiae. A major current concern is the effect of mercury intoxication on the foetus and young children, in whom mercury produces neuropsychological changes. In the USA, the maximum permissible daily allowance of mercury intake is 0.1 µg per kilogram [61]. The US FDA recommends that pregnant women, nursing mothers and young children should avoid predatory fish.

Ethyl-mercury: Thimerosal, used as a preservative in multi-dose vaccination vials, contains ethyl-mercury. Vaccinated infants are therefore at risk, and consequently in the USA, there has been a switch to usage of single-dose vials as a result. The WHO has, however, continued with the use of multi-dose vials, because in many parts of the world infectious diseases remain a major cause of death and disability and ethyl mercury is less toxic than methyl mercury. It has a shorter half-life, allowing excretion of mercury before the next dose.

Other Industry-Related Toxins

Acrylamide Acrylamide, a toxic vinyl monomer, is no longer a commercial product. It is converted to a non-toxic polymer that is used for water purification and waterproofing. Occurrence of peripheral neuropathy due to acrylamide now is vastly reduced. Patients present with moist, peeling hands and feet, ataxia and a large fibre peripheral neuropathy. The chemical interferes with fast, anterograde, axonal transport mechanisms. The pathology consists of swelling along the axon due to accumulation of neurofilament. Interest has been aroused by the finding of acrylamide in connection with the cooking of French fries!

Organo-phosphates: There are thousands of organophosphate compounds, ubiquitously used as pesticides, in plastics and as lubricants for other purposes. Ominously, current interest has been aroused by their usage in chemical warfare. They are absorbed through the skin or any mucosal surface, either accidentally or deliberately. In South Asia they are common suicidal agents.

Acute organophosphate intoxication produces an immediate cholinergic crisis due to inhibition of acetylcholinesterase enzyme, which results in an acute syndrome of excessive parasympathetic activity due to stimulation of muscarinic receptors in bronchi, exocrine glands and the vagus. The crisis consists of excessive gut and lachrymal secretion, excessive gut motility, bradycardia and constriction of the pupils. Within 12-96 hours after injection, it may be followed by a Type II or intermediate syndrome due to post-synaptic excess stimulation of nicotinic receptors found in cholinergic, sympathetic ganglia and in the neuromuscular junction. The syndrome consists of proximal limb, respiratory muscle and neck flexor weakness. The third syndrome that occurs is organo-phosphate-induced delayed peripheral neuropathy (OPIDP), some 2-3 weeks later. It is much less common than the other two types. It consists of a sensorimotor axonal neuropathy due to inhibition of an enzyme called neuropathy target enzyme (NTE). The first symptoms are calf pain and cramps followed by paraesthesiae in a glove and stocking distribution, numbness and later, weakness. It progresses subacutely. The preceeding cholinergic phase may not occur, or may be very subtle. During the recovery phase, upper motor neuron signs due to spinal cord involvement may become more apparent. Once CNS damage has occurred, the prognosis is not so good, as there may be residual spastic paraparesis with distal leg wasting. This clinical pattern, almost like GBS, is seen in the major epidemics due to tri-ortho cresyl phosphate (TOCP) poisoning. One such epidemic was the Jamaica ginger extract (Jake) epidemic, because the chemicals were contaminants in a softdrink called Jamaica ginger or Ginger Jake. It probably affected 50,000-100,000 people in the USA in the early 1930's [44] as quoted by Smith HV & Spalding JMK, 1959 [264]. Another major epidemic occurred in Meknes, Morocco in 1959, when food had been cooked in oil contaminated with aviation fuel containing TOCP, and sold as a cheap brand of olive oil. Over 2000 people were affected [264]. The principles used to detect the cause of this illness demonstrate sound epidemiological methodology. The very rich, the very poor, visitors, soldiers in a garrison, prisoners and non-Muslims were all unaffected. Visitors brought their own food, soldiers and prisoners did not eat in town, the very poor could afford no oil and the rich bought more expensive, unadulterated products. Non-Muslims had their own market. Hence, only poor Muslims were affected. There have been epidemics of TOCP poisoning in other parts of the world due to contamination of cooking oil by aviation fuel, notably in Sri Lanka and Mumbai, India. (256, 295) The latest syndrome described is chronic organophosphate-induced neuropsychiatric disorder, COPIND [180]. This may be due to acute low-level organophosphate exposure, known as Phenomenon 1, or to chronic low-level exposure, Phenomenon 2. Examples are US-Gulf war veterans and British farmers who dipped their sheep. A comprehensive review of the literature by Lotti M, (2002) [180] found no consistent relationship between low-level exposure and neurobehavioural changes or peripheral neuropathy.

When neurobehavioural changes and peripheral neuropathy both occur in the same person, there is no relationship between the two. Other factors are implicated. Organophosphate intoxication may be diagnosed using electrophysiology [27].

Treatment of the Type I syndrome is by atropine and pyridoxine. There is no proven treatment for OPIDP, other than removal from the source of exposure.

Nerve Agents [114,219] are organophosphate liquid compounds, fast-evaporating, water soluble, non-persistent in the environment, which do not accumulate within the body. They are highly toxic. They produce a cholinergic crisis with high immediate mortality. Chronic effects in survivors are hypoxic ischaemic encephalopathy, neuro-behavioural changes and rarely peripheral neuropathy.

Tri-Chloro Ethylene: Tri-chloro ethylene toxicity is uncommon. We mention it because acute industrial exposure has resulted in an unusual cranial nerve syndrome affecting mostly Cr. V, but also other nerves from Cr. II to Cr. VII [93].

Ethylene Oxide (EO) [40]: Ethylene oxide is a gas used to sterilize hospital equipment and supplies. A cluster of 12 cases of ethylene oxide toxicity, occurred among female nurses and operating technicians. It was thought to be due to absorption of the toxin and its byproduct, ethylene chlorohydrin, through the skin or by inhalation. All exposed developed a contact dermatitis. 11 out of 12 had an axonal peripheral neuropathy and 10 out of 12 had memory loss. Although by numbers ethylene oxide does not appear to be of major importance, nevertheless it demonstrates clearly how exposure to toxins can occur inadvertently without the person's knowledge. Any patient presenting with a contact dermatitis should be checked carefully for manifestations of toxicity in other systems.

Dioxins

2,3,7,8 tetrachlorodibenzo-p-dioxin (PCDD)

Dioxin exposure occurs in workers in pesticide plants [283]. In this study, 17.1% of workers who had chloracne, suggestive of high exposure, had sensory neuropathy but only 1.2% of workers without chloracne. In Seveso, Italy, in 1976, an explosion in a chemical manufacturing plant resulted in exposure of townspeople to dioxin. A case-control study in 1982-83 [16] showed no peripheral neuropathy by WHO criteria, but possible peripheral nerve involvement on clinical and electrophysiological investigations. This again raises the crucial issue of definitions, discussed in the introduction to this chapter.

Dioxin is also a contaminant of "Agent Orange," a herbicide that was used from 1962-71 in the Vietnam War. People who complained of being affected were those who did the aerial spraying. Their complaints were of neuropsychiatric disturbance, or of symptoms of peripheral neuropathy. In one study [203], the serum dioxin levels of veterans involved in aerial spraying of the chemical were determined and used as a measure of exposure. Peripheral nerve function was assessed in various ways over a number of years up to 1997. A statistically significant risk of peripheral neuropathy was found in the high exposure category in 1992 and 1997. EMG and NCV were not used in these years, nor was pre-clinical diabetes mellitus looked at. In another study in 1995-6 [153], 1224 Korean, of the Vietnam War veterans and 54 Koreans who were not Vietnam veterans were assessed. Their history of exposure to Agent Orange was determined. When compared with non-Vietnam veterans, the Vietnam veterans had increased frequency of the following: eczema (OR=6.54), radiculopathy (OR= 3.98), diabetes mellitus (OR= 2.69), peripheral neuropathy (OR= 2.39), hypertension (OR= 2.29). A major problem in this study is that peripheral neuropathy has been looked at for the first time decades after the original exposure to dioxin. The Report of the National Academy of Sciences, Institute of Medicine [105], concludes that there is currently insufficient data available to implicate agents like Agent Orange with peripheral neuropathy and other neurological disease.

Animal Toxins

About 100,000 people die annually from animal envenomation and a similar number fall seriously ill following seafood consumption [119].

Envenomation occurs when a person is bitten or stung by a poisonous species. Those that affect the peripheral nervous system are mostly snakes, spiders, scorpions or ticks.

Snakes: Snakebite affects the peripheral nervous system at the neuromuscular junction, either pre-or post-synaptically, by producing a reversible, post-synaptic blockage of receptors (β bungarotoxin) or an irreversible, pre-synaptic block (α bungarotoxin). Both result in neuromuscular weakness, rather similar to myasthenia gravis. Death is due to respiratory failure and peripheral neuropathy has also been reported. In addition to the above, toxins may produce local pain and swelling, may damage muscle and thereby produce necrosis with myoglobinuria, as well as necrosis at the site of the bite, with or without a coagulopathy.

In Sri Lanka in 1999, 32,303 cases of snakebite were reported. The case fatality rate was stated to be 0.6%. 95% of all bites were due to cobra, Russell's viper and krait. Beginning in July of 2000, in Sri Lanka, an 8-month long prospective study of 56 consecutive patients who reached hospital with snakebite and neurological symptoms was conducted. Frequency of findings was as follows: ptosis 85.7%, ophthalmoplegia 75%, limb weakness 26.8%, respiratory failure 17.9%, palatal weakness 10.7%, neck weakness 7.1%, delayed sensory neuropathy 1.8%. One patient died from intracerebral haemorrhage [257].

Treatment is well established, consisting of the appropriate first aid, anti-snake venom and life-support systems when needed. Obvious preventive measures are that all rural workers should wear protective footwear in the fields, avoid placing hands into long grass and between stones, should sleep at night above ground level and if bitten, should be carried to medical help without exerting [18].

Scorpion and Spider Envenomation: These toxins target a variety of ion channels, Na$^+$, K$^+$, Ca^{2+} and Cl$^-$ producing peripheral and autonomic nervous system hyperexcitability. There is intense local pain followed by an adrenergic crisis, which may progress to cardiogenic pulmonary oedema and death. Scorpion stings are second only to snakebites as a cause of envenomation [298]. The red scorpion, Mesobuthus tamulus, found in India, is the most dangerous species. Treatment is by anti-scorpion venom serum and prazosin, a post-synaptic α-adrenergic blocker [17,215]. The use of prazosin was introduced by the Bawaskars, a husband and wife team in rural Maharashtra. They have been able to reduce mortality from 30% to less than 1% with prazosin alone.

Tick Paralysis: Paralysis as a result of tick bite mimics GBS, except that it is a descending rather than an ascending paralysis. Two main species are responsible [94], Dermacentor variabilis in USA and Ixodes holocylus in Australia. The American tick blocks Na$^+$ influx at the nodes of Ranvier and the Australian tick blocks acetylcholine release at the presynaptic membrane, rather like botulinum toxin. Treatment is by removal of the tick, including its mouthparts, and supportive care if required. Symptoms from the American tick reverse rapidly after removal, but those produced by the Australian tick may persist for several days, or even worsen before improvement occurs. It is imperative to "comb for the evidence," especially on the scalp, axilla and perineum, whenever GBS is suspected, as failure to remove the tick in time resulted in death in 11.7% of 332 cases [94].

Seafood Poisoning [227]. Poisoning is due most often to consumption of fish and shellfish, which themselves have consumed primitive marine plants that make a variety of neurotoxins. The most important of these are ciguatoxins, saxitoxins and tetrodotoxin.

Ciguatoxins come from dinoflagellates, which are eaten by herbivorous fish, which are then eaten by carnivorous fish such as barracuda, mackerel, moray eel and coral trout. Humans eating infected fish develop ciguatera, the commonest form of tropical fish poisoning in the Pacific and Caribbean Islands, since the toxin is not destroyed by cooking. The lipophilic toxin causes voltage-gated sodium channels to remain open. Systemic effects include perioral and distal paraesthesiae and a heightened awareness of pain. Cold objects or those at room temperature produce a "burning sensation", whereas warm objects produce a "cold-sharp" feeling. There is muscle pain and weakness, involvement of the autonomic nervous system and an encephalopathy. Although controlled clinical trials show no benefit, case reports suggest that mannitol infusion benefits more than 60% of patients by diminishing swelling of peripheral nerves. Gabapentin is given for pain.

Saxitoxins are also produced by dinoflagellates which are consumed by shellfish off the north-east and north-west coasts of the US and in the Gulf of Mexico. Saxitoxins block the sodium channels, causing reduced action potentials in muscle and nerve. Symptoms are paraesthesiae around the mouth and in the hands, followed by double vision, unsteadiness and respiratory failure. Treatment is supportive for about a week.

There is a symbiotic relationship between the puffer fish eaten in Japan and the marine vibrio which produces tetrodotoxin. Symptoms are similar to those of saxitoxin but a rapidly progressive neuromuscular paralysis can also occur.

Plant Toxins

There are many toxic plants, but the number of species which are neurotoxic and which specifically affect the peripheral nervous system is much fewer. Toxic plants are usually consumed as food or for their medicinal value, although accidental or deliberate consumption also occur.

Cassava root, commonly eaten as a source of calories in Africa, contains cyanide. If inadequately cooked, or consumed in quantity without adequate intake of the sulphur-containing amino acids and/or Vitamin B_{12}, cassava can produce thio-cyanates which can produce a sensory neuronopathy and a spastic paraplegia [223,243].

Lathyrism: (29) Lathyrus sativus, a neurotoxic pulse which is a very hardy plant containing protein, causes a spastic paraplegia in parts of Central India. It was also given to prisoners-of-war in World War II. Some 15% of patients have lower motor neurone involvement [62], and peripheral sensory polyneuropathy occurs in 7% [63].

The climbing lily, gloriosa superba contains colchicine, periwinkle (catharanthus roseus), contains Vinca alkaloids and the May Apple plant (podophyllum peltatum) which contains podophyllin, all produce a sensory-motor axonal neuropathy. In Southern USA and Central America, the seeds of a wild cherry (Karwinskia humboldtiana) can produce a GBS-like syndrome. The toxin is tulidora [45].

NUTRITIONAL PERIPHERAL NEUROPATHIES

Malnutrition and micronutrient deficiencies are estimated to contribute to 17% of the entire global burden of disease and accounted for 6 million deaths in 2000, or 11% of the global total [179]. Less developed regions in Asia, Africa and South America are the worst affected. On the other hand, there is an epidemic of obesity in some of the more developed regions. In the U.S. between 1988 and1994, 20% of men and 25% of women were obese. (278) In 1997, bariatric surgery was performed for morbid obesity in 6.3 / 100,000 people in the U.S.

There are no population based data on the incidence and prevalence of nutritional neuropathy. In developed countries, nutritional neuropathy is uncommon and usually associated with chronic disease, alcoholism, special diets, disorders of digestion and absorption, and disturbances of vitamin metabolism including those caused by drugs such as isoniazid [249*].

Nutritional neuropathies are commoner in clinical practice in developing countries. The causes remain the same, but there are important additional factors, such as a largely vegetarian diet in South Asia and the contribution of toxic factors like cassava.

Early recognition of nutritional neuropathies is important. Their onset is sometimes sudden. There may be cranial nerve involvement. In addition to peripheral nerves, other parts of the nervous system may also be affected. B_{12} and copper deficiency both affect the posterolateral columns of the spinal cord, the cerebrum and to a lesser extent, the optic nerves. Both also produce hematological abnormalities. Vitamin E deficiency affects the spinocerebellar tracts and posterior columns. All such signs are additional clues to diagnosis. Since nutritional neuropathies are axonal, recovery is slow and may be incomplete if treatment is started late.

Thiamine (Vitamin B_1) Deficiency

The fact that thiamine deficiency produces beriberi is a piece of historical epidemiology [49]. In Batavia (Java) between 1890 and 1900 Eijkman noted that chickens fed with polished rice developed a polyneuritis. Giving them the husk of the rice removed by polishing, the 'silverskin', prevented it. (47). Eijkman's colleague, A. G. Voderman, studied 300,000 prisoners and found that only 1 in 10,000 of those who ate unpolished rice had beriberi, but 1 in 39, to whom polished rice had been fed, developed the disease [49]. Casimir Funk termed the protective substance he had isolated from rice polishings 'vitamine' [49]. Body storage of thiamine is low, it has a short half-life and therefore steady intake is necessary. In developed countries, the main causes of deficiency are alcohol abuse, total parenteral nutrition and bariatric surgery.

Cobalamin (Vitamin B_{12}) Deficiency

In the absence of population-based data, among patients presenting to the clinician with peripheral neuropathy, cobalamin deficiency is probably the commonest deficiency neuropathy. In developed countries, the commonest cause is pernicious anaemia (PA) [284]. Incidence of cobalamin deficiency and PA increase with age. In a population survey, 1.9% of those over the age of 60 had PA [46]. Although traditionally PA was thought to occur mainly in Northern Europeans, it is now known to occur in African Americans and people from South America [46]. A study from the UK showed the frequency of PA to be the same in Indians and Caucasians. Contributing factors amongst Indians were a vegetarian diet and intestinal malabsorption (53). The prevalence of cobalamin deficiency is higher in the elderly 7-16% [112], but the percentage of these with clinical manifestations is unknown. In this group, because of the high incidence of cobalamin deficiency if a peripheral neuropathy is present it must be shown to be due to cobalamin deficiency.

Causes of cobalamin deficiency other than a malabsorption syndrome, dietary insufficiency or PA are exposure to nitrous oxide, which deactivates cobalamin, the use of drugs reducing gastric acid secretion and genetic disorders of cobalamin metabolism.

Diagnosis of cobalamin deficiency is not straightforward. Sensitivity and specificity of diagnosis are improved if levels of the cobalamin metabolites, homocysteine and methylmalonic acid, are measured in addition to the serum cobalamin level whenever it is less than 200 µg/ml. In a study of 324 patients with peripheral neuropathy [250], at a specialist centre, 27 (8%) had elevated methylmalonic acid and homocysteine, suggesting cobalamin deficiency. Of these 27, 12 had normal serum cobalamin levels and half of these were found to have PA. Over 17 years at 2 New York hospitals, 143 patients were found to have 153 episodes of cobalamin deficiency [122]. Neuropathy alone was found in 25%, myelopathy in 12% and 41% had both. Whether peripheral neuropathy occurs separately from myelopathy is controversial.

The haematocrit was normal in 27.4% and the mean corpuscular volume in 23% of these episodes. In non-anaemic patients, diagnosis was delayed and neurological manifestations worsened. All patients who were followed up responded to treatment and recovery was complete in 47.1%. Those whose haematological findings were normal fared badly, as did those who had had symptoms for a long time and whose nervous systems had been severely affected prior to commencing treatment.

Pyridoxine (Vitamin B$_6$) Deficiency

Pyridoxine deficiency occurs in chronic alcoholism, patients taking isoniazid for tuberculosis and those on chronic peritoneal dialysis. Excess pyridoxine also produces neuropathy - see section 7 above

Niacin Deficiency

Niacin deficiency produces pellagra, causing diarrhoea, dermatitis, dementia and death. It is still seen in less developed regions of the world, but the peripheral neuropathy is mild compared with the CNS manifestations [249].

Alpha Tocopherol (Vitamin E) Deficiency

Alpha Tocopherol (Vitamin E) deficiency occurs mostly in the context of malabsorption of lipids and can be due to specific transport disorders.

Bariatric Surgery

Gastric surgery for patients with morbid obesity (Bariatric surgery) can result in peripheral neuropathy. In a case-control study using obese patients after bariatric surgery as cases and controls who were obese people after cholecystectomy, the incidence of peripheral neuropathy was found to be 16% in cases but only 3% in controls. The result was considered due to malnutrition [278]. In a review of 556 patients undergoing bariatric surgery at the Mayo Clinic between 1980 and 2003, 8.6% were found to have peripheral neuropathy.

Thiamine (Vitamin B_1) deficiency was thought to be an important factor. Prevention depends on proper post-operative nutritional counseling [279].

Copper Deficiency

Copper (Cu) deficiency, which mimics subacute combined degeneration and also produces a pancytopaenia, is another cause of nutritional neuropathy, but there is no further epidemiological data available [163,123].

Tropical Myeloneuropathy [242]

Ever since Strachan described 810 cases of "a form of multiple neuritis prevalent in the West Indies", there have been many descriptions of possibly different syndromes occurring in different populations at different times under different circumstances. There are two main forms, Tropical Ataxic Neuropathy (TAN) (sensory ataxia, burning feet), and Tropical Spastic Paraplegia (TSP). TAN comprises neuropathy, perhaps with nerve deafness, optic neuropathy and confusional episodes. It has a multifactorial aetiology that includes malnutrition, increased nutritional demands, as in pregnancy and lactation, post-infectious tropical malabsorption and neurotoxic agents present in food, such as cassava. In a population-based, case-control study of TAN, the incidence was found to be 64/10,000 person years, but no relationship was found to intake of cassava or exposure to cyanide [222].

PARANEOPLASTIC NEUROPATHIES

Paraneoplastic neuropathies are due to the remote effects of malignancy and are found in less than 1% of all patients with any cancer [75]. They are often severe and occur before the malignancy becomes apparent. The usual causes of neuropathy in malignancy are malnutrition, leptomeningeal and, less commonly, nerve infiltration and side effects of treatment for the cancer. These are less severe than paraneoplastic neuropathy and become apparent late in the illness when there is significant weight loss [271*]. The study by Elrington et al [90] found 44% of 150 patients presenting to chest physicians had neuromuscular or autonomic deficits. Only one patient had subacute sensory neuropathy and two had the Lambert-Eaton syndrome.

Between 50 and 75% of patients with paraneoplastic neuropathy have small cell lung cancer, making this malignancy its commonest cause [271]. Small cell lung cancer (SCLC) is the most common cancer worldwide and makes up 20% of all lung cancers (Lung cancer facts and figures, CancerLine.com). Lung cancer affects 900,000 men and 330,000 women yearly. Throughout the world in 2000, 10 million people of both sexes were newly affected with cancer and the projection for 2020 is 15 million. (WHO, 2006). Although lung cancer is less common in women, the proportion of women with small cell lung cancer varies in different parts of the world and may even be greater than it is for men [111].

Other malignancies, also associated with paraneoplastic syndromes, are cancers of breast, ovary, prostate, gastro-intestinal tract, the lymphomas and the plasma cell proliferative disorders. In plasma cell proliferative disorders, an excess of abnormal immunoglobulin is found in the blood, hence the term paraproteinemia may be used. Paraproteinemic neuropathies account for 10% of idiopathic polyneuropathies in some studies [244]. Monoclonal gammopathies of uncertain significance (MGUS) are found in two thirds of patients with paraproteinaemic neuropathy. The incidence of peripheral neuropathy is increased in MGUS and the other paraproteinemic disorders. In multiple myeloma, peripheral neuropathy is prominent in 10% of patients and is found in up to 33% if electrophysiological criteria are used. In osteosclerotic myeloma, which is uncommon, being found in only 3-5% of patients with multiple myeloma, peripheral neuropathy is the presenting feature in up to 95% of patients [85]. The syndrome is termed POEMS for polyneuropathy, organomegaly, endocrinopathy, M-protein and skin changes. The incidence of paraproteinemias in the general population is unknown, but probably quite low. The crude incidence of multiple myeloma for males worldwide is 1.5 per 100,000 compared with 30.9 per 100,000 for lung cancer in males (GLOBOCAN 2002, International Agency for Research on Cancer).

Those syndromes of the peripheral nervous system most frequently associated with malignancy are subacute sensory neuronopathy, autonomic neuropathy leading to chronic gastrointestinal pseudo-obstruction and the Lambert-Eaton myasthenic syndrome. These have been defined as "Classical Syndromes" [110]. If any one of them occurs and a malignancy is diagnosed within 5 years of the syndrome being diagnosed, then a definitive diagnosis of paraneoplastic peripheral neuropathy can be made [110]. Other diagnostic criteria are the presence of onconeural antibodies and improvement in the neuropathy after treating the malignancy. Anti-Hu antibodies are those most commonly associated with subacute sensory neuronopathy and small cell lung cancer.

The following is a brief review of subacute sensory neuronopathy.

A good overview of paraneoplastic syndromes of the nervous system may be found In: Cancer of the Nervous System [75] and of paraneoplastic syndromes of the peripheral nerve in a review article by Rudnicki SA & Dalmau J [245*].

Tumor is usually not apparent at the time of 'presentation of neuronopathy' and should be carefully sought at regular intervals until it is detected. In a series of 71 patients with anti-Hu antibody and either paraneoplastic encephalomyelitis or sensory neuronopathy or both, 60% were subsequently found to have a tumour. The tumour was small, localized, and sometimes apparent only at autopsy. In 78% the tumour was a SCLC [74]. In another study, paraneoplastic encephalomyelitis preceded tumour diagnosis in 71% of patients by 6.5 months (range 0.1 to 47 months) [111].

The diagnosis of sensory neuronopathy should be made if the following criteria are met: subacute onset, rapid progression with a Rankin score of 3, i.e. some degree of dependence within 3 months, numbness, pain, proprioceptive sensory loss, asymmetrical onset, especially in the arms, and electro-physiology showing absent sensory action potentials and possibly sensory nerve involvement. Multifocal involvement of motor nerves, the autonomic nervous system and the central nervous system sometimes occurs. It was found in 52 of 71 patients (73%) in the series of Dalmau. et al. [74].

The commonest syndrome was a sensory neuronopathy in 52/71 or 73%, followed by motor nerve dysfunction in 14/71 or 20%, limbic encephalopathy in 14/71 or 20%, cerebellar degeneration in 11/71 or 15%, brainstem encephalitis in 10/71 or 14%, and autonomic nervous system involvement in 7/71 or 10%. Among the 52 with sensory neuronopathy, in 44, it was the predominant feature.

Course and Outcome

The course of paraneoplastic peripheral neuropathy is usually rapidly progressive. In the study by Graus et al [111], 53% of patients were severely disabled, totally dependent on others at the time of diagnosis. Only a minority (5%) had a completely independent existence and remained stable for at least 12 months without treatment. The median survival of the 200 patients was 11.8 months. Factors associated with increased mortality were age over 60 years, Rankin score more than 3, multifocal neurological involvement and lack of treatment. The main cause of death was central or peripheral respiratory failure or autonomic failure [74]. Neither immunosuppression, nor steroids nor plasma exchange improved symptoms [74], but treatment of the tumour, with or without immunotherapy, was thought to improve or stabilize paraneoplastic encephalomyelitis (OR = 4.56, CI =1.62 – 12.86) [111].

Clinicians are also interested in knowing how many patients with neuropathy might have an underlying malignancy and what types of neuropathy have a greater association with cancer. A reference centre data bank from France provides some information, but the highly selected nature of this population should be kept in mind [9]. The incidence of malignancy was highest, 47%, in those with sensory neuronopathy and the usual relationship with onconeural antibodies was found. The incidence of malignancy was up to 15% in vasculitic neuropathy, 10% in CIDP and mononeuritis multiplex, 4.5% in axonal neuropathy, and very low, only 1.5% in GBS. The investigators concluded that such patients should not have in-depth investigation for cancer unless onconeural antibodies were found in the serum or there was clinical evidence of encephalomyelitis or vasculitis.

RELEVANCE OF PERIPHERAL NEUROPATHY TO NEUROLOGICAL SERVICES

The relevance of peripheral neuropathy to neurological services can be considered firstly from the point of view of the burden of disability in the community, secondly in terms of the resources needed for diagnosis, and thirdly from a preventive perspective.

The Burden of Disability

The high prevalence of peripheral neuropathy across the world makes neuropathy an important focus for neurological services. As we have shown, many local factors influence the prevalence of peripheral neuropathies. Service providers must be aware of regional variations in the frequencies of diseases and complications which are related to socio-economic conditions, genetic variations and geographical factors. Thus, for example, poverty is a major determinant of the frequency and associated morbidity of diabetic neuropathy, just as it is of nutritional neuropathies. Similarly, the high cost of antiretroviral therapy means that treatment is more widely used in the more developed economies, which radically alters the epidemiology of antiretroviral toxic neuropathy on the one hand, and of HIV-induced distal sensory polyneuropathy on the other. There are small pockets of especially high prevalence for dominantly inherited genetic neuropathies, and genetically determined variations in susceptibility to the complications of diabetic neuropathy. Economic and geographical factors affect the risk of exposure to environmental toxins such as heavy metals. Similar factors influence the occurrence of infections such as leprosy and the C. jejuni strains which give rise to Guillain-Barré syndrome.

Although the crude prevalence of polyneuropathy can often be shown to be high, data on the epidemiology of neuropathy-related disability are extremely scarce. Thus, for example, the amount of disablement produced by diabetes, one of the most important and best studied causes of neuropathy, is still largely unquantified: the best information concerns the complications of lower limb ulceration and amputation, and even here the specific contribution of neuropathy to this morbidity is uncertain.

Peripheral neuropathy may not have had its fair share of attention from neurological and rehabilitation services on account of the tendency of the associated disabilities to be less salient than those produced by some other neurological conditions. The complications and disabilities associated with peripheral neuropathy are important for neurological services firstly because they are intrinsically distressing for patients and families and secondly because they constitute a very significant proportion of the total economic burden associated with neurological disease. In many cases cost-effective rehabilitation interventions are available, for example for pain (which is under-diagnosed in neurological practice) [76], and also for foot-drop. Orthotics services are underdeveloped in many centers, and more research is needed in order to define the needs of patients with peripheral neuropathies.

Diagnostic and Rehabilitation Assessment

There are many pitfalls in the accurate diagnosis of peripheral neuropathy. Neurological services require robust assessment protocols including systematic questionnaires, quantifiable sensory testing and appropriate support from neurophysiological and pathological services. The latter must include the usual range of biochemical, immunological and hematological tests, and there must also be access to specialized investigations including nerve biopsy and genetic testing. In parallel with these diagnostic assessments there should be provision for equally systematic assessment of pain and disability, to facilitate effective rehabilitation and support.

Prevention

Many of the opportunities for primary prevention of peripheral neuropathy lie within the domain of public health or of internal medicine rather than of neurological services. The greatest impact for the greatest number would come from measures to improve glycemic control in people with diabetes mellitus, which would reliably reduce incidence and severity of diabetic neuropathies. Prevention of Guillain Barre Syndrome through control of C jejuni is a theoretical possibility, but at the public health level the most important targets for infection control will be leprosy and HIV/AIDS.

Neurological services can be more directly involved in prevention of neuropathies due to drugs and environmental agents. Systematic assessment protocols are required, together with reliable reporting systems and effective methods of communication with relevant specialties such as pharmacy, occupational medicine and public health. Individual clinical neurologists have responsibilities in this respect, both for early detection of exposures so as to reduce future disability in individual patients and also for primary prevention of exposure in an at-risk population.

In the same vein, detection of impaired glucose tolerance as well as full diabetes mellitus through thorough investigation of neuropathies makes an important contribution to the prevention of future morbidity in individual patients presenting with either polyneuropathy or autonomic neuropathy – this could be termed secondary prevention.

Finally, neurological services need to be set up for what has been termed tertiary prevention: the anticipation and management of avoidable future disablement in patients presenting with neuropathy. This requires clinicians to be trained in the principles of preventive rehabilitation and is achievable through systematic assessment of risks (for example of skin ulceration, falls, social complications of disability, and so on).

CONCLUSION

This chapter has focused largely on the epidemiology of symmetrical polyneuropathies, which are among the most common neurological disorders in the general population and in neurological practice. Most categories of disease include conditions which cause neuropathy, so that the global and regional epidemiology of neuropathies reflects that of a very wide range of diseases. This heterogeneity limits the number of useful generalizations that can be made about polyneuropathies: in many respects, individual types of neuropathy must be considered separately from one another. However, some aspects of assessment and rehabilitation are common to many types of neuropathy, and these should comprise an important element of neurological services.

As we have shown, a great deal more research evidence is required in order to quantify the burden of disability associated with polyneuropathies and to enable the rehabilitation needs of different populations to be predicted.

ACKNOWLEDGEMENTS

1. Dr. Roberta H. Raven, for her invaluable help in the preparation of the manuscript.
2. Dr. Mary Reilly, for reviewing the genetics section and making useful comments
3. Ms. Aksha Endigeri, for her meticulous typing and formatting of the manuscript

REFERENCES

[1] Abbas ZG. and Archibald LK. (2005). Epidemiology of the diabetic foot in Africa. *Medical Science Monitor; 11(8)*: 262-270

[2] Abbott CA., Garrow AP., Carrington AL., et al. (2005). North-West diabetes foot care study. Foot ulcer risk is lower in South-Asian and African-Caribbean compared with European diabetic patients in the U.K.: the North-West diabetes foot care study. *Diabetes Care; 28(8)*:1869-75

[3] Ahlstrom G., Gunnarsson LG., Leissner P., et al. (1993). Epidemiology of neuromuscular diseases, including the post polio sequelae, in a Swedish county. *Neuroepidemiology; 12(5)*:262-9

[4] Aiyesimoju AB., Osuntokun BO., Bademosi O, et al. (1984). Hereditary neurodegenerative disorders in Nigerian Africans. *Neurology; 34(3)*: 361-2

[5] Albin RL. and Albers JW. (1990). Long-term follow-up of pyridoxine induced acute sensory neuropathy-neuronopathy. *Neurology ;40*:1319

[6] Allen N., Mendell JR., Billmaier DJ., et al. (1975). Toxic polyneuropathy due to methyl n-butyl ketone: an industrial outbreak. *Archives of Neurology; 32*:209

[7] Altenkirch H., Mager J., Stoltenburg G. et al.(1977). Toxic polyneuropathies after sniffing a glue thinner. *Journal of Neurology; 214*:152

[8] Andersson R. (1970). Familial amyloidosis with polyneuropathy. *Acta Medica Scandinavica; 188*: 85–94

[9] Antoine JC., Mosnier JF., Absi L., et al. (1999). Carcinoma associated paraneoplastic peripheral neuropathies in patients with and without anti-onconeural antibodies. *Journal of Neurology Neurosurgery Psychiatry; 67(1)*:7-14.

[10] Apfel SC. (1996). Docetaxel neuropathy. *Neurology ;46*:2

[11] Argyriou AA., Chroni E., Koutras A., et al. (2005) Vitamin E for prophylaxis against chemotherapy-induced neuropathy: a randomized controlled trial. *Neurology;64*:26-31

[12] Asbury AK. and Cornblath DR. (1990). Assessment of current diagnostic criteria for Guillain-Barre syndrome. *Annals of Neurology;27 Suppl*:S21-4.

[13] Ashok S., Ramu M., Deepa R., et al. (2002) Prevalence of neuropathy in type 2 diabetic patients attending a diabetes centre in South India. *Journal of the Association of Physicians of India; 50*:546-50

[14] Bacellar H., Munoz A., Miller EN., et. al. (1994). Temporal trends in the incidence of HIV-1-related neurologic diseases: Multicenter AIDS cohort study, 1985-1992. *Neurology; 44*:1982 – 1900

[15] Bakir F., Damluji SF., Amin-Zaki L., et al. (1973). Methylmercury poisoning in Iraq. *Science; 181*:230

[16] Barbieri S., Pirovano C., Scarlato G., et al. (1988). Long-term effects of 2.3.7.8-tetrachlorodibenzo-p-dioxin on the peripheral nervous system. Clinical and neurophysiological controlled study on subjects with chloracne from the Seveso area. *Neuroepidemiology;7*:29-37

[17] Bawaskar HS. and Bawaskar PH. (1996). Severe envenoming by the Indian red scorpion Mesobuthus tamulus; the use of prazosin therapy. *Quarterly Journal of Medicine; 89*: 701 -704

[18] Bawaskar HS. and Bawaskar PH. (2002). Profile of snakebite envenoming in western Maharashtra, India. *Transactions of the Royal Society of Tropical Medicine and Hygiene; 96*: 79 – 84

[19] Beghi E. and Bogliun G. (1996). The Guillain-Barre Syndrome (GBS). Implementation of a register of the disease on a nationwide basis. Italian GBS Study Group. *Italian Journal of Neurological Sciences; 17(5)*: 355-61

[20] Beghi E., Kurland LT., Mulder DW., et al. (1985). Guillain-Barré syndrome: clinico-epidemiologic features and effect of influenza vaccine. *Archives of Neurology;42*:1053-1057

[21] Behse F and Buchthal F. (1977). Alcoholic neuropathy: clinical, physiological and biopsy findings. *Annals of Neurology;2*:95-110

[22] Belongia EA., Hedberg CW., Gleieh GJ., et al. (1990). An investigation of the cause of the eosinophilia-myalgia syndrome associated with tryptophan use. *New England Journal of Medicine;323*:357

[23] Berger AR, Schaumburg HH., Gourevitch MN., et al. (1999). Prevalence of peripheral neuropathy in injection drug users. *Neurology; 53*: 592-597

[24] Berger AR., Arezzo JC., Schaumburg HH., et al. (1993). 2',3'- Dideoxycytidine (ddC) toxic neuropathy: A study of 52 patients. *Neurology.;43*:358-362

[25] Berger AR., Schaumburg HH., Schroeder C., et al. (1992). Dose response, coasting and differential fiber vulnerability in human toxic neuropathy: a prospective study of pyridoxine neurotoxicity. *Neurology;42*:1367-1370

[26] Bernsen R., de Jager A., Schmitz P., et al. (1999). Residual physical outcome and daily living 3 to 6 years after Guillain-Barre syndrome. *Neurology; 53*: 409-410.

[27] Besser R., Gutmann L., Dillman U., et al. (1989). End-plate dysfunction in acute organophosphate intoxication. *Neurology; 39*: 561

[28] Bharucha EP. and Bharucha NE. (1987) Neurological manifestations among those exposed to toxic gas at Bhopal. *Indian J.Medical Research; 86(Suppl.)*: 59-62

[29] Bharucha NE. (1986). Lathyrism In: Shah SJ (ed.), API text book of Medicine, Bombay, 4th ed: 204-205

[30] Bharucha NE., Bharucha AE. and Bharucha EP. (1991). Prevalence of peripheral neuropathy in the Parsi community of Bombay. *Neurology; 41*:1315-17.

[31] Bharucha NE., Bharucha EP. Dastur HD, et al. (1987). Pilot survey of prevalence of neurologic disorders in the Parsi community of Bombay. *American Journal of Preventive Medicine; 3*: 293-299.

[32] Bihan H., Laurent S.. Sass C., et al. (2005). Association among individual deprivation, glycemic control, and diabetes complications: the EPICES score. *Diabetes Care; 28(11)*: 2680-5

[33] Birouk N., Gouider R., Guern E Le., et al. (1997). Charcot-Marie-Tooth disease type 1A with 17p11.2 duplication. Clinical and electrophysiological phenotype study and factors influencing disease severity in 119 cases. *Brain; 120*: 813-823

[34] Booya F., Bandarian F., Larijani B., et al. (2005). Potential risk factors for diabetic neuropathy: a case control study. *BMC Neurology; 5*:24

[35] Bort S., Sevilla T., Vilchez JJ., et al. (1995). The diagnosis and prevalence of locus CMT1A duplication in Charcot-Marie-Tooth disease type 1. *Medicina Clinica; 104(17)*:648-52

[36] Bosboom WMJ., van den Berg LH., Franssen H. et al. (2001). Diagnostic value of sural nerve demyelination in chronic inflammatory demyelinating polyneuropathy. *Brain; 124*: 2427-2438

[37] Bouchard C., Lacroix C., Plante V., et al. (1999). Clincopathologic findings and prognosis of chronic inflammatory demyelinating polyneuropathy. *Neurology; 52*: 498-503

[38] Boulton AJM., Malik RA., Arezzo JC., et al. (2004). Diabetic somatic neuropathies: Technical Review. *Diabetes Care; 27*: 1458-1486

[39] Boulton AJM., Vinik AI., Arezzo JC., et al. (2005). Diabetic Neuropathies A Statement By The American Diabetes Association. *Diabetes Care; 28*: 956-962

[40] Brashear A., Univerzagt FW., Farber MO. et al. (1996). Ethylene oxide neurotoxicity: a cluster of 12 nurses with peripheral and central nervous system toxicity. *Neurology; 46*:992-8

[41] Brew BJ. (2003). The peripheral nerve complications of human immunodeficiency virus (HIV) infection. *Muscle and Nerve; 28*: 542-552

[42] Brodsky JB., Cohen EN., Brown BW. et al. (1981). Exposure to nitrous oxide and neurologic disease among dental professionals. *Anesthesia and analgesia.; 60*: 297

[43] Bruce DG., Davis WA., Davis TM. (2005). Longitudinal predictors of reduced mobility and physical disability in patients with type 2 diabetes: the Fremantle Diabetes Study. *Diabetes Care; 28(10)*:2441-7

[44] Burley BD. (1932). Journal of American Medical Association; 98: 298 *(as quoted in Smith HV and Spalding JMK. (1959)*

[45] Calderon-Gonzalez R , Rizzi-Hernandez H. (1967). Buckthorn polyneuropathy. *New England Journal of Medicine; 277*:69-71

[46] Carmel R, Johnson CS. (1978). Racial patterns in pernicious anemia. Early age at onset and increased frequency of intrinsic-factor antibody in black women *New England Journal of Medicine ;298(12)*:647-50.

[47] Carpenter KJ and Sutherland B. (1995). Eijkman's contribution to the discovery of vitamins. *Journal of Nutrition.; 125*: 155

[48] Carter GT., Jensen MP., Galer BS., et al. (1998). Neuropathic pain in Charcot-Marie-Tooth disease. *Archives of Physical Medicine and Rehabilitation; 79*:1560-4

[49] Carter KC. (1977). The germ theory, beriberi and the deficiency theory of disease. Medical. *History; 21*: 119

[50] Cavaletti G, Beronio A, Reni L et al. (2004). Thalidomide sensory neurotoxicity a clinical and neurophysiologic study. *Neurology;62*:2291-2293

[51] Cavanagh JB, Fuller NH, Johnson HR., et al. (1974). The effects of thallium salts, with particular reference to the nervous system changes: a report of three cases. *Quarterly.Journal of .Medicine.; 43*:293

[52] Chan TY and Critchley JA. (1996). Usage and adverse effects of Chinese herbal medicines. *Hum. Exp. Toxicology;15*:5

[53] Chanarin I, Malkowska V, O'Hea AM, et al. (1985). Megaloblastic anaemia in a vegetarian Hindu community. *Lancet;2(8465)*:1168-72.

[54] Chang AP, England JD, Garcia CA, et al. (1998). Focal conduction block in n-hexane polyneuropathy. *Muscle Nerve; 21*:964-969

[55] Charness ME, Morady F, Scheinman MM. (1984). Frequent neurologic toxicity associated with amiodarone therapy. *Neurology ;34*:669-671

[56] Chattopadhyay M, Goss J, Wolfe D, et al. (2004). Protective effect of herpes simplex virus-mediated neurotrophin gene transfer in cisplatin neuropathy. *Brain; 127*:929-939

[57] Chaturvedi N. Abbott CA. Whalley A. et al. (2002). Risk of diabetes-related amputation in South Asians vs. Europeans in the UK. *Diabetic Medicine; 19(2)*:99-104

[58] Chaudhry V, Chaudhry M, Crawford TO, et al. (2003). Toxic neuropathy in patients with pre-existing neuropathy. *Neurology; 60*:337-340

[59] Chaudhry V, Cornblath DR, Corse A, et al. (2002). Thalidomide-induced neuropathy. *Neurology ;59*:1872-1875

[60] Chio A, Cocito D, Leone M, et al. (2003). Guillain-Barre syndrome A prospective, population-based incidence and outcome survey. *Neurology; 60*: 1146-50.

[61] Clarkson TW, Magos L. Myers GJ. (2003). The toxicology of mercury: current exposures and clinical manifestations. *N. Engl. J.Med.; 149*:1731-1737

[62] Cohn DF and Striefler M. (1981). Human neurolathyrism: a followup study of 200 patients. *Arch. Suisses Neurol. Neurochir.Psychiatric; 128*:151-156

[63] Cohn DF, Striefler M, Dubash S, et al. (1983). Peripheral nerve changes in chronic neurolathyrism. *Neurology India; 31*:45-51

[64] Combarros O. (2003). Hereditary neuropathies. *Current Opinion in Neurology; 16(5)*:613-22

[65] Combarros O., Calleja J., Polo JM., et al. (1987). (1987). Prevalence of hereditary motor and sensory neuropathy in Cantabria. *Acta Neurologica Scandinavica. 75(1)*:9-12

[66] Conference Proceedings. (1992). Proceedings of a consensus development conference on standardised measures in diabetic neuropathy. *Neurology; 42*:1823-1839

[67] Connolly AM. (2001). Chronic inflammatory demyelinating polyneuropathy in childhood. *Pediatric Neurology; 24(3)*: 177-182

[68] Coppini DV. Wellmer A. Weng C. et al. (2001). The natural history of diabetic peripheral neuropathy determined by a 12 year prospective study using vibration perception thresholds. *Journal of Clinical Neuroscience; 8(6)*:520-4

[69] Cornblath DR and McArthur JC. (1988). Predominantly sensory neuropathy in patients with AIDS and AIDS related complex. *Neurology; 38*: 794 – 796

[70] Cornblath DR, Mellits D, Griffin JW, et al. (1988). Motor conduction studies in Guillain-Barre syndrome: description and prognostic value. *Annals of Neurology; 23*:354-9.

[71]   Cusick M. Meleth AD. Agron E, et al. (2005). Early Treatment Diabetic Retinopathy Study Research Group. Associations of mortality and diabetes complications in patients with type 1 and type 2 diabetes: early treatment diabetic retinopathy study report no. 27. *Diabetes Care;28(3)*:617-25

[72]   da Silveira CM, Salisbury DM, de Quadros CA. (1997). Measles vaccination and Guillian Barre Syndrome. *Lancet; 349(9044)*: 14-6

[73]   Dalakas MC. (2001). Peripheral neuropathy and antiretroviral drugs. *J. Peripheral Nervous System;* 6:14-20

[74]   Dalmau J, Graus F, Rosenblum MK, et al.(1992). Anti Hu-associated paraneoplastic encephalomyelitis/sensory neuronopathy. A clinical study of 71 patients. *Medicine (Baltimore); 71 (2)*: 59-72

[75]   Dalmau J. and Graus F. (1997). Paraneoplastic Syndromes of the Nervous system. In: Cancer of the Nervous System; Black P, Loeffler JS (eds.). *Blackwell Science:* 674-702

[76]   Daousi C ,MacFarlane IA.,Woodward A, et al. (2004). Chronic painful peripheral neuropathy in an urban community: a controlled comparison of people with and without diabetes. *Diabetic Medicine; 21*, 976–982

[77]   Darin N and Tulinius M. (2000). Neuromuscular disorders in childhood: a descriptive epidemiological study from western Sweden. *Neuromuscular Disorders;10*:1-9

[78]   Davis NB, Taber DA, Ansari RH, et al. (2004). Phase II trial of PS-341 in patients with renal cell cancer: a University of Chicago phase II consortium study. *J.Clinical Oncology;22*:115-119

[79]   de la Cour CD and Jakobsen J. (2005). Residual neuropathy in long-term population-based follow-up of Guillain-Barre syndrome. *Neurology; 64*: 246-253

[80]   de la Monte, Gabuzda DH, Ho DD. et al. (1988) Peripheral neuropathy in the acquired immunodeficiency syndrome. *Annals of Neurology; 23*:485

[81]   DeRouen TA, Martin MD, Leroux BG, et al. (2006). Neurobehavioral effects of dental amalgam in children : a randomized clinical trial. *JAMA ; 295(15)*: 1784-92

[82]   Diabetes Control and Complications Trial Research Group. (1995). The effect of intensive diabetes therapy on the development and progression of neuropathy. *Annals of Internal Medicine; 122*:561-568

[83]   Diabetes Control and Complications Trial/Epidemiology of Diabetes Interventions and Complications Research Group Writing Team. (2002). Effect of intensive therapy on the microvascular complications of type 1 diabetes mellitus. *Journal of American Medical Association. 287(19)*:2563-9

[84]   Diabetes Epidemiology Group (1990). Secular trends in incidence of childhood IDDM in ten Countries. *Diabetes;39*: 858-864

[85]   Dispenzieri A, Kyle RA, Lacy MQ, et al. (2003). POEMS syndrome: definitions and long-term outcome. *Blood; 101 (7)*: 2496 – 2506

[86]   Donaghy M. (2004). Genes for peripheral neuropathy and their relevance to clinical practice. *Journal of Neurology and Neurosurgery and Psychiatry; 75*: 1371-1372

[87]   Dray TG, Robinson LR, Hillel AD. (1999). Laryngeal electromyographic findings in Charcot-Marie-Tooth disease type II. *Archives of Neurology;56(7)*:863-5

[88] Dyck PJ, Karnes JL, O'Brien PC, et al. (1992). The Rochester Diabetic Neuropathy Study: reassessment of tests and criteria for diagnosis and staged severity. *Neurology; 42(6)*:1164-70.

[89] Dyck PJ, Kratz KM, Karnes JL, et al. (1993). The prevalence by staged severity of various types of diabetic neuropathy, retinopathy, and nephropathy in a population-based cohort: The Rochester Diabetic Neuropathy Study. *Neurology; 43*:817-824

[90] Elrington GM, Murray NM, Spiro SG, et al. (1991). Neurological paraneoplastic syndromes in patients with small cell lung cancer. A prospective survey of 150 patients. *J Neurol Neurosurg Psychiatry; 54(9)*:764-7.

[91] Emilia-Romagna Study Group on Clinical and Epidemiological Problems in Neurology (1997). A prospective study on the incidence and prognosis of Guillain-Barre syndrome in Emilia-Romagna region, Italy (1992-1993). *Neurology; 48*: 214-221.

[92] Feasby TE, Gilbert JJ, Brown WF, et al. (1986). An acute axonal form of Guillain-Barre polyneuropathy. *Brain;109 (Pt 6)*:1115-26.

[93] Feldman RG. (1979). Trichloroethylene. In Vinken PJ and Bruyn GW (eds.). *Handbook of Clinical Neurology*. Vol.36: Intoxications of the Nervous System. Amsterdam. North Holland. pp. 457

[94] Felz MW, Smith CD, Swift TR. (2000). A six-year-old girl with tick paralysis. *New England Journal of Medicine; 342*: 90-4

[95] Flattors SJ, Bennett GJ. (2004). Ethosuximide reverses paclitaxel and vincristine-induced painful peripheral neuropathy. *Pain;109*:150-161

[96] Fraser AG, McQueen IN, Watt AH, et al. (1985). Peripheral neuropathy during long-term high-dose amiodarone therapy. *J. Neurol. Neurosurg Psychiatry; 48*:576-578

[97] Freccero C. Svensson H. Bornmyr S, et al. (2004). Sympathetic and parasympathetic neuropathy are frequent in both type 1 and type 2 diabetic patients. *Diabetes Care; 27(12)*:2936-41

[98] Freimer ML, Glass JD, Chaudhry V, et al. (1992). Chronic demyelinating polyneuropathy associated with eosinophilia-myalgia syndrome. *J. Neurol. Neurosurg. Psychiatry; 55*: 352

[99] Gaist D, Garcia Rodrigues LA, Huerta C et al. (2001). Are users of food-lowering drugs at increased risk of peripheral neuropathy? *Eur. J.Clin. Pharmacology;56*:931-933

[100] Gaist D, Jeppesen U, Andersen M et al. (2002). Statins and risk of polyneuropathy:a case-control study. *Neurology; 58*:1333-1337

[101] Garcia CA, Malamut RE, England JD, et al. (1995). Clinical variability in two pairs of identical twins with the Charcot Marie Tooth disease type 1A duplication *Neurology; 45*: 2090-2093

[102] Gastaut JL, Gastaut JA, Pellissier JF et al. (1989). Peripheral neuropathies in human immunodeficiency virus infection: a perspective study of 56 patients (in French). *Rev. Neurol. (Paris); 145*: 451

[103] Gedlicka C, Kornek GV, Schmid K, et al. (2003). Amelioration of docetaxel/cisplatin induced polyneuropathy by alpha-lipoic acid. *Ann.Oncology;14*:339-340

[104] Ginsberg L. Malik O, Kenton AR et al. (2003). Coexistent hereditary and inflammatory neuropathy. *Brain; 127*: 193-202

[105] Goetz CG, Bolla KI, Rogers SM. (1994). Neurologic health outcomes and Agent Orange: Institute of Medicine report. *Neurology; 44*: 801-9

[106] Gordois A, Scuffh AM., Shearer A, et al. (2003). The healthcare costs of diabetic peripheral neuropathy in the US. *Diabetes Care; 26*: 1790-1795

[107] Gorson KC and Ropper AH. (2006). Additional causes for distal sensory polyneuropathy in diabetic patients. *Journal of Neurology, Neurosurgery & Psychiatry; 77*:354-8

[108] Gorson KC, Ropper AH, Adelman LS. et al. (2000). Influence of diabetes mellitus on chronic inflammatory demyelinating polyneuropathy. *Muscle nerve; 23*: 37

[109] Govoni V, Granieri E, Casetta I, et al. (1996). The incidence of Gullain Barre syndrome in Ferrara, Italy: is the disease really increasing? *J. Neurol. Sci.; 137*: 62-8

[110] Graus F, Delattre JY, Antoine JC et al. (2004). Recommended diagnostic criteria for paraneoplastic neurological syndromes. *Journal of Neurology neurosurgery psychiatry; 75*: 1135-1140

[111] Graus F, Keime-Giubert F, Reñe R, et al. (2001). Anti-Hu-associated paraneoplastic encephalomyelitis: analysis of 200 patients. *Brain; 124*: 1138-1148

[112] Green R and Kinsella LJ. (1995). Current concepts in the diagnosis of cobalamin deficiency. *Neurology; 45*: 1435 -1440

[113] Griffin JW, Li CY, Ho TW, et al. (1995). Guillain-Barre syndrome in northern China: the spectrum of neuropathologic changes in clinically defined cases. *Brain; 118*: 577-595.

[114] Gunderson CH, Lehmann CR, Sidell FR. et al. (1992). Nerve agents: a review. *Neurology; 42*: 946-50

[115] Gutman L and Johnson D. (1981). Nitrous oxide-induced myeloneuropathy: report of cases. *J.Ann. Dent. Assoc.;103*:239

[116] Hadden RDM, Cornblath DR, Hughes RAC, et al. (1998). Electrophysiological Classification of Guillain-Barre Syndrome: Clinical Associations and Outcome. *Annals of Neurology; 44*: 780-788.

[117] Hagberg B and Westerberg B. (1983). Hereditary motor and sensory neuropathies in Swedish children. 1. Prevalence and distribution by disability groups. Acta Paediatrica Scandinavica; 72: 379-383

[118] Hahn AF, Hartung HP, Dyck PJ. (2005). Chronic inflammatory demyelinating polyradiculoneuropathy. In: Dyck PJ & Thomas PK (eds.): *Peripheral Neuropathy*, 4th ed; Philadelphia: Saunders; chp. 99: 2221-2253

[119] Harris JB and Blain PG. (2004). Neurotoxicology: what the neurologist needs to know. *J. Neurol. Neurosurg. Psychiatry; 75 Suppl.3*:29-34

[120] Harris M. Eastman R. Cowie C. (1993). Symptoms of sensory neuropathy in adults with NIDDM in the U.S. population. *Diabetes Care; 16(11)*:1446-52

[121] Hattori N, Misu K, Koike H et al. (2001). Age of onset influences clinical features of chronic inflammatory demyelinating polyneuropathy. *J. Neurol. Sci.;184*: 57

[122] Healton EB, Savage DG, Brust JC et al. (1991) Neurologic aspects of cobalamin deficiency. *Medicine; 70*: 229

[123] Hedera P, Fink JK and Bockenstedt PL. (2004). Myelopolyneuropathy and pancytopenia due to copper deficiency and high zinc levels of unknown origin: further

support for existence of a new zinc overload syndrome. *Archives of Neurology; 61(4)*: 604-5

[124] Herman WH. and Kennedy L. (2005). Underdiagnosis of peripheral neuropathy in type 2 diabetes. *Diabetes Care:28(6)*:1480-1.

[125] Hertzman PA, Blevins WL, Mayer J et al. (1990). Association of the eosinophilia-myalgia syndrome with the ingestion of tryptophan. *N.Engl. J.Medicine; 322*: 869

[126] Hill AB. (1965). The environment and disease: association or causation? *Proc. R. Soc. Med.;58*:295-300

[127] Hillbom M. and Wennberg A. (1984). Prognosis of alcoholic peripheral neuropathy. *J. Neurol. Neurosurg. Psychiatry; 47(7)*:699-703

[128] Ho TW, Li CY, Cornblath DR, et al. (1997). Patterns of recovery in the Guillain-Barre syndromes. *Neurology; 48*: 695-700.

[129] Ho, TW, Mishu B, Li CY, et al. (1995). Guillain-Barre syndrome in northern China: relationship to Campylobacter jejuni infection and anti-glycolipid antibodies. *Brain; 118*: 597-605.

[130] Hoke A and Cornblath DR. (2005). Peripheral neuropathies in human immunodeficiency virus infection. In: Dyck PJ & Thomas PK (eds.): *Peripheral Neuropathy*, 4th ed. Vol. 2 ; Philadelphia: Saunders: 2129 – 2145

[131] Holmberg BH. (1993). Charcot-Marie-Tooth disease in northern Sweden: an epidemiological and clinical study. *Acta Neurologica Scandinavica; 87(5)*:416-22

[132] Holmgren G. Costa PM. Andersson C. et al. (1994). Geographical distribution of TTR met30 carriers in northern Sweden: discrepancy between carrier frequency and prevalence rate. *Journal of Medical Genetics; 31(5)*:351-4

[133] Hsu WC. Chiu YH. Chiu HC, et al. (2005). Two-stage community-based screening model for estimating prevalence of diabetic polyneuropathy KCIS no. 6. *Neuroepidemiology; 25(1)*:1-7

[134] Hughes RA, Choudhary PP, Osborn M. et al. (1996). Immunization and risk of relapse of Guillian-Barre syndrome or chronic inflammatory demyelinating polyradiculoneuropathy. *Muscle Nerve; 19*: 1230-1231

[135] Hughes RA, Swan AV, Doorn PA. (2003). Chronic drugs and interferons for chronic inflammatory demyelinating polyradiculoneuropathy. *Cochrane Database Syst. Review; 1*: CD003280

[136] Hughes RA, Umapathi T, Gray IA, et al. (2004). A controlled investigation of the cause of chronic idiopathic axonal polyneuropathy. *Brain ;127*:1723-1730

[137] Hughes RAC, Raphaël JC, Swan AV, van Doorn PA. (2006). Intravenous immunoglobulin for Guillain-Barre Syndrome (Cochrane review). *The Cochrane database systematic review; Issue 2*: CD002063.

[138] Hughes RAC, Swan AV, van Koningsveld R, et al. (2006). Corticosteroids for Guillain-Barre Syndrome (Cochrane review). *The Cochrane database systematic review; Issue 2*: CD001446.

[139] Hurwitz ES, Holman RC, Nelson DB, et al. (1983). National surveillance for Guillain-Barre syndrome: January 1978-March 1979. *Neurology; 33*: 150-157.

[140] Ikeda SN. Masamitsu AY. Sobue G. (2002). Familial transthyretin-type amyloid polyneuropathy in Japan: Clinical and genetic heterogeneity. *Neurology; 58*: 1001-1007

[141] Ishibashi S, Yokota T, Shiojiri T, et al. (2003). Reversible acute axonal polyneuropathy associated with Wernicke-Korsakoff syndrome : impaired physiological nerve conduction due to thiamine deficiency. *J.Neurol.Neurosurg.Psychiatry;74*:674-676

[142] Italian General Practitioner Study Group. (1995). Chronic symmetric symptomatic polyneuropathy in the elderly: a field screening investigation into Italian regions. I. Prevalence and general characteristics of the sample. *Neurology; 45*:1832 -1836

[143] Jacobs BC, Endtz H Ph., van der Meche A, et al . (1995). Serum anti GQ1b IgG antibodies recognize surface epitopes on campylobacter jejuni from patients with Miller Fisher Syndrome. *Annals of Neurology: 37*: 260-264

[144] Jacobs BC, Rothbarth PH, van der Meche FGA, et al. (1998). The spectrum of antecedent infections in Guillain-Barre syndrome A case-control study. *Neurology; 51*: 1110-1115.

[145] Jacobs BC, van Doorn PA, Groeneveld JHM, et al. (1997). Cytomegalovirus infections and anti-GM2 antibodies in Guillain-Barre syndrome. *J Neurol Neurosurg Psychiatry; 62*: 641-43.

[146] Jacobs BC, van Doorn PA, Schmitz PIM, et al. (1996). Campylobacter jejuni infections and Anti-GMI antibodies in Gullainn-Barre syndrome. *Annals of Neurology;40*: 181-187

[147] Kane RC, Bross PF, Farrell AT, et al. (2003). Velcade U.S.FDA approval for the treatment of multiple myeloma progressing on prior therapy. *Oncologist;8*:508-513

[148] Kaplan JE, Katona P, Hurwitz ES, et al. (1982). Guillain-Barre syndrome in the United States, 1979-1980 and 1980-81. *JAMA; 248(6)*:698-700.

[149] Kempler P. Tesfaye S. Chaturvedi N, et al. (2002). EURODIAB IDDM Complications Study Group. Autonomic neuropathy is associated with increased cardiovascular risk factors: the EURODIAB IDDM Complications Study. *Diabetic Medicine; 19(11)*:900-9

[150] Kennedy RH, Danielson MA, Mulder DW, Kurland P. (1978). Guillain-Barre syndrome – a 42 year epidemiological and clinical study. *Proc Mayo Clin; 53*: 93-9.

[151] Keshavan MS. Isaac M. Kapur RL. (1980). Ill-defined somatic symptoms in a South Indian rural clinic. Some preliminary clinical observations. *Tropical & Geographical Medicine; 32(2)*:163-8

[152] Khoury SA. (1978). Guillain-Barre syndrome: epidemiology of an outbreak. *Am J Epidemiology; 107(5)*:433-8.

[153] Kim JS, Lim HS, Cho SI, et al. (2003). Impact of Agent Orange exposure among Korean Vietnam veterans. *Ind. Health; 41*: 149-57

[154] King H and Rewers M. (1993). Global estimates for prevalence of diabetes mellitus and impaired glucose tolerance in adults. WHO Ad Hoc Diabetes Reporting Group. *Diabetes Care; 16(1)*:157-77.

[155] Kinnunen E, Färkkilä, Hovi T et. al. (1989). Incidence of Gullain-Barré syndrome a nationwide oral poliovirus vaccine campaign. *Neurology; 39*: 1034 – 1036

[156] Kinnunen E, Junttila O, Haukka J. et al. (1998). Nationwide oral poliovirus vaccination campaign and the incidence of Guillain-Barre Syndrome. *American Journal of Epidemiology; 147(1)*: 69-73

[157] Kinsella LJ and Green R. (1995). "Anesthesia paresthetica": nitrous oxide-induced cobalamin deficiency. *Neurology; 45*: 1608-1610

[158] Klein R. Klein BE. Moss SE. (2005). Ten-year incidence of self-reported erectile dysfunction in people with long-term type 1 diabetes. *Journal of Diabetes and its Complications; 19(1)*:35-41

[159] Koike H, Iijima M, Sugiura M. et al. (2003). Alcoholic neuropathy is clinocopathologically distinct from thiamine-deficiency neuropathy. *Annals of Neurology; 54*:19-29

[160] Koller H, Kieseier BC, Sebastian J. (2005). Chronic inflammatory demyelinating polyneuropathy. *New Eng. J. of Medicine; 352(13)*: 1343 – 1356

[161] Koller H, Schroeter M, Kieseier BC. et al. (2005). Chronic inflammatory demyelinating polyneuropathy – update on pathogenesis, diagnostic criteria and therapy. *Curr. Opin. Neurology; 18*: 273-278

[162] Krajewski KM, Lewis RA, Fuerst DR, et al (2000). Neurological dysfunction and axonal degeneration in Charcot–Marie–Tooth disease type 1A *Brain: 123*:1516-1527

[163] Kumar N, Gross JB and Ahlskog JE. (2004). Copper deficiency myelopathy produces a clinical picture like subacute combined degeneration. *Neurology; 63*: 33-39

[164] Kunel RW, Duncan G, Watson D, et al. (1987). Colchicine-myopathy and neuropathy. *N.Engl.J.Medicine;316*:1562-1568

[165] Kurihara S. Adachi Y. Wada K. et al. (2002). An epidemiological genetic study of Charcot-Marie-Tooth disease in Western Japan. *Neuroepidemiology; 21(5)*:246-50

[166] Kurland LT, faro SN and Siedler H. (1960). Minamata disease: the outbreak of a neurologic disorder in Minamat, Japan and its relationship to the ingestion of seafood contaminated by mercuric compounds. *World Neurology;1*:370

[167] Kuroki S, Saida T, Nukina M, et al. (1993). Campylobacter jejuni strains from patients with Guillain-Barre syndrome belong mostly to Penner serogroup 19 and contain ß-N-acetylglucosamine residues. *Ann Neurology; 33*: 243-247.

[168] Kuwabara S, Misawa S, Mori M et al. (2006). Long term prognosis of chronic inflammatory demyelinating polyneuropathy: a five year follow up of 38 cases. *J.Neurol. Neurosurg. Psychiatry; 77(1)*: 66-70

[169] Kuwabara S, Ogawara K, Koga M, et al. (1999). Hyperreflexia in Guillain-Barre syndrome: with acute motor axonal neuropathy and anti-GM1 antibody. *J Neurol Neurosurg Psychiatry; 67*: 180-184

[170] Landi G, D'Alessandro R, Dossi BC, et al. (1993). Guillain-Barre syndrome after exogenous gangliosides in Italy. *B. Med. Journal; 307*: 1463-4.

[171] Laroche CM, Carroll N, Moxham J, et al. (1988). Diaphragm weakness in Charcot-Marie-Tooth disease. *Thorax; 43(6)*:478-9

[172] Lasky T, Terracciano GJ, Magder L, et al. (1998). The Guillain-Barre syndrome and the 1992-1993 and 1993-1994 influenza vaccines. *N Engl J Medicine; 339*: 1797-802.

[173] Le Quesne PM and McLeod JG. (1977). Peripheral neuropathy following a single exposure to arsenic clinical course in four patients with electrophysiological and histological studies. *J. Neurol. Sci ;32*:437

[174] Leger JM and Behin A. (2005). Multifocal motor neuropathy. *Current. opinion in Neurology; 18*:567-573

[175] Lepore G. Bruttomesso D. Nosari I., et al. (2002). Glycaemic control and microvascular complications in a large cohort of Italian Type 1 diabetic out-patients. *Diabetes, Nutrition & Metabolism - Clinical & Experimental; 15(4)*:232-9

[176] Lipton RB, Apfel SC, Dutcher JP et al. (1989). Taxol produces a predominantly sensory neuropathy. *Neurology;39*:368

[177] Lockwood DN and Kumar B. (2004). Treatment of leprosy. *B. Medical Journal; 328*: 1447-1448

[178] Lockwood DN. (2002). Leprosy elimination – a virtual phenomenon or a reality? *B. Medical Journal; 324*:1516-1518

[179] Lopez A. (2004). Malnutrition and the burden of disease. *Asia Pac. J. Clin. Nutr.; 13* (Suppl):S7

[180] Lotti M. (2002). Low-level exposures to organophosphorus esters and peripheral nerve function. *Muscle Nerve; 25(4)*:492-504

[181] Lunn MPT, Manji H, Choudhary PP. et al. (1999). Chronic inflammatory demyelinating polyradiculoneuropathy: a prevalence study in south east England. *J.Neurol. Neurosurg. Psychiatry; 66*: 677-680

[182] Lyu RK, Tang LM, Cheng SY, et al. (1997). Guillain-Barre syndrome in Taiwan: a clinical study of 167 patients. *J Neurol Neurosurg Psychiatry; 63*: 494-500.

[183] MacDonald B K, Cockerell OC., Sander J W A S. et al. (2000). The incidence and lifetime prevalence of neurological disorders in a prospective community-based study in the UK. *Brain; 123*: 665-676

[184] MacMillan JC and Harper PS. (1994). The Charcot-Marie-Tooth syndrome: clinical aspects from a population study in South Wales, UK. *Clinical Genetics; 45(3)*:128-34

[185] Mandell GL and Sande MA. (1993). Antimicrobial agents drugs used in the chemotherapy of tuberculosis and leprosy. In Goodman and Gilman's *The pharmacological basis of therapeutics*, 8th ed., McGraw-Hill, New York: pp. 1146.

[186] Marques W Jr. Freitas MR. Nascimento OJ. et al. (2005). 17p duplicated Charcot-Marie-Tooth 1A: characteristics of a new population. *Journal of Neurology. 252(8)*:972-9

[187] Martyn CN and Hughes RA. (1997). Epidemiology of peripheral neuropathy. *J Neurol Neurosurg Psychiatry; 62*: 310-8.

[188] Mayeno AN, Belongia EA, Lin F, et al. (1992). 3-(Phenylamino) alanine, a novel aniline-derived amino acid associated with the eosinophilia-myalgia syndrome: a link to the toxic oil syndrome? *Mayo Clinic Proceedings; 67*: 1134

[189] Mbanya JC. and Sobngwi E. (2003). Diabetes in Africa. Diabetes microvascular and macrovascular disease in Africa. *Journal of Cardiovascular Risk; 10(2)*:97-102

[190] McArthur JC, Cohen BA, Selnes OA, et al. (1989). Low prevalence of neurological and neuropsychological abnormalities in otherwise healthy HIV-I infected individuals; Results from the multicenter AIDS cohort study. *Annals of Neurology; 26(5)*: 601-611

[191] McArthur JC, Yiannoustsos C, Simpson DM. et al. (2000). A phase II trial of nerve growth factor for sensory neuropathy associated with HIV infection. AIDS clinical trials group team 291. *Neurology; 54*: 1080 – 1088

[192] McCombe PA, Pollard JD, McLeod JG. (1987). Chronic inflammatory demyelinating polyradiculoneuropathy: A clinical and electrophysiological study of 92 cases. *Brain; 110*:1617-1630

[193] McGann R and Gurd A. (2002). The association between Charcot-Marie-Tooth disease and developmental dysplasia of the hip. *Orthopedics; 25*:337-9

[194] McKhann GM, Cornblath DR, Griffin JW, et al. (1993). Acute motor axonal neuropathy: a frequent cause of acute flaccid paralysis in china. *Annals of Neurology; 33*: 333-342.

[195] McLeod JG, Pollard JD, Macaskill P, et al. (1999). Prevalence of chronic inflammatory demyelinating polyneuropathy in New South Wales, Australia. *Annals of Neurology; 46(6)*: 910-3

[196] McMahon BJ, Helminiak C, Wainwright RB, et al. (1992). Frequency of adverse reactions to hepatitis B vaccine in 43,618 persons. *Am. J Medicine; 92*: 254-6.

[197] Medsger TA. (1990). Tryptophan-induced eosinophilia-myalgia syndrome. *N. Engl.J.Medicine; 322*:926

[198] Mehndiratta MM and Hughes RA. (2002). Corticosteroids for chronic inflammatory demyelinating polyradculoneuropathy. *Cochrane Database Syst. Review; (1)*: CD002062

[199] Mehndiratta MM, Hughes RA, Agarwal P. (2004). Plasmaelectrophoresis for chronic inflammatory demyelinating polyradculoneuropathy. *Cochrane Database Syst. Rev.* 2004; (3): CD003906

[200] Melnick SC and Flewett TH. (1964). Role of infection in the Guillain-Barre syndrome. *J Neurol Neurosurg Psychiatry; 27*: 395-407.

[201] Meretoja P, Silander K, Kalimo H. (1997). Epidemiology of hereditary neuropathy with liability to pressure palsies (HNPP) in south western Finland. *Neuromuscular Disorders; 7*: 529-532

[202] Merkies IS, Schmitz PI, van der Meche FG, et al. (2003). Connecting impairment, disability, and handicap in immune mediated polyneuropathies. *J Neurol Neurosurg Psychiatry; 74*: 99-104.

[203] Michalek JE, Akhtar FZ, Arezzo JC. et al. (2001). Serum dioxin and peripheral neuropathy in veterans of Operation Ranch Hand. *Neurotoxicology; 22*: 479-90

[204] Mishu BC, Patton CM, Blaser MJ. (1993). Microbiologic characteristics of Campylobacter jejuni strains isolated from patients with Guillain-Barre syndrome. *Clin Infect Dis; 17*: 538.

[205] Mohsin F. Craig ME. Cusumano J, et al. (2005). Discordant trends in microvascular complications in adolescents with type 1 diabetes from 1990 to 2002. *Diabetes Care; 28(8)*:1974-80

[206] Monforte R, Estruch R, VallsSole J, et al. (1995). Autonomic and peripheral neuropathies in patients with chronic alcoholism. A dose related toxic effect of alcohol. *Archives of Neurology; 52*:45-51

[207] Mori M, Kuwabara S, Fukutake T, et al. (2001). Clinical features and prognosis of Miller Fisher syndrome. *Neurology; 56*: 1104-6.

[208] Morocutti C. Colazza GB. Soldati G. et al. (2002). Charcot-Marie-Tooth disease in Molise, a central-southern region of Italy: an epidemiological study. *Neuroepidemiology; 21(5)*:241-5

[209] Mostacciuolo ML. Micaglio G. Fardin P. et al. (1991). Genetic epidemiology of hereditary motor sensory neuropathies (type I). *American Journal of Medical Genetics; 39(4)*:479-81

[210] Mostacciuolo ML. Schiavon F. Angelini C. et al. (1995). Frequency of duplication at 17p11.2 in families of northeast Italy with Charcot-Marie-Tooth disease type 1. *Neuroepidemiology; 14(2)*:49-53

[211] Mukherjee S, Chakraborti D, Quamruzzaman Q, et al. (2005). Abstract of the XVIIIth World Congress of Neurology. OPL 194 neurotoxicity in groundwater arsenic contamination in India and Bangladesh with special reference to neuropathy. *J. Neurol. Sci.; 238 (Supp.1)*:S96

[212] Munar-Ques M, Saraiva MJ. Viader-Farre C. et al. (2005). A Genetic epidemiology of familial amyloid polyneuropathy in the Balearic Islands (Spain). *Amyloid; 12(1)*: 54-61

[213] Mygland A and Monstad P. (2001). Chronic polyneuropathies in Vest-Agder, Norway. *Eur J Neurology; 8(2)*:157-65.

[214] Nachamkin I, Allos BM, Ho T. (1998). Campylobacter species and Guillain-Barre syndrome. *Clinical Microbiology Reviews; 11*: 555-567.

[215] Natu VS, Murthy RKK, Deodhar KP. (2006). Efficacy of species specific anti-scorpion venom serum (AScVS) against sever, serious scorpion stings (Mesobuthus tamulus concanesis Pocock) – An experience from Rural Hospital in Western Maharashtra. *JAPI; 54*:283 -287

[216] Nelis E. Van Broeckhoven C. De Jonghe P. et al. (1996). Estimation of the mutation frequencies in Charcot-Marie-Tooth disease type 1 and hereditary neuropathy with liability to pressure palsies: a European collaborative study. *European Journal of Human Genetics; 4(1)*:25-33

[217] Nery Ferreira BE. Silva IN. de Oliveira JT. (2005). High prevalence of diabetic polyneuropathy in a group of Brazilian children with type 1 diabetes mellitus. *Journal of Pediatric Endocrinology; 18*:1087-94

[218] Nevo Y, Pestronk A. Kornberg AJ. et al. (1996). Childhood chronic inflammatory demyelinating neuropathies: Clinical course and long-term follow-up. *Neurology; 47*:98-102

[219] Newmark J. (2005). Nerve agents. *Neurologic clinics; 23*: 623-641

[220] Ng J, O'Grady G, Pettit T, et al. (2003). Nitrous oxide use in first-year students at Auckland University. *Lancet; 361(9366)*:1349-50.

[221] Ng TH, Chan YW, Yu YL, et al. (1991). Encephalopathy and neuropathy following ingestion of a Chinese herbal broth containing podophyllin. *Journal of the Neurological Sciences; 101*:107-113

[222] Oluwole OS, Onabolu AO, Cotgreave IA. et al. (2003). Incidence of endemic ataxic polyneuropathy and its relation to exposure to cyanide in a Nigerian community. *J.Neurology Neurosurgery Psychiatry; 74(10)*: 1417-1422

[223] Oluwole OS, Onabolu AO, Link H, et al. (2000). Persistence of tropical ataxic neuropathy in a Nigerian community. *J Neurology Neurosurgery Psychiatry; 69(1):*96-101.

[224] Ooi WW and Srinivasan J. (2004). Leprosy and the peripheral nervous system: basic and clinical aspects. *Muscle Nerve; 30(4)*:393-409.

[225] Palumbo PJ, Elveback LR, Whisnant JP. (1978). Neurologic complications of diabetes mellitus: transient ishemic attack, stroke, and peripheral neuropathy. In: Schoenberg BS. (eds.): *Advances in Neurology*, vol.19, New York; Raven press: 593-601.

[226] Partanen J, Niskanen L, Lehtinen J, et al. (1995). Natural history of peripheral neuropathy in patients with non-insulin-dependent diabetes mellitus. *New England Journal of Medicine; 333(2)*:89-94.

[227] Pearn J. (2001). Neurology of ciguatera. *J.Neurol. Neurosurg. Psychiatry; 70*:4-8

[228] Postma TJ, Vermoken JB, Liefting AJ., et al. (1995). Paclitaxel-induced neuropathy. *Annals of Oncology; 6*:489

[229] Pradeepa R. Deepa R. Mohan V. (2002). Epidemiology of diabetes in India--current perspective and future projections. *Journal of the Indian Medical Association. 100(3)*:144-8

[230] Pratt RW and Weimer LH. (2005). Medication and toxin-induced peripheral neuropathy. *Seminars in Neurology; 25(2)*: 204 – 216

[231] Radhakrishnan K. el-Mangoush MA. Gerryo SE. (1987). Descriptive epidemiology of selected neuromuscular disorders in Benghazi, Libya. *Acta Neurologica Scandinavica. 75(2):*95-100

[232] Ramachandran A. Snehalatha C. Vijay V. et al. (2002). Impact of poverty on the prevalence of diabetes and its complications in urban southern India. *Diabetic Medicine; 19(2)*:130-5

[233] Ramos-Alvarez M, Bessudo L, Sabin A. (1969). Paralytic syndromes associated with noninflammatory cytoplasmic or nuclear neuronopathy: acute paralytic disease in Mexican children, neuropathologically distinguishable from Landry-Guillain-Barre syndrome. *JAMA; 207*: 1481-92.

[234] Rantala H, Cherry JD, Shields WD, et al. (1994). Epidemiology of Guillian Barre Syndrome in children: relationship of oral polio vaccine administration to occurrence. *The Journal of Pediatrics; 124(2)*: 220-3

[235] Raphaël JC, Chevret S, Hughes RAC, et al. (2006). Plasma exchange for Guillain-Barre Syndrome (Cochrane review). *The Cochrane database systematic review; Issue 2*

[236] Raphael JC, Masson C, Morice V, et al. (1986). The Landry-Guillain-Barre syndrome. Study of prognostic factors in 223 cases. (Article in French). *Rev Neurol (Paris); 142*: 613-624.

[237] Ratnaike RN. (2003). Acute and chronic arsenic toxicity. *Postgraduate Medical Journal; 79*:391-396

[238] Rees JH, Soudain SE, Gregson NA, (1995). Campylobacter jejuni infection and Guillain-Barre syndrome. *New England Journal of Medicine; 333*: 1374-79.

[239] Rees JH, Thompson RD, Smeeton NC. et al. (1998). Epidemiological study of Guillain-Barre syndrome in south east England. *J Neurology Neurosurgery Psychiatry; 64*: 74-77

[240] Reilly MM. Staunton H. Harding AE. (1995). Familial amyloid polyneuropathy (TTR ala 60) in north west Ireland: a clinical, genetic, and epidemiological study. *Journal of Neurology, Neurosurgery & Psychiatry; 59(1)*:45-9

[241] Rogers T, D Chandler, D Angelicheva, et al. (2000). A novel locus for autosomal recessive peripheral neuropathy in the EGR2 region on 10q23. *Am J Hum Genet; 67(3)*:664-71

[242] Roman GC, Spencer PS, Schoenberg BS. (1985). Tropical myeloneuropathies: The hidden endemias. *Neurology; 35*: 1158-1170

[243] Roman GC. (1994). An epidemic in Cuba of optic neuropathy, sensorineural deafness, peripheral sensory neuropathy and dorsolateral myeloneuropathy. *J Neurol Sci.; 127(1)*:11-28.

[244] Ropper AH, Gorson KC. (1998). Neuropathies associated with paraproteinemia. *The New England Journal of Medicine; 338 (22)*: 1601-1607

[245] Rudnicki SA and Dalmau J. (2005). Paraneoplastic syndromes of the peripheral nerves. *Current opinion in Neurology; 18*: 598-603

[246] Rustscheff S & Hulten. (2003). An unexpected and severe neurological disorder with permanent disability acquired during short-course treatment with metronidazole. *Scand J Infect Dis.; 35(4)*:279-80.

[247] Rusyniak DE, Furbee RB and Kirk MA. (2002). Thallium and arsenic poisoning in a small Midwestern town. *Ann. Emerg. Med. ;39*:307

[248] Sander MD. Abbasi D. Ferguson AL. et al. (2005). The prevalence of hereditary neuropathy with liability to pressure palsies in patients with multiple surgically treated entrapment neuropathies. *Journal of Hand Surgery - American Volume; 30(6)*:1236-41

[249] Saperstein DS & Barohn RJ. (2005). Polyneuropathy caused by nutritional and vitamin deficiency. In: Dyck PJ & Thomas PK (eds.): *Peripheral Neuropathy*; 4th ed. Philadelphia: Saunders; chp. 89: 2051 – 2062

[250] Saperstein DS, Wolfe GI, Gronseth GS, et al. (2003). Challenges in the identification of cobalamin-deficiency polyneuropathy. *Arch. Neurology; 60*:1296 - 1301

[251] Savettieri G, Rocca WA, Salemi G, et al. (1993). Prevalence of diabetic neuropathy with somatic symptoms: A door-to-door survey in two Sicilian municipalities. *Neurology; 43*: 1115-1120.

[252] Schaumburg HH. (2000). Human neurotoxic disease; Causation criteria for identification of neurotoxicity: cardinal tenets of neurotoxic disease. In: Spencer PS and Schaumburg HH (eds): *Experimental and clinical neurotoxicology*. New York: Oxford University Press; Chp.2: 55-82

[253] Schifitto G, McDermott, McArthur JC, et al. (2002). Incidence of and risk factors for HIV-associated distal sensory polyneuropathy. *Neurology; 58*:1764 –8

[254] Schoenberg BS. (1978). Epidemiology of Guillain-Barre syndrome. In: Schoenberg BS. (eds.): *Advances in Neurology*; vol. 19, New York; Raven Press:.249-60

[255] Sedano MJ, Calleja J, Canga E. et. al. (1994). Guillain-Barre syndrome in Cantabria, Spain. An epidemiological and clinical study. *Acta Neurol Scand; 89*: 287-92.

[256] Senanayake N. (1981). Tri-cresyl phosphate neuropathy in Sri Lanka: a clinical and neurophysiological study with a three year follow up. *J Neurol Neurosurg Psychiatry; 44(9)*:775-80

[257] Seneviratne U and Dissanayake S. (2002). Neurological manifestation of snake bite in Sri Lanka. *J. Postgrad. Med.; 48*:275-8

[258] Sheikh KA, Nachamkin I, Ho TW, et al. (1998). Campylobacter jejuni lipopolysacharides in Guillain-Barre syndrome Molecular mimicry and host susceptibility. *Neurology; 51*: 371-378.

[259] Simmons Z, Wald JJ and Albers JW. (1997). Chronic inflammatory demyelinating polyradiculoneuropathy in children: II. Long-term follow-up, with comparison to adults. *Muscle Nerve; 20*: 1569

[260] Simpson DM, Olney R, McArthur JC. et al. (2000). A placebo-controlled trial of lamotrigine for painful HIV-associated neuropathy. *Neurology;54*:2115

[261] Singleton JR, Smith AG, Russell J, et al. (2005). Polyneuropathy with impaired glucose tolerance: implications for diagnosis and therapy. *Curr. Treat. Options Neurol.;7*:33-42 (Special Indian Edition)

[262] Skre H. (1974). Genetic and clinical aspects of Charcot Marie Tooth's disease *Clinical Genetics; 6*: 98-118

[263] Smith AG, Albers JW. (1997). n-Hexane neuropathy due to rubber cement sniffing. *Muscle Nerve; 20*: 1445-1450

[264] Smith HV and Spalding JMK. (1959). Outbreak of paralysis in Morocco due to orthocresyl phosphate poisoning. *Lancet; 2*:1019

[265] Smith WC, Anderson AM, Withington SG, et al. (2004). Steroid prophylaxis for prevention of nerve function impairment in leprosy: randomised placebo controlled trial (TRIPOD 1). *BMJ.;328(7454)*:1459

[266] So Yt, Holtzman DM, Abrans DI. et al. (1988). Peripheral neuropathy associated with acquired immunodeficiency syndrome, prevalence and clinical features from a population-based survey. *Arch.Neurol.; 45*:945-948

[267] Soliven B, Dhand UK, Kobayashi K et al. (1997). Evaluation of neuropathy in patients on suramin treatment. *Muscle Nerve ;20*:83-91

[268] Soto O, Hedley-Whyte ET. (2003). Case records of the Massachusetts General Hospital. Weekly clinicopathological exercises. Case 33-2003. A 37 year old man with a history of alcohol and drug abuse and sudden onset of leg weakness. *N. Engl. J. Med.; 349*:1656-1663

[269] Sousa A. Andersson R. Drugge U. et al. (1993). Familial amyloidotic polyneuropathy in Sweden: geographical distribution, age of onset, and prevalence. *Human Heredity; 43(5)*:288-94

[270] Sousa A. Coelho T. Barros J. et al. (1995). Genetic epidemiology of familial amyloidotic polyneuropathy (FAP)-type I in Povoa do Varzim and Vila do Conde (north of Portugal). *American Journal of Medical Genetics; 60(6)*:512-21

[271] Spies JM, McLeod JG. (2005). Paraneoplastic Neuropathy. In In: Dyck PJ & Thomas PK (eds.): *Peripheral Neuropathy*; 4th ed. Philadelphia: Saunders. Vol. 2; 2471-2487

[272] Strumberg D, Brügge S, Kom MW , et al. (2002). Evaluation of long-term toxicity in patients after cisplatin-based chemotherapy for non-seminomatous testicular cancer. *Ann.Oncology;13*:229-336

[273] Sullivan KA, Feldman E. (2005). New developments in diabetic neuropathy. *Current opinion in neurology; 18*: 586-590

[274] Sumner CJ, Sheth S, Griffin JW, et al. (2003). The spectrum of neuropathy in diabetes and impaired glucose tolerance. *Neurology; 60*: 108-111

[275] Swygert LA, Maes EF, Sewell LE, et al. (1990). Eosinophilia-myalgia syndrome : results of national surveillance. *JAMA; 264* :1698

[276] Tagliati M, Grinnel J, Godbold J, et al. (1999). Peripheral nerve function in HIV infection. *Arch. Neurol; 56*:84-89

[277] Teunissen LL, Notermans NC, Franssen H, et al. (2004). Disease course of Charcot-Marie-Tooth disease type 2: a 5-year follow-up study. *Archives of Neurology.;61(9)*:1470

[278] Thaisetthawatkul P, Collazo-Clavell ML, Sarr MG et al. (2004). A controlled study of peripheral neuropathy after bariatric surgery. *Neurology; 63 (8)*: 1462 – 70

[279] Thaisetthawatkul P. (2003). Peripheral neuropathy following gastric bypass surgery. Paper presented at: 55th *Annual meeting of the American Academy of Neurology*: Honolulu, Hawaii; March 29-April 5

[280] The Italian Guillain-Barre Study Group. (1996). The prognosis and main prognostic indicators of Guillain-Barre syndrome A multicentre prospective study of 297 patients. *Brain; 119*: 2053-2061

[281] The Manhattan HIV Brain Bank. (2004). HIV-associated distal sensory polyneuropathy in the era of highly active antiretroviral therapy. *Arch Neurol.; 61(4)*:546-51.

[282] Thi NN. Paries J. Attali JR. et al. (2005). High prevalence and severity of cardiac autonomic neuropathy in Vietnamese diabetic patients. *Diabetic Medicine; 22(8)*:1072-8

[283] Thomke F, Jung D, Besser R, et al. (1999). Increased risk of sensory neuropathy in workers with chloracne after exposure to 2,3,7,8-polychlorinated dioxins and furans. *Acta Neurol.Scand.; 100*:1-5

[284] Toh BH, van Driel IR, Gleeson PA. (1997). Pernicious anemia. *N.Engl. J.Med.; 337*: 14418

[285] Tomlinson D (2002). *Diabetic Neuropathy. International Reviews of Neurobiology.* Amsterdam: Elsevier Press: Vol 50

[286] Vallat JM. Tazir M. Magdelaine C. et al. (2005). Autosomal-recessive Charcot-Marie-Tooth diseases. *Journal of Neuropathology & Experimental Neurology; 64* :363-70

[287] Van Asseldonk JT, Franssen H, Van den Berg RM. et al. (2005). Multifocal motor neuropathy. *Lancet Neurology; 4*: 309-319

[288] Van Brakel WH, Lever P, Feenstra P. (2004). Monitoring the size of the leprosy problem: which epidemiological indicators should we use? *Indian J Public Health; 48(1)*: 5-16

[289] Van Brakel WH. (2000). Peripheral neuropathy in leprosy and its consequences. *Lepr Review;71* Suppl:S146-53

[290] Van Koningsveld R, Van Doorn PA, Schmitz PIM, et al. (2000). Mild forms of Guillain-Barre syndrome in an epidemiologic survey in the Netherlands. *Neurology; 54*: 620-625.

[291] Van Schaik N, Winer B, De Haan R et al. (2002). Intravenous immunoglobulin for chronic inflammatory demyelinating polyradiculoneuropathy. *Cochrane Database Syst. Review; 2*: CD001797

[292] Victor M. (1984). Polyneuropathy due to nutritional deficiency and alcoholism. In: Dick PJ, Thomas PK, Lambert EH and Bunge RP (eds.) *Peripheral neuropathy.* Philadelphia: WB Saunders :pp1899

[293] Visser LH, van der Meche FGA, Meulstee J, et al. (1996). Cytomegalovirus infection and Guillain-Barre syndrome: the clinical, electrophysiologic, and prognostic features. *Neurology; 47*: 668-673.

[294] Vittadini G, Buonocore M, Colli G, et al. (2001). Alcoholic polyneuropathy: a clinical and epidemiological study. *Alcohol Alcohol;36*:393-400

[295] Vora DD, Dastur DK, Braganza BM et al. (1962). Toxic polyneuritis in Bombay due to ortho-cresyl-phosphate poisoning. *J. Neurol. Neurosurg. Psychiatry; 25*: 234 – 242

[296] Vrobel TR, Miller PE, Mostow ND et al. (1989). A general overview of amiodarone toxicity: its prevention, detection and management. *Prog. Cardiovasc. Dis.; 31*: 393

[297] Warner-Smith M, Darke S, Day C. (2002). Morbidity associated with non-fatal heroin overdose. *Addiction; 97*: 963-7

[298] Warrell DA. (1997). Prazosin: scorpion envenoming and the cardiovascular system. Tropical Doctor.; Vol. 27: No. 1

[299] Windebank AJ. (2005). Metal Neuropathy. In: Dyck PJ & Thomas PK (eds.): *Peripheral Neuropathy*; Philadelphia: Saunders; 4th ed. Vol. 2:2527-2551

[300] Windebank AJ: (1993). Polyneuropathy due to nutritional deficiency and alcoholism. In: Dyck P, Thomas P, Lambert E, Bunge R (eds.): *Peripheral Neuropathy.* Philadelphia: WB Saunders:1310 - 1321

[301] Winer JB, Hughes RAC, Anderson MJ, et al. (1988). A prospective study of acute idiopathic neuropathy. II. Antecedent events. *Journal of Neurology, Neurosurgery and Psychiatry ; 51*: 613-618

[302] Winer JB. (2002). Treatment of Guillain-Barre syndrome *Q J Med; 95*:717-721.

[303] Witte DR. Tesfaye S. Chaturvedi N. et al. (2005). EURODIAB Prospective Complications Study Group. Risk factors for cardiac autonomic neuropathy in type 1 diabetes mellitus. *Diabetologia.; 48(1)*:164-71

[304] World Health Organization. (2005). Leprosy: global situation. *Weekly epidemiological record.; 80*: 289-296

[305] Yuki N, Hirata K. (1998). Preserved Tendon Reflexes in Campylobacter Neuropathy. *Annals of Neurology; 43(4)* 546-7.

[306] Yuki N, Takahashi M, Tagawa Y, et al. (1997). Association of Campylobacter jejuni serotype with antiganglioside antibody in Guillain-Barre syndrome and Fisher's syndrome. *Ann Neurol; 42*:28-33.

[307] Yuki N, Yoshino S, Sato S, Miyatake T. (1990). Acute axonal polyneuropathy associated with anti-GM1 antibodies following Campylobacter enteritis. *Neurology; 40*: 1900-1902.

[308] Zgibor JC. Songer TJ. Kelsey SF. et. al. (2002). Influence of health care providers on the development of diabetes complications: long-term follow-up from the Pittsburgh Epidemiology of Diabetes Complications Study. *Diabetes Care. 25(9)*:1584-90

RECOMMENDED FURTHER READING

Books

1. Anderson DW and Schoenberg DG (eds.) (1991). *Neuroepidemiology: A Tribute to Bruce Schoenberg*. Boca Raton, FL: CRC Press
2. Dyck PJ & Thomas PK (eds.): (2005). *Peripheral Neuropathy* (4th ed.). Vol. 1 & 2. Philadelphia: Saunders;
3. Schoenberg BS. (ed.) (1978). *Neuroepidemiology: A tribute to Bruce Schoenberg*. New York: Raven Press
4. Spencer PS and Schaumburg HH (eds.) (2000). *Experimental and clinical neurotoxicology* (2nd ed.). New York: Oxford University Press
5. Continuum - *Tropical Neurology* (Feb. 2002). Vol. 8: No. 1
6. Continuum - *Peripheral Neuropathy*. (Dec. 2003). Vol. 19: No. 6
7. Griffin JW. and Sheikh K. (2005). The Guillain Barré syndromes . In: Dyck PJ & Thomas PK (eds.): Peripheral Neuropathy (4th ed); Philadelphia: Saunders. chapter 98: 2197
8. Herkovitz SH and Schaumburg HH. (2005). Neuropathy caused by Drugs. In: Dyck PJ & Thomas PK (eds.): Peripheral Neuropathy (4th ed); Philadelphia: Saunders. Chapter 114: 2553

Articles in Journals

1. England JD and Asbury AK. (2004). Peripheral Neuropathy. *The Lancet; 363*: 2151 – 2161
2. Grogan PM, Katz JS. (2005). Toxic Neuropathies. *Neurologic Clinics; 23* : 377 – 396
3. Hughes RAC. (2002). Regular review: peripheral neuropathy. *British Medical Journal; 324*: 466 - 469
4. Hughes R. (2005). Treatment of peripheral nerve disorders. *Current Opinion in Neurology; 18*: 554 – 556
5. Lawn ND, Wijdicks EFM. (1999). Fatal Guillain-Barré syndrome. *Neurology; 52* : 635 - 638
6. Luciano CA, Pardo CA and McArthur JC. (2003). Recent developments in the HIV neuropathies. *Current Opinion in Neurology; 16*: 403 – 409
7. Nicholson GA. (2006). The dominantly inherited motor and sensory neuropathies. Clinical and molecular advances. *Muscle Nerve; 33*: 589 - 597
8. Peltier AC and Russell JW. (2002). Recent advances in drug-induced neuropathies. *Current Opinion in Neurology; 15*: 633 – 638
9. Ropper AH. (1992). The Gullain-Barré Syndrome. *The New England Journal of Medicine; 326(17)*: 1130-1136
10. Senviratne U. (2000). Gullain-Barré Syndrome. *Postgraduate Medical Journal; 76* : 774 – 782

11. Shy ME. (2004). Charcot-Marie-Tooth disease: an update. *Current Opinion in Neurology;* *17*: 579-585

12. Umapathi T and Chaudhry V. (2005). Toxic Neuropathy. *Current Opinion in Neurology;* *18*: 574 – 580

13. van Doorn PA and Ruts L. (2004). Treatment of chronic inflammatory demyelinating polyneuropathy. *Current Opinion in Neurology;* *17*: 607 – 613

14. Yuki N and Odaka M. (2005). Ganglioside mimicry as a cause of Guillain-Barré Syndrome. *Current opinion in Neurology;* *18*: 557 - 561

In: Handbook of Clinical Neuroepidemiology
Editors: V. L. Feigin and D. A. Bennett, pp. 301-338

ISBN 978-1-60021-511-7
© 2007 Nova Science Publishers, Inc.

Chapter 9

NEUROMUSCULAR DISORDERS

Daniel Koontz and Bashar Katirji

Neuromuscular Division, Department of Neurology, University Hospitals Case Medical
Center and Case Western Reserve University School of Medicine,
Cleveland, Ohio, USA.

ABSTRACT

This chapter addresses disorders of the motor neuron, the neuromuscular junction, and muscle. These uncommon disorders are highly variable in their onset, progression, degree of ultimate disability, and response to treatment. With potential deleterious effects on ambulation, hand function, speech, swallowing and respiration, they can lead to severe functional burden on patients, as well as financial burden on patients, their families and caregivers, and society. As understanding of these diseases has evolved, especially over the last 2 decades, diagnostic accuracy, prognosis, and treatment have changed, dramatically altering the epidemiology of the disorders. However, epidemiological data are still sparse for many of the less frequent disorders. Here we provide a current review of the most common of the neuromuscular diseases: dystrophinopathies, myotonic dystrophies, amyotrophic lateral sclerosis, myasthenia gravis, and inflammatory myopathies.

AMYOTROPHIC LATERAL SCLEROSIS

Amyotrophic lateral sclerosis (ALS) is the prototypical disease among disorders of the motor neuron. It is a relentlessly progressive, fatal disease caused by degeneration of both upper motor neurons (UMNs) and lower motor neurons (LMNs.) The earliest descriptions of the disease in the early 1800s referred to it as progressive muscular wasting, which later became progressive muscular atrophy. Both terms reflected the fact that the disease was initially thought to be a disorder of muscle. In 1860, Luys in Paris and Lockhart Clarke in

London independently described degeneration of the anterior horn cells of the spinal cord. Charcot then described the pathologic involvement of the corticospinal tract in relation to the clinical symptoms in 1869 and proposed the term ALS [2].

Table 1. Revised El-Escorial criteria for the diagnosis of amyotrophic lateral sclerosis (UMN = upper motor neuron, LMN = lower motor neuron)

FEATURES PRESENT
<ul><li>Evidence of lower motor neuron degeneration by clinical, electrophysiological or pathological examination</li><li>Evidence of upper motor neuron degeneration by clinical examination</li><li>Progressive spread of signs within a region, or to other regions as determined by history or examination</li></ul>
FOUR TOPOGRAPHICAL ANATOMIC REGIONS
<ul><li>Bulbar (Brainstem)</li><li>Three spinal cord regions</li><li>Cervical</li><li>Thoracic</li><li>Lumbosacral</li></ul>
LEVELS OF DIAGNOSTIC CERTAINTY
Definite ALS<ul><li>UMN as well as LMN signs, in the bulbar region and at least two spinal regions; or,</li><li>UMN and LMN signs in three spinal regions</li></ul>Probable ALS<ul><li>UMN and LMN signs in at least two regions with some UMN signs necessarily rostral to the LMN signs</li></ul>Probable ALS-laboratory supported<ul><li>Clinical signs of UMN and LMN dysfunction are in only one region; or,</li><li>UMN signs alone are present in one region; and,</li><li>LMN signs defined by electrophysiologic criteria are present in at least two regions</li></ul>Possible ALS<ul><li>Clinical signs of UMN and LMN dysfunction are found together in only one region; or,</li><li>UMN signs are found in two or more regions; or,</li><li>LMN signs are found rostral to UMN signs</li></ul>

Currently the diagnosis of ALS still rests on clinical evidence of upper and lower motor neuron degeneration. The most widely used criteria for diagnosis are the El Escorial criteria. These criteria were formulated by the World Federation of Neurology Research Group on Motor Neuron Disease in El Escorial, Spain in 1994 and were revised at Airlie House in Warrenton, Virginia in 1998 (Table 1) . They separate cases into definite, probable, possible, or suspected ALS based on whether UMN signs, LMN signs or both are present and if so, in how many regions of the neuraxis. The body is divided into 4 regions: brainstem (bulbar), cervical (upper extremities), thoracic, and lumbosacral (lower extremities.) A definite case must include involvement of at least 3 of these regions. Ancillary testing, aside from electrodiagnostic testing, is primarily used to rule out other disease processes and is often not necessary to make the diagnosis [3]. While the revised El Escorial criteria are the most widely used, they have been criticized for being too restrictive, and their strict application to diagnosis has primarily been used in the setting of clinical trials. A trial in Ireland conducted between 1993 and 1998 found that 165 of 388 patients diagnosed with ALS fell into the possible or suspected group, which would make them ineligible for trials. Of these patients, 67% were trial eligible (either definite or probable ALS) at the time of their last follow up with a mean time from symptom onset to trial eligibility of 13 months [4].

Incidence and Prevalence

The worldwide incidence of adult onset motor neuron disease (MND), based on a review by Chancellor and Warlow, ranged from 0.6 per 100,000 to 2.6 per 100,000 with prevalence rates between 1.5 and 8.5 per 100,000. The differences are likely related to the different methodologies used in case ascertainment in the various studies and that some studies were inclusive of other MNDs (e.g. progressive bulbar palsy and progressive muscular atrophy) while others looked purely at ALS. This supports the widely held belief that MND occurs in a fairly uniform distribution worldwide with no true differences in geographical incidence. The incidence of MND increases to a peak between ages 60 and 75 and then declines sharply thereafter [5,6]. Most epidemiological studies have demonstrated a male predominance in incidence with male to female ratios varying between 1.2:1 and 2.0:1 [5]. There is no consistent evidence to support an increasing incidence of ALS.

Clusters of MND have been found in Guam, the Kii peninsula of Japan, and West New Guinea. Of these, the Guamanian population is the best studied. The incidence of ALS in Guam was reported to be 50-100 times that of the developed world between 1950 and 1969. Since that time, however, incidence rates have decreased dramatically, coinciding with a change in the Guamanian culture toward western society. The cause for the high incidence is unknown, but it is thought to be environmental. Offspring of affected individuals have not shown a higher incidence than those of unaffected people, and residents of neighboring Mariana Islands, despite sharing an original migration pattern, are not afflicted with high incidences. Both of these facts argue against a genetic cause. The latency from exposure to the environmental factor to development of disease is long, based on reports of Chamorro immigrants to the United States [5]. The precise environmental cause has not been identified, but ingestion of the seed of the cycad, used by the Chamorro Indians in making flour, has been implicated.

Natural History

Patients are generally asymptomatic until approximately 80% of motor neurons are lost [6]. After symptom onset, the course is relentlessly progressive and ultimately fatal. Limb onset is the most common presentation, occurring in 65-80% of cases. Weakness is typically asymmetric and distal at onset and is accompanied by muscle atrophy. Bulbar involvement is the first sign of the disease in the remainder of patients, with chief complaints consisting of slurred speech and difficulty swallowing. The degree of bulbar involvement is closely tied to respiratory muscle strength and therefore portends a poorer prognosis [2]. Other factors may also predict a less favorable clinical course (see Table 2).

Table 2. Indicators of prognosis in amyotrophic lateral sclerosis (CMAP = compound muscle action potential; RNS = repetitive stimulation; ALS = amyotrophic lateral sclerosis)

	Better prognosis	Worse prognosis
Age	Younger (<50 years)	Older
Weakness at onset	Limb	Bulbar
Dyspnea at onset	Absent	Present
Time from onset to diagnosis	Long	Short
Progression	Slow	Rapid
Fasciculations	Subtle and restricted	Prominent and widespread
Electrodiagnostic studies	Normal CMAPs No CMAP decrement on slow RNS	Low CMAPs CMAP decrement on slow RNS
General nutrition	Good	Poor
Motor neuron disease form	Primary lateral sclerosis Flail-arm syndrome	Classic ALS Familial ALS

All cases are progressive, and the manner in which loss of function tends to spread from the original site of weakness is often predictable. Patients with unilateral arm onset usually develop contralateral arm symptoms prior to symptoms in the legs. Weakness in one leg at presentation predicts weakness in the contralateral leg and ipsilateral arm prior to involvement of the contralateral arm. Likewise, patients who present with arm weakness often develop bulbar symptoms earlier than patients with leg weakness at onset. While patients with dysarthria at onset can be expected to have swallowing symptoms prior to weakness in the limbs, symptoms do not develop more rapidly in the arms than the legs [7]. Spasticity becomes a major factor late in the disease course and 10% of patients will develop a late dementia with frontal affect. The urinary and anal sphincter muscles are spared entirely or until late stages of the disease. Likewise, extraocular muscle involvement is typically absent or very late [2].

The time from symptom onset to disability due to a specific motor dysfunction follows a general pattern. Gait declines early in the course of the disease while disability as a result of declining arm function or bulbar function occurs later generally. Half of the patients will experience their first fall or report first sustained use of a wheelchair between 30 and 48 months from disease onset. Half of the patients decline to the point of requiring assistance from a caregiver with dressing by 46 to 66 months and with feeding by 90 to 120 months.

The need for speech assistive devices or supplemental nutrition arises in half of the patients by 90 to 120 months, and by 102 and 120 months, respectively [7].

Mortality studies have suffered the same non-uniform data collection that incidence studies have. The worldwide mortality rates from MND range from 0.4 to 0.6 per 100,000 in Japan to 1.6 to 2.8 per 100,000 in Norwegian men [5]. The mortality rates from MND have been increasing worldwide. These mortality rates peak between 60 and 75 years of age and then decline [5]. The average time from *symptom onset* to death in ALS is approximately 3 years, and 50% of patients survived 36 to 48 months from symptom onset (95% CI) [7]. The mean survival from time of *diagnosis* among residents of Olmsted County, Minnesota (USA) is 21 to 41 months in patients under age 60 and 15 to 25 months in patients 60 and older (95% CI) [6]. The mean time from symptom onset to diagnosis in the Olmsted County cohort was 13 months [6].

Risk Factors

Whether or not true risk factors for ALS exist is still an unanswered question. Two groups have been specifically studied recently to attempt to shed light on this subject. The first group at risk for ALS is *military personnel*. The issue was first seriously addressed after an apparent increased incidence in American veterans of the gulf war was noticed. Initial analysis argued against an elevated risk, but a more recent study of 2.5 million eligible military personnel compared those deployed during the Gulf War to those not deployed and found that the age-adjusted risk ratio for the deployed population was 1.92 (95% confidence limits: 1.29, 2.84) [8]. Another study examined, prospectively, ALS mortality of men enrolled in the Cancer Prevention Study II with or without a history of military service. The investigators linked military service to ALS by finding a statistically significant age- and smoking-adjusted relative risk of 1.58 [9].

The second group at risk for ALS is *professional athletes*. The incidence rates of ALS in northern Italy were compared to incidence rates of professional football (soccer) players of Italian origin [10]. While 0.77 cases would have been expected in their cohort of 7325 players, the investigators found 5 athletes with ALS. This translated into a statistically significant standardized morbidity ratio of 6.5. The authors also found that longer careers in professional football conferred a higher risk than shorter careers [10].

Socioeconomic Outcomes

ALS is medically as well as economically devastating, starting with the cost of diagnosis. In 1996, the average cost of diagnosing ALS in the United States was estimated to be between $12,000 and $42,000. After diagnosis the expenditures continue to accumulate: Equipment costs have been estimated to be around $7,300 per year; assistive communication devices cost about $24,200 for the most advanced systems; and percutaneous endoscopic gastrostomy (PEG) placement costs $1800 and is followed by yearly nutritional costs of $7300. While these expenses are not trivial, the majority of money spent on ALS is in the terminal stages, if chronic mechanical ventilation is used. The cost of home-based mechanical ventilation in the United States averages between $160,000 and $179,000 per year, while institution-based ventilation averages $429,000 per year. Considering that the average length of mechanical ventilation is three years, these figures dwarf the early expenditures. Exclusive of mechanical ventilation, annual cost of care in the United Kingdom has been estimated at $2316 over the entire course of the disease, while care in France was reported to total $6017 per year [11].

Caregiver burden is also a major factor in the socioeconomic impact of ALS. Unfortunately, no study has included mechanically ventilated patients. A study of German caregivers' assessment of their burden showed that it was fairly low overall [12]. In comparison to other diseases, such as dementia, mixed neuropsychiatric diseases, and geriatric diseases, ALS caregivers perceived a lower level of burden by Burden Scale for Family Caregivers' score. The authors plausibly attributed this to the unimpaired intellect and personality characteristic of ALS. The areas in which most of the burden was perceived were 'personal and social restrictions' and 'physical and emotional health.' Both of these components as well as the overall Burden Scale for Family Caregivers score correlated inversely with the patient's ALS functional rating scale. The number of hours per day spent caring for the patient correlated positively with the Burden Scale for Family Caregivers' score, but not with any of the components of the Cost of Care Index. The authors of an American study determined that patients with more severe disability, were generally not depressed [13]. Quality of life of both caregivers and patients was moderately high. Likewise patients' perceptions of caregivers' quality of life was high, as was the converse. Perception of emotional support was high for both patients and caregivers. While patients tended to decrease active hobbies such as golf, fishing or bowling, they increased passive hobbies, such as reading, puzzles, or computer activities. Not surprisingly though, the majority of both patients (52%) and caregivers (53%) reported negative lifestyle changes due to an ALS diagnosis.

Prevention

Oxidative stress has been implicated in the pathogenesis of ALS. The demonstration that vitamin E supplementation in mice with the Cu-Zn superoxide dismutase (SOD1) gene, which is responsible for the autosomal dominant form of ALS, delayed the development of clinical disease, raised interest in antioxidant therapy as a preventative for the development of sporadic ALS. The Cancer Prevention Study-II was designed to evaluate the role of vitamins E and C in cancer prevention. Over 1.1 million people were enrolled. Of these, 957,740 were followed for 10 years to attempt to determine whether either or both of these vitamins decrease the risk of ALS [14]. During the follow-up period, 525 patients died of ALS. ALS mortality was found to be 62% lower among regular users of vitamin E for 10 or more years than among non-users, while use of other vitamin supplements, including vitamin C, did not display a significant relationship. Whether or not a given reduction in risk of mortality from a rare disease, such as ALS, from any preventive agent is clinically relevant, must be determined in concert with the risks and benefits that agent confers for more common disorders.

Management

Once a diagnosis is made, the first step in the management of the patient with ALS is breaking the news to the patient and family. The American Academy of Neurology (AAN) quality standards subcommittee issued a wide-ranging practice parameter on the care of the patient with ALS which included the following recommendations: The diagnosis should be given by the physician in person, never over the phone; the implications of the diagnosis should be discussed; printed materials on the disease should be given to the patient, or alternatively, the patient and the patient's family should be given recommendations for reliable online information sites if they have access to the internet; the physician should not withhold the diagnosis, provide insufficient information, create a sense of hopelessness, or deliver the information callously [15].

Treatment options should also be discussed soon after diagnosis. Negative trials have predominated in the search for an effective drug against ALS. Trials involving topiramate, indinavir, thyrotropin-releasing hormone, gabapentin, cyclosporine, intravenous immunoglobulin, plasmapheresis, and several anti-oxidants and nerve growth factors have been disappointing. Trials on interferon, insulin-like growth factor-1, minocycline and coenzyme Q10 are ongoing. Riluzole, the only drug approved by the United States Food and Drug Administration for the treatment of ALS, was found to have a modest effect on survival [16]. Based on two placebo-controlled, double-blind randomized trials, riluzole prolongs survival by a median of approximately 60 days in patients with definite or probable ALS, who have had symptoms for less than five years, have a forced vital capacity of greater than 60% predicted, and who have not required a tracheostomy [17,18]. If the above qualifying conditions are not met, the evidence supporting the use of riluzole is limited to the recommendation of its use by experts in the field. While the drug is generally well-tolerated, the main obstacle to its universal use is cost. The retail monthly cost in 2005 in the United States is in excess of $800. If the patient is treated with riluzole, baseline blood count and transaminases should be monitored monthly for the first three months. After the first three months, transaminases should be checked every three months for another 9 months and periodically thereafter. At any given time, therapeutic research trials are ongoing, and patients should be given the opportunity to participate in these.

The vast majority of the care of the ALS patient is not targeted at the disease but at its symptoms and complications. While major randomized controlled trials are lacking, the AAN's practice parameter addressed many of the issues involved in the long-term care of these patients [15]. The authors divided their recommendations into guidelines (based on strong evidence) or options (based on weaker evidence.) For the control of *sialorrhea*, a cause of social stress to many ALS patients, options for treatment of glycopyrolate, benztropine, transdermal hyoscine, atropine, trihexyphenidyl hydrochloride, or amitriptyline. Thick mucus production, which should be differentiated from sialorrhea, should be optionally treated with a beta blocker, specifically propranolol or metoprolol. The options given for control of *pseudobulbar affect* were amitriptyline and fluvoxamine, but more recently, the combination of dextromethorphan and a low dose of an enzyme inhibitor quinidine, was shown to be effective in reducing the emotional liability associated with this affect. If the patient suffers from both pseudobulbar affect and sialorrhea, amitriptyline is the obvious choice.

Dysphagia not only increases risk for aspiration pneumonia, it also leads to worsening weakness from decreased caloric intake. In the early stages, dysphagia can be managed by altering the types of foods the patient eats and the thickness of liquids he drinks. As the dysphagia progresses, however, PEG must be considered. Most patients are willing to consider the institution of percutaneous nutrition. Fifty-two percent of patients, not yet requiring alternative sources for nutrition, endorsed the idea of PEG, and another 22% were uncertain whether they would eventually elect to have the procedure performed [13]. PEG probably increases overall survival time, but the benefit is modest. Median survival after PEG is approximately 6 months [11], and patients with PEG lived on average 1 to 4 months longer than patients who refused or were ineligible for the procedure [15]. The AAN practice parameter stated that PEG is indicated for patients with "symptomatic dysphagia" and should be considered early. The procedure should be performed, as a guideline, when the patient's vital capacity is greater than 50% of predicted [15].

Spasticity is another complication that adversely affects quality of life in ALS patients. It accelerates contractures, which leads to functional decline and decreases coordination. Muscle relaxants, such as baclofen (oral or intrathecal) and dantrolene have been advocated, but these have the potential to cause more weakness. Exercise has also been suggested, but that too has been implicated in causing a more rapid decline in function. A Cochrane Database review addressed the topic of treatments for spasticity, specifically in ALS patients. The authors found only one randomized, controlled trial that included a primary outcome of reduction in spasticity at three months. While future research is needed to address medical therapies, moderate-intensity, endurance-type exercises for the trunk and limbs can be supported by evidence to reduce spasticity [17].

Dyspnea on exertion, fatigue, and morning headaches can be the harbingers of respiratory insufficiency. When vital capacity dips below 50% of predicted, the patient will likely be symptomatic. Chronic respiratory care is the most controversial subject in the care of the patient with ALS. The subjects of supplementary and mechanical ventilation should be addressed early so that the patient's preferences can be followed. The AAN guidelines are that the practitioner be vigilant for symptoms of hypoventilation and measure pulmonary function serially. The most practical way to do this is by measuring vital capacity. Further, it recommends that non-invasive ventilatory support be offered as an initial therapy for symptomatic chronic hypoventilation. Non-invasive ventilation has been shown to improve quality of life and increase survival. When non-invasive ventilation becomes inadequate, invasive ventilation via tracheostomy should be offered to those patients who wish to prolong their survival after the patient and family are fully informed of its benefits and burdens. The vast majority of patients (97%) early in the course of respiratory failure are willing to consider non-invasive ventilation, such as BI-PAP [13]. In contrast, only 15% of patients with early ALS favored mechanical ventilation in the future [13]. However, among those patients who do eventually elect to receive mechanical ventilation at home or in institutions, the majority are glad to be alive, with home-dwellers reporting a higher quality of life [11]. The patient should always maintain the right to withdraw any treatment, including mechanical ventilation. At which point the patient decides to withdraw ventilation, adequate dosages of opiates and anxiolytics to relieve dyspnea and anxiety should be administered [15].

Palliative care often becomes the focus of care in the terminal stages of ALS. Between 40 and 73% of patients report pain late in their disease course. As an option, the AAN recommends non-narcotic analgesics, anti-inflammatory drugs and antispasticity agents for initial therapy. The use of opioids to treat dyspnea has been endorsed as a guideline by the AAN, since dyspnea occurs in about 50% of patients with ALS, and is relieved by opioids in 81% of hospice patients. Finally, the AAN suggests a referral to hospice as an option in the terminal stages of ALS, citing a retrospective analysis, which attributed a 94% rate of "peaceful and settled" death to patients who died under hospice care [15].

MYASTHENIA GRAVIS

Myasthenia gravis (MG) is the most common neuromuscular junction disorder and perhaps the best studied autoimmune disease. It is characterized by fluctuating fatigue and weakness, often prominently involving ocular muscles. While the first account of a disease process with fluctuating weakness was made by Sir Thomas Willis in 1672, William Erb was the first to describe the characteristic features in 3 patients in 1879 [20]. The clinical features were further characterized and solidified as a distinct disease by Samuel Goldflam 14 years later [21]. The eponym Erb-Goldflam Syndrome is still used synonymously with myasthenia gravis. While countless others have contributed to the understanding of the disease, perhaps the most significant contribution came in 1934 when Mary B. Walker discovered the remarkable effect of physostigmine and, subsequently, neostigmine. She postulated that these drugs' therapeutic effect in MG was grounded in their ability to inhibit acetylcholine esterase [22]. Not only did this represent the first reproducibly successful, albeit temporary, treatment, but it also strongly supported the idea that the pathology lay at the neuromuscular junction.

Incidence and Prevalence

Myasthenia gravis is an uncommon disorder. There is strong evidence, however that its prevalence is increasing, although part of this increase may be attributed to better case recognition, patients' increased life-expectancy, and aging of the population. The prevalence has increased in every decade since the 1950s based on published epidemiological studies. For example, the weighted mean prevalence increased from 22.2 per million in the 1950s to 93.9 per million in studies published from 1990 to 2002, making the more recent prevalence 4.2 times higher [23].

The annual incidence of MG ranges between 1.1 and 6 per million. A large Danish study, designed specifically to clarify the epidemiology of MG in a large and stable population, found an annual incidence of 4.4 per million [24]. Women are affected nearly twice as often as men [24-26]. Most of this difference can be accounted for by the high incidence in women in their teen and early adult years. The relative incidence is highest in women in the third decade of life [24-26], while the incidence in men is more evenly distributed with peaks in the third and sixth decades, the sixth being most common [24-26]. All races are susceptible, but Japanese and Chinese studies have shown a higher incidence of acquired infantile cases, and the Chinese population has a higher proportion of cases presenting before puberty [25].

While the role of the acetylcholine receptor antibody assay in diagnosis of MG is not disputed, not all patients are seropositive. Data from 756 Italian patients showed 73% had a positive titer at the time of diagnosis [26]. A Serbian study, in which the assay was performed at a random point during the disease process, found 221 of 276 patients (80%) harbored the antibody [27]. Many of the so-called seronegative patients likely carry a different serum antibody directed at different end plate antigens. Among them, the muscle specific tyrosine kinase (MuSK), a protein that is expressed exclusively at the neuromuscular junction and is closely related to the acetylcholine receptor, was recently recognized. It is present in 40 to 70% of patients who are seronegative to the acetylcholine receptor antibody [27-29]. The exact role of MuSK in adult muscle is still unknown. In the developing muscle, MuSK is essential for aggregating the acetylcholine receptors and is activated by nerve-derived agrin.

Natural History

The natural history of MG has changed markedly since it was initially recognized. As intensive care and disease-modifying treatments have advanced, this once truly grave disease has become distinctly treatable. However, the clinical course still varies widely between patients. The MG Foundation of America clinical classification scheme is used to rate the severity of disease (Table 3). Generally, there are four broad categories of acquired MG: generalized MG with onset before age 50, generalized MG with onset after age 50, generalized MG associated with thymoma, and ocular MG. The most common presenting symptom at onset is diplopia and/or ptosis due to weakness of extra-ocular muscles or lid elevators, respectively. This represents at least part of the symptom complex in 85-90% of patients. The number of patients with isolated ocular MG has varied widely in published reports over time, ranging from 15-59% [30]. This broad range is probably related to the definition of ocular MG since adequate time from onset must be given before the disease is categorized as such. Clearly, the longer the interval from symptom onset, the less likely the patient with purely ocular disease is to generalize. A reasonable limit is 3 years, as only 3-10% of patients who have not generalized within 3 years will go on to do so [25]. Historical estimates have listed ocular MG patients comprising 15% of the total MG population, and recent reports approximate this figure [31,32].

Patients are considered to have generalized MG once they have muscle weakness beyond the ocular muscles. Behind diplopia and ptosis, bulbar presentation accounts for approximately 20% of cases and dysarthria is the most common bulbar initial symptom, occurring in isolation in 7% [25]. Bulbar weakness is a major contributor to disability throughout the course of the disease. Weakness of facial muscles may cause labial dysarthria, decreased facial expression, inability to purse the lips, or inability to fully close the eyelids.

Dysphagia may be labial, lingual, pharyngeal, or a combination of the three, and is seen in over 30% of patients [31]. It correlates with weight loss [25] and, when severe, can lead to drooling, aspiration, atelectasis or respiratory failure. Bulbar weakness can also manifest with weakness of the sternocleidomastoids or muscles of mastication (jaw drop).

Weakness of the limbs is seen as the initial symptom in 20% of patients [25]. This often starts as early fatigability and may affect either distal or proximal muscles. Muscle atrophy is the exception rather than the rule, reported in 8-12% of a large patient population [25], and, when prominent, should raise suspicion for another diagnosis. Respiratory weakness is an uncommon initial symptom, but most patients display decreased vital capacity compared to age-matched controls [25].

Table 3. Myasthenia Gravis Foundation of America Clinical Classification

Class I	Any ocular muscle weakness May have weakness of eye closure All other muscle strength is normal
Class II	Mild weakness affecting other than ocular muscles May also have ocular muscle weakness of any severity
II a	Predominantly affecting limb, axial muscles or both May also have lesser involvement of oropharyngeal muscles
IIb	Predominantly affecting oropharyngeal, respiratory muscles, or both May also have lesser involvement of limb, axial muscles, or both
Class III	Moderate weakness affecting other than ocular muscles May also have ocular muscle weakness of any severity
IIIa	Predominantly affecting limb, axial muscles or both May also have lesser involvement of oropharyngeal muscles
IIIb	Predominantly affecting oropharyngeal, respiratory muscles, or both May also have lesser involvement of limb, axial muscles, or both
Class IV	Severe weakness affecting other than ocular muscles May also have ocular muscle weakness of any severity
IVa	Predominantly affecting limb, axial muscles or both May also have lesser involvement of oropharyngeal muscles
IVb	Predominantly affecting oropharyngeal, respiratory muscles, or both May also have lesser involvement of limb, axial muscles, or both
Class V	Defined by intubation, with or without mechanical ventilation, except when employed during routine postoperative management. The use of a feeding tube without intubation places the patient in class IVb.

Myasthenic crisis, defined as an MG exacerbation, which results in acute respiratory failure, is the primary life-threatening complication. The mortality associated with crisis has declined sharply in the last half century, dropping from 75% to between 4 and 8% [33-35]. Overall, the current annual MG-related mortality rate is estimated at 1.4 per million [32]. Most deaths are not directly due to the crisis, rather they are from other medical problems associated with critical illness, primarily sepsis from ventilator-associated pneumonia [33,34]. Approximately 20% of patients will experience crisis, usually within the first two years of the disease [24,33,34]. The most common precipitating factor is infection of the respiratory tract. The median duration of crisis is 11 days, based on a retrospective study of patients treated with either intravenous immunoglobulin (IVIG) or plasma exchange [33].

The incidence of thymoma in patients with MG is approximately 15%. This should be differentiated from thymic hyperplasia, which is more common. Thymoma is seen most often in the older-onset group. Patients with thymoma have a relatively more severe course and experience crisis with greater frequency than those without thymoma. Kuks and Oosterhuis reported a 16% MG-related death rate and a 45% remission rate in their 138 thymoma patients versus a 2.8% MG-related death rate and 38% remission rate in their 537 non-thymoma patients. They point out, though, that all of the deaths within the thymoma group were prior to 1984 and propose that the natural course of the disease in patients with thymoma is more severe than those without, but the outcome with immunomodulation is the same [25].

Risk Factors

Other autoimmune diseases commonly coexist with MG, but the reported frequencies have been highly variable, ranging from 2.3 to 24% [25]. The younger-onset group (age less than 50) carries other autoimmune diagnoses most often [31]. On the other hand, older-onset and thymoma groups are more likely to harbor anti-ryanodine receptor and anti-titin antibodies, which have been linked to a more severe disease course, independent of the presence of thymoma [36,37]. Acquired MG is seen in patients' family members more often than the general public. In Kuks and Oosterhuis's 800 patients, 14 (1.7%) were found to have an affected family member [25].

Socioeconomic Outcomes

No large studies have addressed the financial burden of myasthenia gravis. Besides, the relevance of any such study at present would have to be questioned, given the recent changes in the natural course of the disease and newer treatment options. The therapies used to treat myasthenic crisis are expensive. The cost of IVIG is approximately $35 to $50 per gram, meaning the average treatment course for a 70 kg patient would cost between $9800 and $14,000. Plasma exchange is similar in cost in the United States, but may be a cheaper alternative in areas where technical fees to cover the much more complex administration of this treatment are lower. While prednisone is inexpensive, many of the immunomodulators are not. In the United States, the cost of a standard monthly dose of generic azathioprine is $139.21, cyclosporine $299.98, and mycophenolate mofetil $645.62 (prices as of November, 2005 from drugstore.com).

The psychosocial effect of MG has been assessed. While patients may exhibit more vegetative symptoms of depression, which may be related to fatigue, they generally do not tend to have depressed mood more often than the general public [38]. In a prospective Italian study, those with MG were found to have a poorer health-related quality of life than controls [39]. Further, the health-related quality of life was worse in those patients with higher Osserman scale scores (Table 4.) Another study, which was not prospective, corroborated that health-related quality of life suffered in MG patients, but overall quality of life did not suffer substantially [40]. Both studies also showed that mental health, as perceived by the patients, was not adversely affected.

Table 4. Osserman Classification for MG

0	Asymptomatic
1	Ocular signs and symptoms
2	Mild generalized weakness
3	Moderate generalized weakness, bulbar dysfunction, or both
4	Severe generalized weakness, respiratory dysfunction, or both

Management

Once a diagnosis of MG is made, the patient should be educated with regard to the treatable nature of the disease, the potential complications, and the typically good prognosis. A screen for other autoimmune conditions should be performed, especially in younger patients with generalized disease. Additionally, either a contrasted CT scan or MRI of the chest should be ordered to evaluate for thymoma. Then the discussion about medical therapy should begin. Pyridostigmine (Mestinon) is the mainstay of medical therapy, but may not be necessary for all patients. For instance, some patients with isolated unilateral ptosis may prefer a ptosis crutch added to their glasses rather than taking medication several times daily. Pyridostigmine is an acetylcholinesterase inhibitor and, as such, is purely a symptomatic treatment. It is typically started at 30-60 mg per dose, administered approximately every 4-6 hours. The effect starts within 30 minutes with a peak effect around 2 hours [41]. It does not carry the same adverse effects as prednisone or other immunomodulators, but, with its muscarinic actions, it commonly produces gastrointestinal symptoms including nausea, vomiting, diarrhea, and cramps. Pyridostigmine can also cause increased secretions, which can exacerbate dysphagia or dyspnea. Most side effects may be combated with glycopyrrolate, atropine, or other anticholinergics. Patients typically adjust their doses and dosing intervals to balance their myasthenic symptoms versus the cholinergic side effects.

When symptoms are not adequately controlled with AChE inhibitors, corticosteroids are the most rapidly effective therapy. After a review of the potential benefits and side effects, which include weight gain, osteoporosis, hyperglycemia, edema, and psychiatric disturbances, the patient should be given the option of starting oral steroid therapy. *Prednisone* at daily adult doses of 50-80 mg is recommended [41,42]. It should be started at a dose of 15-20 mg daily and titrated up by 5 mg every second or third day [41]. Alternatively, patients with moderately severe generalized weakness may be admitted for initiation of high-dose steroids, which has the benefit of more rapid improvement in weakness [42]. Approximately 50% of patients will worsen in the first few days to weeks of corticosteroid initiation. Starting at the lower dose and gradually increasing it reduces the severity of the initial deterioration [41]. Improvement of MG symptoms starts by 2-4 weeks in most patients, with maximal benefit being reached at 6-12 months. At this point, the dose may be tapered, but can rarely be eliminated. In addition to the immunosuppressive benefits of corticosteroids, one relatively small retrospective study of 94 patients showed that patients with ocular MG who received prednisone had a decreased risk of developing generalized MG at 2 years (odds ratio: 0.13) [43].

Given the long list of adverse effects of steroids and the high proportion of patients who suffer from them, other immunomodulators are favored for chronic treatment of MG (Table 5.) To date none of the so-called "steroid-sparing" drug has been found to be superior to corticosteroids in a large randomized trial, and the two are often used in combination. A small trial with initial randomization assessed the effect of *azathioprine* compared to prednisone and found no difference in the two groups [44]. There was a suggestion that treatment failure was higher in the prednisone group, but those who failed either treatment were likely to respond to combination therapy of azathioprine and prednisone. This study was followed up by a small double-blind, randomized trial comparing prednisolone and azathioprine in combination versus prednisolone alone [45]. Fewer treatment failures and longer remissions were found in the group on combination therapy. While this treatment method seems to defeat the steroid-sparing purpose, the authors did find that side effects were seen less often in the azathioprine-treated patients, and a lower dose of prednisolone was necessary to maintain remission.

Table 5. Immunomodulating drugs and doses used for MG

Prednisone	50-80 mg/day* (may be dosed every other day)
Azathioprine	1-3 mg/kg/day
Cyclosporine	2-3 mg/kg/day
Mycophenolate mofetil	1 g twice a day

* tapered to lowest dose needed to maintain remission, if achieved

Data in support of the other commonly used immunomodulators are also, at best, from small, randomized trials, and one cannot be confidently recommended over another. One small double-blind, randomized, placebo-controlled trial examined the effect of *cyclosporine* in patients who failed cholinesterase inhibitors [46]. The patients in this study showed statistically significant improvement in weakness at 6 and 12 months with fewer treatment failures and a trend toward reduction in anti-acetylcholine receptor antibodies. A more recent study of cyclosporine showed either remarkable benefit or remission in over 50% of patients who had failed cholinesterase therapy, thymectomy, corticosteroids, and azathioprine [47]. The primary side effect, which requires laboratory monitoring, is renal insufficiency. Other side effects include hypertension and gingival hyperplasia in addition to the numerous drug-drug interactions [42].

The use of *cyclophosphamide* has been based on scattered case reports [42,47,48]. Its side effect profile, which includes frequent alopecia, hemorrhagic cystitis, gastrointestinal symptoms, and increased risk of malignancy with long-term treatment, has prevented its wide use. Intravenous pulsed cyclophosphamide (initial dose of 500 mg/m^2) given monthly over nine months was effective and allowed reduction of systemic steroids usage and had only few adverse effects [47]. Interest in the drug has recently been rekindled since Drachman et al. reported its use in "rebooting" the immune system. They used a high dose (50 mg/kg/day) of intravenous cyclophosphamide for 4 days with the intent of ablating the immune system, but leaving the hematopoietic stem cells intact. This treatment led to marked improvement in the three patients treated, and it was well tolerated. The effect in these refractory patients continued through 3.5 years of follow-up [48].

Mycophenolate mofetil has also been studied as a treatment for MG. The largest series included 85 patients and, while not controlled, showed that 73% improved on the treatment and only 6% discontinued it because of side effects [49]. Its side effects include anemia, leukopenia, and gastrointestinal upset. Monthly blood counts should be monitored. The mean time to improvement with this drug was found to be 10.7 weeks, with mean maximal improvement not occurring for 6 months [49]. This highlights the importance of an extended trial for any immunomodulator prior to considering a patient a treatment failure.

In patients with severe symptoms or myasthenic crisis, where rapid improvement is necessary, two options are available: plasma exchange (also known as plasmapheresis) and intravenous immunoglobulin (IVIG). *Plasma exchange* has been used as the standard therapy for severe MG exacerbations and crisis, but only uncontrolled studies support its use. The outcome is better when it is combined with immunosuppressant therapy, as this leads to a lower risk of rebound phenomenon [42]. The primary side effects with plasma exchange are access-related complications, since a large-bore double-lumen catheter in a central vein is often required. These include hematomas, line sepsis, and thrombotic events. *Intravenous immunoglobulin* may be used as an alternative to plasma exchange. The standard dose used has been 2 g/kg divided over 5 daily doses, although a recent randomized, double-blind trial showed no difference between 1g/kg and 2 g/kg dosing [50]. Two trials that compared IVIG and plasma exchange, one of which was randomized [51], found similar efficacy of both treatment modalities, but IVIG was associated with fewer side effects. IVIG carries a risk of hypercoagulability, potentially leading to stroke, myocardial infarction, deep venous thrombosis or pulmonary embolus. This risk can be reduced by using a more dilute solution – typically 5%. Renal failure is also a risk as is fluid overload, especially in patients with congestive heart failure.

Perhaps the most controversial area in MG management is *thymectomy* in patients without thymoma. There are many different theories regarding who should have the procedure and which approach is best. Overall, thymectomy is widely recommended by the vast majority of experts for young, otherwise healthy adult patients with generalized MG. This treatment modality is thought to give those patients the best chance of remission. Unfortunately, no properly designed, large trial has evaluated this. An international, multi-center trial is underway to attempt to evaluate the efficacy of thymectomy in non-thymomatous and seropositive patients, but the results would be, at best, several years away [52].

DYSTROPHINOPATHIES: DUCHENNE AND BECKER MUSCULAR DYSTROPHY

The dystrophinopathies are a group of disorders characterized by absent, reduced, or abnormal Dystrophin in skeletal muscle. Dystrophin is a subsarcolemmal cytoskeletal protein encoded by a large gene on the X chromosome at position Xp21. The two major dystrophinopathy phenotypes are Duchenne Muscular Dystrophy (DMD) and Becker Muscular Dystrophy (BMD). DMD results from absence or near absence of dystrophin, whereas BMD is caused by reduced amounts or abnormally-sized dystrophin. Accordingly, DMD is the more severe form of dystrophinopathy.

The phenotype, now known as DMD, was first described by Meryon in 1851 [53], and subsequently by Duchenne, after whom the disease is named, in 1861 [54]. Over 100 years after Meryon's report, Becker and Kiener described in 1955 a benign X-linked variant of DMD [55]. While the X-linked recessive inheritance pattern immediately implicated the X chromosome as the mode of transmission, the causative gene product was not known until the late 1980s when Hoffman, Brown and Kunkel isolated a 3685 amino acid protein, given the name dystrophin [56].

Incidence and Prevalence

Duchenne muscular dystrophy is the most common neuromuscular disease of childhood, affecting almost exclusively boys. Rarely, girls with Turner syndrome or other X chromosome abnormalities will manifest the full phenotype. The incidence is between 1 in 3500 to 1 in 3000 live male births with an estimated worldwide prevalence of 63 per million [57,58]. BMD accounts for far fewer cases of dystrophinopathy. Historically its incidence has been estimated to be 6 – 20% that of DMD, but these data may underestimate the true incidence, as these statistics were gathered prior to the identification of the dystrophin protein and its gene. More recently, the incidence of BMD in Wales has been reported as 1 in 18,450 live male births, which was approximately one third the incidence of DMD, and corresponded to a prevalence of 24.8 per million [59]. Elsewhere, prevalence has been reported between 12 to 27 per million [60]. Approximately 5 – 10% of female carriers of the dystrophin gene will manifest a milder form of disease symptoms [57]. Populations at higher risk for the disease are those in which consanguineous breeding is common, as is the case in Tunisia [61].

Natural History

DMD is a relentlessly progressive and uniformly fatal disease. Although it can be detected by high serum creatine kinase (CK) levels in the neonatal period, the first symptoms are not usually noted until at least the second or third year of life with developmental motor delay, inability to run or climb stairs, and frequent falls. Between the ages of 3 and 6, weakness is noted in the muscles of the proximal lower extremities and torso. This leads to a lordotic gait and the pathognomic Gower's sign. The classic pseudohypertropy of the calf muscles is also present by this age. Less marked, but also present at this stage are enlarged deltoid, infraspinatus, gluteal, and vastus lateralis muscles. While the muscles of the upper extremities are affected early, their functional limitation is minimal early in the disease. The extraocular muscles, muscles supplied by the facial nerve, and the external anal sphincter are spared throughout the disease process. Intellectual development is often affected, and mean IQ has been reported to be 83, with approximately 20% achieving a score of 70 or lower [54,61].

As the child grows, limb and torso muscle strength continues to decline, and contractures start to develop. Between the ages of 6 and 10, 70% of patients will have significant contractures in the iliotibial bands, hip flexors, and heel cords. On exam, proximal muscles continue to be weaker than distal in general, and by age 10 approximately 50% of patients have lost biceps, triceps, and patellar tendon reflexes, while ankle jerks often persist. Between 7 and 11 years of age patients lose the ability to climb stairs, stand from a supine position, and eventually walk even short distances [57]. By age 12 most are wheelchair-bound. Weakness, rather than contractures, seems to be the cause of loss of ability to ambulate [59]. Contractures of the elbow and wrists accelerate in the wheelchair-bound patients [62,63]. Respiratory muscle weakness, which can be detected by decreased vital capacity and negative inspiratory force, begins to develop as early as age 8 or 9 years [57], but it usually is not symptomatic till after the age of 13-15 years.

Cardiac involvement due to the lack of dystrophin expression in the heart is extremely common in DMD, and is evidenced by degenerative changes in muscle fibers of the ventricles, atria and conduction system. Sinus tachycardia is usually the only manifestation of cardiac involvement for the majority of the patient's life. A characteristic EKG pattern is seen in 90% of patients: sinus tachycardia with increased R/S amplitude ratio in lead V_1, deep Q waves in left V_5 and V_6 leads. Intra-atrial conduction disturbances are more frequent than atrio-ventricular and ventricular conduction defects. Echocardiography often reveals hypokinesis of the posterobasal portion of the ventricular wall, but ejection fraction is reduced, usually slightly, in only 20 percent of patients. The cardiac abnormalities, unlike the skeletal muscle pathology, progress much more slowly and remain asymptomatic in the majority of children, likely due to lack of exercise [57].

The teen years usually herald the onset of scoliosis, which typically develops between the ages of 13 and 15 [59]. The degree of thoracic scoliosis, in turn, correlates with the extent of respiratory failure. Approximately 40 percent of patients eventually succumb to respiratory failure. Many of these patients have concomitant respiratory infections. Another 10 to 40 percent die of cardiac failure, which may be related to ventilatory failure and pulmonary hypertension [57].

Life span in DMD is increasing with more aggressive ventilation therapy. A recent study revealed that the mean age of death increased from 14.4 years in the 1960s to 25.3 since 1990 [64]. In that study the mean age of death for non-ventilated patients from 1967 to 2002 was 19.3 [64]. The amount of residual dystrophin predicts survival, although no critical level has been identified [57]. Respiratory parameters can also predict negative outcome with forced vital capacity (FVC) being the most reliable; An FVC of less than 1 liter predicts a mean survival of 3.1 years and a 5-year survival of 8% [65].

BMD has a much less predictable course than DMD. The mean age of onset of symptoms is 12 years. While initial presentation can occur as late as age 70 years, nearly 90 percent of patients will have symptoms by age 20 years. Lower extremity weakness starts at a mean age of 11 years, whereas upper extremity weakness is not noted until a mean age of 31 years. Patients lose the ability to ambulate, on average, in their thirties, but the range stretches from early adolescence to late seventies. EKG abnormalities are similar to those observed in DMD, although less prevalent. Unlike DMD, which exhibits small ventricles, BMD may be associated with dilated cardiomyopathy. IQ is generally low normal, and lower IQ tends to correlate with earlier presentation. The age at death is on average 42 years, but like other characteristics of this disease, displays a wide range [57].

Medical and Socioeconomic Outcomes

Similar to the medical outcomes of the dystrophinopathies, the socioeconomic outcomes vary with phenotype. Population-based studies are more easily undertaken for the more common and more uniform DMD phenotype. Since DMD is primarily a disease of childhood, the economic burden is placed primarily on the patient's parents. Mothers of affected children in France were found to spend an average of 1.5 hours per day on medical and paramedical activities, which took away from all other activities and leisure time. Other studies have shown out-of-pocket expenses for medical care by families of disabled children came to 12.5% of their total income. This does not include the cost of diagnosis, which in 1991 was estimated to be $2800 [61].

A study of Medicaid patients in the state of Washington (USA) evaluated expenditures for children with chronic illnesses, including the muscular dystrophies. The study, which included 170 patients with muscular dystrophy (not stratified by specific subtype), found that muscular dystrophy is one of the most costly chronic diseases of childhood, second only to chronic respiratory disease. The cost was higher than cerebral palsy, cystic fibrosis, spina bifida, or malignancy. The average total Medicaid payments per patient in 1993 were $16,684. As would be expected, the highest segment of cost came from home health services, totaling 40% of total care. Compared to other chronic diseases, the percent spent on inpatient care of the muscular dystrophy patient was relatively low at 27%. Physician services, outpatient services, drugs, equipment, and other providers' services comprised about 10% of total care costs [66].

In the final stages of the illness, the majority of cost is associated with mechanical ventilation, should the patient, family and physician choose to pursue it. Studies have shown that physicians and other healthcare workers tend to place an undue weight on mechanical ventilation as an indicator of quality of life and patients generally find their quality of life acceptable or improved on long-term mechanical ventilation [65]. This highlights the importance of educating the patient in treatment options and expectations and allowing him to decide whether or not to pursue this treatment option. The setting of mechanical ventilation has a huge impact on cost. Home-based ventilation has been reported to be 77% less expensive than care in a long-term care facility [61].

Prevention

Carrier detection is the basis of prevention of the dystrophinopathies. The simplest method for identifying a carrier female was devised by Milhorat and Goldstone in 1965, a method which is still widely accepted. A *definite carrier* is a female with an affected son and an affected brother or maternal uncle, or with an affected son and a sister with an affected son. A female without affected male relatives but with two or more affected sons, or with an affected son and at least one affected grandson is a *probable carrier*. Finally, a female is classified as a *possible carrier* if she has only one affected son or if she does not have an affected son but has an affected male sibling, maternal uncle, maternal cousin or son of a sister [57].

Laboratory testing has become increasingly more important in carrier detection. While CK testing is abnormal in 45 – 70% of carriers, serum levels tend to decrease with age and during pregnancy and its use in carrier detection is limited [57]. Multiplex polymerase chain reaction (PCR) analysis of carrier DNA can detect evidence of deletions in the dystrophin gene in heterozygotes. Retrospective studies have reported carrier detection frequencies as high as 100% using PCR [67]. Should this method fail to detect carrier status in a case in which suspicion is high, fluorescence in situ hybridization (FISH), using a set of exon-specific cosmid DNA probes can be employed. Further testing, including analysis of dystrophin mRNA and analysis of genetic markers, is available prior to proceeding to muscle biopsy, which is not reliably diagnostic in carriers.

Management

Management can be broken down into four major categories of therapy: pharmacologic, rehabilitative, surgical, and respiratory. Proper care mandates a multi-disciplinary approach, which includes specialists in neurology, cardiology, orthopedics, pulmonology, and physical medicine and rehabilitation, as well as social work, mental health, and physical and occupational therapy.

Pharmacologic therapy centers primarily on corticosteroids. Several studies have demonstrated their short-term benefit on muscle strength, pulmonary function, and slowing progression of the disease. Recently, the American Academy of Neurology (AAN) issued a practice parameter endorsing the use of oral prednisone at a dose of 0.75 mg/kg/day in all patients with Muscular dystrophy [68]. This was based on evidence of its benefit from 7 class I (prospective, randomized, controlled) clinical trials. Per the recommendations of this practice parameter, the dosage above should be maintained unless side effects dictate otherwise. In that case, the dosage should be decreased first to 0.5 mg/kg/day, and if adverse effects persist, the dose can be further reduced to 0.3 mg/kg/day, a dose which has shown to be still significantly effective. Potential side effects that should be monitored and would warrant decreasing the dose include weight gain, cushingoid appearance, cataracts, a decrease in growth rate, gastrointestinal symptoms, and behavioral changes. No studies are available to evaluate the sequelae of long-term corticosteroid therapy on children with DMD. Deflazacort, an oxazoline analogue of prednisone which is not available in the United States, was evaluated by two class I trials that demonstrated benefit in muscle strength and function. It was recommended by the AAN as an alternate therapy, at a recommended dose of 0.9 mg/kg/day. Side effects were similar to prednisone and included weight gain and asymptomatic cataracts. Data comparing deflazacort to prednisone are insufficient to evaluate whether a favorable side effect profile could be attributed to either therapy [68].

Rehabilitation management aims to prolong independence, maintain locomotion, and prevent physical deformity. A multi-disciplinary approach is necessary involving parents, physicians, nurses, therapists, social workers, psychologists and counselors. Exercise should be approached cautiously in patients with dystrophinopathy as exercise-induced muscle injury is a risk. Contractures tend to develop as a result of immobility of the limbs and often accelerate shortly after wheel-chair reliance [62]. Static stretching and splinting are recommended for prevention of contracture. Prevention of contractures, in isolation, prevents deformity but does not prolong ambulation, which is more dependent on muscle strength. Bracing, on the other hand, has been shown to prolong ambulation [62,63], and may also delay scoliosis. Other equipment of benefit to a patient's quality of life at various stages of the disease include a properly-fitted wheelchair, a pressure-relieving mattress, a hand-held shower, a shower chair, grab bars, a raised toilet seat or bedside commode, and a wheelchair ramp [60].

Surgical therapy is primarily aimed at limb contractures and spinal deformity. Contractures at the hip and ankle are released by subcutaneous tenotomy. This procedure is combined with early post-operative rehabilitation and lightweight ankle-foot orthoses [62]. This approach is best applied before the patient loses mobility and results in a prolongation of the ability to walk by an average of 2 years. Spinal surgery is indicated when rapidly evolving scoliosis is threatening pulmonary compromise and before scoliosis reaches more than 40 degrees. Segmental spine stabilization with and without bone fusion have been advocated, but comparative trials of the two approaches are lacking. Benefits of spinal surgery include improved ability to sit, amelioration of pain, and decreased dependence on braces [57].

Respiratory care is an ongoing concern, although much more so after wheelchair confinement. Baseline pulmonary function testing should be performed on all DMD children and the family should be educated with regards to the potential respiratory complications of the disease. The American Thoracic Society's consensus statement in 2004 recommended periodic (twice per year) respiratory care after wheelchair confinement, after a fall of vital capacity below 80% predicted, or after the age of 12 years regardless of symptoms [65]. Daytime ventilation should be considered when waking pCO_2 exceeds 50 mm Hg or when hemoglobin oxygen saturation persists below 92% while awake. This can be accomplished initially with noninvasive intermittent positive pressure ventilation. Discussions about chronic mechanical ventilation should take place well before the need arises. If mechanical ventilation is instituted, patients should be followed by a pulmonologist, and pneumococcal and annual influenza vaccinations are advised [60].

MYOTONIC DYSTROPHIES

Myotonic dystrophy is the second most common muscular dystrophy overall and the most common adult-onset muscular dystrophy. First described by Steinert (hence the name Steinert disease) and by Batten and Gibb in 1909, it is notable for its wide variation in clinical presentation. Typically, it is a slowly progressive disease characterized by muscle weakness, clinical myotonia, and a wide range of involvement other organ systems, including the eyes, heart, lungs and endocrine system.

The inheritance pattern of the disease was observed shortly after recognition of the disease entity to be autosomal dominant. The discovery of the causative mutation was shown in 1992 to be an expansion of a trinucleotide repeat in the 3' untranslated region of the DMPK (myotonic dystrophy protein kinase) gene on chromosome 19. The repeat is a CTG repeat that can vary widely in affected individuals from approximately double the normal number of 30 repeats to several thousand repeats [69]. The muscle weakness is most notable in the distal muscles of the extremities and the facial muscles. Clinical myotonia can usually be observed, most reliably in the hands. Severe congenital and early childhood-onset forms of myotonic dystrophy are common [69].

In 1994 Ricker, et al. described a group of patients with similar disorder with muscle weakness that was predominantly proximal, myotonia that was primarily subclinical, and milder systemic abnormalities. The patients also lacked the CTG repeat on chromosome 19 [70]. This group of patients was labeled as having proximal myotonic myopathy (PROMM). In 1998-1999, Day and Ricker's groups mapped the genetic abnormality in DM2 to chromosome 3 and demonstrated that the abnormality is a tetranucleotide expansion in an intron of the zinc finger protein 9 (ZNF9) [71-73], thus solidifying the distinction between classical myotonic dystrophy, now known as myotonic dystrophy type 1 (dystrophia myotonica type 1, DM1) and PROMM, a term that has been used interchangeably with myotonic dystrophy type 2 (dystrophia myotonica type 2, DM2). In contrast to DM1, DM2 does not have a congenital form and anticipation is not prominent.

Incidence and Prevalence

Incidence and prevalence studies of myotonic dystrophy must be interpreted cautiously, as the clinical manifestation vary widely, discovery of the gene responsible for the disorder has only recently been made, and the distinction between DM1 and DM2 has only been made recently. Harper reported an incidence of 1 in 8,000 with a prevalence rate of 5 to 20 per 100,000 in Western Europe [74]. Emery reported a worldwide prevalence range of 1 – 10 per 100,000 [75]. A more recent report attempted to incorporate genetic diagnosis in the estimations of DM1 prevalence in Italy [76]. This report drew attention to the possibility that the true prevalence of the disease may have been underestimated in the past. Whereas the investigators found a prevalence rate of 9.3 per 100,000 in their study population of Northeastern and Central Italy, previous epidemiological studies performed in the same regions in 1975 and 1981 had shown rates less than half of this value. No epidemiological studies exist to date on the recently described DM2, although the prevalence of the disease is likely underestimated because of the absence of a congenital form. DM2 is most common in Northern Europeans, and may be as common as DM1 in Germany [77].

Unlike the dystrophinopathies, the distribution of myotonic dystrophy is not uniform over all ethnic groups. A Japanese study (conducted before the discovery of the CTG repeat) found an incidence of 1 in 20,000 – less than half the incidence in Western Europe [78]. In ethnic Africans, Southeast Asians and Australian Aborigines, the disease is thought to be exceedingly rare. A survey study found no cases of myotonic dystrophy in 3 centers in South Africa, representing a population of over 30 million. Likewise no cases were reported among 53 million ethnic Thai. Only one affected family was reported among 120 million Nigerians. In contrast, the incidence in the Saguenay-Lac-Saint-Jean region of Quebec, Canada is 162 per 100,000. All of the cases in this remote community of 30,000 have been linked to a single common ancestor [74]. While the true incidence in these different regions may be influenced by referral bias, this was unlikely because the reporting of the incidence of Duchenne muscular dystrophy, used as a control, was similar to expected values [79].

Natural History

The clinical manifestations of DM1 range from death during infancy to complete lack of symptoms until the eighth decade of life. There is a rough correlation between the number of repeats and the age at onset of symptoms and the severity of muscle disease. The median age at onset is between 20 and 25 years. The most common presenting symptoms are muscle weakness, the initial complaint of 60% of patients, and muscle stiffness due to myotonia in 36%. Other presenting symptoms, in descending order of frequency, include mental retardation, cataracts, and neonatal respiratory distress [74]. Thirty-one percent have no complaint, but the diagnosis is made by studying family members of a patient with known DM1.

The pattern of muscle weakness in DM1 separates it from other forms of muscular dystrophy. It primarily affects muscles of the head and neck and distal muscles of the extremities. The sternocleidomastoid muscle and neck flexors are often affected, and typically to a greater degree than neck extensors. Facial muscle weakness, while representing a nearly constant feature of the disease, is not marked. Often the patients show inability to whistle. A minor degree of symmetrical ptosis is characteristic. These features, along with hollowing of the temples from temporalis wasting, create the typical facies of early DM1. Later, the frequent development of masseter weakness, which leaves the lower jaw hanging slightly open, and frontal balding complete the unmistakable facial appearance (Hatchet facies). In more advanced cases, weakness of the palate puts the patient at risk for aspiration and, in combination with the facial weakness and myotonia of the tongue, contributes to dysarthria. In the limbs, distal muscle weakness is more common than proximal. Weakness of intrinsic hand muscles is a common early finding, but is not as marked as that seen in other distal myopathies, and wasting of these muscles occurs later. It is usually accompanied by weakness of the wrist and anterior compartment calf muscles. Although the weakness does generalize as the disease progresses, the patient usually maintains the ability to ambulate until very late in the disease course [74]. The average time from onset of illness to wheelchair-dependence is 27 years [80], and approximately half will require at least some wheelchair assistance in the years prior to death [81].

Myotonia is the most distinguishing feature of the disease, yet patients often do not complain of it. Clinical myotonia, defined as failure of the muscle to relax after cessation of voluntary contraction, is most easily elicited in the hand muscles after a forceful grip (grip myotonia). Percussion myotonia, elicited on percussion of the thenar muscles or the tongue (using a tongue depressor), is also a common finding. As the muscle weakness progresses, clinical and percussion myotonia actually diminishes, and myotonia rarely contributes significantly to disability.

The central nervous system (CNS) is often involved. The typical affect of those patients in whom the CNS is involved is blunted and apathetic. Overt mental retardation, seen mostly in congenital or early-childhood forms, is uncommon in the adult-onset form. Hypersomnia is another common feature.

The range of systemic manifestations in DM1 is wide. Cardiac involvement is common and is a frequent cause of death. Although most patients do not have symptoms, electrocardiographic abnormalities occur in up to 90%. Cardiac involvement include conduction system abnormalities, supraventicular and ventricular tachyarrythmias and, less often, myocardial dysfunction. The most frequent abnormality is first-degree heart block with a prevalence that ranges between 20-40%. Wide QRS complex, such as due to a right or left bundle branch block, is common. Cardiac arrhythmias, including atrial flutter or fibrillation and ventricular tachycardia or fibrillation, also occur but do not correlate with severity of neuromuscular disease. In contrast to its effects on the conduction system, overt cardiomyopathy is unusual. Both myotonia and weakness may affect the diaphragm, which in turn leads to alveolar hypoventilation, the hallmark of respiratory involvement in DM1. Smooth muscle is also involved, primarily evidenced by swallowing disturbances, which lead to aspiration, and, less commonly colonic involvement, which commonly leads to constipation but may cause megacolon or pseudo-obstruction. Most patients with DM1 have some abnormality in the smooth muscle of the gastrointestinal tract [69]. The endocrine system is thoroughly involved as well. Most patients show hyperinsulinism without diabetes, implicating an insulin-receptor defect. Sixty to eighty percent of males with DM1 exhibit testicular atrophy with slightly reduced testosterone levels. Women, while not symptomatic with respect to secondary sexual characteristics, have a high rate of fetal loss. Pituitary involvement is suggested by high follicle-stimulating hormone levels. Ocular involvement is most characteristically marked by early cataracts. Slit-lamp examination shows multicolored subcapsular opacities – the so-called "Christmas tree" cataracts. Less common ocular abnormalities include retinal degeneration, ptosis, low intraocular pressure, blepharitis, corneal lesions, and extraocular muscle involvement.

Life expectancy in DM1 is mildly reduced compared to the general population. The median survival is about 60 years, with the majority dying between ages 50 and 65 of age, about 70% from complications of DM1. There is a weak inverse correlation between CTG repeat length and survival. The most common cause of death is pneumonia, accounting for the primary cause in 31% and the secondary cause in another 11%. Cardiac arrhythmia is the second leading cause of death (29%), and is usually due ventricular fibrillation (that may lead to sudden death at home) or embolic events related to atrial fibrillation [81].

The congenital form of DM1 does not show clinical myotonia in the first year of life as a rule, which differentiates it from myotonia congenita, and electrical myotonia is also uncommon. Ninety percent have facial weakness, the most frequently occurring symptom. Over half will also exhibit hypotonia, delayed motor development, mental retardation (a stark contrast to the adult form of the disease), poor sucking and swallowing, talipes, and/or neonatal respiratory distress that may require respiratory support. Neonatal mortality is high in this severe form of DM1, but no epidemiological studies currently provide a precise estimation. If the affected individual survives through infancy, the prognosis improves considerably. Hypotonia generally improves as the features of the adult-onset form arise, and patients are generally more limited by mental handicap than physical [74].

The natural course of DM2 is not well known, owing to its fairly recent recognition as a disease entity. The age at onset of symptoms has ranged from 13 to 67 years, and there has been no congenital form. Muscle symptoms are the most common presenting complaints and include weakness, stiffness, myotonia, and pain. The pattern of weakness is different from that seen in DM1. Neck flexors, elbow extensors, thumb and deep finger flexors, and hip flexors and extensors are commonly involved, whereas ankle dorsiflexors and facial muscles are not commonly involved. Fluctuating muscle pains are seen in the majority of patients over age 50. Systemic manifestations, including cataracts and cardiac conduction defects, are indistinguishable from DM1. Primary male hypogonadism is seen in the majority of patients, and most exhibit insulin insensitivity [77].

Risk Factors

Early studies of patients with DM1 had indicated that the disease has a variable penetrance and its severity typically increased in subsequent generations within a family, a phenomenon referred to as anticipation. The anticipation observed in DM1 families is more evident with maternal transmission than following paternal transmission. These phenomena (variable penetrance, anticipation and a maternal transmission bias) are best explained by the trinucleotide repeat expansion in DM1. The penetrance in DM1 is not precisely known but, when accounting for very mild cases, is near complete and likely correlates with the CTG expansion size of the parent. The risk of an individual with a known affected parent for developing symptomatic myotonic dystrophy varies based on the age of that individual and the profile of the affected parent. An asymptomatic adult over the age of 20 has at most a 5% percent risk of manifesting clinically significant disease, and the risk declines as years pass without symptom-onset [74]. It is also now known that there is a fair correlation between the repeat length on one hand and age of symptom onset and disease severity on the other. This correlation is best with relatively short CTG repeats, while it is not very strong with for very long repeats (more than 400).

Given the wide variation of phenotypes in DM1, the ability to predict the severity of illness in the offspring of an affected individual is often as important as or more important than whether the disease will manifest. The risk of congenital myotonic dystrophy is very low in offspring of affected males. This is in part attributable to the lack of fertility in males with severe disease. The risk of congenital disease in the offspring of a woman depends on her disease profile. She confers a 10-30% risk of congenital or severe childhood-onset disease to her offspring if she has significant disease. However, her offspring has a slightly higher (10-50%) risk of congenital or severe childhood-onset disease if she has already had one child with the congenital form or she, herself, had childhood-onset disease [74].

Socioeconomic Outcomes

Presymptomatic testing has been available since 1988. In contrast to Huntington's disease, in which an asymptomatic adult has a risk of developing a rapidly progressive fatal disease, myotonic dystrophy that manifests in adulthood is typically not devastating. Thus, the considerations of those pursuing testing are different. The primary reason for testing is risk-determination for offspring. The psychosocial impact of this practice has been examined in the Saguenay-Lac-Saint-Jean region of Quebec, Canada, which carries the world's highest concentration of DM1 patients [82]. The practice in this region, as used in most parts of the world, is to test only adults, who wish to be tested. The findings in the Saguenay-Lac-Saint-Jean region indicate that most subjects who were at risk and were tested, whether found to be carriers or not, endorsed the idea and recommended it to family members. Just over half of carriers perceived some negative impact on their life, including their self esteem, concerns about their future, and concerns about their children. Just over a third of that group, 20% of all carriers, regretted having the testing done overall.

The economic impact of myotonic dystrophy is difficult to measure as the duration of the disease is often decades of adult life, throughout which disability proceeds slowly. One study addressed employment in chronic neuromuscular disorders with viability into adulthood [83]. Comparing to limb-girdle muscular dystrophy, facioscapulohumeral dystrophy, Becker muscular dystrophy, spinal muscular atrophy, and Charcot-Marie-Tooth disease, only the latter had a lower employment rate than myotonic dystrophy. Myotonic dystrophy patients had an employment rate of 31%, while 49% of the combined patients with the other diseases were working. In addition, 80% of employed patients with myotonic dystrophy were industrial or "service/clerical/sales" workers. The IQ and education of myotonic dystrophy patients were thought to affect both employment status and the occupation: The mean IQ of patients with myotonic dystrophy (92.4) was significantly lower than that of the other neuromuscular diseases, and only 47% of patients graduated high school, and 9% finished college.

Prevention

As with other inherited autosomal dominant disorders, prevention relies on genetic counseling. The data listed in the Risk Factors section above may be used to guide potential parents. An asymptomatic woman with an affected parent may wish to be screened prior to having children, and this option should be offered. Given the lower socioeconomic status of this patient population, however, genetic testing is often not possible. Prenatal testing by mutational analysis is also available, and large expansions, usually indicating more severe disease, can be detected. This correlation is not certain, but, generally, finding over 1000 repeats predicts a severe case while finding fewer than 100 predicts a low likelihood of severe disease.

Management

Perhaps no other neuromuscular disease requires the level of multi-disciplinary care that myotonic dystrophy does. For the neurologist, myotonia is usually very treatable; however, myotonia is often either not disabling or not bothersome enough for patients to remain compliant with therapy. Mexiletine, phenytoin, tocainide, quinine, and procainamide have all been used. Though mexiletine and tocainide are the most effective [84], tocainide is not recommended any longer because of potentially serious hematological side effects. Therefore, mexiletine, at a smaller dose than that used for arrhythmias, is the recommended first line.

Whereas myotonia may go nearly unnoticed by patients, muscle weakness can be very disabling. Physical therapy can be helpful for this. One small study of DM1 patients observed that after 12 weeks of aerobic exercise found that patients' oxidative capacity and fitness improve and their mean muscle fiber area increased [85]. The problem encountered with physical therapy, however, is that patient-compliance is low, especially in the long term. Routine breathing exercises can combat hypoventilation and reduce the accumulation of secretions [74]. This may also improve the characteristic somnolence. Modafinil is effective in reducing excessive somnolence and the Epworth sleepiness scale scores, and it improves mood significantly [86].

From a cardiac perspective, arrhythmias should be sought. All patients should have a routine electrocardiogram at least yearly. A 24 hour holter-monitor should be obtained whenever fainting spells, palpitations, or syncope are elicited by taking a careful cardiac history. An echocardiogram and signal-averaged ECG should complete the initial evaluation. More detailed cardiac electrophysiological studies are recommended based on clinical symptoms, family history and initial cardiograms (Table 6). The need for pacemaker placement is common, but the degree of heart block that warrants the procedure is still debated [87]. An ophthalmologic exam should be part of the standard care of myotonic dystrophy patients, both initially and through follow-up. Patients generally achieve good results after surgical cataract extraction. Hypergylcemia, when requiring treatment, can be controlled with metformin or thiazolidinediones. Finally, gastroparesis may be helped by metoclopramide.

Table 6. Suggested indications for cardiac electrophysiological study in DM1 patients. (adapted from Pelargonio, G., Della Russo, A., Sanna, T., et al. (2002) 'Myotonic dystrophy and the heart' *Heart* 665-670.)

Suggestive symptoms	• Syncope • Palpitations • Dizziness
Family history	• Sudden death • Ventricular fibrillation • Sustained ventricular tachycardia • Pacemaker implant
EKG findings	• Left bundle branch block • Right bundle branch block and left anterior fasciular block • Right bundle branch block and left posterior fasciular block • First degree AV block and PR >240 ms, left anterior fasciular block or left posterior fasciular block • Second or third degree AV block
Holter monitor findings	• Sinus pause >3 seconds • Sinus bradycardia <40 /min • Frequent ventricular premature beats • Non-sustained ventricular tachycardia • Sustained ventricular tachycardia

INFLAMMATORY MYOPATHIES

The inflammatory myopathies are a group of acquired muscle diseases that includes polymyositis, dermatomyositis, and inclusion body myositis (IBM). The three diseases can be difficult to distinguish clinically, especially when presentations are not classical. In addition, the pathologic criteria for biopsy diagnosis are complicated by non-uniform involvement of muscle, which leads to sampling error. For these reasons, present epidemiologic data cannot be considered precise. Furthermore comparison between studies is difficult because different classification schemes have been used to separate patients. When this class of diseases was first described in the mid-1800s, no attempt at distinction was made. They were thought to be a single disease entity, marked by severe weakness, progressing over months, and, in some cases, a rash. Over time, dermatomyositis was distinguished by its rash, and the rest of cases were all labeled polymyositis [88]. In 1967 a case of chronic polymyositis was reported with inclusions, which were thought to be viral particles [89]. The term inclusion body myositis was first used in 1971 [90], thus completing the division of inflammatory myopathies into the three diseases recognized today.

The first major attempt at diagnostic criteria was made in 1975 by Bohan and Peter [91,92]. They addressed only polymyositis and dermatomyositis. Using clinical, pathologic, serologic, and electrophysiological criteria (see Table 7), cases were categorized as polymyositis and, if they also have skin changes, as dermatomyositis. No distinction was made pathologically between the two diseases and IBM was neglected entirely. While this categorization is still widely used, recently more emphasis has been placed on pathologic differentiation between the three disorders. Dermatomyositis has two characteristic histological patterns caused by primary abnormality of blood vessels causing ischemic injury to muscle fibers. These include perifascicular atrophy and, less commonly, wedge-shaped microinfarcts. Also, criteria for inclusion body myositis, which encompass clinical, serologic, and pathologic criteria, are established. A definite diagnosis cannot be made without each of the three following biopsy findings: 1. An inflammatory myopathy characterized by mononuclear cell invasion of non-necrotic muscle fibers. 2. Vacuolated fibers. 3. Either (a) intracellular amyloid deposits or (b) 15-18 nm tubulofilaments by electron microscopy [93]. Other diagnostic classification schemes exist, but these are used for inclusion or exclusion by the vast majority of epidemiological studies.

Table 7. Bohan and Peter Classification System[4,5]

Clinical	Chronic or subacute symmetric proximal
Pathological	Muscle fiber necrosis with presence of regenerating fibers and interstitial mononuclear infiltrate
Laboratory	Elevated CK with frequent elevations of transaminases, lactate dehydrogenase and aldolase
Electrophysiological	Increased insertional activity, fibrillation potentials and/or positive sharp waves, and small, polyphasic motor units
Skin	Heliotrope rash around the eyelids with periorbital edema and Gottron's signs (erythematous rash over the knuckles, elbows, and knees)

- All of the first 4 criteria: definite polymyositis.
- Three of the first 4 criteria: probable polymyositis.
- Two of the first 4 criteria: possible polymyositis.
- Three or 4 criteria plus skin changes: definite dermatomyositis.
- Two criteria plus skin change: probable dermatomyositis
- One criterion plus skin changes: possible dermatomyositis.

Incidence and Prevalence

The average annual incidence of the inflammatory myopathies, as a group, is 2.2 to 7.7 per million based on a recent review that included fifteen individual studies [94]. Overall, the incidence in polymyositis and dermatomyositis is higher in women, while that of IBM is higher in men. Polymyositis and, more commonly, dermatomyositis may occur in children, while IBM occurs only in adults, typically middle-aged or older. A recent study found that from 1995 to 1998 in the United States, the annual incidence of juvenile dermatomyositis ranged from 2.5 to 4.1 (average 3.2) per million. Incidence by race showed 3.4 for white non-Hispanic, 3.3 for African-American, and 2.7 for Hispanic. Girls were affected more than twice as often as boys [95]. Most studies have found that the incidence of both polymyositis and dermatomyositis increases with age, with a peak in the late 6th or 7th decade [94].

The prevalence is less relevant for polymyositis and dermatomyositis because they are treatable conditions. However, IBM which is a chronic and progressive condition, has a prevalence that ranges from 4.9 to 10.7 per million. In the population older than 50, the prevalence ranges from 16 to 35.3 per million [94], rendering IBM the most common myopathy in this age group.

A caveat must be rendered that these data are subject to error in the form of misdiagnosis. As mentioned above, most studies for polymyositis and dermatomyositis used the Bohan and Peter classification of 1975. More recent evidence indicates that the three disease processes are distinct and that there are histopathological and pathophysiological differences between the three. A recent study proposed that polymyositis is overdiagnosed when using the older criteria [96]. This retrospective study of 165 patients with myositis of subacute onset found only 2% to have definite polymyositis. The diagnosis of polymyositis in this study was based on serum CK elevation of twice normal and strict biopsy evidence of mononuclear cells, located in the endomysium, and surrounding (and preferably invading) non-necrotic muscle fibers. The findings in this study were in stark contrast to prior studies, which have shown frequencies of 30-60% of polymyositis among those with subacute myositis.

Natural History

Polymyositis and dermatomyositis typically progress over several weeks to months. They are both marked by proximal muscle weakness, including the limb girdle muscles and neck flexors. Muscles of respiration and swallowing may also be involved. Aside from striated muscle, other systems may be involved, most notably the pulmonary system. Interstitial lung disease (ILD) occurs in 5-10% of patients radiographically and in as many as 40% by pulmonary function testing. The anti-Jo-1 antibody, seen in 20% of dermatomyositis and polymyositis patients, predicts the presence of ILD, as it is seen over half of the ILD cases. Cardiac involvement has also been reported, although it is rarely symptomatic. Nonetheless EKG abnormalities may be seen in up to 40%, the most common of which are nonspecific ST-T wave changes. Clinically, dermatomyositis is differentiated from polymyositis by the presence of a rash which often precedes muscle weakness. It is an erythematous, edematous rash that is found over the extensor surfaces of the elbow, finger and knee joints, as well as the chest, back and shoulders, and the bridge of the nose. In addition to this rash, a heliotrope rash, which is a purplish discoloration around the eyelids, with periorbital edema is often observed and helps to solidify the diagnosis. Finally, violaceous raised papules, called Gottron papules, are often seen in a symmetric distribution over the knuckles or, less commonly, the extensor surfaces of other joints [98].

Inclusion body myositis presents more slowly, progressing over months to years. While proximal muscle weakness is also common in IBM, it has a characteristic distribution of weakness that differentiates it from the other inflammatory myopathies. Typically, the quadriceps muscles are weak out of proportion to the hip flexors, and distal weakness, notably in the finger and wrist flexors and, sometimes, in ankle dorsiflexion, is prominent.

Dysphagia is more frequent in IBM, compared to the other inflammatory myopathies, occurring in 60%. As a rule, other organ systems outside of skeletal muscle are not affected [98].

Risk Factors

Both polymyositis and dermatomyositis have been associated with malignancy, although the veracity of the association is still debated. Reports of the incidence malignancy have varied from 4% to 42% with dermatomyositis being the higher. In a review of 7 studies that reported malignancy in myositis, all groups showed an increased standard incidence ratio except for the polymyositis group in one study [94]. The diagnosis of cancer may precede, be concurrent with, or follow the diagnosis of myopathy. In those patients with myositis, malignancy becomes less probable as time passes with the highest risk in the first 3 years [94]. Another association that has been reported is with connective tissue diseases. A connective tissue disease is coincident with 11-40% of polymyositis or dermatomyositis cases. Females outnumber males in this subgroup by 9 to 1 [94]. Associations between IBM and malignancy, connective tissue disease, or other disorders have not been consistently reported, and age greater than 50 seems to be the only true risk factor.

Management

The therapies for the inflammatory myopathies are mainly immunosuppressant and immunomodulatory treatment. Empiric data would suggest that dermatomyositis is more responsive to treatment than polymyositis. Both diseases are treated with similar medications at similar doses. Prednisone is generally used as a first line drug, generally started at 1g/kg/day for 4-8 weeks followed by a slow taper. Alternatively IVIG may be used as first line or for prednisone-failures. This is usually given as 2g/kg and often divided over 2-5 days. Steroid-sparing agents include methotrexate (7.5-25 mg weekly) and azathioprine (3-5 mg daily). One trial that included 15 total patients and compared a 3 month course of IVIG to placebo in dermatomyositis showed a statistically significant benefit over placebo based on the assessment of strength at 6 months [99]. Plasma exchange was found to be ineffective in a randomized, controlled trial and therefore is not recommended [88].

A recent Cochrane systematic review of the literature examined the existing literature regarding treatment of polymyositis and dermatomyositis [100]. It included only 6 randomized or quasi-randomized trials. Of these, only 4 were judged to be adequate with respect to avoidance of bias, and only three of these were placebo-controlled. Overall, the trials for these diseases suffer from the same problem encountered with other rare diseases: they are underpowered and do not have long enough follow-up periods. The review concluded that there is inadequate evidence to support the use of immunosuppressants, fully recognizing that many clinicians' experience shows these medications to be useful. An international consensus on primary end points for future clinical trials has been published [101].

Inclusion body myositis has proven to be resistant to immunomodulatory therapy. Experts are divided on whether attempts at treatment, outside of trials, should be made at all. Clearly one of the benefits of making the diagnosis of IBM is saving the patient from the potential side effects of the immunomodulators, particularly prednisone. Intravenous immunoglobulin is perhaps the best studied therapy for this disease. High-dose IVIG was compared to placebo, and did not demonstrate a significant difference in muscle strength, but did appear to improve some components of weakness, including dysphagia [102]. Compared to placebo in patients simultaneously treated with prednisone, IVIG also failed to show a statistically significant difference in muscle strength, although endomysial inflammation was significantly reduced in the IVIG group [103]. A randomized, double-blind placebo controlled trial of methotrexate found no benefit in muscle strength, but the methotrexate group did show significantly decreased creatine kinase levels compared to placebo [104].

CONCLUSION

The depth and breadth of information regarding neuromuscular diseases has grown dramatically in the past 2 decades. A similar review of available evidence 20 years ago would not include the genetic causes for disease in the dystrophinopathies or the myotonic dystrophies. In fact there would be no mention at all of DM1 or DM2, as DM2 would not have been described. At that time there would have been no successful treatment trials in ALS or DMD, and treatment options would be much more limited for the inflammatory myopathies and MG.

These advances, however, highlight some of the difficulty with epidemiological data in the face of ever-changing diagnostic techniques, treatment options, and prognoses combined with improved general medical care. Comparison of incidence and, to an even greater extent, prevalence between different eras must take these considerations into account. Another problem with interpretation of epidemiological data is assuring proper case ascertainment. Different diagnostic criteria have been used with different studies, and these affect not only incidence and prevalence but also response to treatment in clinical trials. Despite the recent progress, further research is necessary. This research must be collaborative between major centers, as these diseases are rare, and small numbers of patients lead to underpowered studies. Further, agreement must be reached on standardized inclusion and exclusion criteria for both clinical trials and epidemiological studies, so the resultant data can be interpreted accurately.

REFERENCES

[1]   Brown, R. H., Meininger, V. & Swash M. (eds.) (2000). *Amyotrophic Lateral Sclerosis.* London: Martin Dunitz Ltd.

[2]   Swash M. 'Clinical features and diagnosis of amyotrophic lateral sclerosis' in Brown, et al. (eds.), (2000). *Amyotrophic Lateral Sclerosis.* London: Martin Dunitz Ltd, pp: 3-30.

[3]   World Federation of Neurology website (1998). 'El Escorial revisited: Revised criteria for the diagnosis of amyotrophic lateral sclerosis.' www.wfnals.org/-guidelines/1998elescorial/elescorial1998criteria.htm.

[4]   Traynor, B. J., Codd, M. B., Corr, B., et al. (2000). 'Clinical features of amyotrophic lateral sclerosis according to the El Escorial and Airlie House diagnostic criteria: a population-based study.' *Archives of Neurology 57*, 1171-1176.

[5]   Chancellor, A. M. & Warlow, C. P. (1992). 'Adult onset motor neuron disease: worldwide mortality, incidence and distribution since 1950.' *Journal of Neurology, Neurosurgery, and Psychiatry 55*, 1106-1115.

[6]   Sorenson, E. J., Stalker, A. P., Kurland, L. T., et al. (2002). 'Amyotrophic lateral sclerosis in Olmsted County, Minnesota, 1925 to 1998.' *Neurology 59*, 280-282.

[7]   Brooks, B. R., Sanjak, M., Belden, D., et al. 'Natural history of amyotrophic lateral sclerosis – impairment, disability, handicap' in Brown, et al. (eds.), (2000). *Amyotrophic Lateral Sclerosis.* London: Martin Dunitz Ltd , pp: 31-58.

[8]   Horner, R. D., Kamins, K. G., Feussner, J. R., et al. (2003). 'Occurrence of amyotrophic lateral sclerosis among Gulf War veterans.' *Neurology 61*, 742-749.

[9]   Weisskopf, M. G., O'Reilly, E. J., McCullough, M. L., et al. (2005). 'Prospective study of military service and mortality from ALS.' *Neurology 64*, 32-37.

[10] Chiò, A., Benzi, G., Dossena, M., et al. (2005). 'Severely increased risk of amyotrophic lateral sclerosis among Italian professional football players.' *Brain 128*, 472-476.

[11] Ginsberg, G & Lowe, S. (2002). 'Cost effetiveness of treatments for amyotrophic lateral sclerosis: a review of the literature.' *Pharmacoeconomics 20*, 267-387.

[12] Hecht, M. J., Graesel, E., Tigges, S., et al. (2003). 'Burden of care in amyotrophic lateral sclerosis.' *Palliative Medicine 17*, 327-333.

[13] Trail, M., Nelson, N. D., Van, J. V., et al. (2003). 'A study comparing patients with amyotrophic lateral sclerosis and their caregivers on measures of quality of life, depression, and their attitudes toward treatment options.' *Journal of the Neurological Sciences 209*, 79-85.

[14] Ascherio, A., Weisskopf, M. G., O'Reilly, E. J., et al. (2005). 'Vitamin E intake and risk of amyotrophic lateral sclerosis.' *Neurology 57*, 104-110.

[15] Miller, R. G., Rosenberg, J. A., Gelinas, D. F., et al. (1999). 'Practice parameter: The care of the patient with amyotrophic lateral sclerosis (an evidence based review)' *Neurology. 52,*1311-1323.

[16] Quality Standards Subcommittee of the American Academy of Neurology (1997). 'Practice advisory on the treatment of amyotrophic lateral sclerosis with riluzole: Report of the Quality Standards Subcommittee of the American Academy of Neurology' *Neurology. 49,* 657-659.

[17] Bensimon G, Lacomblez L, Meininger V, and the ALS/Riluzole Study Group (1994). A Controlled Trial of Riluzole in Amyotophic Lateral Sclerosis. *N Eng J Med.; 330*:587-591.

[18] Lacomblez L, Bensimon G, Leigh PN, et al (1996). Dose ranging Study of riluzole in amyotrophic lateral sclerosis. *Lancet. 347*:1425-1431.

[19] Ashworth, N. L., Satkunam, L. E., & Deforge, D. (2005). 'Treatment for spasticity in amyotrophic lateral sclerosis/motor neuron disease' *The Cochrane Database of Systematic Reviews.* 2.

[20] Erb, W. H. (1883). *Handbook of electrotherapeutics* New York: William Woods.

[21] Goldflam, S. (1893). 'Ueber einen scheinbar heilbaren bulbärparalytischen symptomencomplex mit betheiligung der extremitäten' *Deutschen Z Nervenheilkunde 4*, 312-352.

[22] Walker, M. B. (1934). 'Treatment of myasthenia gravis with physostigmine' *Lancet 1*, 1200-1201.

[23] Phillips, L. H. (2003). 'The epidemiology of myasthenia gravis' *Annals of the New York Academy of Sciences 998*, 407-412.

[24] Somnier, F. E., Keiding, N. & Paulson, O. B. (1991). 'Epidemiology of myasthenia gravis in Denmark' *Archives of Neurology 48*, 733-739.

[25] Kuks, J. B. M.& Oosterhuis, H. J. G. H. (2003). 'Clinical presentation and epidemiology of myasthenia gravis' in Kaminski, H. J. (ed.) (2003). *Myasthenia Gravis and Related Disorders* Totowa, NJ: Humana Press, Inc. pp. 93-113.

[26] Mantegazza, R., Baggi, F., Antozzi, C., et al. (2003). 'Myasthenia gravis: Epidemiological data and prognostic factors' *Annals of the New York Academy of Sciences 998*, 413-423.

[27] Lavrnic, D., Losen, M., Vujic, A., et al. (2005). 'The features of myasthenia gravis with autoantibodies to MuSK' *Journal of Neurology, Neurosurgery, and Psychiatry 76*, 1099-1102.

[28] Hoch, W., McConville, J., Helms, S., et al. (2001). 'Autoantibodies to the receptor tyrosine kinase MuSK in patients with myasthenia gravis without acetylcholine receptor antibodies' *Nature Medicine 7*, 365-368.

[29] Ohta, K., Shigemoto, K., Kubo, S., et al. (2004). 'MuSK antibodies in AChR Ab-seropositive MG vs AChR Ab-seronegative MG' *Neurology 62*, 2132-2133.

[30] Daroff, R. B. (2003). 'Ocular Myasthenia' in Kaminski, H. J. (ed.) (2003). *Myasthenia Gravis and Related Disorders* Totowa, NJ: Humana Press, Inc. pp. 115-128.

[31] Beekman, R., Kuks, J. B. M., Oosterhuis, H. J. G. H. (1997). 'Myasthenia gravis: diagnosis and follow-up of 100 consecutive patients' *Journal of Neurology 244*, 112-118.

[32] Christensen, P. B., Jensen, T. S., Tsiropoulos, I., et al. (1998). 'Mortality and survival in myasthenia gravis: a Danish population based study' *Journal of Neurology, Neurosurgery, and Psychiatry 64*, 78-83.

[33] Murthy, J. M., Meena, A. K., Chowdary, G. V. & Naryanan J. T. (2005). 'Myasthenic crisis: Clinical features, complications and mortality.' *Neurology India 53*, 37-40.

[34] Qureshi, A. I., Choudhry, M. A., Akbar, M. S., et al. (1999). 'Plasma exchange versus intravenous immunoglobulin treatment in myasthenic crisis' *Neurology 52*, 629-632.

[35] Gracey, D. R., Divertie, M. B. & Howard, F. M., Jr. (1983). 'Mechanical ventilation for respiratory failure in myasthenia gravis: Two-year experience with 22 patients' *Mayo Clinic Proceedings 58*, 597-602.

[36] Romi, F., Gilhus, N. E. & Aarli, J. A. (2005). 'Myasthenia gravis: clinical, immunological, and therapeutic advances' *Acta Neurologica Scandinavica 111*, 134-141.

[37] Romi, F., Skeie, G. O., Aarli, J. A. & Gilhus, N. E.(2000). 'The severity of myasthenia gravis correlates with the serum concentration of titin and ryanodine receptor antibodies' *Archives of Neurology 57*, 1596-1600.

[38] Paul, R. H. & Gilchrist, J. M. (2003). 'Psychological and social consequences of myasthenia gravis' in Kaminski H. J. (Ed.) (2003). *Myasthenia Gravis and Related Disorders* Totowa, NJ: Humana Press, Inc. pp. 355-371.

[39] Padua, L., Evoli, A., Aprile, I., et al. (2001). 'Health-related quality of life in patients with myasthenia gravis and the relationship between patient-oriented assessment and conventional measures' *Neurological Sciences 22*, 363-369.

[40] Paul, R. H., Nash, J. M., Cohen R. A., et al. (2001) 'Quality of life and well-being of patients with myasthenia gravis' *Muscle and Nerve 24*, 512-516.

[41] Drachman, D. B. (1997). 'Myasthenia Gravis' *New England Journal of Medicine 330*, 1797-1810.

[42] Kaminski, H. J. (2003). 'Treatment of myasthenia gravis' in Kaminski H. J. (Ed.) (2003). *Myasthenia Gravis and Related Disorders* Totowa, NJ: Humana Press, Inc. pp. 355-371.

[43] Kupersmith, M. J., Latkany, R. & Homel, P. 'Development of generalized disease at 2 years in patients with ocular myasthenia gravis' *Archives of Neurology 60*, 243-248.

[44] Myasthenia Gravis Clinical Study Group (1993). 'A randomised clinical trial comparing prednisone and azathioprine in myasthenia gravis. Results of the second interim analysis.' *Journal of Neurology, Neurosurgery, and Psychiatry 56*, 1157-1163.

[45] Palace, J., Newsom-Davis, J., Lecky, B. (1998) 'A randomized double-blind trial of prednisolone alone or with azathioprine in myasthenia gravis. Myasthenia Gravis Study Group. *Neurology 50*, 1778-1783.

[46] Tindall, R. S., Rollins, J. A., Phillips, J. T., et al. (1987) 'Preliminary results of a double-blind, randomized, placebo-controlled trial of cyclosporine in myasthenia gravis' *New England Journal of Medicine 316*, 719-724.

[47] De Feo LG, Schottlender J, Martelli NA, Molfino NA. (2002) Use of intravenous pulsed cyclophosphamide in severe, generalized myasthenia. *Muscle and Nerve 26*, 31-36.

[48] Drachman, D. B., Jones, R. J., Brodsky, R. A. (2003) 'Treatment of refractory myasthenia: re-booting with high-dose cyclophosphamide' *Annals of Neurology 53*, 7-9.

[49] Meriggioli, M. N., Ciafaloni, E., Al-Hayk, K. A., et al. (2003) 'Mycophenolate mofetil for myasthenia gravis: an analysis of efficacy, safety and tolerability' *Neurology 61*, 1438-1440.

[50] Gajdos, P., Tranchant, C., Clair, B., et al. (2005) 'Treatment of myasthenia gravis exacerbation with intravenous immunoglobulin' *Archives of Neurology 62*, 1689-1693.

[51] Qureshi, A. I., Choudhry, M. A., Akbar, M. S., et al. (1999) 'Plasma exchange versus intravenous immunoglobulin treatment in myasthenic crisis' *Neurology 52*, 629-632.

[52] Wolfe, G. I., Kaminski, H. J., Jaretzki, A. 3rd, et al. (2003) 'Development of a thymectomy trial in nonthymomatous myasthenia gravis patients receiving immunosuppressive therapy' *Annals of the New York Academy of Sciences 998*, 473-480.

[53] Meryon E. On granular and fatty degeneration of the voluntary muscles (1852). *Med Chir Trans* 35:73.

[54] Duchenne de Boulogne GBA (1861). De l'electrisation localisee et de son application a la pathologie et a la therapeutique. Paris: Bailiere & Fils.

[55] Becker PE, Kiener F. Eine neue X-chromosomale muskeldystrophie (1955). *Arch Psychiatr Z Neurol* 193:427.

[56] Hoffman EP, Brown RH, Jr., Kunkel LM (1987). Dystrophin: the protein product of the Duchenne muscular dystrophy locus. *Cell 51*:919-928.

[57] Engel, A. G., Yamamoto, M. & Fischbeck, K. H. (2004). 'Dystrophinopathies' in Engel, A. G. & Franzini-Armstrong, C. (eds.) (2004). *Myology* (3rd edn.). New York: McGraw Hill, Inc. pp. 961-1025.

[58] Emery, A. E. (1991). 'Population frequencies of inherited neuromuscular diseases - a world survey' *Neuromuscular Disorders 1*, 19-29.

[59] Bushby, K. M. D. , Thambyayah, M. & Gardner-Medwin, D. (2002). 'Prevalence and incidence of Becker muscular dystrophy' *Lancet 337*, 1022-24.

[60] Carter, G. T. (1997). 'Rehabilitation management in neuromuscular disease' *Journal of Neurologic Rehabilitation 11*, 69-80.

[61] Fardeu-Gautier, M. & Fardeu, M. (1994). 'Socioeconomic aspects of neuromuscular disease.' In in Engel, A. G. & Franzini-Armstrong, C. (eds.) (2004). *Myology* (3rd edn.). New York: McGraw Hill, Inc. pp: 739-745.

[62] Vignos PJ, Wagner MB, Gashgarian B, Katirji B (1996). Evaluation of a Program for Long-Term Treatment of Duchenne Muscular Dystrophy. *J Bone Joint Dis 78(A)*:1844-1852.

[63] Wagner MB, Vignos PJ, Carlozzi C, Hull AL (1993). Assessment of hand function in Duchenne muscular dystrophy. *Arch Phys Med Rehabil 74*:801-804

[64] Eagle, M., Baudouin, S. V., Chandler, C., et. al. (2002). 'Survival in Duchenne muscular dystrophy: improvements in life expectancy since 1967 and the impact of home nocturnal ventilation' *Neuromuscular Disorders 12*, 926-9.

[65] American Thoracic Society (2004) 'Respiratory care of the patient with Duchenne muscular dystrophy: ATS consensus statement' *American Journal of Respiratory and Critical Care Medicine 170*, 456-65.

[66] Ireys, H. T., Anderson, G. F., Shaffer, T. J., et. al. (1997) 'Expenditures for care of children with chronic illnesses enrolled in the Washington state Medicaid program, fiscal year 1993' *Pediatrics 100*, 197-204.

[67] Moxley, R. T. 3rd, Ashwal, S., Pandya, S., et. al. (2005) 'Practice parameter: corticosteroid treatment of Duchenne dystrophy' *Neurology 64*, 13-20.

[68] Joncourt, F., Neuhaus, B., Jostarndt-Foegen, K., et al. (2004) 'Rapid identification of female carriers of DMD/BMD by quantitative real-time PCR' *Human Mutation 23*, 385-391.

[69] Harper, P. S. & Monckton, D. G. (2004). 'Myotonic Dystrophy' in Engel, A. G. & Franzini-Armstrong, C. (eds.) (2004). *Myology* (3rd edn.). New York: McGraw Hill, Inc. pp: 1039-1076.

[70] Ricker, K., Koch, M. C., Lehmann-Horn, F., et al. (1994). 'Proximal myotonic myopathy: A new dominant disorder with myotonia, muscle weakness, and cataracts' *Neurology 44*, 1448-1452.

[71] Ranum, L. P. W., Rasmussen, P., Benzow, K., et al. (1998). 'Genetic mapping of a second myotonic dystrophy locus' *Nature Genetics 19*, 196-198.

[72] Day JW, Roelofs R, Leroy B, et al. (1999). 'Clinical and genetic characteristics of a five-generation family with a novel form of myotonic dystrophy: DM2' *Neuromuscular Disorders 9*, 19-27.

[73] Ricker K, Grimm T, Koch M, et al. (1999). 'Linkage of proximal myotonic myopathy to chromosome 3q' Neurology *52*, 170-171.

[74] Harper, P. S. (2001). *Myotonic Dystrophy* (3rd Edn.) London: W. B. Saunders.

[75] Emery, A. E. (1991). 'Population frequencies of inherited neuromuscular diseases - a world survey' *Neuromuscular Disorders 1*, 19-29.

[76] Siciliano, G., Manca, M. L., Gennarelli, M., et al. (2001). 'Epidemiology of myotonic dystrophy in Italy: re-appraisal after genetic diagnosis' *Clinical Genetics 59*, 344-349.

[77] Day, J. W., Ricker, K, Jacobsen, J. F., et al. (2003). 'Myotonic dystrophy type 2: molecular, diagnostic and clinical spectrum' *Neurology 60*, 657-664.

[78] Osame, M. & Furusho, T. (1983). 'Genetic epidemiology of myotonic dystrophy in Kagoshima and Okinawa districts of Japan' *Clinical Neurology 23*, 1067-1071.

[79] Ashizawa, T. & Epstein, H. F. (1991). 'Ethnic distribution of myotonic dystrophy gene' *Lancet 338*, 642-643.

[80] Mathieu, J., De Braekeleer, M., Prevost, C, & Boily, C. (1992). 'Myotonic dystrophy: clinical assessment of muscular disability in an isolated population with presumed homogeneous mutation' *Neurology 42*, 203-308.

[81] de Die-Smulders, C. E. M., Höweler, C. J., Thijs, C., et al. (1998). 'Age and cause of death in adult-onset myotonic dystrophy' *Brain 121*, 1557-1563.

[82] Prevost, C., Veillette, S., Perron, M., et al. (2004). 'Psychosocial impact of predictive testing for myotonic dystrophy type 1' *American Journal of Medical Genetics 126A*, 68-77.

[83] Fowler, W. M., Abresch, R. T., Koch, T. R., et al. (1997). 'Employment profiles in neuromuscular diseases' *American Journal of Physical Medicine & Rehabilitation 76*, 26-32.

[84] Kwiecinski H., Ryniewicz B. & Ostrzycki A. (1992) 'Treatment of myotonia with antiarrhythmic drugs' *Acta Neurologica Scandinavica 86*, 371-375.

[85] Ørngreen, M. C., Olsen, D. B. &Vissing, J. (2005) 'Aerobic training in patients with myotonic dystrophy type 1' *Annals of Neurology 57*, 754-757.

[86] MacDonald, J. R., Hill, J. D. & Tarnopolsky, M. A. (2002) 'Modafinil reduces excessive somnolence and enhances mood in patients with myotonic dystrophy' *Neurology 59*, 1876-1880.

[87] Pelargonio, G., Della Russo, A., Sanna, T., et al. (2002) 'Myotonic dystrophy and the heart' *Heart* 665-670.

[88] Bromberg, M. B. (2005). 'Advances in diagnosis and management of inflammatory myopathies' *Journal of Clinical Neuromuscular Disease 6*, 167-179.

[89] Chou, S. (1967). 'Myxovirus-like structures in a case of human chronic polymyositis' *Science 158*, 1453-1455.

[90] Yunis, E. & Samaha, F. (1971). 'Inclusion body myositis' *Laboratory Investigation 25*, 240-248.

[91] Bohan, A. & Peter, J. B. (1975). 'Polymyositis and dermatomyositis (first of two parts)' *New England Journal of Medicine 292*, 344-347.

[92] Bohan, A. & Peter, J. B. (1975). 'Polymyositis and dermatomyositis (second of two parts)' *New England Journal of Medicine 292*, 403-407.

[93] Griggs, R. C., Askanas, V., DiMauro, S., et al. (1995). 'Inclusion body myositis and myopathies' *Annals of Neurology 38*, 705-713.

[94] Mastaglia, F. L. & Phillips, B. A. (2002). 'Idiopathic inflammatory myopathies: epidemiology, classification, and diagnostic criteria' *Rheumatic Disease Clinics of North America 28*, 723-741.

[95] Mendez, E. P., Lipton, R., Ramsey-Goldman, R., et al. (2003). 'US incidence of juvenile dermatomyositis, 1995-1998: results from the national institute of arthritis and musculoskeletal and skin diseases registry' *Arthritis and Rheumatism 49*, 300-305.

[96] Van der Meulen, M. F. G., Bronner, I. M., Hoogendijk, J. E., et al. (2003). 'Polymyositis: an overdiagnosed entity' *Neurology 61*, 316-321.

[97] Katirji, B., Kaminski, H. J., Preston, D. C., et al. (eds.) (2002). *Neuromuscular Disorders in Clinical Practice*. Boston: Butterworth-Heinemann.

[98] Chad, D. A. (2002). 'Inflammatory myopathies' in in Katirji, et al. (Eds.), *Neuromuscular Disorders in Clinical Practice*. Boston: Butterworth-Heinemann. pp: 1169-1180.

[99] Dalakas, M. C., Illa, I., Dambrosia, J. M., et al. (1993). A controlled trial of high-dose intravenous immune globulin infusions as treatment for dermatomyositis. *N Engl J Med 329*: 1993-2000.

[100] Choy, E. H. S., Hoogendijk, J. E., Lecky, B. & Winer, J. B. (2005). 'Immunosuppressant and immunomodulatory treatment for dermatomyositis and polymyositis' *Cochrane Database of Systematic Reviews 4*.

[101] Rider, L., Giannini, E., Brunner, H., et al. (2004). 'International consensus on preliminary definitions of improvement in adult and juvenile myositis' *Arthritis and Rheumatism 50*, 2281-2290.

[102] Dalakas, M. C., Sonies, B., Dambrosia, J., et al. (1997). 'Treatment of inclusion body myositis with IVIg: a double-blind, placebo-controlled study' *Neurology 48*, 712-716.

[103] Dalakas, M. C., Koffman, B., Fujii, M., et al. (2001). 'A controlled study of intravenous immunoglobulin combined with prednisone in the treatment of IBM' *Neurology 56*, 323-327.

[104] Badrising, J. A., Maat-Schieman, M. L., Ferrari, M. D., et al. (2002). 'Comparison of weakness progression in inclusion body myositis during treatment with methotrexate or placebo' *Annals of Neurology 51*, 369-372.

RECOMMENDED FURTHER READING

1. Brown RH Jr, Swash M, Pasinelli P (Editors.). *Amyotrophic Lateral Sclerosis.* 2nd Edition, London: Informa Healthcare, 2006.

2. Kaminski H. J. (Editor). *Myasthenia Gravis and Related Disorders* Totowa, NJ: Humana Press, Inc., 2003.

3. Katirji B, Kaminski HJ, Preston DC, Ruff RL, Shapiro BE (Editors). *Neuromuscular Disorders in Clinical Practice* Boston: Butterworth-Heinemann, 2002.

4. Engel AG and Franzini-Armstrong C. (Editors). *Myology.* 3rd Edition, New York: McGraw Hill, Inc., 2004.

5. Harper PS. *Myotonic Dystrophy.* 3rd Edition, London: W. B. Saunders, 2001.

6. Emery AE. 'Population frequencies of inherited neuromuscular diseases - a world survey' *Neuromuscular Disorders* 1, 19-29, 1991.

In: Handbook of Clinical Neuroepidemiology
Editors: V. L. Feigin and D. A. Bennett, pp. 339-389

ISBN 978-1-60021-511-7
© 2007 Nova Science Publishers, Inc.

Chapter 10

CENTRAL NERVOUS SYSTEM INFECTIONS

H. T. Chong and C. T. Tan

Department of Medicine, Faculty of Medicine, University of Malaya,
Kuala Lumpur 50603, Malaysia.

ABSTRACT

This chapter reviews the incidence and prevalence of central nervous system infections in developed and developing countries. It showed that the prevalence of bacterial meningitis is influenced by geography, age group, socioeconomic factors, seasonality and vaccination program. The commonest causes of bacterial meningitis are *H. influenzae b* (Hib), *Streptococcus pneumoniae* and *Neisseria meningitides,* streptococcus sp., *Listeria monocytogenese,* and *Escherichia coli.* In developed countries which have introduced Hib vaccination program, the incidence of Hib meningitis has dropped precipitously. In some developing countries such as China, India and Indonesia, tuberculous meningitis remains the commonest cause of meningitis, especially among children. Fungal meningitis is uncommon, except for cryptococcal meningitis. It is common among the immunosuppressed in developed countries, but equally common among the non-immunosuppressed in developing countries. The enteroviruses are probably the commonest cause of aseptic meningitis, which occurs mainly in children and are self-limiting. World-wide, Japanese encephalitis and herpes simplex encephalitis are the two most important cause of encephalitis. This chapter also reviews the salient clinical features, management and prevention strategies of these infections, as well as the neurological complications of various infections, such as enterovirus 71, malaria and HIV. Particular emphasis is paid to the emerging and re-emerging causes of central nervous system infections, namely enterovirus 71, West Nile and Nipah viruses.

INTRODUCTION

Central nervous system infection is an important aspect of neurology for many reasons. Worldwide it is one of the most prevalent neurological diseases; and in many, especially developing, countries, it is the commonest neurological disorder. The presentations of central nervous system infection are varied, and depended on both microbial and host factors, making precise clinical diagnosis difficult. Even with advanced molecular diagnostic tools, such as polymerase chain reactions, many patients had no definitive microbiological diagnosis upon discharge. Apart from bacterial infection, there is also a lack of effective therapeutic agents, and what are available are generally out of reach of the many in the poor countries who are most at risk. The important and prevalent causative agents varied from place to place, and so localized preventive measures are necessary for the control of the disease. The epidemiology of many infections are also rapidly changing, with emergence of new diseases, such as Nipah encephalitis in Malaysia and Bangladesh, and the spreading of previously known viruses to new areas, such as West Nile virus to the North America and Japanese encephalitis to Papua New Guinea and Australia. On the other hand, the incidence of bacterial meningitis is falling due to successful vaccination programs in developed countries. This chapter will look at bacterial, viral and various other infections of the nervous system.

BACTERIAL MENINGITIS

Bacterial meningitis is an uncommon disease. The causative agents are similar worldwide, with *H. influenzae* type b, *S. pneumoniae* and *N. meningitides* being the commonest in most regions. The exceptions are discussed below.

Epidemiology

Bacterial meningitis occurs at a baseline endemic rate that varies from place to place and from season to season, with occasional or rare outbreak (epidemic) of meningococcal disease. The peak incidence during the endemic period is seldom more than 2 or 3 times the trough incidence, but during epidemics or hyperepidemics of meningococcal disease, the rates may be 100 times or more of the peak endemic incidence. Specific incidence rates of various regions are shown in table 1. In some areas such as Hong Kong [59] and the Western Cape region of South Africa [39], however, the commonest cause of endemic non-viral meningitis was tuberculous meningitis. Tuberculous meningitis also constituted a significant burden of disease in some regions – in Swaziland 21% of meningitis was caused by *M. tuberculosis* [60] while in Egypt the percentage was up to 23% [35]. In most other countries, it was important in patients with HIV.

Table 1. Worldwide epidemiology of bacterial meningitis

Regions	Years	Age, yrs	Isolates in confirmed cases, $/10^5$ and/or %			
			H. inf. b	S. pneu.	N. Men.	Other
Canada* & US [1-5]	1964-1996	Mainly ≤ 16	$0.2\text{-}4.3/10^5$ 0*-66%	$0.9\text{-}2.3/10^5$ 11-27%	$0.8\text{-}2.1/10^5$ 2.5*-19%	$0.3\text{-}2.7/10^5$ 12-50%
Brazil & Chile [7-10]	1988-2001	Mainly < 20	$\sim 4.1/10^5$ 9.9-44.2%	$\sim 3.3/10^5$ 4.2-15.4%	$\sim 8.4/10^5$ 10-52.1%	$\sim 3.5/10^5$ ~22.1%
Europe [13-29]	1975-2002	All	$0.08\text{-}7.6/10^5$ 0-41%	$0.8\text{-}3.5/10^5$ 5.5-49%	$0.83\text{-}22/10^5$ 5.2-66%	$\sim 0.38/10^5$ 2-27.2%
Africa, meningitic belt [30-32]	1981-1996	All	2-42%	0-50%	3-95%	0.2-27%
Africa, non-meningitic belt [30-39]	1958-2000	All	4-57%	3.6-59%	0-82%	0-49%
Asia, Middle East [35, 40-44]	1981-1999	Mainly < 13	$\sim 16.88/10^5$ 28-66%	$\sim 9.69/10^5$ 11-35%	$\sim 10.77/10^5$ 0-29.6%	6-23%
Asia, South [45, 46]	1987-2001	All	3.6-47%	32-60%	~37%	-
Asia, East [47-51]	1984-2001	≤ 15	$\sim 6/10^5$ 35-60%	$\sim 2.1/10^5$ 8.3-20%	~ 38.3%	9-45%
Asia, Southeast [52-55]	1975-2000	All	0-53%	15-22.2%	0.6-12%	12.4-54.4%

*After H. influenzae type b vaccination.

~ Estimates based on small number of studies or subjects

Natural History and Outcomes

Patients with bacterial meningitis often present with fever, headache, meningism, impaired consciousness and focal neurological deficits. With the advent of antibiotic mortality has been reduced from over 70% to less than 20% in most countries. The overall mortality ranged from 3% – 19.8% [23,61] and 4.1% - 38% [10,62] of survivors had neurological deficits. Countries in Africa, except South Africa, however, consistently reported higher mortality and morbidity rates, with mortality ranged from 17% to 41% and 12.9% to 23.5% of survivors had neurological deficits.

Besides geography, mortality depended on several other factors; age, pathogen and concomitant medical conditions. Neonates with bacterial meningitis had mortality at least double of that of older children – in Japan, neonatal mortality was 8.2% compared with 4.1% of older patients [48], in Jordan 32% [63] compared with 12% [30], in Thailand 45% compared with 17% [54] and in Gambia 37% compared with 17% [64]. Patients with S. pneumoniae suffered from higher mortality than those with N. meningitides and H. influenzae meningitis, a difference noted consistently across many regions. Other poor prognostic factors included age over 60 years, presence of other medical conditions such as diabetes mellitus and malignancy, high white cell count in the cerebrospinal fluid, seizure, bacteremia, severe neurological deficits on the first day and coma at presentation [65-68].

A quarter to a third of survivors suffered from neurological deficits, which included hearing impairment (10-14%), motor deficits such as weakness or spasticity (3.5 – 30%), subdural effusion (23%), seizure (4 – 10%), developmental delay in children (9%), hydrocephalus (6%) and mental retardation (4%) [42,67].

Risk Factors

The incidence of bacterial meningitis is influenced by various factors such as sex, age, vaccination status, contact geography, socioeconomic situation and seasonal variation. Male is 1.7 to 2.4 times more likely than female to contract meningitis in most studies. Age is another important factors; neonates have much higher risk of developing meningitis than older children and adults, and the risk decreases with age [4,8]. Group B streptococcus and gram negative bacilli such as *E. coli, Pseudomonas* species, *Salmonella* species, and gram positive cocci such as *Staphylococcus epidemidis* are the common causes in neonates, while in children between 1 month and 5 years old *H. influenzae* type b was the commonest among those not vaccinated against the disease; in children and young adult from 5 to 29 years old, *N. meningitides* was the commonest; while in those older than 30 years old *S. pneumoniae* was the commonest. *Listeria monocytogenes* is an important cause in the extremes of age. Successful vaccination programs had dramatically reduced the incidence of *H. influenzae* type b meningitis in North American and some Western European countries (see section on Prevention below). Household contact is a well known risk factor for *H. influenzae* and *N. meningitides* diseases.

The incidence of various pathogens varies from place to place. From a worldwide perspective, *H. influenzae* is the commonest pathogen in Asia, *N. meningitides* in Europe, South America and the African meningitis belt countries, while *S. pneumoniae* in the rest of Africa and North America. The meningitic belt countries in Africa experience epidemics of meningococcal disease every 8 to 10 years since at least 1900. Estimates of endemic incidence of meningococcal meningitis during non-epidemic years in Niger yield a means annual rate of $45/10^5$ population, and this rose to $550/10^5$ population during epidemic years. [30,31] This is contrasted with an estimated annual incidence of all meningitides of $61/10^5$ population in Saudi Arabia, $9.3/10^5$ in Hefei, China, $5.5/10^5$ in Denmark and $2.32/10^5$ in Aichi, Japan [12,41,46,47].

Socioeconomic situations, such as household crowding, educational status and income, may be important risk factors for meningitis. In the United States, Afro-Americans were 2.1 – 2.6 times more likely to suffered from *S. pneumoniae, N. meningitides* and group B streptococcal meningitis compared with the whites [4]; and *H. influenzae* disease was commoner among the black and Asians in the United Kingdom [16]. Rarely, *Streptococcus suis* may cause meningitis in those coming into contact with pigs [56,57].

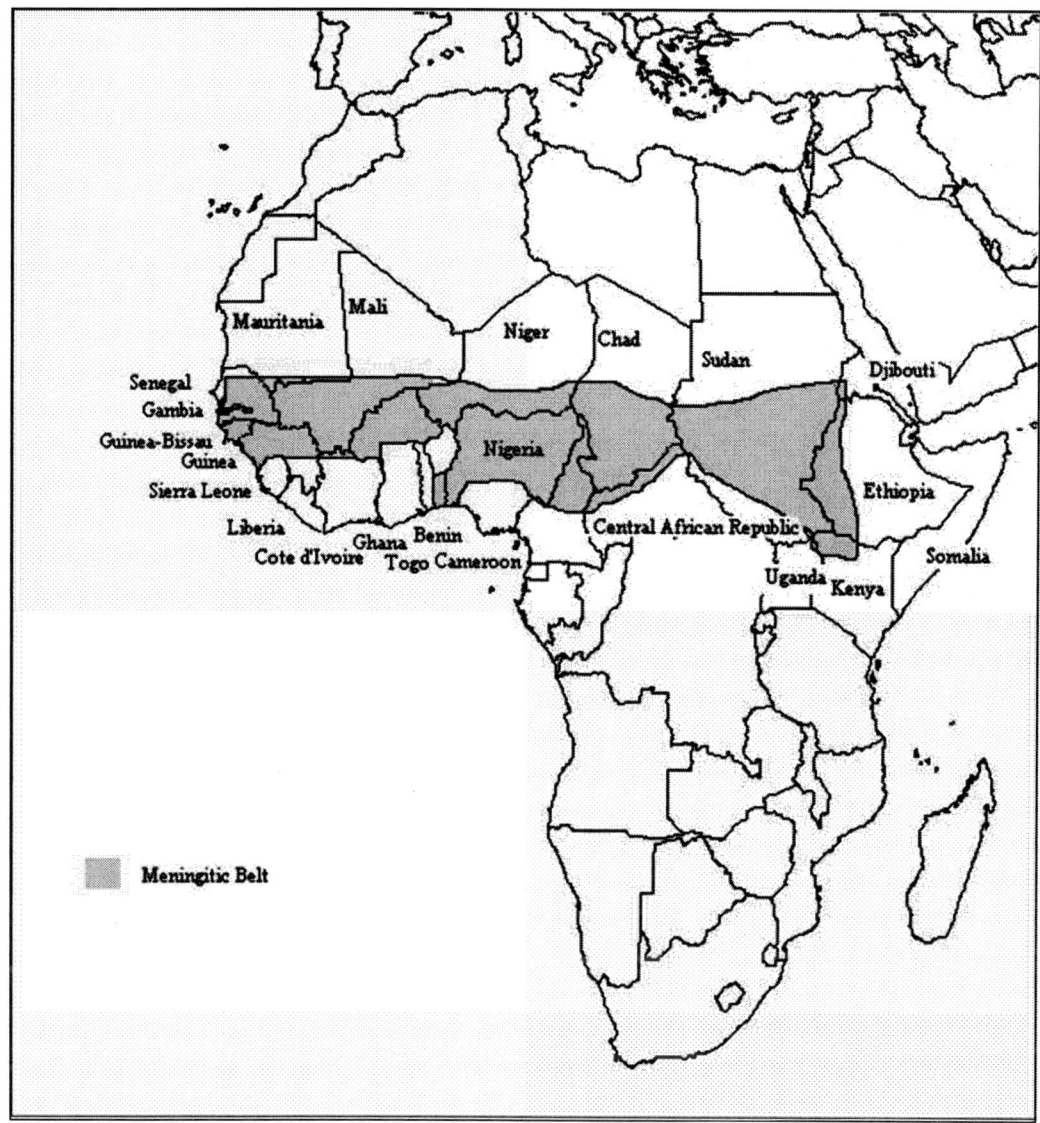

Figure 1. The Meningitic Belt of Africa

In North America and Europe, meningitis shows seasonal variation; meningococcal and pneumococcal diseases were common in the first quarter of the year, and hemophilus disease during the last quarter; while in the non-meningitic areas in Africa, meningococcal and pneumococcal disease peaked from February to April in the Northern Hemisphere and in the Southern Hemisphere, September and October. In Africa meningitic belt countries, meningitis occurred during the dry season (January to May). Seasonal variation was observed in the Saudi Arabia, with *H. influenzae* disease peak in March to May and September to November, but no seasonal variation was seen in China and Papua New Guinea.

Prevention

Successful vaccination program dramatically reduced the incidence of *H. influenzae* type b disease; in the United Kingdom, vaccination reduced the number of *H. influenzae* meningitis by 87% in the North East Thames region [16] and by 92% in Scotland [15]; while the United States, the proportion of *H. influenzae* meningitis had dropped from 66% to 12% of all meningitic cases. Similar trend was observed in Chile, with a drop from 36.4% to 9.9% [9]. In some areas, the fall in *H. influenzae* disease was accompanied by a rise in meningococcal disease [9,15], though such trend was not observed in other studies [2,16].

Pneumococcal vaccine is indicated in three groups of patients; adults older than 65 year-old, adults with chronic underlying diseases such as cardiopulmonary or renal diseases, diabetes mellitus, splenectomy and cerebrospinal fluid fistula, and immunocompromised patients older than 10 year-old, including individuals with HIV infections [68].

Tetravalent meningococcal or serogroup C polysaccharide vaccines are indicated in high risk groups, such as college freshmen [68] or population in high risk areas, such as the meningitic belt countries in Africa [69].

Family contacts of patients with meningococcal or *H. influenzae* meningitis should be given prophylactic antibiotic using rifampicin at a does of 20 mg/kg (maximum of 600 mg per-dose) for duration of 2 days to 4 days.

Management

The two epidemiologic trends that are important in considering antibiotic treatment of bacterial meningitis are firstly, the worldwide increase in infection with antibiotic-resistant strains of *S. pneumoniae* and secondly, the dramatic decline in *H. influenzae* disease in countries with successful vaccination program. In these countries, often *S. pneumoniae* and *N. meningitides* became the predominant causative agents. Treatment with empirical antibiotics should be instituted early, and guided by the patient's age and medical conditions (see Table 2).

Four double-blind randomized controlled trials in children older than 2 months had shown that dexamethasone therapy substantially reduced audiologic and neurologic complications. However, the majority of children enrolled in these trials suffered from *H. influenzae* meningitis. A more recent trial showed reduction of audiologic and neurologic complications in children with *S. pneumoniae* meningitis but the difference was not statistically significant [70]. Therefore, in children older than 2 months thought to have *H. influenzae* meningitis should be given dexamethasone slightly before or together with antibiotic therapy at a dose of 0.15 mg/kg every 6 hours for two to four days.

A recent double-blind randomized controlled trial showed that early adjunctive dexamethasone at a dose of 10 mg intravenous every 6 hour for 4 days reduced mortality due to *S. pneumoniae* meningitis in adults by more than 50% with no significant increase in adverse events. There was no significant reduction in neurologic or audiologic complications noted [71].

Table 2. Antibiotic treatment of bacterial meningitis

	Suggested antibiotic	
Patient condition	*Empirical Treatment*	
Preterm or low birth weight infants less than 1 month old	Broad spectrum third generation cephalosporin* and Vancomycin 15 mg/kg intravenous q6hr adjusted to therapeutic blood levels.	
Less than 3 months old	Broad spectrum third generation cephalosporin* and Ampicillin 100 mg/kg i.v. q8hr	
3 months to 50 years old	Broad spectrum third generation cephalosporin*	
Above 50 years old or patients with impaired cellular immunity	Broad spectrum third generation cephalosporin* and Ampicillin 2 g intravenous q4hr	
Neurosurgical or head trauma patients	Broad spectrum third generation cephalosporin* and Vancomycin adjusted to therapeutic blood levels.	
On Gram staining	*Choice of antibiotic*	
Gram positive cocci	Broad spectrum third generation cephalosporin* and Vancomycin15 mg/kg intravenous q6hr for 2 days	
Gram negative cocci	Penicillin G 300,000 units/kg/day up to 24 million units/day intravenous or Broad spectrum third generation cephalosporin* for resistant strains	
On culture		*Duration*
S. pneumoniae	Broad spectrum third generation cephalosporin* and Vancomycin 15 mg/kg intravenous q6hr for 2 days	10 – 14 days
H. influenzae	Ceftriaxone*	7 days
N. meningitides	Penicillin G 300,000 units/kg/day up to 24 million units/day intravenous or Broad spectrum third generation cephalosporin* for resistant strains	7 days
L. monocytogenes	Ampicillin 100 mg/kg intravenous q8hr of pediatric patients or 2 g intravenous q4hr for adults and Gentamicin	14 – 21 days
S. agalactiae	Penicillin G with or without gentamicin for the first 72 hours until bacterial susceptibility test is completed. If susceptible to penicillin, stop gentamicin and complete 10 – 14 days of penicillin G.	14 – 21 days
Enterobactericeae	Broad spectrum third generation cephalosporin* and Gentamicin	21 days
Pseudomonas aeruginosa or acinetobacter	Ceftazidime 50 – 100 mg/kg up to 2 g intravenous q8hr and Aminoglycoside	21 days

*Broad spectrum third generation cephalosporin – such as ceftriaxone 50 – 100 mg/kg for pediatric patients or 2 g for adults intravenous q12hr; or cefotaxime 50 mg/kg for pediatric patients or 2 g for adults intravenous q6hr. In neonates and patients with impaired cellular immunity, the preferred choice is cefotaxime; in others, ceftriaxone. Adapted from Quagliarello VJ and Scheld WM. 'Treatment of bacterial meningitis' *NEJM*, March 6, 1997. 336(10):708-716.

Apart from antimicrobial therapy, supportive therapy plays an important role. Patients with bacterial meningitis should ideally be monitored in the intensive care unit. Mechanical ventilatory support may be required in patients with impaired consciousness or respiratory complications. Seizure is common, occuring in, for example, 15% of patients with pneumococcal meningitis. Seizures need to be controlled rapidly, preferably with intravenous agents such as lorazepam or phenytoin. Hyponatraemia, often due to the Syndrome of Inappropriate Antidiuretic Hormone secretion, is also relatively common; and fluid and electrolytes balance needs careful attention. Unconscious patients are at risk of developing deep vein thrombosis and pulmonary embolism, and prophylactic subcutaneous heparin therapy may be indicated in immobile patients, except in patients who are septicaemic and have disseminated intravascular coagulopathy, and those with meningococcaemia are at particular risk. In patients with signs of raised intracranial pressure, such as abnormal doll eyes reflexes, bilateral Babinski's sign or rapidly worsening of conscious state, urgent scan of the brain is indicated as complications such as epidural effusion, intracranial abscess formation, obstructive hydrocephalus or hemorrhage need to be treated surgically. If the raised intracranial pressure is due to cerebral edema, raising the patient's head to 30°, hyperventilation and osmotic agent such as mannitol may be indicated. In patients with refractory raised intracranial pressure due to cerebral oedema, surgical decompression may be helpful. Other complications include secondary infections of the skin, genitourinary or respiratory tract, and complications of long term mechanical ventilation should ideally be prevented by meticulous nursing care and early tracheostomy.

VIRAL MENINGITIS AND ENCEPHALITIS

There is a long list of viral agents that cause central nervous system infections. Except for neonates, viral infections of the central nervous systems are far more common and varied than bacterial infection, but fortunately with much better outcomes. In the United Kingdom, neonatal viral meningitis had an incidence of 0.11/1000 live births, while bacterial meningitis had an incidence of 0.25/1000 live births [72]. In another study in Northern Finland, 12,000 children born in 1966 were followed up from birth to 14 year-old. The annual incidence of bacterial infection of the central nervous system was $36.3/10^5$, while that of viral was $688/10^5$. While 14.5% of children with bacterial meningitis died, only 4.5% of those with viral infection died; and 30.9% of children developed neurological sequelae after bacterial infection, only 8.1% developed such deficits after viral infection. Central nervous system infections caused 7.6% of all death from 28 days to 14 years old, 6.6% of hearing deficits and 3% of neurological deficits [73]. There is an overlap of both the etiologic agents and clinical features between viral meningitis and encephalitis; and in meningoencephalitis, both pathologic processes may coexist. Enteroviruses, though commonly cause aseptic meningitis, may cause encephalitis in about 3% of patients; West Nile virus causes encephalitis in about half the patients and aseptic meningitis in a quarter of the patients. Patient with meningitis or encephalitis have fever, headache, impaired conscious state and seizure. Meningitis and encephalitis are discussed here separately because the bulk of the epidemiologic studies focus on either one or the other, and the fact that aseptic meningitis carries a better prognosis.

Epidemiology

The commonest cause of viral meningitis worldwide is the enteroviruses. They are small, positive sense RNA viruses. There are more than 60 distinct serotypes of enteroviruses divided into 5 subgroups: the polioviruses (3 serotypes), coxsackievirus A (23 serotypes), coxsackievirus B (6 serotypes), echoviruses (31 serotypes) and enteroviruses (10 serotypes). In 55% - 70% of presumed viral meningitis, a specific viral pathogen is identified; and non-polio enteroviruses account for 85% - 95% of all cases [74]. This means that the enteroviruses account for a third to half of the presumed viral meningitis, a figure that is consistent in many, though not all countries. 63.4% of childhood viral meningitis in Tunisia was caused by enteroviruses [75], so was 45.3% of childhood aseptic meningitis in Singapore [76], 45.2% in France [77], 26.3% in Spain [78], 27% in South Africa [79], and 24% - 61.3% in the United States [74].

Human is probably the only significant natural host for the enteroviruses. They are spread by fecal-oral, and occasionally, by respiratory droplet transmission. In temperate countries, the spread is facilitated by the warm weather and enteroviral infection peaks in summer to fall. In warm countries, the incidence is high all year round. Although there are over 60 serotypes of enteroviruses, often only a few serotypes dominate. In the United States, the 15 most common serotypes account for more than 85% of all enteroviral isolates. The predominate serotypes were probably endemic in a particular geographical location, and cause cyclical outbreaks depending on a variety of factors, including the availability of new, susceptible host populations, who are often young children. Non-endemic serotypes or serotypes that have been absent for several years, once introduced into a particular community, are more likely to cause epidemics or even pandemic infection affecting older children or adults [74].

Some serotypes of enteroviruses are more likely to cause meningitis than others; in the United States, the six commonest serotypes were echovirus 11, 9, coxsackievirus B5, echovirus 30, 4 and 6. A survey of 49 outbreaks reported throughout the world since 1974 revealed that echovirus 30, 4, 18, 13 and 16 were the most commonly reported causes of aseptic meningitis outbreaks (in decreasing order). The other coomon serotypes included echovirus 6, 7, 9, 11, 18, 33, and coxsackievirus A9, B4, B5. Most of the outbreaks involved less than 300 patients [74,80-122].

Prior to the introduction of the live attenuated mumps vaccine, mumps meningitis was one of the commonest causes of aseptic meningitis. Cerebrospinal fluid pleocytosis occurred in half of the patients with mumps parotitis, though most were asymptomatic. Symptoms of meningitis were reported in up to 30% of all patients with mumps parotitis by 4 to 10 days of illness, though meningitis may precede parotitis by up to 7 days, and half or more of mumps meningitis may not be associated with parotitis at all. 4 – 35% of patients with parotitis develop encephalitis. The incidence of mumps before vaccination was $76.3/10^5$ in the United States in 1968 and $21/10^5$ in the United Kingdom in 1987. After the widespread use of the live attenuated vaccine, the incidence dropped to $0.66/10^5$ in the United States in 1993 and less than $1/10^5$ in the United Kingdom in 1997. Similar findings were noted in Finland [74,123].

The commonest syndrome of herpes simplex meningitis occur concomitant with or shortly after primary HSV-2 genital infection. More than a third of women and 11% of men develop aseptic meningitis after primary HSV-2 genital infection, while primary HSV-1 is less often associated with aseptic meningitis and non-primary genital infection with either HSV type rarely results in meningitis. Overall HSV causes 1-3% of all cases of aseptic meningitis.

Other viruses that commonly cause aseptic meningitis include arboviruses, Epstein-Barr virus, influenza virus and in the seroconversion illness caused by human immunodeficiency virus.

The commonest cause of encephalitis varies from place to place. In developed regions, such as Western Europe, Northern America and some parts of Asia, the herpesviruses are the commonest cause of encephalitis – in children, the varicella zoster virus causes 22% - 35% [123,124] of encephalitis with a diagnosis, while in adults, the herpes simplex virus causes 16% - 24% [125,126] of encephalitis. In less developed regions, the arboviruses are the commonest cause; in Eastern Europe, Central European tick-borne encephalitis is responsible for 29% - 53% of encephalitis with a diagnosis [127,128]; while Japanese encephalitis causes 18% - 22% of encephalitis in Southeast Asia; among children the proportion is even higher, from 31% to 67% [129-131]. Worldwide, Japanese encephalitis is numerically the most important cause, with an estimated 20 000 – 50 000 cases, and a mortality of 15 000 deaths per annum. It causes more mortality and morbidity than all the other arboviruses combined. [132,133] However, only 40% - 69% of encephalitis had a definitive diagnosis, [134,135] and it is estimated that even in developed regions, only a small proportion all encephalitis is caused by herpes simplex virus (about 10% - 32% of all encephalitis) with the larger undiagnosed proportion presumably caused by arboviruses [134,136,137].

The overall incidence of viral encephalitis is $1/10^5$ to $7.4/10^5$; but is higher among children; in those from 1 to 2 years old the incidence is as high as $16.7/10^5$ per-annum [138]. The incidence of herpes simplex encephalitis ranges from 0.1 to $0.84/10^5$ per-annum [134,139]. Other common causes of encephalitis include other herpesviruses (human herpes virus type 6 and 7, B virus, and in the immunosuppressed, cytomegalovirus and Epstein-Barr virus), rabies, coxsackievirus type B, other non-polio enteroviruses, adenovirus, and in areas without adequate immunization programs, mumps, measles and rubella in the newborn.

Enteroviral infection of the central nervous system is usually mild except for enterovirus serotype 71 (EV71). It was first isolated in California in 1969 from a child with aseptic meningitis and outbreaks of EV71 infection have since occurred in the United States [140], Australia, Sweden, Japan, Malaysia, Singapore and Taiwan. In 1975 it caused an outbreak in Bulgaria with 705 cases of poliomyelitis-like illness; 93% of which occurred in children under five year-old, and the death of 44 people [141]. In 1986, it caused an outbreak of hand, foot and mouth disease and herpangina in southeast Australia which primarily affected children under 5 years of age, and half of those affected had severe symptoms of central nervous system involvement [116]. In recent years, it has caused recurrent outbreaks in the Asia Pacific region. The first of these recent outbreaks occurred in Sarawak, Malaysia, in 1997; which was then followed by smaller outbreaks in Malaysia and Japan. In 1998 the outbreaks continued in Singapore and Taiwan, and here in Taiwan the largest outbreak was recorded. Epidemiologic study indicated that the approximately 130 000 reported cases probably represented less than 10% of the estimated total number of cases. 400 of these children were admitted into hospital with central nervous system involvement and 78 died of brainstem encephalitis and neurogenic pulmonary edema. In 1999 a hand-foot-and-mouth disease outbreak occurred in Perth, Western Australia, and in 2000 outbreaks occurred in Korea, Japan, Singapore, Taiwan and Peninsular Malaysia with patients presenting with a range of clinical manifestation that included aseptic meningitis, encephalitis, poliomyelitis-like disease and hand-foot-and-mouth disease. Molecular epidemiology study suggested that the source country of these outbreaks is probably Malaysia, where 4 subgenogroups co-circulated from 1997 to 2000 and some of these subgenogroups subsequently circulated to other Asia Pacific countries causing outbreaks [141].

Among the 533 arboviruses and zoonosis that have been identified worldwide, more than 20 of these cause encephalitis in humans. Fortunately most of these have restricted geographical distribution. Japanese encephalitis and West Nile encephalitis viruses are the two exceptions. Japanese encephalitis was first described in Japan in the 1870's. Since then it has spread to China, Far East Russia, Korea, Southeast and South Asia, the Philippines, New Guinea, Guam Island and Northern Australia. Japanese encephalitis virus is transmitted by Culex mosquitoes between birds and pigs, both of which develop high viraemia and are important in maintaining, amplifying and spreading the virus to new areas or transmission to human. Human does not develop significant viraemia, and is thus a dead-end host. Human become infected when living close to the enzootic cycle of the virus; therefore cases are found in the rural areas and city edges. As the Culex mosquitoes breed in pools of stagnant water, their numbers increase tremendously after the monsoon rain, and human infection soon follows. In northern areas, from Far East Russia to Thailand and northern India, huge epidemics occur during the summer months, while in southern areas (south Thailand and South Vietnam, Malaysia, Philippines, Sri Lanka and Indonesia), it is endemic with sporadic cases occurring throughout the year. Climatic data suggests that the number of infection follows temperature closely; with a sharp rise in cases during summer months with temperature above 20°C, possibly reflecting longer mosquito larval development time and longer extrinsic incubation period of the virus in cool temperature, thus reducing transmission rate. It is mainly a disease of children and young adults. However, when epidemics affected new areas, adults were also affected, perhaps more severely so than patients from endemic areas. The reasons for the spread of Japanese encephalitis across the vast geographical regions in Asia and Asia Pacific and the falling number of cases in developed countries are not completely understood; changes in agricultural practices, increasing irrigation, animal husbandry, mass vaccination program and even weather conditions have all been attributed to the changing pattern of Japanese encephalitis infection [133].

West Nile virus is a flavivirus closely related to Japanese encephalitis and St Louis encephalitis viruses. It was first identified to cause human disease in 1937 in Uganda. The reservoir is birds and the Culex mosquitoes transmit it. Migratory birds are probably important in transporting the disease throughout the endemic regions in Africa, the Mediterranean countries and the Middle East, where it often causes meningitis in humans. Cases have been recorded as far as Australia. Severe encephalitis cause by West Nile virus was seen in the 1950 outbreak in Israel [132]. The first major epidemic outside the previous geographical location occurred in Romania in 1996, where 393 patients were affected, most of whom had meningoencephalitis and a case fatality rate of 4.3% was reported, mostly among those over 50 years of age [142,143]. In summer 1999, 102 patients from the Volgograd and Krasnodar regions in Russia suffered from an epidemic of meningitis and meningoencephalitis, which was retrospectively diagnosed to be West Nile encephalitis [144]. In August the same year, an epidemic of West Nile virus affecting 62 patients with 7 mortality occurred in New York, marking the first appearance of this virus in the western hemisphere [139]. By 2002, West Nile virus has spread to the Pacific coast with cumulative human cases numbered 3900 and more than 250 deaths [145]. In the United States, the epidemic typically occurs from July to December, peaking in late August and early September. Even though the vast majority of human infections are transmitted by infected mosquitoes, transmissions through organ transplantation, transfusion of blood products and vertically, either transplacentally or through breast milk have been documented.

An outbreak of new, fatal, encephalitis caused by a novel paramyxovirus, later named Nipah virus, occurred among pig farmers in Malaysia from September 1998 to May 1999. Subsequently, the same virus was found to cause outbreaks with prominent respiratory involvement in Bangladesh, affecting mainly children. The natural reservoir and host of the Nipah virus is believed to be the fruit bats (*Pteropus hypomelanus* and *Pteropus vampyrus*). In the Malaysian outbreak, it is believed deforestation and industrial plantation led to substantial reduction in the fruit bats habitat. In 1997/1998, slush-and-burn agricultural practice caused severe haze in most of the Southeast Asia. Coupled with the severe drought brought on by the El-Nino Southern Oscillation, there was an acute reduction in the flowering and fruiting of trees in forest foraged by the fruit bats. Intensive farming practices, where fruit trees were planted within the compound of large pig farms to supplement income attracted the fruit bats. The virus is excreted in the bats urine and saliva; and the pigs probably contracted the virus through exposure to the bats urine or saliva on half eaten fruits. Transmission between pigs and from pigs to human occurred through contact with bodily excretion of infected pigs. Human to human transmission was documented in nosocomial contact, though rarely. [146] The first outbreak occurred in Perak, affecting only a small number of pigs and pig farmers. Subsequent transportation of infected pigs spread the virus to the largest pig farm area in Malaysia in Bukit Pelanduk, culminating in the outbreak that affected a total of 265 patients with 105 deaths. Culling of over a million pigs in the area finally brought the outbreak under control [147]. Nipah outbreaks recurred in Bangladesh in 2001 and 2003 but did not involve pigs. It was believed that the patients in Bangladesh contracted the virus directly from bats [148], even though a previous study suggested that bat to human transmission is probably inefficient [149]. Human to human transmission too was thought to be important in the Bangladesh outbreak as relatives with close contact with patients became ill, in keeping with documented cases of nosocomial transmission of the virus during the Malaysian outbreak [146]. As the outbreak was recurrent in Bangladesh, and fruit bats from as far as Cambodia were shown to be seropositive to Nipah or Nipah-like virus, there is a risk of wider geographical recurrence of Nipah infection in South and Southeast Asia.

Rabies virus continues to be endemic worldwide except Antarctica and some island populations, such as New Zealand, Britain, Japan and Hawaii. Over 35 000 people die of rabies each year, and an estimated 25 000 of these in India alone. In most countries in Asia,

Africa and South America, dogs are the major reservoir of rabies; dogs and cats bites account for over 90% of all human rabies infection. In some countries, other animals are important reservoir; such as raccoons on the East Coast and skunks and foxes in the rest of North America, mongooses and meerkats in South Africa, jackals in Southeast Asia, and cattle and vampire bats in South America. Rarely rabies can be transmitted by corneal transplantation and possibly by respiratory droplets. [132] The incidence of rabies is between 0.1 to $1/10^5$ in most Asian countries, and less than $0.1/10^5$ in South America, depending on the incidence of dog bites. [150]

In the New World, common causes of encephalitis, besides herpes simplex virus, are the California serogroup encephalitis, St. Louis encephalitis, Western, Eastern and Venezuelan equine encephalitides. Among the 15 viruses in the California serogroup of bunyaviruses, 5 are known to cause human illness, though almost all human cases of encephalitis are caused by LaCrosse virus. The principle vector of LaCrosse virus is the *Aedes triseriatus* mosquitoes, and the main amplifying hosts are chipmunks and squirrels, with humans as the incidental dead-end hosts. More than 90% of California serogroup encephalitis had occurred in Minnesota, Wisconsin, Iowa, Illinois, Indiana and Ohio. LaCrosse virus encephalitis is endemic, with 70 – 100 cases reported annually. Incidence peaks in summer, with approximately 90% of infection affecting children less than 15 years old, and nearly twice as many boys as girls are affected.

St. Louis viral encephalitis is the second commonest type of arboviral encephalitis in the United States. It affects the Ohio-Mississippi valley, Minnesota, eastern Texas, Louisiana, Florida, Kansas, Colorado and California. The principle vector is the *Culex* species of mosquitoes, and the virus is amplified in small perching and pigeon-like birds, such as sparrows, robins and doves. When conditions are optimal for viral transmission, the virus spills out of enzootic cycle and infects human incidentally. Since first described in 1933, multi-states epidemics of St. Louis encephalitis had been documented approximately every 10 years. Patients of all age groups are susceptible in epidemics, though the elderly is often the first to be affected [68,137].

Western equine encephalitis affects mainly the western states. It is mainly transmitted by the *Culex tarsalis* mosquitoes, the same vector as St. Louis virus. This species of mosquitoes switches its feeding preference from avians in early summer to mammals in the mid-to-late summer; therefore, equine and human diseases peak in August and September. Because of shrinking number of horses, the availability of equine vaccine and improved vector control, the incidence has fallen steadily. Since 1988, an average of less than 5 cases has been reported annually. In human, infants are more susceptible to encephalitis, and about 20% of patients are younger than 1 year old [68,137].

Eastern equine encephalitis is the most lethal arboviral encephalitis in the United States. It occurs almost exclusively along the Atlantic and Gulf coasts, with single cases occurring farther inland. The chief vector is the *Culiseta melanura* mosquitoes, a strictly ornithophilic mosquitoes that breed in highly specific microenvironment, resulting in its confined geographical spread. Human disease occurs when less specific mosquitoes ventured into its ecologic domain [68,137].

Venezuelan equine encephalitis affects South and Central America and Florida. The principle vectors are the *Aedes* and *Culex* mosquitoes, and small rodents as the mammalian hosts. Humans are infected when venture into the territory. Venezuelan equine encephalitis occurs in both the endemic and the epidemic forms [132].

Tick-borne encephalitis is caused by a number of antigenically related flaviviruses, which infects tick populations throughout the northern woodlands of the world. These viruses are distributed widely, from Siberia across to Scandinavia, the Vienna Woods, the Black Forest of Europe, to Belgium, Scotland, Northern Ireland, the Canadian forest, northern United States and Japan. These groups of viruses include the Western and Eastern tick-borne encephalitis viruses which are distributed in western and Eastern Europe, and Siberia and Northern Asia respectively, Negishi virus in Japan, Powassan virus in North America, and Kyasanur forest virus in Mysore, India [68]. These viruses are transmitted by the *Ixodes* ticks, and tick-borne encephalitis is endemic in the northern woodlands. Since the 1990's the incidence of Western tick-borne encephalitis has increased dramatically in western and eastern Europe. In Baden-Wurttemberg, Germany, the incidence is $1.2/10^5$ per annum, and in Lithuania, the incidence peaked at 1997 at $17.4/10^5$ per annum. The increase is probably due to the increase in the tick population [151,152].

Besides the herpesviruses (herpes simplex virus type 1 and 2, Epstein-Barr virus, cytomegalovirus, human herpes virus 6 and 7 and Herpes B virus), arboviruses, enterovirus and zoonotic viruses, the other viruses that are common causes of viral encephalitis include rabies, mumps and measles viruses. The human immunodeficiency virus also causes an infectious encephalopathy. Other conditions that may mimic viral encephalitis are neurosyphilis, tuberculous meningitis, rickettsial infection, trypanosomiasis, acute disseminated encephalomyelitis, pseudomigraine with pleocytosis, central nervous system vasculitis, multiple micrometastasis from distant malignancy and paraneoplastic limbic encephalitis.

Natural History and Outcomes

The clinical features of central nervous system infection depend on the anatomic localization of the infection. If the infection is limited to the meninges and the ependymal surfaces, the clinical manifestations are limited to fever, headache, neck stiffness, meningism and cerebrospinal fluid pleocytosis; clinically recognized as meningitis. If the infection involves the brain parenchymal, there are often signs of confusion, impaired consciousness, focal neurological deficits and even seizure, which are clinically recognized as encephalitis. The intimate anatomic and vascular relationship in the central nervous system, however, determines a degree of associated inflammatory involvement of the meninges in encephalitis and *vice versa*. Therefore the term meningoencephalitis is often used. Encephalopathy, disruption of the brain function not directly due to infection, may also occur. This can be either caused by prolonged seizures, vascular supply compromise (such as in meningovascular syphilis), or metabolic disturbances (hypoglycemia in malaria). The clinical manifestation, natural history and outcomes also depend on the etiologic agent, the host's age and immune status.

Enteroviral infections presents with a spectrum of severity depending on host factors. In neonates, enteroviral infections often cause a systemic illness in which meningoencephalitis is commonly a part. Depending on the serotypes of the virus, meningitis or meningoencephalitis affects 27% to 75% of neonates. The patients often present with fever, anorexia, vomiting, rash and respiratory findings. Systemically, there are often signs of meningitis or meningoencephalitis, with seizure and focal neurological deficits, often indistinguishable from herpes simplex encephalitis. The infection then could progress on to myocarditis, hepatitis or hepatic necrosis, necrotizing enterocolitis and even disseminated intravascular coagulopathy. Morbidity and mortality are as high as 74% and 10% respectively [74].

In older infants, the outcome is better; though the short term morbidity may still be substantial and the duration prolonged. Constitutional symptoms such as fever, headache and myalgia; gastrointestinal complaints such as anorexia, vomiting, diarrhea and respiratory complaints are common. About half has meningism. Certain serotypes are associated with particular clinical features, such as EV 71 causing herpangina, hand-foot-and-mouth disease and fatal rhombencephalitis in children under the age of 5; maculopapular rash in Echovirus serotype 9 and myocarditis in coxsackieviruses. Older children and adults often present with fever, headache, and mild meningism. The illness lasts 1 to 2 weeks and the prognosis is good. Since enteroviruses are cleared from the host by antibody-mediated immunity, patients with agammaglobulinemia may develop chronic meningitis or meningoencephalitis, which could last many years and often ends fatally [74].

Aseptic meningitis caused by other viruses is typically mild and undifferentiated by clinical features. HSV-2, and occasionally HSV-1 and EBV, may cause benign, recurrent aseptic meningitis with symptom-free intervals, called Mollaret's meningitis [74].

Herpes simplex encephalitis, almost always caused by HSV type 1, is one of the commonest causes of endemic encephalitis worldwide. It is also among the most severe human central nervous system infections. Patients with herpes simplex encephalitis present with several days history of fever, headache, alter mentation, impaired consciousness, personality change, memory loss, focal neurological deficits, seizures and papilloedema. On magnetic resonance imaging, T2 weighted and FLAIR images often show hyperintensity on the medial and basal temporal lobe extending up to the insula. Electroencephalogram show unilateral or bilateral temporal lobe periodic sharp-and-waves. Cerebrospinal fluid examination shows raised opening pressure, a lymphocytic pleocytosis of 5 to 500 cells/mm^3, though often less than 200 cells/mm^3; a mild to moderate elevation in protein level and a normal or mildly reduced sugar level. There may be red cells or xanthochromia reflecting the hemorrhagic nature of the encephalitis. Viral culture is almost always negative, and brain biopsy, though specific, is neither sensitive nor without complication. Polymerase chain reaction with or without concurrent serological study on the cerebrospinal fluid has largely supplanted brain biopsy in the investigation of herpes simplex encephalitis as it is rapid, has a sensitivity of 95% and specificity of close to 100% [153]. The outcome of herpes simplex encephalitis is poor. In untreated or inappropriately treated patients, mortality is over 70%; and only 2.5% of all patients (9.1% of survivors) return to normal function after recovery [154]. Important prognostic factors include the age of the patients (patients less than 30 years of age have better prognosis), the level of consciousness at the onset of disease, the adequacy of therapy and the number of viral DNA copies in the cerebrospinal fluid [154,155].

Only 1 in 25 to 1 in 1000 of human Japanese encephalitis infections is symptomatic. Patients with Japanese encephalitis usually present with a few days history of constitutional, respiratory and gastrointestinal symptoms; specifically there is fever, coryza, diarrhea, headache, vomiting, followed by seizures, especially in younger children, and impaired consciousness. In older children and in adults, abnormal behavior may be the only initial sign. A proportion of patients make a rapid and spontaneous recovery. Other may present with aseptic meningitis without features of encephalitis. In patients with encephalitis, seizure occurs in 85% of children and 10% of adults. Generalized tonic-clonic seizure is commoner than focal motor seizures, and in a proportion of children, subtle motor seizure with twitching of a finger, eyelid, mouth, or eye deviation, nystagmus, salivation or irregular breathing pattern may occur. Multiple seizure and status epilepticus are associated with poor outcome. On examination, the classical features of Japanese encephalitis are extrapyramidal signs, which include a dull, flat, mask-like facies, tremor, cogwheel rigidity and hypertonia. Head nodding, pill-rolling tremor, choreathetosis, facial grimacing and lip smacking are often present as well. Though seen in 70 – 80% of adults American service personnel, these features are only seen in 20-40% of Indian children. Other signs include upper motor neuron facial nerve palsy, present in about 10% of children which may be intermittent and subtle, and flaccid paralysis in 5 – 20% of patients. A subgroup of patients may present first with acute flaccid paralysis after a short febrile illness, and though 30% of them eventually develop encephalitis, in the majority, acute flaccid paralysis is the only feature. Signs that herald poor prognosis include opisthotonus and rigidity spasms (which occurs in up to 15% of patients), changes of respiratory pattern, flexor or extensor posturing, pupillary or oculocephalic reflex abnormality. On investigation, peripheral blood neutrophilia and hyponatraemia due to SIADH may be present. Cerebrospinal fluid examination shows that the opening pressure is increased in half of the patients; there is typically a moderate pleocytosis of 10 – 100 cells/mm^3 of predominantly lymphocytes, mild increase in protein (50 – 200 mg/dl) and normal sugar levels. Computerized tomography scan of the brain showed non-enhancing hypodensity in the basal ganglia, thalamus and brainstem in half of the patients. Magnetic resonance imaging is more sensitive, showing T2 weighted images hypointense lesions more extensively, in the above areas, as well as in the cerebral hemispheres and cerebellum. Electroencephalographic abnormalities are varied, and include alpha, theta or delta coma, burst suppression pattern, epileptiform activities and/or diffuse slowing. After the first few days of illness, IgM detection by ELISA in the cerebrospinal fluid has a sensitivity and specificity of more than 95%. Polymerase chain reaction to detect viral RNA is available, though its reliability has not been tested. Mortality is about 30%, and 50% of survivors has significant neurological. About 30% of survivors have motor deficits, which include weakness, hypertonia, fixed deformities of limbs and extrapyramidal signs. 20% of survivors have severe cognitive impairment. Children are more likely than adults to have neurological deficits upon recovery. Among the other 50% of patients who have good recovery, half have subtle neurological deficits, such as learning disability, behavioral problems and mild neurological signs [133].

In West Nile infection, only 1: 140 to 1:320 of the patients infected is symptomatic. In the Romanian, Russian and the United States outbreaks in 1996 and 1999 the commonest presentation was meningoencephalitis. Prior to this, the virus is known to cause benign febrile illness with arthralgias in much of Africa and Middle East and encephalitis was rare. The encephalitic patients present after an incubation period of 2 - 14 days with acute onset of fever, headache, sore throat, malaise, myalgias, nausea, abdominal pain, diarrhea, vomiting, arthralgias and lymphadenopathy. Half has maculopapular rash. Less than 15% of patients progressed to encephalitis, but those who do has impaired conscious state, disorientation and focal neurological deficits, such as limb weakness, cranial nerve palsies, seizures, abnormal movements, sensory deficits and abnormal reflexes. Acute flaccid paralysis of the limbs, respiratory and bulbar muscles due to anterior horn cells involvement are common, and may occur without features of encephalitis. In those under 18, the illness is less common and milder. Investigation showed cerebrospinal fluid lymphocytic pleocytosis and IgM antibody captured ELISA is positive in the cerebrospinal fluid for up to 500 days [156,157]. Mortality rate is approximately 12%, with those over the age of 68 accounted for all death in the recent North American outbreak. Among the survivors of meningitis or encephalitis, persistent fatigue, myalgias, headache, poor memory, myoclonus of the upper limb or face, postural or kinetic tremor and parkinsonism were common, though the latter is usually mild. Most patients recovered sufficiently well to be discharged, and more than two thirds were functioning independently. Patients with acute flaccid paralysis, however, often show no improvement in limb function, though sphincteric functions recovered well. Electromyography in these patients showed persistent, chronic denervation changes [158].

Only 15% of victims bitten by rabid dogs developed rabies. The likelihood of developing rabies after rabid animal bites depends on the species of animal, location and severity of the bite, and whether the bite is through clothing that mechanically removes saliva from the teeth. The incubation period of human rabies is generally between 15 days and 1 year, though incubation period of up to 6 years had been documented. The clinical manifestations of rabies are varied. Clinical rabies starts with prodrome of malaise, anorexia, fever and headache. More than half of the patients complained of pain and paraesthesiae at the site of bite 1 to 14 days before the onset of other signs. The encephalitic form of rabies (so called "furious rabies") starts with anxiety, nervousness, and within hours or days, the patient becomes confused with alternating lucid intervals, and developed bizarre behavior with prominent autonomic signs such as mydriasis and piloerection. As the disease progresses, periods of severe agitation and aggressiveness alternate with drowsiness, and aerophobia and hydrophobia with pharyngeal and diaphragmatic spasms in almost all patients. These signs abate when the patient becomes comatose and die. In about 20% of patients, especially in those with bat-transmitted disease, the paralytic form (so called "dumb rabies") may develop. These patients develop fever and a Guillian-Barre-like syndrome of progressive flaccid paralysis and respiratory failure. Classical rabies encephalitic features are absent. The difference in clinical manifestations is probably due to host immune response 132].

In the outbreak of Nipah virus infection in Malaysia in 1998 – 1999, about 75% of patients suffered from a systemic infection with prominent encephalitic features, while the other 25% were asymptomatic. After an incubation of 2 – 14 days (ranges from 1 to 32 days), the patient presents with fever, headache, chills and rigors, myalgia, dizziness, anorexia, vomiting and cough. Clinically the patient is often drowsy, confused with generalized hyporeflexia. Over the next few days, segmental myoclonus involving the diaphragm, limb and facial muscles soon develops. This is followed by severe dysautonomia, with severe hyperthermia, tachycardia, hypertension, and signs of brainstem involvement. The patient then rapidly decompensates and dies of severe, irreversible shock. In the Malaysian outbreak 57% of patients had abnormal chest x-ray, most of whom had lobar consolidation. Blood tests showed lymphopaenia, thrombocytopaenia and elevated liver enzymes. Cerebrospinal fluid examination showed abnormality in 75 – 81% of patients, which mainly consisted of mildly elevated protein, sugar levels and white cell counts. Magnetic resonance imaging showed widespread hyperintense focal lesions in the subcortical and deep white matter on T2 weighted images. Electroencephalogram showed diffuse slow waves with sharp waves in 56% of the patients. IgM against Hendra virus was positive in 31 - 58% of the patients' cerebrospinal fluid samples and 76 – 81% of the patients' serum samples, depending on the duration of the illness. Mortality is 32 – 41%; and 15 – 19% recovered with neurological deficits. A past history of diabetes mellitus, severe dysautonomia, brainstem involvement and the presence of virus in the cerebrospinal fluid are poor prognostic features [159-162]. In the Malaysian outbreak, 9% of patients recovered from symptomatic infection and 3.4% of asymptomatic patients subsequently developed relapse. In between relapses the patients were well, and some had multiple relapses. Patients with relapse Nipah infection presented either with seizure or focal neurological deficits. Magnetic resonance imaging showed patchy areas of confluent cortical lesions, while necropsy showed focal encephalitis with presence of Nipah virus antigen. Mortality of relapse Nipah is about 18%, while the survivors are mostly well [163,164]. Nipah virus infection reemerged in Bangladesh in 2001 and 2003, where local *pteropus* bats were found to have antibodies against Nipah virus. The clinical features were similar to that in the Malaysian outbreak [165].

The New World encephalitides include California encephalitis, in which LaCrosse virus accounts for nearly all of the cases, St. Louis encephalitis, Western, Eastern and Venezuelan equine encephalitis. LaCrosse and St. Louis encephalitides are the commonest causes of arbovirus encephalitis in the United States. Patients with LaCrosse encephalitis present with fever, headache, vomiting and about half of the patients have seizure, altered consciousness or meningism. In adults, the infection is either asymptomatic or it causes a benign febrile illness or aseptic meningitis. The mortality is less than 0.5%, though 75% of children have abnormal electroencephalogram 3 – 4 years later, 10 – 15% of survivors have significant neurological deficits and 6 – 15% of survivors have symptomatic epilepsy [68,137,139].

The ratio of symptomatic to asymptomatic St. Louis virus infection is 1:100. The majority of symptomatic patients develop encephalitis, with the elderly being the most at risk. Aseptic meningitis accounts for 15% of all symptomatic cases, though in children the proportion is as high as 35-60%, as the disease is milder in children. In the elderly, aseptic meningitis is uncommon, and accounts for 5% or less of the cases. 85% of elderly patients manifest the disease as encephalitis. The encephalitis is preceded by a prodrome of flu-like illness of fever, myalgias, nausea and vomiting, followed by headache, confusion, disorientation, irritability, impaired consciousness, tremors, seizures, and in some, a central form of Syndrome of Inappropriate Antidiuretic Hormone secretion (SIADH) [68]. The case fatality is 2% in young adult and 22% in the elderly [137].

In Western equine encephalitis virus infection, asymptomatic infections are commoner than symptomatic ones, and infants are particularly susceptible to encephalitis. Encephalitic patients presents with fever, myalgias, malaise, pharyngitis, vomiting, lethargy, irritability, seizures and coma. The overall case fatality is 5%, though higher in patients older than 55 years. Most adults recover fully; however serious sequelae are common in infants younger than 1 years of age, with 56% of infants under 1 month of age, 16% of infants between 1 and 2 months of age, and 11% of patients between 2 and 3 months of age had severe impairment of the motor or cognitive functions, resulting in permanent disabilities [68,137].

Eastern equine encephalitis is the deadliest encephalitis in North America. Almost all infections result in clinical illness. Patients often presents with fever, headache, vomiting, lethargy; though more typically, they have abrupt onset of high fever, rapid deterioration of conscious state from drowsy to being comatose, with focal neurological deficits and focal seizures. On MRI, focal abnormalities are seen in the basal ganglia and the thalami, similar to those seen in patients with Japanese encephalitis, and disseminated lesions in the brainstem. Like Western equine encephalitis, young children are more susceptible to infections; they have less frequent prodrome, a higher case-to-infection ratio, and more severe sequelae. The extremes of age suffer from higher mortality; overall case fatality rate is 30%, while 70% of surviving children have serious sequelae [68,137,166].

Venezuelan encephalitis typically causes mild infection with headache, fever, myalgias and pharyngitis. Encephalitis is uncommon and mild, and mortality rare [68,139].

Western tick-borne encephalitis classically presents as a biphasic illness. After an incubation period of about 5 to 17 days, and up to 28 days, the patients often present with prodrome of fever, headache, malaise, upper respiratory and abdominal symptoms such as diarrhea, which lasts about 1 to 7 days. Laboratory investigations show elevated liver enzymes, mild to moderate thrombocytopenia and leucopenia. Most patients then recover from the prodrome for about 1 to 3 weeks. After this, 50% of the patients develop meningitis, 40% develop meningoencephalitis, and 10% meningoencephalomyelitis. These patients present with impaired conscious states, coma, seizures, dysphasia, limb weakness, cranial nerve palsies and bulbar palsy, dysaethesiae, respiratory insufficiency and extrapyramidal signs of tremor, ataxia and dysdiadochokinesia. Cerebrospinal fluid findings were similar to other aseptic meningitis, and MRI shows thalamic lesions in most patients; and in some patients further lesions are found in the cerebellum, brainstem and caudate nucleus. Adults, as compared with adolescents, and patients with monophasic illness have more severe form of the illness. Case fatality is low at 1%, and a half to three quarters of the patients recovers fully, while the rest mainly suffers from persistent limb weakness or cognitive impairment. Other long term sequelae include the complaints of emotional lability, tiredness, headache, poor memory, poor concentration, and mood and sleep disturbance [151,152].

Risk Factors

Contact with the source of infection is the most important risk factor of acquiring most central nervous system infections. Among the commonest infections, such as those caused by herpesviruses, enteroviruses, mumps virus, adenovirus and HIV, contact with human carrier is the most important risk factors. With other infections, contact with either the vectors, such as mosquitoes and ticks, or with sick animals is the most important risk factors. Since many of the viruses are limited geographically, traveling to these places is an obvious risk factor.

Apart from environmental risk factors, the most important host risk factors include age, gender and host immune status. The elderly population is at risk of St. Louis, and West Nile encephalitis, while the very young is at risk of Eastern and Western equine encephalitis and the more severe forms of herpes simplex encephalitis and enteroviral meningitis or encephalitis. Like many bacterial meningitis, males are at higher risk of developing certain viral central nervous system infections, especially among children [167], even though among adults, the overall hospitalization rates for male and female were similar [134]. This partly related to exposure, such as occupational exposure to Nipah encephalitis in the pig farm industry where the male to female patients ratio was 5:1 in the Malaysian outbreak [159,160], and partly related to greater outdoor exposure among the males; for example, males are more likely to suffer from Japanese encephalitis and twice as likely to suffer from Western tick-borne encephalitis [152,131]. However, in many instances the reason is poorly understood. Males are at least 1.5 times more likely than female in acquiring enteroviral meningitis; and in mumps infection, males are twice as likely as female to be symptomatic and three times as likely to have central nervous system involvement [74]. The immune status of the patient is another important risk factor. In fact, this could explain much of the difference in the risk of acquiring central nervous system infections in the extreme-of-age populations. Patients with immunosuppression or impaired blood brain barrier are more at risk of acquiring severe West Nile encephalitis; and patients with diabetes mellitus has a 123% increase in mortality in Nipah encephalitis [162]. Cytomegalovirus, varicella zoster virus, measles virus and adenovirus infections, progressive multifocal leucoencephalopathy (caused by JC virus), chronic enteroviral meningitis and the more severe form of herpes simplex encephalitis were either seen almost exclusively or occur more commonly in the immunocompromised patients [74,155,168].

Prevention

Generally speaking there are three strategies in the prevention of viral infection of the central nervous system; animal exposure prevention, vector exposure control and vaccination program. In animal exposure prevention, the animal hosts are separated from humans. In Japanese encephalitis, for example, pigs are the chief amplifying hosts of the virus, and in some areas, pig infection by the virus approaches 100% during seasonal epidemics. Centralization of pig farming has been effective in reducing the incidence of human Japanese encephalitis in Korea and Japan [137]. The Nipah encephalitis outbreak in Malaysia was only brought under control after massive culling of approximately a million pigs in the outbreak areas [145]. Restriction of stray dogs has been used in controlling rabies in the United States [150] and other countries.

Since many of the viral encephalitides were transmitted by mosquitoes or ticks, vector exposure control has been advocated in the control of these infections, notably in the control of Japanese encephalitis, West Nile encephalitis, LaCrosse encephalitis, St. Louis encephalitis and the equine encephalitides. Personal protection from vector, such as reducing the number of mosquitoe bites in areas endemic of Japanese encephalitis and West Nile encephalitis by minimizing outdoor exposure at dusk and dawn, wearing clothing with minimal skin exposure, sleeping under bed nets and using DEET (N, N-diethyl-3 methylbenzamide) were advice routinely given though remains impractical for local residents. Measures to control vector breeding, such as using larvacides in rice fields or insecticides spraying, have also been proved ineffectual in controlling Japanese encephalitis, as it was estimated that a single rice field could breed over 30 000 mosquitoes in a day [131,133].

Vaccination remains the most effective control measures. Currently vaccines are available for rabies, Japanese encephalitis, Western tick-borne encephalitis, varicella zoster virus, mumps, measles and rubella in the form of the MMR vaccine, and poliomyelitis. Widespread administration of inactivated Japanese encephalitis vaccine, given to children in three doses at 0, 7 and 30 days, has significantly reduced the number of clinical cases in Taiwan, Japan, South Korea and the People Republic of China. [131] A recently introduced live attenuated virus has also been shown effective in only two doses and could be administered at shorter interval of 1 and 2.5 months. [133] Orally absorbed animal vaccine against rabies, distributed by hand and by aircraft, have controlled rabies in parts of Europe, particularly in Switzerland, Germany, Belgium and France.[150] The MMR vaccine has also dramatically reduced the incidence of measles encephalitis from being one of the commonest viral encephalitides to less than $1/10^5$ annually. [74,123]

In spite of these successes, the cause of most meningitides and encephalitides are not known, and effective control measures remain elusive. [134]

Management

Over the last four decades, the number of effective antiviral therapies has increased dramatically. The first antiviral trial for herpes simplex encephalitis was done in the 1960's using idoxuridine. Though ultimately found to be ineffective and too toxic, subsequent trials found vidarabine and acyclovir to be effective. Acyclovir reduced mortality from 70% to 19% and increased the number of patients with little or no sequelae from 2.5% to 38%. Acyclovir has also been shown to be more effective than vidarabine. In patients presenting with encephalitis, it is an accepted clinical practice to start acyclovir therapy (at 30 mg/kg/day in three divided doses, or double in neonates) before the results of definite investigation becomes available, mainly because of the relatively high incidence of herpes simplex encephalitis, its severe consequences especially if effective antiviral is started late, and the relative low side effect profile of acyclovir. Since more than 80% of acyclovir is excreted unchanged by the kidneys, patients with renal impairment may rapidly develop acyclovir toxicity. Relapse of herpes simplex encephalitis may occur if treatment with acyclovir is stopped after 10 days, but is rare after 2 weeks of treatment (5%), and does not occur if high dose of acyclovir is used for 3 weeks. Vidarabine is used rarely in patients who cannot tolerate acyclovir. Acyclovir in similar doses is effective in varicella zoster encephalitis. Combination therapy of ganciclovir (10 mg/kg/day in two divided doses) and foscarnet (180 mg/kg/day in 2 or 3 divided doses) is used for cytomegaloviral encephalitis. Though unproven, patients with B virus (herpes simae or cercopithecine herpes virus) infection should be given acyclovir or ganciclovir treatment because of the high mortality rate. Pleconaril is used for chronic or recurrent enteroviral meningitis or in immunosuppressed patients. [168,169] Ribavirin has been tested in a historical control trial and was shown to reduce mortality in Nipah encephalitis from 54% to 32% and improve outcomes in survivors. [170] Ribavirin, immunoglobulin and α-interferon have been tested in open labeled trials in West Nile encephalitis, but more definitive evidence is needed to determine their efficacy. Steroid has been used in raised intracranial pressure and varicella zoster vasculitis though evidence for its efficacy is lacking. [156,169]

Apart from antiviral therapy, supportive measures are the cornerstone in the management of these patients. All patients should be admitted into hospital, and those critically ill should be admitted into intensive care unit equipped with mechanical ventilators. Seizures should be controlled rapidly, preferably with intravenous phenytoin or lorazepam. Careful monitoring is required for fluid and electrolytes balance, respiration, blood pressure and cardiac rhythm. Complications that could arise include vasculitic cerebral infarction, cerebral venous thrombosis, syndrome of inappropriate ADH secretion, deep vein thrombosis, aspiration pneumonia, urinary tract infection, skin pressure sores, upper gastrointestinal tract bleeding, and disseminated intravascular coagulopathy. [169]

HUMAN IMMUNODEFICIENCY VIRUS

The human immunodeficiency virus (HIV) is the most prevalent infection of the nervous system worldwide and has been associated with the widest clinical spectrum of neurological diseases. The neurological diseases that are directly related to HIV infection are HIV dementia, vacuolar myelopathy and peripheral neuropathy. The most frequent central nervous system infections associated with HIV are cerebral toxoplasmosis, cryptococcal meningitis, progressive multifocal leucoencephalopathy (PML), tuberculous meningitis, cytomegaloviral encephalitis and polyradiculomyelitis, and primary central nervous system lymphoma.

Epidemiology

About 75% of HIV transmission worldwide occurred heterosexually. Communicability of HIV infection is remarkably low compared with other sexually transmitted diseases; it is estimated that transmission occurs in 1 in 100 anal receptive intercourses, 1 in 500 male to female vaginal spread and 1 in 1000 female to male vaginal spread. Transmission risk is increased by the number of partners, the presence of other sexually transmitted diseases and the lack of circumcision in male. Approximately 10% of infections are transmitted by contaminated needles and syringes used by intravenous drug users. Aspirating blood into the syringe before injection ("booting") increases the risk of transmission. Medical needle stick injury in hospital personnel occurs in about 1 in 1000 exposures. Transmission across placenta and by breast feeding has been documented, as well as transmission from baby to mother via breast feeding. Up to 42% of HIV infected mother transmit the virus to their infants.

Globally, the magnitude of the epidemic is staggering. It is estimated that there are at least 40 million people living with HIV or acquired immunodeficiency syndrome (AIDS) and 95% of these are living in developing world. The disease has caused more than 20 million deaths worldwide. More than 25 million of these are living in Sub-Saharan Africa, where the disease is the leading cause of death, and where it is spreading most rapidly. The epidemic has caused great disruption to health care services, economic and social structures by depleting the labor force and health care resources as well as leaving over a million orphans. Heterosexual transmission and contaminated blood and blood products are the two main routes of spread in this region. There are 5.8 million people living with HIV/AIDS in South and Southeast Asia. The virus is transmitted by heterosexual, homosexual and contaminated syringes and needles in this region, as well as by contaminated blood and blood products in South Asia. The largest increase in seroconversion rates are also seen here, up to 5% among intravenous drug users in Thailand. There are 1.4 million people living with HIV/AIDS in South America and another 400 000 in the Caribbean, where the transmission pattern is similar to that in Southeast Asia. In North America, there are 1.2 million people living with HIV/AIDS and about 500 000 have developed AIDS. The number of AIDS death decreased for the first time in 1996 in North America. There has also been dramatic decrease in seroconversion among homosexual men, though in other risk groups, especially among intravenous drug users and their partners, the rate continues to rise. There are about 700 000 people living with HIV/AIDS in Central and Eastern Europe, 640 000 in East Asia, 540 000 in Western Europe, 400 000 in North Africa and the Middle East and 15 000 in the Oceanic countries.

The epidemiology study of HIV infection has been complicated by the genetic diversity of the virus. HIV-1 and HIV-2 are two distinct viruses that cause similar clinical manifestations and are spread by the same means. HIV-1 is responsible for the majority of clinical infections worldwide, and HIV-2 is restricted to West Africa or people of West African origin. The transmission of HIV-2 is less efficient than that of HIV-1 both sexually as well as from mother to baby. HIV-1 has been divided into 10 subtypes or clades according to the differences in the *env* gene. The *env* gene shows up to 50% differences in isolates found in different parts of the world and viruses with 20% or more differences are classified into different clades. The A, C and D clades are common in Sub-Saharan Africa, while in North America and Western Europe, the B clade causes almost all the infections. The C clade is dominant in India, Brazil, as well as in Central and South Africa. The A clade is dominant in Thailand, and the A and E recombinant clade is causing unprecedented heterosexual spread in Thailand (see figure 2). [132]

The proportions of HIV patients who develop various complications vary from study to study, depending on local pattern of infection and the availability of treatment. [176] Generally, about half of the patients develop fever and headache during acute seroconversion illness and a small percentage develop aseptic meningitis. Acute encephalitis is uncommon. Neurologic manifestations during seroconversion illness, however, are associated with accelerated progression to AIDS. Later on in the illness, 7 to 24% of patients develop HIV dementia, and the risk is higher in children. About 20% develop vacuolar myelopathy, while the incidence of symptomatic distal sensory polyneuropathy is 36% a year, though another

26% develop asymptomatic polyneuropathy a year. At autopsy, 95% of patients dying of AIDS had histopathological abnormalities in the peripheral nerves.

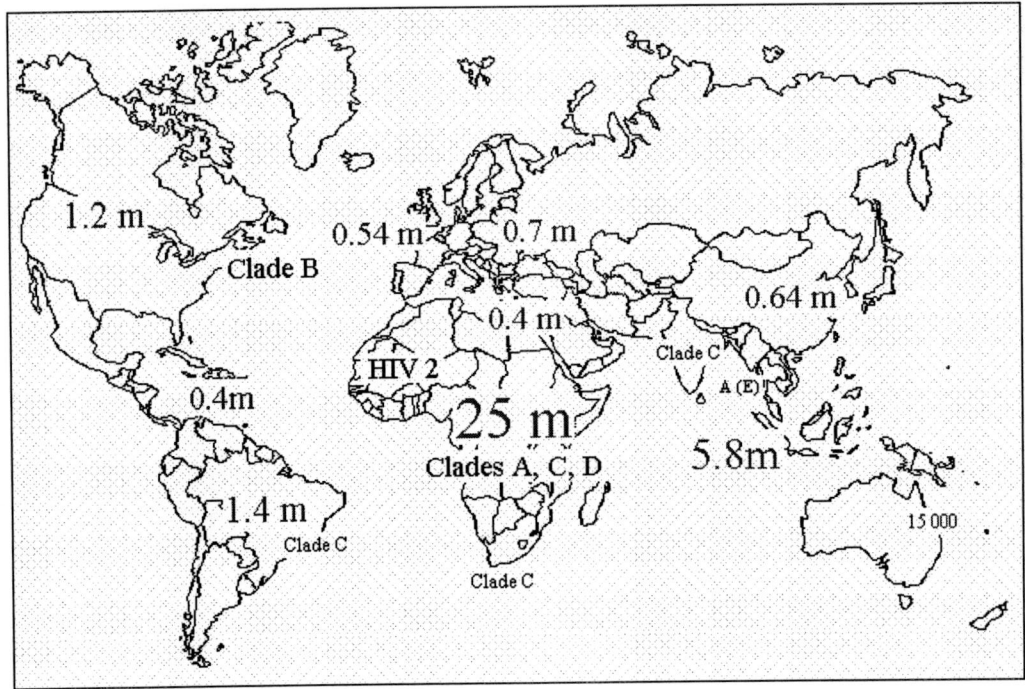

Figure 2. The Worldwide Distribution of HIV Infections and HIV virus clades

In the developed world, 18-19% of patients develop cytomegaloviral encephalitis, 11-12% develop primary central nervous system lymphoma, 7-9% develop toxoplasma encephalitis and 1-8% develop cryptococcal meningitis. In some developing countries, however, cryptococcal meningitis is more common. For example, in Sub-Saharan Uganda, the incidence of cryptococcal meningitis was 40.4/1000 person-years, and it was associated with 17% of all HIV death. [177] In Thailand, 75% of central nervous system infections in HIV patients are due to cryptococcal meningitis. [178]

Natural History and Outcome

The clinical manifestations of HIV infection is highly variable, and is determined largely by the patient's immune status, mirrored by peripheral blood CD4 counts. One to three weeks after the infection, half of the patients develop a mononucleosis-like illness with fever, headache, lymphadenopathy, maculopapular rash and myalgia. Laboratory investigations showed thrombocytopaenia and leukopenia, with rapid decrease in CD4 counts, but raised CD8 count. This lasts 3 days to 3 weeks, but may be extended for months. There is viraemia, and antibody conversion occurs by two to six weeks. With seroconversion and the development of CD8 cytotoxic cells, viraemia becomes intermittent and the CD4 count is reestablished to normal or near normal level. During this period, the patient may develop aseptic meningitis, and rarely, encephalitis, cranial nerve palsies, Guillian-Barre syndrome and acute disseminated encephalomyelitis.

The patient then enters a long asymptomatic phase which may lasts from months to up to 15 years. During this period, there is rapid viral production, mainly from the CD4 cells, which slowly decline in number over the subsequent years before a precipitous fall and the development of AIDS. Patients are often relatively well during this period, though aseptic meningitis, encephalitis and Guillian-Barre syndrome have been described in these patients. The patient's CD4 count often ranges from 500 – 1000 cells/mm^3.

The CD4 lymphocytes gradually deplete over time, due to the cytopathic effect of the virus, decrease in CD4 production, and possibly to autoimmune destruction. Eventually, the control of HIV replication collapse in over 90% of patients, with recurrence of explosive viraemia, and the patient develops full blown AIDS. Clinically, the patient develops generalized lymphadenopathy, mononeuritis multiplex, tuberculous meningitis and in some, HIV dementia. The CD4 counts often ranges from 200 – 500 cells/mm^3.

With further depletion of the CD4 count to below 200 cells/mm^3, the patient is prone to develop opportunistic infections, such as toxoplasma encephalitis and cryptococcal meningitis, and other manifestations of HIV infection, such as HIV dementia, vacuolar myelopathy and distal sensory polyneuropathy. In the pre-terminal stage, when the CD4 count drops below 50 cells/mm^3, the patient is at risk of cytomegaloviral retinitis and encephalitis and primary central nervous system lymphoma.

HIV dementia is a syndrome of progressive deterioration in cognitive functions seen in late stage of HIV infection. Clinically it is characterized by mental apathy, memory impairment, poor attention and concentration, abulia with loss of fine motor control, tremor and unsteady gait. The dementia progresses rapidly, and the patient may develop mutism, incontinence, and generalized spasticity and eventually die after months. It is often seen in patients with CD4 count of less than 200 cells/mm^3, though since the introduction of HAART, the proportion of new HIV dementia patients with CD4 counts between 200 and 350 cells/mm^3 may be increasing.

Vacuolar myelopathy often presents with progressive posterolateral mid-thoracic spinal cord syndrome. The patient presents with progressive spastic paresis of the lower limbs with loss of proprioception and bladder involvement. A sensory level is often not evident, and the upper limbs are often spared as well.

The peripheral nerves are affected in three different mechanisms in HIV. Early on during the asymptomatic phase, the patient may develop an autoimmune form of acute inflammatory demyelinating polyneuropathy, also known as Guillian-Barre syndrome. Later on the patient may develop mononeuritis multiplex due to vasculitic lesions in individual nerves. The commonest form of peripheral nerve disease is a painful axonal sensory polyneuropathy which presents as distal painful dysaesthesiae, glove-and-stocking paraesthesiae and loss of deep tendon reflexes. The autonomic system may be involved with postural hypotension, sphincteric dysfunction, resting tachycardia and cardiac conduction abnormalities. In patients with more severe disease, the gracile tracts in the posterior column of the spinal cord may be involved with loss of axon and myelin sheaths. The differential diagnosis of a painful sensory polyneuropathy is toxic neuropathy caused by didanosine (ddI), zalcitabine (ddC) and stavudine (d4T).

Primary infection by *Toxoplasma gondii* is asymptomatic or causes a mononucleosis-like illness with fever and lymphadenopathy in 90% of immunocompetent hosts, though the organisms persists as cysts for life in many. In most patients toxoplasma encephalitis is caused by reactivation of infection when the host immune system is impaired. The patient presents subacutely over days with fever, headache, confusion, impaired conscious state, seizures and focal neurological deficits. CT scan shows isodense or hypodense contrast-enhancing ring lesions in the basal ganglia and cortico-medullary junction. MRI is more sensitive and shows hypointense lesions in the same regions. Often it is difficult to differentiate toxoplasma lesions from primary central nervous system lymphoma. Since the vast majority of HIV patients have positive anti-toxoplasma IgG, and patients with toxoplasmosis with severe immunosuppression may be seronegative, serologic test is often not helpful in diagnosis. A presumptive clinical diagnosis may be made if the patient responds to treatment within 2 weeks. Radiological response lags behind clinical improvement, and may not be evident for 2 to 3 months.

Cryptococcal meningitis is caused by encapsulated yeast found ubiquitously in the environment, *Cryptococcus neoformans*. In HIV patients, the presentation is often less acute. The symptoms consist of fever, headache, nausea, vomiting and cognitive impairment. Signs of focal neurological deficits and meningism are uncommon. In over half of the patients, the infection may involve other system, most commonly the lungs. Contrasted CT or MRI scan may show dilated Virchow-Robin spaces, gelatinous pseudocysts, cryptococcomas in the basal ganglia region, and/or hydrocephalus. Cerebrospinal fluid analysis shows normal or slightly elevated lymphocyte counts, elevated opening pressure and protein level, and low sugar level. The encapsulated yeast may be seen with Indian ink preparation, and cryptococcal antigen test is positive in about 95% of patients.

Progressive multifocal leukoencephalopathy (PML) is cause by a papovavirus, the JC virus. The infection is acquired in childhood and the virus remains latent in the kidneys. With immunosuppression the infection is reactivated. The patient either presents with focal neurological deficits, often localized to the posterior cerebrum, or with non-specific symptoms and signs suggestive of dementia or psychiatric illness. Seizures occur rarely. The progress is slow but relentless. CT scan may be normal or show multiple low density white matter lesions with little or no mass effect in the occipito-parietal regions.

Cytomegalovirus (CMV) causes infections late in the course of AIDS, often when the patient's CD4 count drops below 50 cells/mm^3. Besides retinitis, CMV causes three other common neurological manifestations, which are encephalitis, radiculomyelitis and multifocal neuropathy. Patients with CMV encephalitis present subacutely over a few weeks with memory and attention deficits, headache, unsteadiness, and in a third of patients, fever. Clinical signs include memory impairment, psychomotor retardation, and unlike HIV dementia, signs localized to the posterior fossa. About 40% of patients have cranial nerve palsy, internuclear ophthalmoplegia, nystagmus, deafness, vertigo and ataxia. The course is rapid and relentless; patients often develop dementia and succumb in weeks. Patients with CMV radiculomyelitis present with painful lower motor neuron lesion subacutely over weeks. The common clinical features are painful lower limb weakness with hyporeflexia, loss of sphincteric control and sensory loss, especially over the sacral region. Early treatment often leads to stabilization of the disease; while if left untreated, the disability progresses rapidly leading to death. CMV multifocal neuropathy occurs very late in the course of AIDS, and patients often have other manifestations of CMV infection. The patients often present with acute or subacute asymmetrical axonal or mixed axonal and demyelinating lesions of the cranial or peripheral nerves. Diagnosis is made by polymerase chain reaction for detection of CMV DNA in the cerebrospinal fluid.

Risk Factor

HIV is a blood borne and sexually transmitted disease. The three main routes of transmission are sexual intercourse, vertical transmission from mothers to children, and exposure to contaminated blood or blood products. Therefore, those with HIV infected sexual partners, children born to mothers with HIV infection, intravenous drug users who share needles with other users with HIV infection and people receiving inadequately screened blood or blood products are at the highest risk of acquiring the infection. Meta-analysis showed that the presence of other sexually transmitted diseases (STD's), both ulcerative and non-ulcerative forms, increases both the infectiousness and susceptibility to HIV infection in sexual intercourse and so increases the risk of infection by 2 to 5 times. [179] Genetic factors, however, may protect against HIV infection or the progression of disease. The absence of CCR5 due to homozygous δ-32 deletion in the coding region protects against HIV-1 transmission, while heterozygosity delays disease progression. Similarly, the chemokine receptor, CCR2 allele, also protects against disease progression. [180]

The strongest risk factor associated with invasive cryptococcosis, symptomatic CMV disease, toxoplasmosis and progressive multifocal leukoencephalopathy (PML) is immunesuppression, especially HIV infection and transplantation. In the United States, for example, the annual incidence among people not infected with HIV is $0.2 - 0.9/10^5$, and 1700 $- 6600/10^5$ among patients with HIV infection. Comparatively, among transplant patients the annual incidence is $300 - 6000/10^5$, and among cancer patients, $0.5/10^5$. In developed countries 20 – 30% of patients with invasive cryptococcosis had no other discernible medical illness. [181] HIV infection, therefore, has caused substantial increase in the incidence of cryptococcal meningitis. In Thailand, for example, the epidemic of HIV infection led to 10 fold increase in the incidence of cryptococcal meningitis. [182] Similarly, symptomatic CMV infection is extremely rare in immunocompetent individuals, with only approximately 34 cases reported worldwide. Among HIV patients the annual incidence is 12% among patients with CD4 count less than 50 cells/mm^3. [181] The incidence of toxoplasmosis among the HIV patients before the HAART era was $5.4/10^5$ and that of PML $2.0/10^5$, and less than 10% of toxoplasmosis occurred in patients without HIV infection. [134,176,181]

Prevention and Management

The HIV virus is transmitted vertically from mothers to babies, by sexual contact and via contaminated blood and blood products. In sexual contact, the transmission and susceptibility of HIV infection are both increased by the presence of STD. Primary prevention strategies therefore include proper usage of condom, implementation of stringent blood procurement and transfusion procedures, needle exchange program for recreational drug users, treatment of STD, peripartum prophylaxis with antiretroviral drug and sexual health education. The proper usage of male condoms has been shown in many observational studies to effectively reduce the risk of acquiring HIV infection by 2 to 10 times. [183] Targeted, frequent treatment of symptomatic STD in areas of evolving epidemics of HIV may reduce the incidence of HIV infection. [179,184] In a meta-analysis of 27 observation studies, male circumcision is shown to half the risk of HIV infection in man. [185] Placebo controlled trials have shown that antiretroviral drugs reduced the maternal-fetal transmission of HIV. Without treatment; 20% to 30% of babies acquire the virus from their mothers. Zidovudine alone reduces the risk by 28% to 60%. Combining zidovudine and lamivudine or nevirapine alone further reduces the risk by 40% to 50%. [186]

HAART consists of three nucleoside reverse transcriptase inhibitors (NRTI's) or two nucleoside reverse transcriptase inhibitors (NRTI's) with either a non-nucleoside reverse transcriptase inhibitor (NNRTI) or a protease inhibitor (PI) (table 3). The introduction of HAART has drastically reduced the incidence of many of the complications and opportunistic infections in HIV patients. In developed countries, the epidemiology of HIV infection, especially that of related opportunistic infections, has been altered by the introduction of HAART. After the introduction of HAART, the incidence of any HIV defining illness has decreased from approximately 50/100 person-years in 1994 to 13.3/100 person-years in 1997. In France, the incidence of HIV dementia has dropped from 1.6/100 person-years in 1994 to 0.5/100 person-years in 1996, while in the United States, the incidence had dropped from 21.1/1000 person-year in the 1990-1992 period when monotherapy was first introduced, to 10.5/1000 person-year in the 1996-1998 period when HAART was introduced. Similarly, the incidence of cryptococcal meningitis had dropped from 5.0/1000 person-year to 1.5/1000 person-year over the same period, and primary central nervous system lymphoma from 2.8/1000 person-year to 0.4/1000 person-year. The incidence of both cryptococcal meningitis and PML had also showed decreasing trend over the same period, from 5.0/1000 person-year to 1.5/1000 person-year and 2.0/1000 person-year to 1.5/1000 person-year respectively, though these were not statistically significant. [176] For individual patient, secondary prophylaxis of opportunistic infections can be discontinued if HAART brings about an increase in CD4 count to above 200 cells/mm^3 for 3 months or more. [187]

The introduction of HAART though often results in reduction of plasma viral load to undetectable levels, does not effect total removal of the virus especially from cellular reservoirs. In the central nervous system, HIV persists in microglial cells, astrocytes and monocytes. HIV encephalitis is still common in patients treated with HAART, and was found in up to 25% of autopsy brains of such patients in one study. A subtle form of cognitive impairment is also prevalent in the treated patients, and increasingly, HIV dementia is no longer observed only in patients with very low CD4 counts, but also in patients with higher CD4 counts. [188] The treatment of various opportunistic infections in HIV is detailed in table 4.

Table 3. Clinically significant drug interaction with highly active anti-retroviral therapy

Agent and dosage		Interaction
Nucleoside reverse transcriptase inhibitors (NRTI's)		
Zidovudine (AZT)	600 mg/d in 2 or 3 divided doses	Ribavirin, rifampicin, rifabutin, nelfinavir, lamivudine, didanosine, zalcitabine.
Stavudine (d4T)	30 mg[a] or 40 mg[b] bd	Nelfinavir, lamivudine, didanosine, zalcitabine.
Lamivudine (3TC)	150 mg bd	Zidovudine and stavudine
Didanosine (ddI)	125 mg[a] or 200 mg[b] bd; or 400 mg daily	Quinolones, zidovudine and stavudine
Zalcitabine (ddC)	0.75 mg bd	Zidovudine and stavudine
Abacavir	300 mg bd	
Tenofovir		
Non-nucleoside reverse transcriptase inhibitors (NNRTI's)		
Nevirapine	200 mg daily for 2 weeks; then 200 mg bd	Opiates, indinavir, saquinavir and delavirdine.
Efavirenz	600 mg nocte	Amprenavir, indinavir, saquinavir,
Delavirdine	400 mg tds	Alprazolam, midazolam, triazolam, astemizole, terfenadine, clarithromycin, dihydropyridine Ca^{++} blockers, ergot alkaloids, quinidine, rifampicin, warfarin, grapefruit juice (>200 ml/day), indinavir, ritonavir, saquinavir and nevirapine.
Protease Inhibitors (PI's)		
Indanavir	800 mg q8hr	Benzodiazepine, astemizole, terfenadine, statins, rifampicin, rifabutin, sildanefil, grapefruit juice (>200 ml/d), amprenavir, nelfinavir, ritonavir, saquinavir, efavirenz, delavirdine and nevirapine.
Saquinavir	600 mg or 1200 mg q8h	Barbiturates, carbamazepine, clonazepam, astemizole, terfenadine, statins, rifampicin, rifabutin, sildanefil, grapefruit juice (>200 ml/d), indinavir, ritonavir, efavirenz, delavirdine and nevirapine.
Ritonavir	300 mg q12h increase over 2 weeks to 600 mg bd	Barbiturates, carbamazepine, benzodiazepine, H_1 histamine antagonists, all Ca^{++} blockers, oral contraceptive pills, statins, rifampicin, rifabutin, sildanefil, indinavir, nelfinavir, saquinavir and delavirdine.
Nelfinavir	750 mg q8h	Barbiturates, carbamazepine, benzodiazepine, astemizole, terfenadine, oral contraceptive pills, statins, rifampicin, rifabutin, sildanefil, indinavir, ritonavir, saquinavir, efavirenz and delavirdine.
Amprenavir	1200 mg bd	Statins, rifampicin, rifabutin, sildanefil, indinavir, nelfinavir and efivirenz.
Lopinavir	400 mg bd	

Notes: [a]For weight less than 60 kg; [b] for weight more than 60 kg.

Table 4. Treatment of Opportunistic Infections in HIV Patients

Infection	Treatment
Cerebral toxoplasmosis	Pyrimethamine 200mg load then 50mg/day with Sulfadiazine 1g qid (or clindamycine 600mg qid) and Folinic acid 10mg/d. OR
	Trimethoprim/sulfamethoxazol 2.5-5mg/kg qid po or iv OR
	Pyrimethamine 200mg load then 50mg/d with either: (a). clarithromycin 1g bd or (b). Azithromycin 600 – 1800 mg/d or (c). Dapsone 100 mg/d OR
	Atovaquone 750 mg qid po
Cryptococcal meningitis	Amphotericin B 0.7 mg/kg/d iv ($\pm$ flucytosine 100 mg/kg/d po) for 2 weeks then fluconazole or itraconazole 400 mg/d for 10 weeks AND
	Repeated spinal tap, spinal drain or shunting to treat severely raised intracranial pressure.
	Secondary prophylaxis: fluconazole 200 mg/d po
Progressive multifocal leucoencephalopathy	HAART arrests or remits half of PML and prolong survival in these patients.
	Cidofovir (5 mgk/kg iv once weekly) may offer additional benefit
CMV encephalitis or polyradiculomyelitis	Ganciclovir 5mg/kg iv bd or Foscarnet 90mg/kg bd iv or Cidofovir 5mg/kg iv weekly two doses then fortnightly. Maintenance dose: ganciclovir 5mg/kg/d.
Tuberculous meningitis	Isoniazid, rifampicin, ethambutol & pyrazinamide. Ethambutol can be replaced by streptomycin or amikicin
	Dexamethasone 0.4 mg/kg/d iv for 1 week, reduce by 0.1 mg/kg/d every week, then 4 mg/d po reduce by 1 mg every week.
Primary CNS lymphoma	HAART with either one of: a. Whole brain irradiation and corticosteroid b. Methotrexate iv then whole brain irradiation c. Methotrexate, thiotepa, procarbazine iv with intrathecal methotrexate
HIV dementia or myelopathy	HAART (note: most NRTI's and NNRTI's penetrate well into the CSF; most protease inhibitors do not)
HIV sensory polyneuropathy	Symptomatic relieve with either: a. Amitriptylene 25 – 100 mg/d b. Tramadol 150 – 400 mg/d c. Carbamazepine 200 mg tds - qid

OTHER INFECTIONS

Tuberculous Meningitis

Globally, more than 7 million people develop tuberculosis every year. The incidence of tuberculous infection is highest in Africa and Southeast Asia, with annual incidences of $270/10^5$ and $192/10^5$ respectively. Annually there are 3 million deaths due to tuberculosis, with over a million in Southeast Asia alone. [189] About 1% of patients of patients with tuberculous infection has tuberculous meningitis. [190] There are 6 000 to 9 000 cases of tuberculous meningitis diagnosed yearly in the United States giving an annual incidence of 2 to $3/10^5$. Tuberculous meningitis is among the commonest causes of meningitis in some regions. In Hong Kong, it is the commonest cause of meningitis, accounting for 15.3% of meningitis admitted. [59] The incidence of tuberculous meningitis in Hong Kong, however, has fallen from $1.8 / 10^5$ in 1965 to $0.43 / 10^5$ in 1984. [191] In Taiwan, 8% of all meningitis is due to *Mycobacterium tuberculosis*, [135] in Malawi, 8.8%, [37] in Iraq, 5%, [192] and in Indonesia 5.7% . In China, the incidence of tuberculous meningitis ranges from $0.9 - 17.2 / 10^5$. [191]

Tuberculosis affects the central nervous system in a variety of ways. Patients with tuberculous meningitis present with fever, anorexia, night sweat, lethargy, stiff neck, headache, which progresses to confusion, altered consciousness and drowsiness over 4 to 8 weeks. A fourth of the patients had cranial nerve palsy, and less than half had concurrent pulmonary tuberculosis. In patients with HIV, the progression is often more rapid. In children the disease presents more insidiously with personality change, irritability, listlessness, fever, anorexia, nausea, vomiting, and seizures. Headache is less likely. [193] The outcome is poor; in developing countries, for example, the overall mortality is about 30% and up to 18% suffered from severe disability. Mortality is higher in patients with HIV infection (up to 68%) and low Glasgow Coma Scale scores (up to 60%) upon admission. [194] In the spinal cord, tuberculosis could cause spondylitis with compression of the spinal cord, inflammatory thrombosis of the anterior spinal artery and spinal cord infarct, intramedullary granulomatosus or tuberculomas, and rarely, polyradiculomyelitis and syrinx formation. Up to 39% of intramedullary granuloma and 7% of tuberculomas occur without bony lesions. [195]

The most important risk factor for acquiring tuberculous meningitis is HIV infection. In Gabon, Africa, for example, tuberculous meningitis was only seen in HIV infection one study; and among the HIV patients presenting with meningitis, 35.8% had tuberculous meningitis. [196] Other important risk factors including age, alcoholism, malnutrition, drug abuse and homelessness. [193]

The treatment of tuberculous meningitis is similar in both HIV and non-HIV patients. Isoniazid (5-10 mg/kg/d, maximum 300 mg/d) and pyrazinamide (15-30 mg/kg/d, maximum 2.5 g/d), ethambutol (15-25 mg/kg/d, maximum 1.6 g/d) and rifampicin (10-20 mg/kg/d, maximum 600 mg/d) are initiated for 2 months. Dexamethasone may be added for the initial 2 months especially in patients with mild disease. If the clinical response is good, pyrazinamide and ethambutol can be discontinued together with steroid, and isoniazid and rifampicin continued for another 7 to 10 months.

Malaria

At any one time, 5% of the world population is affected by malaria, giving rise to $300 - 500$ million cases worldwide and $0.5 - 2.75$ million deaths every year. Children from Sub-Saharan Africa account for 90% of these deaths, and $75 - 90\%$ of all pediatrics death in this region is due to malaria. Malaria is caused by the 4 species of *Plasmodium* parasites – *P. falciparum, P. ovale, P. vivax* and *P. malaria*, but almost all deaths are due to *P. falciparum*. Most malaria infections occurs between the latitude of 39°N and 29°S and 4 regions within this area account for more than two thirds of the malaria infections in the world – Sub-Saharan Africa, India-Sri Lanka, Vietnam, Papua New Guinea-Solomon Islands, and central to northern South America from Belize to Peru. [197-199]

In adult, cerebral malaria is defined as unarousable coma, as evident by non-localizing motor response to noxious stimuli and incomprehensible vocal response, with the finding of asexual forms of *P. falciparum* in the blood film, and the exclusion of other causes of encephalopathies. Cerebral malaria is the commonest manifestation of severe malaria in adults, especially in Southeast Asia and the Pacific islands. Half of the adult patients with severe malaria from Thailand and Vietnam and 17% of those from Papua New Guinea had cerebral malaria. Adults with cerebral malaria present dramatically with generalized seizure followed by persistent unconsciousness. On examination, there is often neck stiffness, papilloedema, retinal exudates, and in 15% of patients, retinal hemorrhage. Although brainstem reflexes are preserved except in deep coma, conjugate eye movement is often impaired, usually manifests as divergent response to oculocephalic ("doll's eye") and oculovestibular (caloric) reflexes, convergence spasm, ocular blobbing, horizontal and vertical nystagmus, and sixth nerve palsy. Other findings include jaundice, bruxism, pout reflex, spastic quadriplegia and various abnormal posturing, such as extensor, decorticate or decerebrate postures, and opisthotonus. Seizure, often generalized tonic-clonic, occurs in 20% of adults. Overall mortality of cerebral malaria in adult is about 20%, but ranges from 8% in patients with cerebral malaria without other organ impairment to 50% if there is coexisting renal failure and metabolic acidosis. Most deaths occur within 48 hours of presentation. [198,200]

Children with cerebral malaria present with short duration of fever - on average of about 48 hours - with anorexia, vomiting, diarrhoea, vomiting and seizure. Hepatosplenomegaly, abnormal posturing, abnormal eye movement, bruxism, impaired brainstem reflexes and retinal abnormalities are common. Abnormal posturing occurs in up to 30 - 50% of children, and may manifest as decorticate (in half of these patients), decerebrate (in a third), opisthotonic, flexor, or rarely hypotonic posturing. Eye movement abnormalities include divergence gaze, disconjugate eye movement, vertical nystagmus, ocular blobbing and sustained upward deviation. Retinal haemorrhage is seen in 6 - 37% of patients; other retinal abnormalities include exudates in about 5% of children, papilloedema in 8%, retinal whitening in up to 30%, and retinal vessel abnormalities. Convulsion is common, affecting 15 – 100% of children with cerebral malaria depending on case definition, and manifests either as generalized or focal seizure, or as non-convulsive status epilepticus, in which the patient show only jerky eye movement, excessive salivation or irregular breathing pattern. Neurological sequelae are seen in 3 - 29% of survivors, and mortality ranges from 4 - 38%. The most important prognostic factors for mortality are impaired consciousness, respiratory distress, hypoglycemia and jaundice. Children with recurrent seizure, prolonged and deep coma and hypoglycemia are more likely to have residual neurological deficits. Common neurological deficits such as ataxia, monoparesis, hemiparesis or cortical blindness are often transient or improve over months. Other deficits include dysarthria, dysphasia, cognitive impairment, behavioral problems, hearing loss and epilepsy. [198,201-203]

Like many other central nervous system infections, cerebral malaria is a medical emergency. Treatment of hypovolemia, hypoglycemia, seizure, acute renal failure, disseminated intravascular coagulopathy and pulmonary edema, often in intensive care setting, are important aspects of management. Specific antimalarial treatment depends on local resistance pattern. Chloroquine (600 mg base immediately, followed by 300 mg base every 6 to 8 hours for 48 hours, or in children, 10 mg base/kg immediately followed by 5 mg base/kg over 36 hours in 4 doses) is still useful in Central American countries and Turkey. In most other areas, chloroquine resistance is widespread and quinine is the mainstay of treatment. Quinine hydrochloride is given intravenously or deep intramuscularly with a loading dose of 20 mg/kg and a maintenance dose of 10 mg/kg over 4 hour every 8 to 12 hours. Hypoglycemia and QT prolongation are common side effects. In areas where quinine resistance is common, such as Southeast Asia, artemisinin derivatives are useful alternatives. Artesunate is given intravenously, and artemether intramuscularly, with a loading dose of 3.2 mg/kg and maintenance dose of 1.6 mg/kg every 12 – 24 hours. As soon as the patient is able to swallow orally, a 7-day course of either sulfadoxine and pyrimethamine, or doxycycline/tetracycline (clindamycin for pregnant women or children) is started to ensure complete cure. In patients with parasitaemia greater than 5%, or those with respiratory failure, fulminant renal failure, disseminated intravascular coagulopathy or coma, exchange transfusion can rapidly decrease the parasite load. Exchange transfusion should be discontinued once the parasite load falls below 1-5%. [198,199]

Syphilis

Syphilis is caused by *Treponema pallidum,* a spiral, motile, slender spirochete. It is transmitted via an active lesion to mucus membrane or skin, or by contaminated blood products, or in utero. Syphilis was a highly prevalent disease less than a century ago; in the Western World, it affected 8 – 10% of the adult population. During the Second World War, the incidence of syphilis in the United States was $90 / 10^5$. With the advent of antibiotics, the incidence dropped to about $7 / 10^5$ in the 1960's, and rebounded slightly in the next two decades to about $11 / 10^5$. The incidence rose again since the outbreak of HIV infections. The incidence of syphilis in other Western countries in the 1970's and 1980's remained low at $0.18 – 4 / 10^5$. [1,204-206] Among the HIV patients, prospective surveys showed that the prevalence of HIV varies from 1.8% in Miami, Florida, [207] to 3.1% in Spain, [208] 31% in New Orleans [209] and part of Germany.[210] The prevalence of neurosyphilis remained low at 1% - 2.9% in HIV patients. [208,209]

Historically, syphilitic infection has been divided into five stages – primary, secondary, early latent, late latent and tertiary – even though the underlying pathological process represents a continuum of spirochetal invasion. Soon after inoculation, a spirochetemia develops, leading to widespread vasculitis and in some, aseptic meningitis. As the host cellular immunity response develops, the infection is brought under control. In patients with impaired cellular immunity, such as those with malnutrition, HIV infection or during late pregnancy, the infection is not controlled, leading to the development of obliterative endarteritis and local tissue invasion, causing gumma formation, and in the central nervous system, meningovascular syphilis, myelitis, encephalitis, cerebral atrophy, and optic atrophy.

Spirochetal invasion of the central nervous system occurs in at least 40% of the patients in early syphilis, but fortunately, only 25% of patients develop meningitis, and only 4 – 8% of untreated patients develop more advance form of neurosyphilis. Many of the patients with initial, untreated, syphilitic invasion of the central nervous system remit spontaneously. In others, aseptic meningitis develops, which could remain asymptomatic, and is diagnosed only by positive serologic tests or spirochetal isolation from the cerebrospinal fluid, or become symptomatic, or progress to chronic meningitis. The chronic meningitis could remain asymptomatic or progress to tissue invasion, evolving into the myriad of manifestations of neurosyphilis.

In surveys of HIV patients with neurosyphilis, 24 – 33% of patients were found to be in early phase, 32 – 34% in early latent or asymptomatic phase, and 5 – 42% in late phase. [211,212] In another survey, 13% of HIV patients with neurosyphilis were asymptomatic, 4% had acute meningitis. 23% had meningovascular syphilis, 12% had spinal cord disease, 8% had cranial nerve palsies, 17% had general paresis, 6% had seizures, and 4% each had eye involvement, parkinsonism or tabes dorsalis. [213]

Acute aseptic meningitis is the earliest manifestation of neurosyphilis; occurring within the first 12 months of inoculation. It presents as low grade fever, headache, mild photophobia, neck stiffness, and in some, an encephalitic picture with confusion, seizure, acute hydrocephalus, papilloedema and focal neurological deficits, which may include lower cranial nerve palsies, sensorineural deafness, hemiplegia or dysphasia. Acute optic neuritis, either unilateral or one after another, may occur in isolation or together with syphilitic meningitis. The cerebrospinal fluid is almost always abnormal. With adequate treatment, most patients recover within days or weeks. If left untreated, some would progress to other form of neurosyphilis.

If the infection is not controlled, chronic meningitis and obliterative endarteritis may develop in the medium or large arteries. This may lead to parenchymal infarction, or the so-called meningovascular syphilis. In the cerebral cortex or brainstem, this manifests clinically as headache, dizziness, poor memory, or focal neurological deficits, depending on the site of infarct. Hemiparesis, dysphasia, cranial nerve palsies, visual loss and sensory loss are all common. In the spinal cord, it manifests as either syphilitic meningomyelitis or acute syphilitic transverse myelitis. Syphilitic meningomyelitis begins gradually with asymmetrical weakness or numbness of the lower limbs, and progresses to spastic paraplegia, double incontinence, loss of proprioception and vibrational sense. Acute syphilitic transverse myelitis presents as acute, though often incomplete, transection of the thoracic spinal cord with flaccid paraparesis, sensory level, loss of proprioception and vibrational sense, which later evolves into spastic paraparesis.

With chronic cerebral parenchymal invasion, the patient develops progressive dementia with prominent psychiatric features, known as "general paresis of the insane". Depending on locality, about 0.1 - 3% of patients admitted into psychiatric hospitals had a final diagnosis of neurosyphilis. [214,215] The clinical features include emotional lability; an irritable, paranoid personality; apathy, inappropriate behavior, hallucinations, grandiose delusion, memory loss, which leads to disorientation and learning disability; loss of insight; a thick slurred speech, Argyll-Robertson pupil, tremor of the tongue, face and hand, and hyperreflexia.

15 – 30 years after the initial infection, tabes dorsalis may develop and cause lancinating pain, visceral crisis, Argyll-Robertson pupil, ptosis, ophthalmoplegia, optic atrophy, sensory ataxia, areflexia, Charcot joints, urinary overflow incontinence, constipation and megacolon, and impotence. The eyes may be involved in any stage of the infection, and may occurs in isolation (such as iritis, anterior uveitis, optic neuritis), or in association with other manifestations, such as the Argyll-Robertson pupil, ptosis, ophthalmoplegia or optic atrophy.

Neurosyphilis is treated with intravenous penicillin G 3 – 4 million units every 4 hourly for 10 – 14 days or intramuscular procaine penicillin 2.4 million units daily together with probenecid 500 mg qid for 10 days. Intravenous or intramuscular ceftriaxone 2 g daily for 14 days is a useful alternative, though a failure rate of up to 23% has been reported. In patients who are allergic to penicillin, desensitization to penicillin before treatment with the above regimes could be attempted. Alternatively, erythromycin or tetracycline in doses of 500 mg every 6 hourly for 20 to 30 days can be tried, though the failure rate is high. The patients should be reviewed and the cerebrospinal fluid re-examined every 6 monthly until the patient is symptom-free and the cerebrospinal fluid abnormalities reversed. Otherwise another full course of penicillin should be given.

The primary prevention of syphilis include health education and counseling to promote behavior change, such as the reduction of sexual partners and the avoidance of high risk sexual practices, especially in population with high risk behavior; and increase in condom accessibility and use. Secondary prevention strategies include improvement in the quality, accessibility and acceptability of sexually transmitted disease clinics and care; screening of high risk population, partner notification, reporting to notifiable diseases centre, financial incentives to modify health seeking behavior and perhaps mass treatment. [216]

CONCLUSION

Central nervous system infection is one of the most important neurological diseases globally. Even though bacterial meningitis is on the retreat in many developed countries, it is still a major health concern in many poor countries, especially in the African meningitic belt. Viral encephalitides, on the other hand, have become a major concern; flaviviruses which were geographically localized in the past have spread to almost global proportion, and new viruses continued to be discovered. Above and beyond this, the HIV continues to scourge especially the poorer countries. In the future when degenerative and congenital diseases are better understood and managed, infectious diseases may return yet again to be the main cause of mortality and morbidity.

REFERENCES

[1]   Wenger JD and Broome CV. 'Bacterial meningitis: Epidemiology' In Lambert HP (ed)
        Infections of the Central Nervous System: Kass Handbook of Infectious Diseases.
        London: BC Decker, 1991. 16 – 31.

[2]   Dawson KG. Emerson JC and Burns JL. 'Fifteen years of experience with bacterial
        meningitis' *The Paediatrics Infectious Disease Journal.* 1999 September. 18(9); 816-
        822.

[3]   Enders PJ. Trepka MJ. Davis JP. 'Impact of Haemophilus influenzae type b (Hib)
        conjugate vaccines on Haemophilus influenzae meningitis in Wisconsin' *WMJ,* 2000
        Aug. 99(5):45-8.

[4]   Schuchat A. Robinson K. Wenger JD. Harrison LH. Farley M. Reingold AL. Lefkowitz
        L. Perkins BA. 'Bacterial meningitis in the United States in 1995. Active Surveillance
        Team.' *New England Journal of Medicine,* 1997 Oct 2. 337(14):970-6.

[5]   Hussein AS. And Shafran SD. 'Acute bacterial meningitis in adults: A 12-year review.'
        Medicine 2000 November. 79(6); 360-8.

[6]   Nascimento-Carvalho CM. Moreno-Carvalho OA 'Etiology of bacterial meningitis in a
        cohort from Salvador, Bahia' *Arquivos de Neuro-Psiquiatria. 56(1):*83-7, 1998 Mar.

[7]   Nascimento-Carvalho CM. Moreno-Carvalho OA. 'Etiology of bacterial meningitis
        among children aged 2-59 months in Salvador, Northeast Brazil, before and after
        routine use of Haemophilus influenzae type B vaccine.' *Arquivos de Neuro-Psiquiatria,*
        2004 Jun. 62(2A):250-2.

[8]   Weiss DP. Coplan P. Guess H. 'Epidemiology of bacterial meningitis among children
        in Brazil, 1997-1998.' *Revista de Saude Publica,* 2001 Jun. 35(3):249-55.

[9]   Diaz JM. Catalan L. Urrutia MT. Prado V. Ledermann W. Mendoza C. Topelberg S.
        'Trends of etiology of acute bacterial meningitis in Chilean children from 1989 to
        1998. Impact of the anti-H influenzae type b vaccine' *Revista Medica de Chile,* 2001
        Jul. 129(7):719-26.

[10]   Boehme C. Soto L. Rodriguez G. Serra J. Illesca V. Reydet P. 'Three years of acute
        bacterial meningitis in the pediatric service at the Temuco Regional Hospital' *Revista
        Medica de Chile,* 1993 Jun. 121(6):633-8.

[11]   Barboza AG. Ioli P. Zamarbide I. Estrago MI. Castineiras F. de Wouters L. 'A study of
        the incidence and a descriptive analysis of adult non-tuberculous primary bacterial
        meningitis in a population in Argentina' *Revista de Neurologia,* 2002 Sep 16-30.
        35(6):508-12.

[12]   Hansen B. Black FT. Andersen PL 'Purulent meningitis at the Marselisborg Hospital
        1980-1990' [Danish] *Ugeskrift for Laeger, 1994 Nov 21.* 156(47):7049-57.

[13]   Handberg J. Prio TK. Rohde K. Antonsen A. Hansen M. 'Purulent meningitis among
        adults in the county of Frederiksborg. Therapeutic results in the period 1 January 1980-
        -31 December 1990' Ugeskrift for Laeger, 1993 Oct 25. 155(43):3452-5.

[14]   Sigurdardottir B. Bjornsson OM. Jonsdottir KE. Erlendsdottir H. Gudmundsson S.
        'Acute bacterial meningitis in adults. A 20-year overview' *Archives of Internal
        Medicine, 1997 Feb 24.* 157(4):425-30.

[15] Kyaw MH. Christie P. Jones IG. Campbell H. 'The changing epidemiology of bacterial meningitis and invasive non-meningitic bacterial disease in Scotland during the period 1983-99.' *Scandinavian Journal of Infectious Diseases, 2002.* 34(4):289-98.

[16] Urwin G. Yuan MF. Feldman RA. 'Prospective study of bacterial meningitis in North East Thames region, 1991-3, during introduction of Haemophilus influenzae vaccine' *BMJ, 1994 Nov 26.* 309(6966):1412-4.

[17] Perrocheau A. Georges S. Laurent E. 'Epidemiology of bacterial meningitis in France in 2002]' *Revue du Praticien, 2004 May 15.* 54(9):945-50.

[18] Syrogiannopoulos GA. Mitselos CJ. Beratis NG. 'Childhood bacterial meningitis in Southwestern Greece: a population-based study' Clinical Infectious Diseases, 1995 Dec. 21(6):1471-3.

[19] Fernandez-Lopez M. Martinez-Hornos M. Navarro J. Cintado C. 'Bacterial meningitis in the health sector of Virgen del Rocio, Spain' *Enfermedades Infecciosas y Microbiologia Clinica, 1998 Dec.* 16(10):449-52.

[20] Morant A. Diez J. Gimeno C. de la Muela N. Pereiro I. Brines J. 'Epidemiology of Haemophilus influenzae type b, Neisseria meningitidis, and Streptococcus pneumoniae in children in the Valencia Community, Spain. Acute diseases study group' *Revista de Neurologia, 1998 Jan.* 26(149):34-7.

[21] Casado Flores J. Garcia Teresa MA. Cambra F. Pilar Orive J. Teja JL. Rodriguez Nunez A. Quiroga E. Calvo C. Ruiz Extremera MA. Perez Navero J. Melendo J. Soult JA. 'Multicenter prospective study on severe bacterial meningitis in children' Comment in: *An Esp Pediatr.* 1998 Aug;49(2):209.

[22] Ara JR. Cia P. Arribas JL. Aguirre JM. de Juan F. Marco Tello A. 'Clinico-epidemiologic study of bacterial meningitis in Aragon' Medicina Clinica 1994 Nov 12. 103(16):611-4.

[23] Fernandez-Jaen A. Borque Andres C. del Castillo Martin F. Pena Garcia P. Vidal Lopez ML. 'Bacterial meningitis in pediatrics. Study of 166 cases' *Anales Espanoles de Pediatria, 1998 May.* 48(5):495-8.

[24] Roca J. Campos J. Monso G. Trujillo G. Riverola A. Suris JC. Garcia-Tornel S. Barnadas M. 'Meningitis in pediatrics. Clinical and epidemiological study of 173 cases' *Enfermedades Infecciosas y Microbiologia Clinica, 1992 Feb.* 10(2):79-88.

[25] Rosinska M. Zielinski A. 'Meningitis and encephalitis in Poland in 2002' *Przeglad Epidemiologiczny, 2004.* 58(1):57-65.

[26] Hudeckova H. Novakova E. Olear V. 'Analysis of bacterial meningitis in the Slovak Republic 1991-1998. *Epidemiologie, Mikrobiologie, Imunologie, 2000 Aug.* 49(3):130-5.

[27] Van Hoeck KJ, Mahieu LM, Vaerenberg MH and Van Acker KJ. 'A retrospective epidemiological study of bacterial meningitis in an urban area in Belgium' *European Journal of Paediatrics,* 1997. 156: 288-291.

[28] Salmaso S. Mastrantonio P, Scuderi G, Congiu ME, Stroffolini T, Pompa MG and Squarcione S. 'Pattern of bacterial meningitis in Italy, 1994' *European Journal of Epidemiology,* 1997. 13:317-321.

[29] Luca V. Gessner BD. Luca C. Turcu T. Rugina S. Rugina C. Ilie M. Novakova E. Vlasich C. 'Incidence and etiological agents of bacterial meningitis among children <5

years of age in two districts of Romania.' *European Journal of Clinical Microbiology & Infectious Diseases,* 2004 Jul. 23(7):523-8.

[30] Peltola H. 'Burden of meningitis and other severe bacterial infections of children in Africa: Implications for prevention' *Clinical Infectious Diseases,* 2001; 31:64-75.

[31] Campagne G. Schuchat A. Djibo S. Ousseini A. Cisse L. Chippaux JP. 'Epidemiology of bacterial meningitis in Niamey, Niger, 1981-96.' *Bulletin of the World Health Organization,* 1999. 77(6):499-508.

[32] Ahmed AA. Salih MA. Ahmed HS. 'Post-endemic acute bacterial meningitis in Sudanese children.' *East African Medical Journal,* 1996 Aug. 73(8):527-32.

[33] Bernardino L. Magalhaes J. Simoes MJ. Monteiro L. Bacterial meningitis in Angola. [Letter] *Lancet, 2003 May 3. 361(9368):1564-5.*

[34] Fonkoua MC. Cunin P. Sorlin P. Musi J. Martin PM. 'Bacterial meningitis in Yaounde (Cameroon) in 1999-2000' *Bulletin de la Societe de Pathologie Exotique,* 2001 Nov. 94(4):300-3.

[35] Youssef FG, El-Sakka H, Azab A, Eloun S, Chapman GD, Ismail T, Mansour H, Hallaj Z and Mahoney F. 'Etiology, antimicrobial susceptibility profiles, and mortality associated with bacterial meningitis among children in Egypt.' *Annals of Epidemiology* 2004. 14:44-48.

[36] Migliani R. Clouzeau J. Decousser JW. Ravelomanana N. Rasamoelisoa J. Rabijaona H. Dromigny JA. Pfister P. Roux JF. 'Non-tubercular bacterial meningitis in children in Antananarivo, Madagascar' *Archives de Pediatrie,* 2002 Sep. 9(9):892-7.

[37] Gordon SB. Walsh AL. Chaponda M. Gordon MA. Soko D. Mbwvinji M. Molyneux ME. Read RC. 'Bacterial meningitis in Malawian adults: pneumococcal disease is common, severe, and seasonal.' *Clinical Infectious Diseases,* 2000 Jul. 31(1):53-7.

[38] Akpede O. Abiodun PO. Sykes M. Salami CE. 'Childhood bacterial meningitis beyond the neonatal period in southern Nigeria: changes in organisms/antibiotic susceptibility' *East African Medical Journal,* 1994 Jan. 71(1):14-20.

[39] Donald PR. Cotton MF. Hendricks MK. Schaaf HS. de Villiers JN. Willemse TE. 'Pediatric meningitis in the Western Cape Province of South Africa.' *Journal of Tropical Pediatrics,* 1996 Oct. 42(5):256-61.

[40] Daoud AS. al-Sheyyab M. Batchoun RG. Rawashdeh MO. Nussair MM. Pugh RN. 'Bacterial meningitis: still a cause of high mortality and severe neurological morbidity in childhood.' *Journal of Tropical Pediatrics,* 1995 Oct. 41(5):308-10.

[41] Al-Mazrou YY. Al-Jeffri MH. Al-Haggar SH. Musa EK. Mohamed OM. Abdalla MN. 'Haemophilus type B meningitis in Saudi children under 5 years old.' *Journal of Tropical Pediatrics,* 2004 Jun. 50(3):131-6.

[42] Almuneef M. Memish Z. Khan Y. Kagallwala A. Alshaalan M.'Childhood bacterial meningitis in Saudi Arabia.' *Journal of Infection,* 1998 Mar. 36(2):157-60.

[43] Srair HA. Aman H. al-Madan M. al-Khater M. 'Bacterial meningitis in Saudi children.' *Indian Journal of Pediatrics,* 1992 Nov-Dec. 59(6):719-21.

[44] Mahmoud R, Mahmoud M, Badrinath P, Sheek-Hussein M, Alwash R and Nicol AG. 'Pattern of meningitis in Al-Ain medical district, United Arab Emirates – a decadal experience (1990-1999)' *Journal of infection,* 2002. 44:22-25.

[45] Saha SK. Rikitomi N. Ruhulamin M. Watanabe K. Ahmed K. Biswas D. Hanif M. Khan WA. Islam M. Matsumoto K. Nagatake T. 'The increasing burden of disease in Bangladeshi children due to Haemophilus influenzae type b meningitis.' *Annals of Tropical Paediatrics*, 1997 Mar. 17(1):5-8.

[46] Shaikh S. Shaikh RB. Faiz MS. 'Seasonal paradox in acute meningitis at Nawabshah.' *Journal of the College of Physicians & Surgeons - Pakistan*, 2003 Apr. 13(4):207-9.

[47] Yang Y. Leng Z. Shen X. Lu D. Jiang Z. Rao J. Fan X. Liu J. Shen Y. 'Acute bacterial meningitis in children in Hefei, China 1990-1992.' *Chinese Medical Journal*, 1996 May. 109(5):385-8.

[48] Ishikawa T. Asano Y. Morishima T. Nagashima M. Sobue G. Watanabe K. Yamaguchi H. 'Epidemiology of bacterial meningitis in children: Aichi Prefecture, Japan, 1984-1993.' *Pediatric Neurology*, 1996 Apr. 14(3):244-50.

[49] Sakata H. Maruyama S. 'A study of bacterial meningitis in Hokkaido between 1994 and 1998' *Kansenshogaku Zasshi - Journal of the Japanese Association for Infectious Diseases*, 2000 Apr. 74(4):339-44.

[50] Kamiya H, Uehara S, Kato T, Shiraki K, Togashi T, Morishima T, goto Y, Satoh O and Standaert S. 'Childhood bacterial meningitis in Japan' *The Paediatric Infectious Disease Journal*, 1998 September. 17(9) Supplement; S183-5.

[51] J. S. Kim, Y. T. Jang, J. D. Kim, T. H. Park, J. M. Park, P. E. Kilgore, W. A. Kennedy, E. Park, B. Nyambat, D. R. Kim, P. H. Hwang, S. J. Kim, S. H. Eun, H. S. Lee, J. H. Cho, Y. S. Kim, S. J. Chang, H. F. Huang, J. D. Clemens and J. I. Ward 'Incidence of Haemophilus influenzae type b and other invasive diseases in South Korean children' *Vaccine*, 2004. 22: 3952-62.

[52] Navaratnam P and Puthucheary S. 'The bacteriology of acute meningitis in the University Hospital Kuala Lumpur.' *ASEAN Journal of Clinical Sciences*, June 1988. 8(2):59-63

[53] Chan YC. Wilder-Smith A, Ong BKC, Kumarasinghe G and Wilder-Smith E. 'Adult community acquired bacterial meningitis in a Singaporean teaching hospital. A seven-year overview.' *Singapore Medical Journal*, 2002. 43(12):632-636.

[54] Chotpitayasunondh T. 'Bacterial meningitis in children: etiology and clinical features, an 11-year review of 618 cases.' *Southeast Asian Journal of Tropical Medicine & Public Health*, 1994 Mar. 25(1):107-15.

[55] Tran TT. Le QT. Tran TN. Nguyen NT. Pedersen FK. Schlumberger M. 'The etiology of bacterial pneumonia and meningitis in Vietnam.' *Pediatric Infectious Disease Journal*, 1998 Sep. 17(9 Suppl):S192-4.

[56] Matsuo H. Sakamoto S. 'Purulent meningitis caused by Streptococcus suis in a pig breeder' *Kansenshogaku Zasshi - Journal of the Japanese Association for Infectious Diseases*, 2003 May. 77(5):340-2.

[57] Tarradas C. Luque I. de Andres D. Abdel-Aziz Shahein YE. Pons P. Gonzalez F. Borge C. Perea A. 'Epidemiological relationship of human and swine Streptococcus suis isolates.' *Journal of Veterinary Medicine Series B*, 2001 Jun. 48(5):347-55.

[58] Campagne G. Chippaux JP. Djibo S. Issa O. Garba A. 'Epidemiology and control of bacterial meningitis in children less than 1 year in Niamey (Niger)' *Bulletin de la Societe de Pathologie Exotique*, 1999 May. 92(2):118-22.

[59] Sung RY. Senok AC. Ho A. Oppenheimer SJ. Davies DP. 'Meningitis in Hong Kong children, with special reference to the infrequency of haemophilus and meningococcal infection.' *Journal of Paediatrics & Child Health*, 1997 Aug. 33(4):296-9.

[60] Ford H. Wright J. 'Bacterial meningitis in Swaziland: an 18 month prospective study of its impact.' *Journal of Epidemiology & Community Health*, 1994 Jun. 48(3):276-80.

[61] Gomes I. Lucena R. Melo A. 'Clinical and laboratory characteristics of pyogenic meningitis in adults' *Arquivos de Neuro-Psiquiatria*, 1997 Sep. 55(3B):584-7.

[62] Fernandez-Crehuet Navajas R. Martinez de la Iglesia J. Serrano del Castillo A. Perula de Torres L.' Clinical-epidemiological assessment of bacterial meningitis in the province of Cordoba (1983-1989)*Revista de Sanidad e Higiene Publica*, 1991 Mar-Apr. 65(2):127-35.

[63] Daoud AS. al-Sheyyab M. Abu-Ekteish F. Obeidat A. Ali AA. el-Shanti H. 'Neonatal meningitis in northern Jordan.' *Journal of Tropical Pediatrics*, 1996 Oct. 42(5):267-70.

[64] Palmer A. Weber M. Bojang K. McKay T. Adegbola R. 'Acute bacterial meningitis in The Gambia: a four-year review of paediatric hospital admissions.' *Journal of Tropical Pediatrics*, 1999 Feb. 45(1):51-3.

[65] Tang LM. Chen ST. Hsu WC. Lyu RK. 'Acute bacterial meningitis in adults: a hospital-based epidemiological study.' *Qjm*, 1999 Dec. 92(12):719-25.

[66] Molyneux E. Walsh A. Phiri A. Molyneux M. 'Acute bacterial meningitis in children admitted to the Queen Elizabeth Central Hospital, Blantyre, Malawi in 1996-97.' *Tropical Medicine & International Health, 1998 Aug.* 3(8):610-8.

[67] Baraff LJ. Lee SI. Schriger DL. 'Outcomes of bacterial meningitis in children: a meta-analysis.' *Pediatric Infectious Disease Journal*, 1993 May. 12(5):389-94.

[68] Roos KL. 'Acute bacterial meningitis' *Seminar in neurology*, 2000. 20(3): 293-306.

[69] Chippaux JP. Campagne G. Djibo S. Cisse L. Hassane A. Kanta I. 'Preventive immunisation could reduce the risk of meningococcal epidemics in the African meningitis belt.' *Annals of Tropical Medicine & Parasitology*, 1999 Jul. 93(5):505-10.

[70] Quagliarello VJ and Scheld WM. 'Treatment of bacterial meningitis' *New England Journal of Medicine*, March 6, 1997. 336(10):708-716.

[71] De Gans J and Van de Beek D for the European Dexamethasone in adulthood bacterial meningitis study investigators. 'Dexamethasone in adults with bacterial meningitis' *New England Journal of Medicine*, November 14, 2002. 347 (20): 1549 – 1556.

[72] Hristeva L. Booy R. Bowler I. Wilkinson AR. 'Prospective surveillance of neonatal meningitis' *Archives of Disease in Childhood*, 1993 Jul. 69(1 Spec No):14-8.

[73] Rantakallio P. Leskinen M. von Wendt L. 'Incidence and prognosis of central nervous system infections in a birth cohort of 12,000 children.' *Scandinavian Journal of Infectious Diseases, 1986.* 18(4):287-94.

[74] Rotbart HA. 'Viral meningitis'. *Seminars in Neurology*, 2000. 20(3): 277-292.

[75] Jaidane H. Chouchane C. Gharbi J. Chouchane S. Merchaoui Z. Ben Meriem C. Aouni M. Guediche MN. 'Neuromeningeal enterovirus infections in Tunisia: epidemiology, clinical presentation, and outcome of 26 pediatric cases' *Medecine et Maladies Infectieuses*, 2005 Jan. 35(1):33-8.

[76] Tee WS. Choong CT. Lin RV. Ling AE. 'Aseptic meningitis in children--the Singapore experience.' *Annals of the Academy of Medicine*, Singapore, 2002 Nov. 31(6):756-60.

[77] Chambon M. Archimbaud C. Bailly JL. Henquell C. Regagnon C. Charbonne F. Peigue-Lafeuille H. 'Circulation of enteroviruses and persistence of meningitis cases in the winter of 1999-2000.' *Journal of Medical Virology*, 2001 Oct. 65(2):340-7.

[78] Valdezate S. Mesa F. Otero JR. 'Meningitis caused by enterovirus in a pediatric hospital: experience in 1996' *Enfermedades Infecciosas y Microbiologia Clinica*, 1998 Mar. 16(3):135-7.

[79] McIntyre JP. Keen GA. 'Laboratory surveillance of viral meningitis by examination of cerebrospinal fluid in Cape Town, 1981-9.' *Epidemiology & Infection*, 1993 Oct. 111(2):357-71.

[80] Karte H. Wecker I. 'Echovirus 30 epidemic' *Deutsche Medizinische Wochenschrift* 14 July 1978. 103(28):1136-8.

[81] Todd WT. MacMillan MJ. Gray JA. 'ECHO virus type 30 meningitis in Edinburgh.' *Scottish Medical Journal* April 1983. 28(2):160-3.

[82] Mori I. Matsumoto K. Hatano M. Sudo M. Kimura Y. 'An unseasonable winter outbreak of echovirus type 30 meningitis.' *Journal of Infection* November 1995. 31(3):219-23.

[83] Rodriguez RS. Gomez-Barreto D. Pallansch M. Vazquez J. Karabatsos N. 'Epidemic outbreak of viral meningitis caused by type 30 ECHO virus' *Boletin Medico del Hospital Infantil de Mexico* July 1992. 49(7):412-5.

[84] Tang RB. Chen SJ. Wu KG. Lee BH. Hwang B. 'The clinical evaluation of an outbreak of aseptic meningitis in children.' *Chung Hua i Hsueh Tsa Chih - Chinese Medical Journal* February 1996. 57(2):134-8.

[85] Majda-Stanislawska E. Kuydowicz J. Bartczak D. 'Epidemic of ECHO type 30 virus meningitis in children from the Lodz region in the years 1995 and 1996.' *Przeglad Epidemiologiczny*. 51(3):267-74, 1997.

[86] Schumacher JD. Chuard C. Renevey F. Matter L. Regamey C. 'Outbreak of echovirus 30 meningitis in Switzerland.' *Scandinavian Journal of Infectious Diseases* 1999. 31(6):539-42.

[87] Chambon M. Bailly JL. Beguet A. Henquell C. Archimbaud C. Gaulme J. Labbe A. Malpuech G. Peigue-Lafeuille H. 'An outbreak due to echovirus type 30 in a neonatal unit in France in 1997: usefulness of PCR diagnosis.' *Journal of Hospital Infection* Sep 1999. 43(1):63-8.

[88] Bernit E. de Lamballerie X. Zandotti C. Berger P. Veit V. Schleinitz N. de Micco P. Harle JR. Charrel RN. 'Prospective investigation of a large outbreak of meningitis due to echovirus 30 during summer 2000 in Marseilles, France.' *Medicine* Jul 2004. 83(4):245-53.

[89] Hauri AM. Schimmelpfennig M. Walter-Domes M. Letz A. Diedrich S. Lopez-Pila J. Schreier E 'An outbreak of viral meningitis associated with a public swimming pond.' *Epidemiology & Infection* Apr 2005. 133(2):291-8.

[90] Wang JR. Tsai HP. Huang SW. Kuo PH. Kiang D. Liu CC. 'Laboratory diagnosis and genetic analysis of an echovirus 30-associated outbreak of aseptic meningitis in Taiwan in 2001.' *Journal of Clinical Microbiology*, Dec 2002. 40(12):4439-44.

[91] Mohle-Boetani JC. Matkin C. Pallansch M. Helfand R. Fenstersheib M. Blanding JA. Solomon SL. 'Viral meningitis in child care center staff and parents: an outbreak of echovirus 30 infections.' *Public Health Reports*, 1999 May-Jun. 114(3):249-56.

[92] Gorgievski-Hrisoho M. Schumacher JD. Vilimonovic N. Germann D. Matter L. 'Detection by PCR of enteroviruses in cerebrospinal fluid during a summer outbreak of aseptic meningitis in Switzerland.' *Journal of Clinical Microbiology*, 1998 Sep. 36(9):2408-12.

[93] Henigst W. Abar B. Wagner D. Paulig R. 'Virologic and serologic findings in an epidemic of abacterial meningitis of unknown origin' *Klinische Padiatrie*, 1975 Jul. 187(4):314-22.

[94] Gartner H. Sonntag HG. 'Epidemiological studies after an outbreak of meningitis' *Zentralblatt fur Bakteriologie, Parasitenkunde, Infektionskrankheiten und Hygiene - Erste Abteilung Originale - Reihe B: Hygiene, Praventive Medizin*, 1977 Dec. 165(5-6):548-56.

[95] Sumaya CV. Corman LI. 'Enteroviral meningitis in early infancy: significance in community outbreaks.' *Pediatric Infectious Disease*, 1982 May-Jun. 1(3):151-4.

[96] Kinnunen E. Hovi T. Stenvik M. Hellstrom O. Porras J. Kleemola M. Kantanen ML. 'Localized outbreak of enteroviral meningitis in adults.' *Acta Neurologica Scandinavica*, 1987 May. 75(5):346-51.

[97] Ashwell MJ. Smith DW. Phillips PA. Rouse IL. 'Viral meningitis due to echovirus types 6 and 9: epidemiological data from Western Australia.' *Epidemiology & Infection*, 1996 Dec. 117(3):507-12.

[98] Hamasaki M. Kajiwara J. Ishibasi T. Chijiwa K. Otsu R. Mori R. 'An epidemic of aseptic meningitis caused by echoviruses in Fukuoka Prefecture during April 1997 to August 1998' *Kansenshogaku Zasshi - Journal of the Japanese Association for Infectious Diseases*, 1999 Feb. 73(2):138-43.

[99] Jaidane H. Chouchane C. Gharbi J. Chouchane S. Merchaoui Z. Ben Meriem C. Aouni M. Guediche MN. 'Neuromeningeal enterovirus infections in Tunisia: epidemiology, clinical presentation, and outcome of 26 pediatric cases' *Medecine et Maladies Infectieuses*, 2005 Jan. 35(1):33-8.

[100] Reznik VI. Zdanovskaia NI. Sokur IV. Pereskokova MA. Esakova MA. 'Characteristics of the epidemic process in enterovirus infections in relation to the study of a serous meningitis outbreak' *Voprosy Virusologii*, 1980 Sep-Oct. (5):620-3.

[101] Aleraj B. Kruzic V. Borcic B. 'Epidemiology of enteroviral meningitis in Croatia 1958-1988 with special emphasis on the great epidemic of 1988' *Lijecnicki Vjesnik*, 1990 Sep-Oct. 112(9-10):305-9.

[102] Lasarte Velillas JJ. de Juan Martin F. Omenaca Teres M. Lalana Josa MP. Olivan Otal MP. Castillo Laita JA. Aldea Aldanondo MJ. 'Type 4 echovirus meningitis in childhood. Epidemiologic and clinical aspects apropos of an epidemiologic outbreak' *Anales Espanoles de Pediatria*, 1992 Jan. 36(1):29-33.

[103] Freire MC. Cisterna DM. Rivero K. Palacios GF. Casas I. Tenorio A. Gomez JA. 'Analysis of an outbreak of viral meningitis in the province of Tucuman, Argentina (erratum appears in Rev Panam Salud Publica. 2003 Jul;14(1):24) *Pan American Journal of Public Health*, 2003 Apr. 13(4):246-51.

[104] Handsher R. Shulman LM. Abramovitz B. Silberstein I. Neuman M. Tepperberg-Oikawa M. Fisher T. Mendelson E. 'A new variant of echovirus 4 associated with a large outbreak of aseptic meningitis.' *Journal of Clinical Virology*, 1999 Jun. 13(1-2):29-36.

[105] Gallacher K. Ghosh K. Patel A. Walker E. 'An outbreak of echovirus type 4 infections and its implications for diagnosis and management in general practice.' *Journal of Infection*, 1993 May. 26(3):321-4.

[106] Wilfert CM. Lauer BA. Cohen M. Costenbader ML. Myers E. 'An epidemic of echovirus 18 meningitis.' *Journal of Infectious Diseases*, 1975 Jan. 131(1):75-8.

[107] Miyamura K. Yamashita K. Yamadera S. Kato N. Akatsuka M. Yamazaki S. 'An epidemic of echovirus 18 in 1988 in Japan--high association with clinical manifestation of exanthem. A report of the National Epidemiological Surveillance of Infectious Agents in Japan.' *Japanese Journal of Medical Science & Biology*, 1990 Apr. 43(2):51-8.

[108] McLaughlin JB. Gessner BD. Lynn TV. Funk EA. Middaugh JP. 'Association of regulatory issues with an echovirus 18 meningitis outbreak at a children's summer camp in Alaska.' *Pediatric Infectious Disease Journal*, 2004 Sep. 23(9):875-7.

[109] Miwa C. Watanabe Y. 'Epidemic of infectious disease with echovirus type 16--epidemic in Tono area, Gifu Prefecture in 1984' *Kansenshogaku Zasshi - Journal of the Japanese Association for Infectious Diseases*, 1990 Jul. 64(7):809-14.

[110] Sarmiento L. Mas P. Goyenechea A. Palomera R. Morier L. Capo V. Quintana I. Santin M. 'First epidemic of echovirus 16 meningitis in Cuba.' *Emerging Infectious Diseases*, 2001 Sep-Oct. 7(5):887-9.

[111] Narkeviciute I. Vaiciuniene D. 'Outbreak of echovirus 13 infection among Lithuanian children.' *Clinical Microbiology & Infection*, 2004 Nov. 10(11):1023-5.

[112] Tsutsui H. Hamano T. Toho M. Nakamura M. Hayashi K. Yamamura O. Nakagawa H. Fujiyama J. Yoneda M. Kuriyama M. 'Adult cases of viral meningitis caused by echovirus type 13' *Rinsho Shinkeigaku - Clinical Neurology*, 2003 Jun. 43(6):363-5.

[113] Olejnik T. 'Epidemic of lymphocytic cerebrospinal meningitis in the fall of 1974 at Grudziadz' *Neurologia i Neurochirurgia Polska*, 1975 Nov-Dec. 9(6):723-5.

[114] Bowen GS. Fisher MC. DeForest A. Thompson CM Jr. Kleger B. Friedman H. 'Epidemic of meningitis and febrile illness in neonates caused by ECHO type 11 virus in Philadelphia.' *Pediatric Infectious Disease*, 1983 Sep-Oct. 2(5):359-63.

[115] Miwa C. Watanabe Y. 'Epidemic of aseptic meningitis with echovirus type 7 in Gifu prefecture in 1986' *Kansenshogaku Zasshi - Journal of the Japanese Association for Infectious Diseases*, 1989 Jun. 63(6):584-92.

[116] Gilbert GL. Dickson KE. Waters MJ. Kennett ML. Land SA. Sneddon M. 'Outbreak of enterovirus 71 infection in Victoria, Australia, with a high incidence of neurologic involvement.' *Pediatric Infectious Disease Journal*, 1988 Jul. 7(7):484-8.

[117] Miwa C. Sawatari S. 'Epidemic of aseptic meningitis with echovirus type 6 in Gifu Prefecture in 1992' *Kansenshogaku Zasshi - Journal of the Japanese Association for Infectious Diseases*, 1994 Sep. 68(9):1063-7.

[118] Cobos PV. Gutierrez Melendez P. Yanez Ortega JL. Rodrigo Palacios J. Macarron Vicente JL. Montero Alonso MR. Lozano A. 'Epidemiologic study of an outbreak of

echovirus type-9 meningitis' *Revista de Sanidad e Higiene Publica*, 1994 Sep-Dec. 68(5-6):607-15.

[119] Kimura H. Minakami H. Sakae K. Ohbuchi M. Kuwashima M. Otsuki K. 'Outbreak of echovirus type 33 infection in Japanese school children.' [Letter] *Pediatric Infectious Disease Journal*, 1997 Jan. 16(1):83-4.

[120] Valassina M. Cuppone AM. Bianchi S. Santini L. Cusi MG. 'Evidence of Toscana virus variants circulating in Tuscany, Italy, during the summers of 1995 to 1997.' *Journal of Clinical Microbiology*, 1998 Jul. 36(7):2103-4.

[121] Obernikowicz B. 'Clinical observations in the enterovirus cerebrospinal meningitis outbreak in the Plotsk region in the fall of 1995' *Przeglad Epidemiologiczny*, 1998. 52(4):483-90.

[122] Ramelli GP. Simonetti GD. Gorgievski-Hrisoho M. Aebi C. Bianchetti MG. 'Outbreak of coxsackie B5 virus meningitis in a Scout camp.' [Letter] *Pediatric Infectious Disease Journal*, 2004 Jan. 23(1):86-7.

[123] Koskiniemi M, Korppi M, Mustonen K, Rantala H, Muttilainen M, Herrgard E, Ukkonen P, Vaheri A. 'Epidemiology of encephalitis in children. A prospective multicentre study.' *European Journal of Paediatrics*. 1997. 156: 541-545.

[124] Iff T, Donati F, Vassella F, Schaad UB, Bianchetti MG. 'Acute encephalitis in Swiss children: aetiology and outcome.' *European Journal of Paediatric Neurology* 1998. 2: 233-237.

[125] Rantalaiho T. Farkkila M. Vaheri A. Koskiniemi M. 'Acute encephalitis from 1967 to 1991.' *Journal of the Neurological Sciences,* 2001 Mar 1. 184(2):169-77.

[126] Koskiniemi M. Manninen V. Vaheri A. Sainio K. Eistola P. Karli P. 'Acute encephalitis. A survey of epidemiological, clinical and microbiological features covering a twelve-year period.' *Acta Medica Scandinavica,* 1981. 209(1-2):115-20.

[127] Mickiene A. Laiskonis A. Gunther G. Vene S. Lundkvist A. Lindquist L. 'Tickborne encephalitis in an area of high endemicity in lithuania: disease severity and long-term prognosis.' *Clinical Infectious Diseases*, 2002 Sep 15. 35(6):650-8.

[128] Cizman M. Jazbec J. 'Etiology of acute encephalitis in childhood in Slovenia.' *Pediatric Infectious Disease Journal*, 1993 Nov. 12(11):903-8.

[129] Chhour YM. Ruble G. Hong R. Minn K. Kdan Y. Sok T. Nisalak A. Myint KS. Vaughn DW. Endy TP. 'Hospital-based diagnosis of hemorrhagic fever, encephalitis, and hepatitis in Cambodian children.' *Emerging Infectious Diseases*, 2002 May. 8(5):485-9.

[130] Srey VH, Sadones H, Ong S, Mam M, Yim C, Sor S, Grosjean P and Reynes J. 'Etiology of encephalitis syndromes among hospitalized children and adults in Takeo, Cambodia, 1999-2000.' *American Journal of Tropical Medicine and Hygiene*, 2002. 66(2):200-207.

[131] Lowry PW. Truong DH. Hinh LD. Ladinsky JL. Karabatsos N. Cropp CB. Martin D. Gubler DJ. 'Japanese encephalitis among hospitalized pediatric and adult patients with acute encephalitis syndrome in Hanoi, Vietnam 1995.' *American Journal of Tropical Medicine & Hygiene*, 1998 Mar. 58(3):324-9.

[132] Johnson RT. *Viral infections of the nervous system* (2nd ed). Lippincott-Raven, Philadephia. 1998.

[133] Solomon T, Nguyen MD, Kneen R, Gainsborough M, Vaughn D and Vo TK. 'Japanese encephalitis' *Journal of Neurology, Neurosurgery and Psychiatry*, 2000. 68:405-415.

[134] Khetsuriani N. Holman RC. Anderson LJ. 'Burden of encephalitis-associated hospitalizations in the United States, 1988-1997.' *Clinical Infectious Diseases*, 2002 Jul 15. 35(2):175-82.

[135] Lee TC. Tsai CP. Yuan CL. Wei CY. Tsao WL. Lee RJ. Cheih SY. Huang IT. Chen KT. 'Encephalitis in Taiwan: a prospective hospital-based study.' *Japanese Journal of Infectious Diseases*, 2003 Oct-Dec. 56(5-6):193-9

[136] Koskiniemi ML. Vaheri A. 'Acute encephalitis of viral origin.' *Scandinavian Journal of Infectious Diseases*, 1982. 14(3):181-7.

[137] Lowry P. 'Arbovirus encephalitis in the United States and Asia.' *Laboratory and Clinical Medicine*, April 1997. 129(4):405-411.

[138] Koskiniemi M. Rautonen J. Lehtokoski-Lehtiniemi E. Vaheri A. 'Epidemiology of encephalitis in children: a 20-year survey.' *Annals of Neurology*, 1991 May. 29(5):492-7.

[139] Whitley RJ and Gnann JW. 'Viral encephalitis: familiar infections and emerging pathogens' *The Lancet*, February 9, 2002. 359:507-514.

[140] Alexander JP Jr. Baden L. Pallansch MA. Anderson LJ. 'Enterovirus 71 infections and neurologic disease - United States, 1977-1991.' *Journal of Infectious Diseases*, 1994 Apr. 169(4):905-8.

[141] Herrero LJ, Lee CSM, Hurrelbrink RJ, Chua BH, Chua KB and McMinn PC. 'Molecular epidemiology of EV71 in Peninsular Malaysia, 1997-2000'. Archives of Virology, 2003. 148: 1369-1385.

[142] Marra CM. 'Encephalitis in the 21st Century.' *Seminars in Neurology*, 2000. 20(3): 323-327.

[143] Ceausu E. Erscoiu S. Calistru P. Ispas D. Dorobat O. Homos M. Barbulescu C. Cojocaru I. Simion CV. Cristea C. Oprea C. Dumitrescu C. Duiculescu D. Marcu I. Mociornita C. Stoicev T. Zolotusca I. Calomfirescu C. Rusu R. Hodrea R. Geamai S. Paun L. 'Clinical manifestations in the West Nile virus outbreak.' *Romanian Journal of Virology*, 1997 Jan-Dec. 48(1-4):3-11.

[144] L'vov DK. Butenko AM. Gaidamovich SIa. Larichev VF. Leshchinskaia EV. Zhukov AN. Lazorenko VV. Aliushin AM. Petrov VR. Trikhanov ST. Khutoretskaia NV. Whishkina EO. Iashkov AB. 'Epidemic outbreak of meningitis and meningoencephalitis, caused by West Nile virus, in the Krasnodar territory and Volgograd region (preliminary report)' *Voprosy Virusologii*, 2000 Jan-Feb. 45(1):37-8.

[145] McCarthy M. 'Newer viral encephalitides' *The Neurologist*, 2003, 9:189-199.

[146] Tan CT and Tan KS. 'Nosocomial transmissibility of Nipah virus' (letter) *Journal of Infectious Disease*, 2001. 184:1367.

[147] Chua KB. 'Nipah virus outbreak in Malaysia' *Journal of Clinical Virology*, 2003. 26: 265-275.

[148] Hsu VP, Hossain MJ, Parashar UD, Ali MM, Ksiazek TG, Kuzmin I, Niezgoda M, Rupprecht C, Bresee J and Breiman RF. 'Nipah virus encephalitis reemergence, Bangladesh' *Emerging Infectious Diseases*, 2004. 10(12):2082-2087.

[149] Chong HT, Tan CT, Goh KJ, Lam SK and Chua KB. 'The risk of human Nipah virus infection directly from bats (*Pteropus hypomelanus*) is low.' *Neurological Journal of Southeast Asia*, 2003. 8:31-34.

[150] Fishbein DB and Robinson LE. 'Current concepts: Rabies' *New England Journal of Medicine*, 1993. 329 (22): 1632-1638.

[151] Mickiene A, Laiskonis A, Funther G, Vene S, Lundkvist A and Lindquist L. 'Tickborne encephalitis in an area of high endemicity in Lithunia: disease severity and long term prognosis.' *Clinical Infectious Diseases*, 2002. 35:650 – 658.

[152] Kaiser R. 'The clinical and epidemiological profile of tick-borne encephalitis in southern Germany 1994-1998.' *Brain*, 1999. 2067-2078.

[153] Hinson VK and Tyor WR. 'Update on viral encephalitis.' *Current Opinion in Neurology*, 2001. 14:369-374.

[154] Whitley RJ and Kimberlin DW. 'Herpes simplex encephalitis: Children and adolescents' *Seminar in Paediatrics Infectious Diseases*, 2005. 16:17-23.

[155] Redington JJ and Tyler KL. 'Viral infections of the nervous system, 2002.' *Archives of Neurology*, May 2002. 59:712-718.

[156] Solomon T. 'Exotic and emerging viral encephalitides' *Current Opinion in Neurology*, 2003. 16:411-418.

[157] Watson JT and Gerber SI. 'West Nile virus: a brief review' *Concise Reviews of Pediatrics Infectious Diseases*, 2004. 23:357-358.

[158] Sejvar JJ, Haddah MB, Tierney BC, Campbell GL, Marfin AA, Van Gerpen JA, Fleischauer A, Leis AA, Stokic DS and Petersen LR. 'Neurologic manifestations and outcome of West Nile virus infection' *Journal of American Medical Association*, 2003. 290(4):511-515.

[159] Goh KJ, Tan CT, Chew NK, Tan PSK, Kamarulzaman A, Ahmad Sarji S, Wong KT, Abdullah BJJ, Chua KB and Lam SK. 'Clinical features of Nipah virus encephalitis among pig farmers in Malaysia.' *New England Journal of Medicine*, 2000. 342:1229-1235.

[160] Chong HT, Kunjapan SR, Thayaparan T, Tong JMG, Petharunam V, Jusoh MR and Tan CT. 'Nipah encephalitis outbreak in Malaysia, clinical features in patients from Seremban.' *Neurological Journal of South East Asia*, 2000. 5:61-67.

[161] Chua KB, Lam SK, Tan CT, Hooi PS, Goh KJ, Chew NK, Tan KS, Kamarulzaman A and Wong KT. 'High mortality in Nipah encephalitis is associated with presence of virus in cerebrospinal fluid' *Annals of Neurology*, 2000. 48:802-805.

[162] Chong HT, Tan CT, Goh KJ, Chew NK, Kunjapan SR, Petharunam V and Thayaparan T. 'Occupational exposure, age, diabetes mellitus and outcome of acute Nipah encephalitis.' *Neurological Journal of Southeast Asia*, 2001. 6:7-11.

[163] Tan CT, Goh KJ, Wong KT, Sazilah AS, Chua KB, Chew NK, Paramsothy M, Loh YL, Chong HT, Tan KS, Thayaparan T, Shalini K, Mohd Rani J. 'Relapsed and late-onset Nipah encephalitis'. *Annals of Neurology*, 2002;51:703-8.

[164] Chong HT and Tan CT. 'Relapsed and late onset Nipah encephalitis: a report of three cases.' *Neurological Journal of Southeast Asia*, 2003. 8:109-112.

[165] Hsu VP, Hossain MJ, Parashar UD, Ali MM, Ksiazek TG, Kuzmin I, Niezgoda M, Rupprecht C, Bresee J and Breiman RF. 'Nipah virus encephalitis reemergence, Bangladesh' *Emerging Infectious Diseases*, 2004. 10(12):2082-2087.

[166] Chaudhauri A and Kennedy PGE. 'Diagnosis and treatment of viral encephalitis' *Postgraduate Medicine,* 2002. 78: 575-583.

[167] Tobias I, Donati F, Vassella F, Schaad UB and Bianchetti MG. 'Acute encephalitis in Swiss children: aetiology and outcome' *European Journal of Paediatrics Neurology,* 1998. 2:233-237.

[168] Sawyer, MH. 'Enterovirus infection: diagnosis and treatment' *Current Opinion in Paediatrics*, 2001. 13:65-69

[169] Steiner I, Budka H, Chaudhuri A, Koskiniemi M, Sainio K, Salonen O and Kennedy PGE. 'Viral encephalitis: a review of diagnostic methods and guidelines for management' *European Journal of Neurology*, 2005. 12: 331-343.

[170] Chong HT, Tan CT, Kamarulzaman A, Tan CT, Goh KJ, Thayaparan T, Sree Raman K, Chew NK, Chua KB and Lam SK. 'Ribavirin in Acute Nipah Encephalitis.' *Annals of Neurology* 2001;49:810-813.

[171] Melnick J. 'Current status of poliovirus infections.' *Clinical Microbiology Review* 1996. 9(3):293-300.

[172] Feki I. Marrakchi C. Ben Hmida M. Belahsen F. Ben Jemaa M. Maaloul I. Kanoun F. Ben Hamed S. Mhiri C. 'Epidemic West Nile virus encephalitis in Tunisia.' *Neuroepidemiology*, 2005. 24(1-2):1-7.

[173] Asnis DS. Conetta R. Teixeira AA. Waldman G. Sampson BA. 'The West Nile Virus outbreak of 1999 in New York: the Flushing Hospital experience.' [erratum appears in Clin Infect Dis 2000 May;30(5):841]. *Clinical Infectious Diseases*, 2000 Mar. 30(3):413-8.

[174] L'vov DK. Butenko AM. Gaidamovich SIa. Larichev VF. Leshchinskaia EV. Zhukov AN. Lazorenko VV. Aliushin AM. Petrov VR. Trikhanov ST. Khutoretskaia NV. Whishkina EO. Iashkov AB. 'Epidemic outbreak of meningitis and meningoencephalitis, caused by West Nile virus, in the Krasnodar territory and Volgograd region (preliminary report)' *Voprosy Virusologii*, 2000 Jan-Feb. 45(1):37-8.

[175] Burton JM. Kern RZ. Halliday W. Mikulis D. Brunton J. Fearon M. Pepperell C. Jaigobin C. 'Neurological manifestations of West Nile virus infection' *Canadian Journal of Neurological Sciences*, 2004 May. 31(2):185-93.

[176] Sacktor N, Lyles RH, Skolasky R, Kleeberger C, Selnes OA, Miller EN, Becker JT, Cohen B, McArthur JC and the Multicenter AIDS Cohort Study. 'HIV-associated neurologic disease incidence changes: Multicenter AIDS Cohort Study, 1990-1998'. *Neurology*, 2001. 56: 257-260.

[177] French N, Gray K, Watera C, Nakiyingi J, Lugada E, Moore M, Lallo D, Whitworth JAG and Gilks CF. 'Cryptococcal infection in a cohort of HIV-1-infected Ugandan adults'. *AIDS*, 2002. 16:1031-1038.

[178] Likittanasombut P. 'Opportunistic central nervous system infection in human immunodeficiency virus infected patients in Thammasat Hospital, Thailand' *Neurology Asia*, 2004. 9:29-32.

[179] Fleming DT and Wasserheit JN. "From epidemiological synergy to public health policy and practice: the contribution of other sexually transmitted diseases to sexual transmission of HIV infection' *Sexually Transmitted Infections*, 1999. 75:3-17.

[180] Tardieu M. 'HIV-1-related central nervous system diseases' *Annals of Internal Medicine,* 1994. 169: 765-785.

[181] Sepkowitz KA. 'Opportunistic infections in patients with and patients without acquired immunodeficiency syndrome' *Clinical Infectious Diseases*, 2002. 34:1098-1107.

[182] Tunlayadechanont S, Viranuvatti K, Phuapradit P, Sathapatayavong B, Tantirittisak T and Bongird P. 'Cryptococcal meningitis in patients with non-HIV and HIV infection: a clinical study'. *Neurological Journal of Southeast Asia*, 1997. 2: 45-50.

[183] Cates WJ. 'Review of non-hormonal contraception (condoms, intrauterine devices, nonoxyl-9 and combos) on HIV acquisition' *Journal of Acquired Immunodeficiency Syndrome*, 2005. 38(Suppl. 1): S8-S10.

[184] Sangani P, Rutherford G and Wilkinson D. 'Population based interventions for reducing sexually transmitted infections, including HIV infection' *The Cochrane Library*, 2005. 3 [no page number]

[185] Weiss HA, Quigley MA and Hayes RJ. 'Male circumcision and risk of HIV infection in sub-saharan Africa: a systematic review and meta-analysis'. *AIDS*, 2000. 14:2361-2370.

[186] Mofenson LM and Munderi P. 'Safety of antiretroviral prophylaxis of perinatal transmission for HIV-infected pregnant women and their infants' *Journal of Acquired Immunodeficiency Syndrome*, 2002; 30: 200-215.

[187] Portegies P, Solod L, Cinque P, Chaudhuri A, Begovac J, Everall I, Weber T, Bojar M, Martinez-Martin P and Kennedy PGE. 'Guidelines for the diagnosis and management of neurological complications of HIV infection' *European Journal of Neurology*, 2004. 11:297-304.

[188] Bell JE. 'An update on the neuropathology of HIV in the HAART era' *Histopathology*, 2004. 4:549-559.

[189] Zumla A, Malon P, Henderson J and Grange JM. 'Impact of HIV infection on tuberculosis.' *Postgraduate Medical Journal*, 2000. 76:259-268.

[190] Kassubek J, Zucker B, Oehm E, Serr A, Arnold M, Lucking CH and Els T. 'Tuberculous meningoencephalitis in HIV-seronegative patients: variety of clinical presentation and impact on diagnostic and treatment' *Acta Neurologic Scandinavian*, 2001. 104: 389-396.

[191] Teoh R and Humphries M. 'Tuberculous meningitis' IIn Lambert HP (ed) *Infections of the Central Nervous System: Kass Handbook of Infectious Diseases.* London: BC Decker, 1991.189-206.

[192] Al-Abbasi AM. 'Tuberculous meningoencephalitis in Baghdad, 1993-99: a clinical study of 224 cases' *Eastern Mediterranean Health Journal, 2002.* 8(2-3):330-337.

[193] Roos KL. '*Mycobacterium tuberculosis* meningitis and other etiologies of the aseptic meningitis syndrome' *Seminars in Neurology*, 2000. 20(3): 329-335.

[194] Thwaites GE, Nguyen DB, Nguyen HD, Hoang TQ, Do Thi TO, Nguyen TCT, Nguyen QH, Nguyen TT, Nguyen NH, Nguyen TNL, Nguyen NL, Nguyen HD, Vu NT, Cao HH, Tran THC, Pham PM, Nguyen TD, Stepniewska K, White NJ, Tran TH and Farrar

JJ. 'Dexamethasone in the treatment of tuberculous meningitis in adolescents and adults' *New England Journal of Medicine*, 2004. 351: 1741-1751.

[195] Berger JR and Sabet A. 'Infectious myelopathies' *Seminars in Neurology*, 2002. 22(2): 133-141.

[196] Nkoumou MO, Betha G, Kombila M and Clevenbergh P. 'Bacterial and mycobacterial meningitis in HIV positive compared with HIV negative patients in internal medicine ward in Liberville, Gabon' *Journal of Acquired Immunodeficiency Syndromes*, 2003. 32(3):345-346.

[197] Marsh K, Forster D, Waruiru C, Mwangi I, Winstanley M, Marsh V, Newton C, Winstanley P, Warn P, Peshu N, Pasvol G and Snow R. 'Indicators of life-threatening malaria in African children.' *New England Journal of Medicine*, 1995. 332: 13990-1404.

[198] Newton CRJC, Tran TH and White N. 'Cerebral malaria' *Journal of Neurology, Neurosurgery and Psychiatry*, 2000. 69:433- 441.

[199] Birnbaumer DM and Rutkowski A. 'Malaria – a comprehensive review for the emergency physician' *Tropical Emergency Medicine*, 2003. 25(1): 2-12.

[200] World Health Organization 'Severe falciparum malaria' *Transactions of the Royal Society of Tropical Medicine and Hygiene*, 2000. 94 Supplement 1.

[201] Waller, D, Krishna S, Crawley J, Miller K, Nosten F, Chapman D, ter Kuile FO, Craddock C, Berry C, Holloway PAH, Brewster D, Greenwood BM and White NJ. 'Clinical features and outcomes of severe malaria in Gambian children' *Clinical Infectious Diseases*, 1995. 21:577-587.

[202] Bondi FS. 'The incidence and outcome of neurological abnormalities in childhood cerebral malaria: a long term follow up of 62 survivors' *Transactions of the Royal Society of Tropical Medicine and Hygiene*, 1992. 86:17-19.

[203] Allen SJ, O'Donnell A, Alexander NDE and Clegg JB. 'Severe malaria in children in Papua New Guinea' *Quarterly Journal of Medicine*, 1996. 89: 779-788.

[204] Alani S and Millac P. 'Neurosyphilis in the Leicester area' *Postgraduate Medical Journal*, 1982. 58(685):685-687.

[205] Hillbom M and Kinnunen E. 'New cases of neurosyphilis in Finland' *Acta Medica Scandinavica*, 1982. 211(1-2):55-58.

[206] Nordenbo AM and Sorensen PS. 'The incidence and clinical presentation of neurosyphilis in Greter Copenhagen 1974 through 1978.' *Acta Neurologica Scandinavica*, 1981. 63(4):237-246.

[207] Berger JR. 'Neurosyphilis in human immunodeficiency virus type 1 positive individuals. A prospective study.' *Archives of Neurology*, 1991. 48(7):700-702.

[208] Bordon J, Martinez-Vazquez C, Alvarez M, Miralles C, Ocampo A, de la Fuente-Aguado J and Sopena-Perez Arguelles B. 'Neurosyphilis in HIV-infected patients' *European Journal of Clinical Microbiology and Infectious Diseases*, 1995. 14(10):864-869.

[209] Brandon WR, Boulos LM and Morse A. 'Determining the prevalence of neurosyphilis in a cohort co-infected with HIV' *International Journal of STD & AIDS*, 1993. 4(2):99-101.

[210] Malessa R, Agelink MW, Hengge U, Mertins L, Gastpar M and Brockmeyer NH. 'Oliogosymptomatic neurosyphilis with false negative CSF-VDRL in HIV-infected individuals' *European Journal of Medical Research*, 1996. 1(6):299-302.

[211] Rompalo AM, Joesoef MR, O'Donnell JA, Augenbraun M, Brady W, Radolf JD, Johnson R and Rolfs RT. 'Clinical manifestations of early syphilis by HIV status and gender: results of the syphilis and HIV study' *Sexually Transmitted Diseases*, 2001. 28(3): 158-165.

[212] Flood JM, Weinstock HS, Guroy ME, Bayne L, Simon RP and Bolan G. 'Neurosyphilis during the AIDS epidemic, San Francisco, 1985-1992' *Journal of Infectious Diseases*, 1998. 177(4):931-940

[213] Solaro C, De Maria A and Primavera A. 'Trends in HIV, gonorrhoea, and syphilis. Screening for neurosyphilis is recommended' *British Medical Journal*, 2002. 325(7362): 494.

[214] Saik S. Kraus JE. McDonald A. Mann SG. Sheitman BB. 'Neurosyphilis in newly admitted psychiatric patients: three case reports.' *Journal of Clinical Psychiatry*, 2004. 65(7):919-21.

[215] Takada LT. Caramelli P. Radanovic M. Anghinah R. Hartmann AP. Guariglia CC. Bahia VS. Nitrini R. 'Prevalence of potentially reversible dementias in a dementia outpatient clinic of a tertiary university-affiliated hospital in Brazil.' *Arquivos de Neuro-Psiquiatria*, 2003. 61(4):925-9.

[216] St Louis ME. 'Strategies for syphilis prevention in the 1990's' *Sexually Transmitted Diseases*, 1996. 23(1): 58-67.

RECOMMENDED FURTHER READING

1. Johnson RT. *Viral infections of the nervous system* (2nd ed). Lippincott-Raven, Philadephia. 1998.

2. Roos KL. 'Acute bacterial meningitis' *Seminar in neurology*, 2000. 20(3): 293-306.

3. Quagliarello VJ and Scheld WM. 'Treatment of bacterial meningitis' *New England Journal of Medicine*, March 6, 1997. 336(10):708-716.

4. De Gans J and Van de Beek D for the European Dexamethasone in adulthood bacterial meningitis study investigators. 'Dexamethasone in adults with bacterial meningitis' *New England Journal of Medicine*, November 14, 2002. 347 (20): 1549 – 1556.

5. Koskiniemi M, Korppi M, Mustonen K, Rantala H, Muttilainen M, Herrgard E, Ukkonen P, Vaheri A. 'Epidemiology of encephalitis in children. A prospective multicentre study.' *European Journal of Paediatrics*. 1997. 156: 541-545.

6. Peltola H. 'Burden of meningitis and other severe bacterial infections of children in Africa: Implications for prevention' *Clinical Infectious Diseases*, 2001; 31:64-75.

7. Rotbart HA. 'Viral meningitis'. *Seminars in Neurology*, 2000. 20(3): 277-292.

8. Solomon T, Nguyen MD, Kneen R, Gainsborough M, Vaughn D and Vo TK. 'Japanese encephalitis' *Journal of Neurology, Neurosurgery and Psychiatry*, 2000. 68:405-415.

9. Lowry P. 'Arbovirus encephalitis in the United States and Asia.' *Laboratory and Clinical Medicine*, April 1997. 129(4):405-411.

10. Solomon T. 'Exotic and emerging viral encephalitides' *Current Opinion in Neurology*, 2003. 16:411-418.

In: Handbook of Clinical Neuroepidemiology
Editors: V. L. Feigin and D. A. Bennett, pp. 391-427

ISBN 978-1-60021-511-7
© 2007 Nova Science Publishers, Inc.

Chapter 11

CENTRAL NERVOUS SYSTEM TUMORS

James L. Fisher[1,2], Judith A. Schwartzbaum[2-4],
Margaret Wrensch[5] and E. Antonio Chiocca[2,6]

[1]The Arthur G. James Cancer Hospital and Richard J. Solove Research Institute,
Columbus, Ohio USA;
[2]Comprehensive Cancer Center at The Ohio State University, Columbus, Ohio USA;
[3]Division of Epidemiology, College of Public Health, The Ohio State University,
Columbus, Ohio USA;
[4]Institute of Environmental Medicine, Karolinksa Institute, Stockholm, Sweden;
[5]Departments of Neurological Surgery and Epidemiology and Biostatistics, University of
California, San Francisco, San Francisco, California USA;
[6]Dardinger Neuro-oncology Center, Department of Neurological Surgery, The Ohio State
University Medical Center, Columbus, Ohio USA.

ABSTRACT

Increasing incidence rates of CNS tumors probably result from use of new neuroimaging techniques. Established risk factors include exposure to ionizing radiation, rare mutations of penetrant genes, and familial history of CNS tumors, but these factors explain only a small proportion of tumors. Ongoing research focuses on identifying genetic polymorphisms that, in conjunction with environmental carcinogens, increase tumor risk, investigating the inverse association between allergic conditions and glioma, and validating the relationship between cellular telephone use and acoustic neuroma. Although chemotherapy for glioblastoma multiforme and oligodendroglioma improves survival time for some patients, survival time has remained relatively constant over the past 25 years.

INTRODUCTION

Primary central nervous system (CNS) tumors are classified by the World Health Organization (WHO) on the basis of histopathology into the following types: tumors of neuroepithelial tissue (including astrocytoma [grade II], anaplastic astrocytoma [grade III], glioblastoma multiforme [GBM, grade IV], oligodendroglioma and ependymoma), tumors of cranial and spinal nerves (or tumors of peripheral nerves that affect the CNS), tumors of the meninges (including meningioma and hemangioblastoma), CNS lymphomas, germ cell tumors, and tumors of sellar region (including pituitary tumors and craniopharyngioma). We review the incidence of CNS tumors in terms of changes over time, variation according to demographic factors, and geographic variation. We summarize the incidence and survival probability of CNS tumors using information from the Central Brain Tumor Registry of the United States (CBTRUS) [1,2] and the Surveillance, Epidemiology, and End Results (SEER) Program of the National Cancer Institute [3,4]. We review the literature pertaining to risk and prognostic factors, and we refer to several recent published reviews of the literature that provide thoughtful interpretations and critiques. In addition, we describe the standard treatment options for CNS tumors.

Primary CNS tumors, and especially primary brain tumors, are characterized by their histologic heterogeneity so that when definitions and classifications of tumors differ among studies, comparisons are difficult to make. Although the literature concerning most prognostic indicators often makes distinctions between histologic types and grades, only recently has variation in risk factors been addressed according to histologic subtypes. Therefore, in the present review, we are not always able to report findings in refined histologic categories. We present information pertaining to *primary* CNS tumors, and we do not present information pertaining to local extensions from regional tumors or unclassified tumors. Because approximately 85 to 90 percent of all primary CNS tumors occur in the brain, we focus on these more common tumor types, especially tumors of neuroepithelial tissue and the meninges, as they make up approximately 75 to 80 percent of all primary CNS tumors. When there is unusual variation in incidence or clear evidence of a risk or prognostic factor, we also discuss these for less common tumor types.

INCIDENCE BY TIME, SEX, AGE, RACE/ ETHNICITY, AND GEOGRAPHY

The CBTRUS estimates that more than 359,000 people in the United States (US) were living with a diagnosis of a primary CNS tumor, either malignant or non-malignant, in the year 2000 [2]. During the years 1997 to 2001, the average annual rate of occurrence of incident (newly diagnosed) primary malignant CNS tumors in the US was 7.31 per 100,000 persons, and, for primary benign CNS tumors and CNS tumors of uncertain behavior, was 6.80 per 100,000 persons [2]. During that same period, the average annual rate of incident primary malignant and non-malignant CNS tumors, combined, was 14.1 per 100,000 persons

[2]. The incidence of CNS tumors has varied over time, and differs according to sex, age, race and ethnicity.

Incidence over Time

Based on nine geographic areas surveyed by the US SEER Program since 1973, the age-adjusted incidence rate for malignant CNS tumors has increased among both males (from 6.3 per 100,000 males in 1973 to 7.7 per 100,000 males in 2001) and females (from 4.3 per 100,000 females in 1973 to 5.2 per 100,000 females in 2001) [3]. Examination of 10 years (1985 to 1994) of incidence data from CBTRUS revealed a slight but statistically significant average annual percentage change in incidence (0.9 percent) [1]. However, it is likely that most, if not all, of this increase is attributable to improvements in diagnostic imaging (as in computerized topography and magnetic resonance imaging), increased availability of medical care and neurosurgeons, changing approaches in the medical treatment of older patients, and changes in the classifications of specific histologies of CNS tumors, especially brain tumors, from benign to malignant [5-7].

Incidence by Sex

For all CNS tumors, the age-adjusted average annual (1997 to 2001) incidence rate for females (14.27 per 100,000 person-years) is slightly greater than that for males (13.92 per 100,000 person-years) [2]. Table 1 shows the average annual (1997 to 2001) age-adjusted incidence rate and median age at diagnosis for the major histologic groupings and selected common histologic subtypes.

As shown in Table 1, tumors of neuroepithelial tissue, CNS lymphomas and germ cell tumors are more common among males, whereas meningioma are more common among females. The sex difference for meningioma and astrocytoma may result from a positive association between estrogen and meningioma risk and a protective effect of estrogen on astrocytoma risk [7-11], but the causes for these regularly observed sex differences have not been established.

Incidence by Age

In the US, the median age at diagnosis among all patients with a primary CNS tumor between 1997 and 2001 was 56 years [2]. As shown in Table 1, pilocytic astrocytoma and germ cell tumors have a younger median age at diagnosis, and GBM and meningioma have an older median age at diagnosis. Figure 1 shows average annual incidence rates of the major histologic groupings according to age at diagnosis from 1997 to 2001.

Table 1. Median age at diagnosis and age-adjusted average annual (1997-2001) incidence rates[a] of primary CNS tumors (major histologic groupings and selected histologic subtypes) according to sex. Central Brain Tumor Registry of the United States (CBTRUS), reported in: CBTRUS Statistical Report: Primary Brain Tumors in the United States, 1997-2001 [2]

Histologic Group	Number of Cases	Median Age at Diagnosis (Years)	Rate[a]	Male Rate[a]	Female Rate[a]
Tumors of Neuroepithelial Tissue	26,660	54	6.34	7.35	5.32
Pilocytic Astrocytoma	1,378	12	0.32	0.33	0.31
Diffuse Astrocytoma	436	45	0.10	0.12	0.08
Anaplastic Astrocytoma	2,002	51	0.47	0.56	0.40
Glioblastoma	12,377	64	3.01	3.75	2.40
Oligodendroglioma	1,585	41	0.37	0.40	0.34
Anaplastic Oligodendroglioma	738	48	0.17	0.19	0.16
Ependymoma/Anaplastic Ependymoma	1,083	39	0.25	0.29	0.22
Tumors of Cranial and Spinal Nerves	4,672	52	1.11	1.12	1.11
Tumors of Meninges	17,956	63	4.36	2.76	5.72
Meningioma	17,204	64	4.18	2.57	5.56
CNS Lymphomas	1,966	59	0.47	0.56	0.39
Germ Cell Tumors	361	17	0.08	0.11	0.05
Tumors of Sellar Region	3,908	48	0.92	0.95	0.91

a. Rates are per 100,000 population, age-adjusted to the 2000 US (19 age groups) standard, and based on data from the following registries: Arizona, Colorado, Connecticut, Delaware, Idaho, Maine, Massachusetts, Minnesota, Montana, New Mexico, New York, North Carolina, Texas, Utah and Virginia.

In general, incidence rates of all major histologic groupings, except those of germ cell tumors, increase with advancing age group, and begin to decline after age 75. Figures 2 and 3 show average annual incidence rates, according to age at diagnosis, for selected histologies common among adults and children/adolescents (ages 0 to 19), respectively.

Among adults (Figure 2), incidence rates of meningioma and GBM increase with advancing age, except for a decline in the incidence rate of GBM among people age 85 years or older. Among children/adolescents (Figure 3), incidence rates of embryonal/primitive/medulloblastoma, pilocytic astrocytoma, malignant glioma, NOS, ependymoma/anaplastic ependymoma, and neuronal/glial, neuronal and mixed tumors decrease through childhood and adolescence, while the incidence of germ cell tumors reaches a peak during the adolescent years. (Note that a different logarithmic scale is used for Figure 3, so that variation by histology can be displayed.) It should be noted that some of the variation in incidence according to histologic type might reflect diagnostic practices and access to diagnoses in different age groups rather than actual biological variations of the tumors with age.

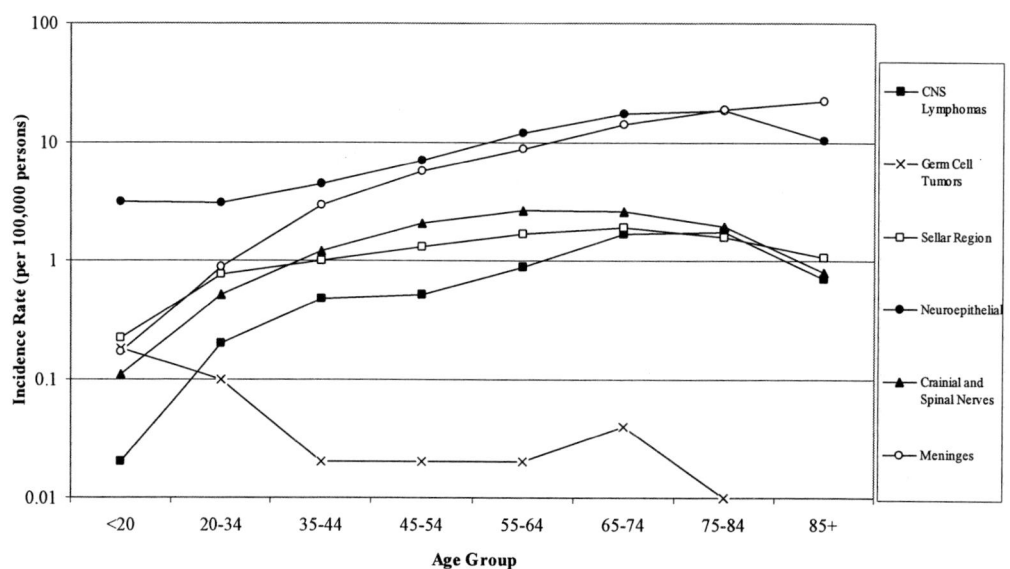

Figure 1. Age-specific incidence rates of primary CNS tumors, 1997-2001, according to major histologic groupings, Central Brain Tumor Registry of the United States (CBTRUS), reported in tabular form in: CBTRUS (2004) Statistical Report: Primary Brain Tumors in the United States, 1997-2001.

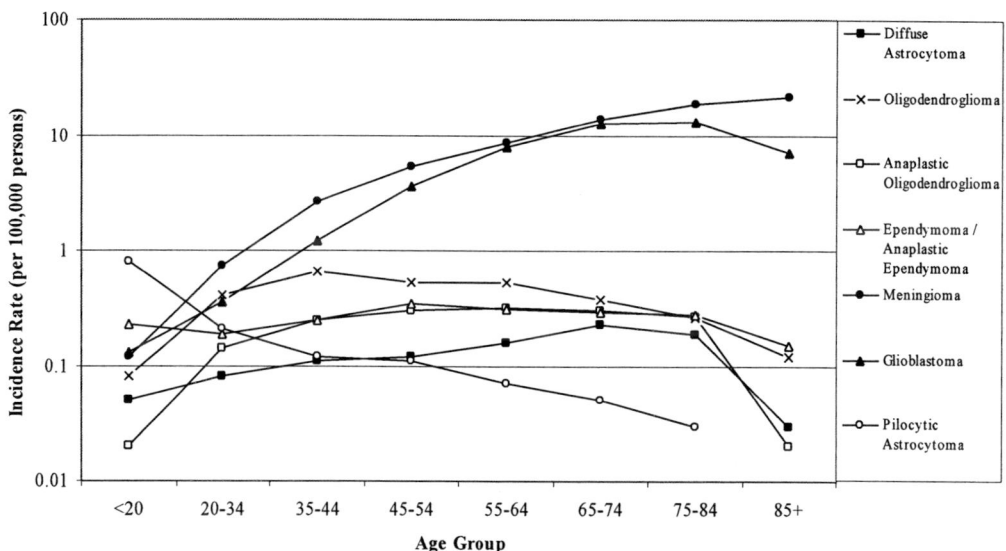

Figure 2. Age-specific incidence rates of primary neuroepithelial brain tumors and meningioma, 1997-2001, Central Brain Tumor Registry of the United States (CBTRUS), reported in tabular form in: CBTRUS (2004) Statistical Report: Primary Brain Tumors in the United States, 1997-2001.

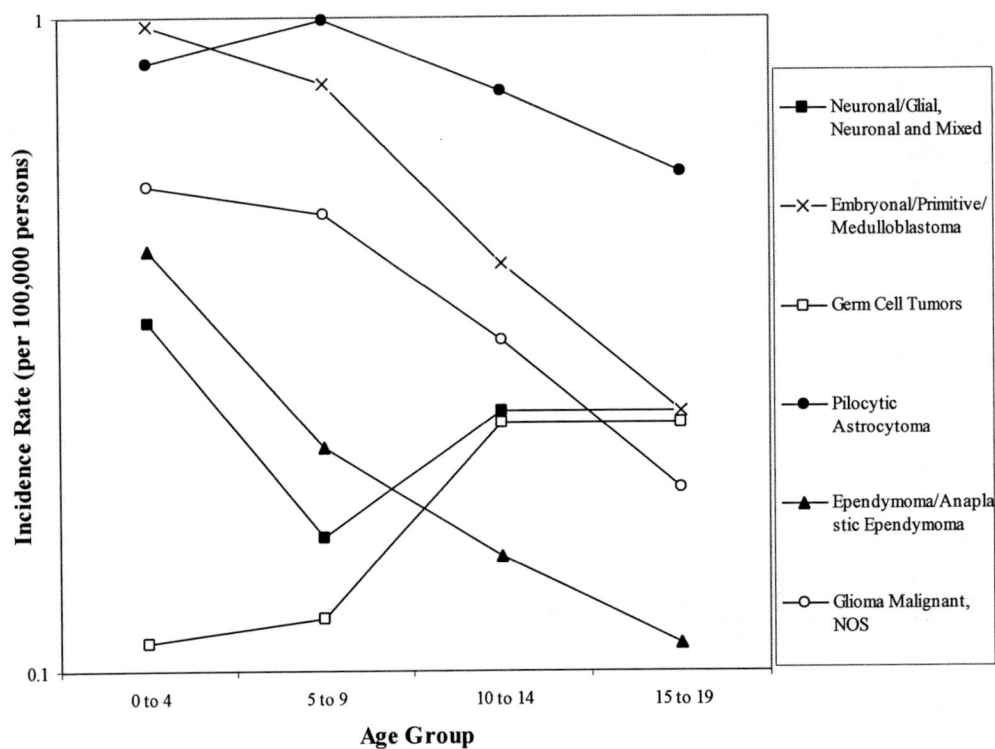

Figure 3. Age-specific incidence rates of primary CNS histologies more common among children, 1997-2001, Central Brain Tumor Registry of the United States (CBTRUS), reported in tabular form in: CBTRUS (2004) Statistical Report: Primary Brain Tumors in the United States, 1997-2001.

Incidence by Race and Ethnicity

Table 2. Age-adjusted average annual (1997-2001) incidence rates[a] of primary malignant CNS tumors according to race and sex. Surveillance, Epidemiology, and End Results (SEER) Program (www.seer.cancer.gov) SEER*Stat Database: Incidence - SEER 11 Regs + AK Public-Use, Nov 2003 Sub for Expanded Races (1992-2001), National Cancer Institute, DCCPS, Surveillance Research Program, Cancer Statistics Branch, released April 2004, based on the November 2003 submission

Race	Male	Female	Total
White	8.4	6.0	7.1
Black	4.6	3.4	4.0
American Indian/Alaska Native	3.0	2.3	2.5
Asian or Pacific Islander	4.0	2.7	3.3

a. Rates are per 100,000 population, age-adjusted to the 2000 US (19 age groups) standard.

In the US, the age-adjusted average annual (1997 to 2001) incidence rate of primary CNS tumors for Whites (14.44 per 100,000 person-years) is greater than that for Blacks (10.24 per 100,000 person-years) [2]. Tumors of neuroepithelial tissue are approximately twice as common among Whites as compared to Blacks, as are tumors of cranial and spinal nerves and germ cell tumors. The incidence of meningioma among Whites is nearly identical to that among Blacks. Table 2 shows the age-adjusted average annual (1997 to 2001) incidence of malignant CNS tumors according to race/ethnicity and sex [4].

Geographic Variation in Incidence

Based on the cancer registries contributing information to the CBTRUS, there is moderate variation in CNS tumor incidence in the US based on geography [2]. The lowest age-adjusted average annual (1997 to 2001) incidence of CNS tumors was in Virginia (8.84 per 100,000 person-years), and the highest was in Colorado (20.99 per 100,000 person-years) [2]. For malignant CNS tumors, a similar degree of variation is reported among the geographic SEER regions [4]. There is also worldwide geographic variation in the incidence of CNS tumors; for example, malignant brain tumors occur in Japan with less than half the frequency of that in Northern Europe. Countries reporting a high incidence of malignant brain tumors include Australia, Canada, Denmark, Finland, Sweden, New Zealand, and the US, whereas areas of the world with a lower incidence - such as Rizal, Philippines and Bombay, India - have an incidence approximately one-fourth that of the high-incidence countries [7,12]. Differences in diagnostic practices and completeness of reporting make all geographic, and especially international, comparisons difficult [7]. In addition, higher incidence rates appear in countries - and within the US, perhaps in states - with greater access to health care and better medical care [7,12]. Results of an interesting study by Singh and Siahpush [13] suggest that, although US immigrants have a lower risk of death from all causes, their risk of death from brain cancer is greater as compared to their US-born counterparts, suggesting that country of birth alters risk, or that potential exposure(s) occurring early in life afford protection to the US-born, or that potential early exposure(s) in non-US countries increase brain tumor risk.

NATURAL HISTORY: SURVIVAL PROBABALITY AND PROGNOSTIC FACTORS

Nearly all CNS tumors have treatment recommendations that prolong survival time (albeit modest for more aggressive tumors, such as GBM), and nearly all patients diagnosed with CNS tumors, especially brain tumors, receive some form of treatment; however, a recent study suggests that only 54 percent of patients diagnosed with malignant glioma receive chemotherapy [14]. Our discussion of the natural history of CNS tumors will focus on survival probability and prognostic factors.

Survival time after diagnosis of a CNS tumor varies greatly by histologic type and age at diagnosis. The relative two-year and five-year survival probabilities associated with primary malignant CNS tumors are 37.3 percent and 29.3 percent, respectively [4]. For the period 1973 to 2001, the two-year relative survival probability for males (37.1 percent) was slightly less than that for females (37.5 percent) [4]. Although the prognosis is poor for many patients with malignant brain tumors, two-year survival probability, for all patients with malignant brain tumors, has increased from 31.0 percent in 1975 to 40.4 percent in 2000 [4]. Much of this increase occurred among patients younger than 65 years of age who were diagnosed with tumors other than anaplastic astrocytoma and GBM. There has been little change in the survival probability for patients diagnosed with tumor histologies typically having a poor prognosis, such as GBM.

Survival time for patients with malignant brain tumors is related to age at diagnosis and histology. Two-year relative survival probabilities are shown in Figure 4 according to age at diagnosis and histology [2].

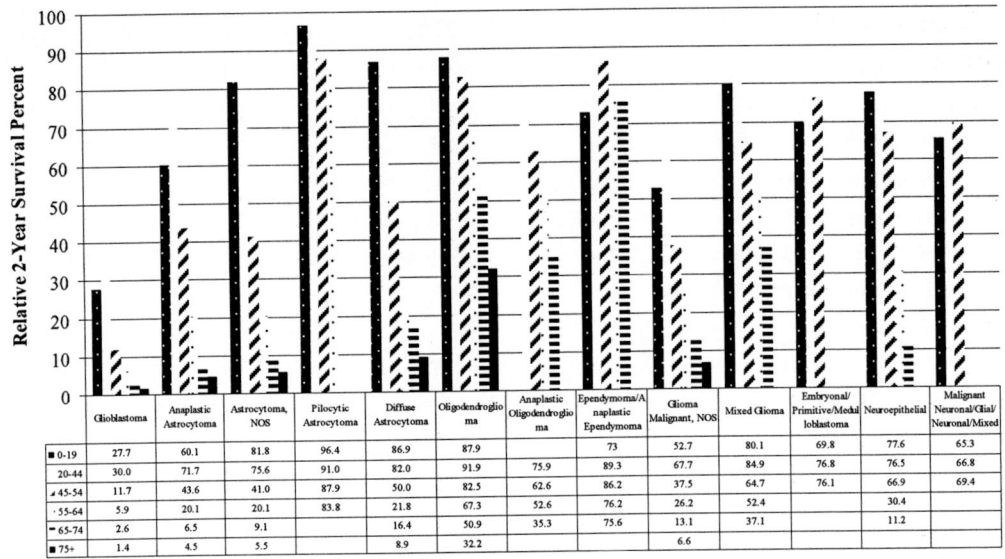

	Glioblastoma	Anaplastic Astrocytoma	Astrocytoma, NOS	Pilocytic Astrocytoma	Diffuse Astrocytoma	Oligodendroglioma	Anaplastic Oligodendroglioma	Ependymoma/Anaplastic Ependymoma	Glioma Malignant, NOS	Mixed Glioma	Embryonal/Primitive/Medulloblastoma	Neuroepithelial	Malignant Neuronal/Glial/Neuronal/Mixed
0-19	27.7	60.1	81.8	96.4	86.9	87.9		73	52.7	80.1	69.8	77.6	65.3
20-44	30.0	71.7	75.6	91.0	82.0	91.9	75.9	89.3	67.7	84.9	76.8	76.5	66.8
45-54	11.7	43.6	41.0	87.9	50.0	82.5	62.6	86.2	37.5	64.7	76.1	66.9	69.4
55-64	5.9	20.1	20.1	83.8	21.8	67.3	52.6	76.2	26.2	52.4			30.4
65-74	2.6	6.5	9.1		16.4	50.9	35.3	75.6	13.1	37.1			11.2
75+	1.4	4.5	5.5		8.9	32.2			6.6				

Histologic Type

Figure 4. Two-year relative survival probabilities of primary malignant CNS tumors according to age at diagnosis and histologic type, based on the follow-up of individuals diagnosed between 1973 and 2001, Surveillance, Epidemiology and End Results (SEER), compiled by the Central Brain Tumor Registry of the United States (CBTRUS) and reported in tabular form in: CBTRUS (2004) Statistical Report: Primary Brain Tumors in the United States, 1997-2001.

For each age group, relative survival probability is lowest for patients with GBM. In general, within each histologic type, except malignant neuronal/glial, neuronal and mixed tumors, survival probability is lowest for those in older age groups.

In addition to age at diagnosis and histology, sex and Karnofsky performance status, aspects of the tumor (location, size, extent of resection), and molecular and genetic markers may be important determinants of survival probability. The potential survival advantage for women, compared to men, has been investigated in many studies. Among patients diagnosed with glioma, Diete et al. [15] reported that the difference between males and females was apparent among patients with grade III astrocytoma, but not among those with GBM. Sant et al. [16] found that the five-year survival probability for women diagnosed with malignant primary brain tumors was 20 percent, whereas the probability for men was 17 percent, and this difference was relatively consistent across 17 European countries. Overall, results from studies regarding sex differences in survival times are mixed, and positive results suggest only slightly longer survival times for women.

Survival Probability and Prognostic Factors for Glioblastoma

Because of the poor prognosis for patients with GBM - median survival time is approximately one year or less in many studies - investigators have sought to determine factors associated with better survival. Lacroix et al. [17] found five independent predictors of survival among 416 study participants with GBM. They were: age, Karnofsky Performance Scale (KPS) score, extent of resection, degree of necrosis, and enhancement on preoperative magnetic resonance imaging studies [17]. Results from other studies have suggested that percent of resection, volume of residual disease, therapeutic approach, larger tumor size, larger postoperative tumor size, capacity for total resection, deterioration of the patient, and condition before radiation therapy were each related to GBM survival. Further, non-central tumor location (defined as infiltration of splenium, basal ganglia, thalamus, or midbrain) [18] has been associated with a shorter survival time, whereas frontal tumors (as opposed to non-frontal tumors) and tumors smaller than 4 cm have been associated with longer survival times [19]. An interesting prognostic factor was reported by Schwartzbaum et al. [20], who found that lower presurgical serum albumin values were strongly related to a shorter survival time in patients with GBM, suggesting systemic effects of an acute phase response associated with growth of GBM.

Recent efforts to identify prognostic factors for GBM and other brain tumors have focused on genetic and molecular markers. Among these are hepatocyte growth factor (HGF), and epidermal growth factor receptor. Higher tumor levels of HGF (a cytokine with multiple functions, including promoting cell proliferation) have been associated with a poorer prognosis in patients diagnosed with malignant glioma, and with recurrence in patients diagnosed with meningioma [21] p53 is a tumor-suppressor gene whose functional loss is thought to result in a growth advantage for astrocytomas. There are inconsistent results regarding associations between survival time from astrocytoma (or its subtypes, including GBM) and both (t)p53 mutation and (t)p53 protein expression. There are also inconsistent results for EGFR expression or amplification, as they relate to survival from astrocytoma, and especially GBM. Simmons et al. [22] showed a complex relationship of survival with age at diagnosis and the tumor p53 and EGFR characteristics among GBM patients. As in many previous studies, there was no difference in survival based on p53 mutation, EGFR expression, or p53 immunopositivity; however, among patients younger than the median age, there was a shorter survival time among younger patients whose tumors overexpressed EFGR but had normal p53 immunohistochemistry [22]. There is additional evidence that p53 protein expression decreases with advancing age, and the association between p53 expression and survival from GBM may be hidden when confounding by age is statistically adjusted. In addition to HGF, p53 and EGFR, loss of heterozygosity on chromosome 10q has been associated with shorter duration of survival from GBM [23]. A recent study reported a strong association between different genotypes of human telomerase MNS16A and GBM survival time (24.7 months median survival time for the SS-genotype, compared to 14.0 months and 13.1 months for the SL- and LL-genotypes, respectively [24]. These results are promising because this is the strongest known finding associating a genetic factor to GBM survival, and because human telomerase MNS16A may be exploitable as a biomarker of potential treatment success.

Survival Probability and Prognostic Factors for Tumors of the Meninges

For benign CNS tumors, such as meningioma, there are currently no estimates of US population-based survival probability, because these tumors were not registered as part of the SEER program until recently. However, population-based data from Norway and Finland suggest an increase in survival time for patients diagnosed with meningioma in Norway from 1963 to 1992 [25], and in Finland from 1953 to 1984 [26]. To estimate the probability of surviving meningioma in the US, McCarthy et al. [27] used data from the National Cancer Database, a collaborative effort of approximately 1,000 hospitals. Five-year survival probability was 69 percent, and varied by age - 81 percent among patients of ages 21 to 64 years and 56 percent among those 65 years of age or older [27]. Patients with benign meningiomas had a five-year survival probability of 70 percent, whereas the five-year survival probability for patients with malignant meningiomas was 55 percent [27].

Prognostic factors for patients with meningioma have not been thoroughly studied. However, results from one very large study from the National Cancer Database, which comprised 9,000 cases of meningioma, revealed that the following factors affected survival from benign meningioma: age at diagnosis, tumor size, and surgical and radiation treatments; in contrast, for malignant meningioma, the prognostic factors included only age and surgical and radiation treatments [27]. For the period 1953 to 1984 in Finland, Sankila et al. [26] found that meningioma prognosis was associated with age at diagnosis, surgical treatment, and period of diagnosis.

There are very few known studies of prognostic factors for tumors of cranial and spinal nerves, CNS lymphomas, germ cell tumors, and tumors of sellar region. In general, we know very little about what differentiates CNS tumor survivors from non-survivors, or about what determines their length of survival. Age at diagnosis and histology remain the only known strong determinants of CNS tumor survival probability. More studies are needed to examine other potentially important factors, especially as they relate to survival from tumors with shorter durations of survival time, such as GBM.

RISK FACTORS

Risk factors for CNS tumors are discovered by conducting analytic epidemiologic studies, which usually compare either CNS tumor risk in participants with or without certain characteristics (cohort studies), or the histories of participants with or without CNS tumors (case-control studies). In the present review, the relevant distinction between a cohort study and a case-control study is that results from a cohort study can provide evidence that a potentially modifiable or varying cause (risk factor) preceded the CNS tumor; whereas, results from a case-control study cannot address temporality. However, some factors of interest, such as constitutive genetic polymorphisms, do not change over time; as a result, case-control studies are just as useful as cohort studies in examining such factors.

We use principles from evidence-based medicine to evaluate the CNS tumor risk factor literature. Because the scheme used to classify levels of evidence in traditional evidence-based medicine was designed, and is predominantly used, for studies intended to examine the efficacy of treatments, the highest traditional level of evidence quality (level 1) is assigned to a well-designed prospective, randomized, controlled, clinical trial. However, the primary goal of analytic epidemiology is to understand causes or risk factors for diseases. Because it is unethical to assign study participants to a potentially harmful exposure, clinical trials are not used to evaluate factors that may increase CNS tumor risk. As a result, there is no 'Level 1' level of evidence quality, *per se*, for CNS tumor risk factors. Therefore, a well-designed cohort study, in which groups of participants with and without the potential risk factor are followed over time for the occurrence of CNS tumors, may be considered the highest level of *obtainable* evidence. We adapted the levels of evidence quality scheme to consider our goal of understanding the causes of CNS tumors. The primary difference in this adapted scheme is removal of the randomized, controlled, clinical trial; the level of evidence from the well-designed cohort study is, in our adapted scheme, the superior source of evidence.

We evaluate epidemiologic evidence for CNS tumors risk factors as follows: 1) identify epidemiologic studies that address the associations of interest by searching PubMed [28] for reports of relevant epidemiologic and laboratory studies; 2) for each study, examine the estimated magnitude and precision of the effect (usually a risk or odds ratio), and its validity based on the relative strengths and weaknesses of the study design, and potential sources of error and bias in the analysis; 3) assign a level of evidence quality to each study; and 4) assign a grade of recommendation to evaluate the potential association between the risk factor and CNS tumor risk. We characterize the overall likelihood of a true association between the risk factor and CNS tumor risk (high, moderate or low) based on the following criteria: homogeneity of results among epidemiologic studies, magnitude of the potential effect, level of evidence for each epidemiologic study, and thoroughness of the epidemiologic literature in addressing the potential association. (These likelihoods are displayed in Table 3.) We discuss risk factors in decreasing order of likelihood of association.

We do not discuss literature on occupational risk factors because it is vast and inconclusive; Wrensch et al. [7] recently summarize the literature.

Genetic and Familial Factors

Most CNS tumors are thought to develop through the progressive accumulation of genetic and/or epigenetic alterations that permit cells to evade normal regulatory mechanisms and escape destruction by the immune system. The epidemiologic information available concerning genetic factors and CNS tumor risk is derived from studies related to the following: 1) CNS tumor risk associated with rare mutations in penetrant genes; 2) patterns of CNS tumors in families (suggesting potential inheritance), and 3) genetic polymorphisms or variability. Most studies of genetic and familial factors and CNS tumor risk concern astrocytic tumors and meningioma; therefore, our discussion is focused on these major histologic groups.

Table 3. Potential primary CNS tumor risk factors and corresponding likelihood of true association based on findings from epidemiologic studies[a]

Potential Primary CNS Tumor Risk Factor	Likelihood
Diseases/syndromes associated with rare mutations	High
Familial aggregation (glioma)	High
Ionizing radiation	High
Epilepsy and seizures (glioma) (probably not causal)	High
Allergies and immune-related conditions (glioma)	High/Moderate
Familial aggregation (meningioma)	Moderate
Epilepsy and seizures (meningioma)	Moderate
Estrogen and reproductive and menstrual factors (astrocytic tumors and meningioma)	Moderate
Head injury and trauma (intravascular brain tumors)	Moderate
Cellular telephone use (acoustic neuroma)	Moderate
Calcium intake (glioma)	Moderate
Maternal N-nitroso compound and antioxidant intakes (childhood brain tumors)	Moderate
Maternal folate supplementation (primitive neuroectodermal tumors)	Moderate
Paternal preconceptional smoking (childhood brain tumors)	Moderate
Genetic polymorphisms (glioma and meningioma)	Low
Mutagen sensitivity (glioma)	Low
Infections (glioma, meningioma and childhood CNS tumors)	Low
Head injury and trauma (non-intravascular brain tumors)	Low
N-nitroso compounds (glioma and meningioma)	Low
Antioxidant intake (glioma)	Low
Tobacco smoking (glioma and meningioma)	Low
Alcohol (glioma, meningioma and childhood brain tumors)	Low
Cellular telephone use (non-acoustic neuroma brain tumors)	Low
Allergies and immune-related conditions (meningioma)	Low
Electromagnetic fields (brain tumors and childhood brain tumors)	Low

a. Likelihoods shown here reflect only the current state of knowledge. Some associations, especially those listed with a low likelihood of association, may require additional study before a thorough assessment of likelihood can be made.

RISK FACTORS WITH STRONG EVIDENCE OF ASSOCIATION WITH CNS TUMORS

Diseases/Syndromes Associated with Rare Mutations and Brain Tumors

Several diseases or syndromes associated with rare mutations in highly penetrant genes increase brain tumor risk. However, in a population-based study of 500 adults with glioma in San Francisco [29], fewer than 1 percent had a known hereditary syndrome. While it is thought that genetic predisposition is influential in relatively few brain tumors (5 to 10 percent), the proportion may be underestimated because some hereditary syndromes are not readily diagnosed and because patients with brain tumors are not routinely referred to a clinical geneticist.

In general, there is strong evidence that some genetic diseases or syndromes increase brain tumor risk [7,30]. Among these, the following have been associated with an increased brain tumor risk: tuberous sclerosis complex, neurofibromatosis types 1 and 2, nevoid basal-cell carcinoma syndrome, syndromes related to adenomatous polyps, and Li-Fraumeni cancer family syndrome [7,30]. Inherited p53 germline mutations, characteristic of Li -Fraumeni syndrome, are central in the development of many cancers, including brain tumors. In addition, germline p53 mutations have been found more frequently in patients who have multifocal glioma, glioma and another primary malignancy, or a family history of cancer than in patients with other brain tumors.

Familial Aggregation and Glioma

Findings from epidemiologic studies of familial aggregation and glioma risk are relatively consistent, although the estimates of the magnitude of increased risk as a result of first-degree relation are widely variable. Five case-control studies suggest the presence of familial aggregation of glioma or glioma subtypes, whereas the results from one case-control study suggest otherwise. The finding of an increased astrocytoma or glioma risk as a result of familial aggregation is also supported by the analyses of six Swedish cohorts, although it should be noted that these studies contain overlapping populations. Malmer et al. [31] suggest that approximately 2 percent of glioma cases may be explained by an autosomal recessive gene, although a polygenic model could not be rejected; and that approximately 5 percent of glioma cases are familial [32]. In a population-based case-control study, Malmer et al. [33] reported that, among 37 familial glioma cases, as compared to 58 sporadic glioma controls with no family history of glioma, a greater proportion of the familial cases had tumors that did not overexpress p53, based on immunohistochemistry. Segregation analyses of families of more than 600 adult patients with glioma showed that a polygenic model best explained the pattern of occurrence of brain tumors [34]. Although the strength of association for familial aggregation of glioma or its subtypes varies among studies, evidence for the presence of familial aggregation has been observed consistently in both cohort and case-control studies.

Because it is possible that common environmental exposures experienced by families, in addition to their genetic characteristics, may result in a greater familial brain tumor risk, several studies have tried to determine whether genetic or environmental factors explain the increased familial risk. Grossman et al. [35] showed that brain tumors occur in families with no known predisposing hereditary disease, and that the pattern of occurrence in many families suggests environmental causes. However, results from a cohort study conducted by Malmer et al. [36] suggest that first-degree relatives, and not spouses, have a significantly increased brain tumor risk. Therefore, it is likely that both genetic and environmental characteristics play a role in familial aggregation of astrocytoma. However, the first molecular genetic evidence for familial aggregation of glioma was recently submitted by Paunu et al. [37], whose results suggest a novel low-penetrance locus at 15q23-q26.3 among people with familial gliomas in Western Finland.

Ionizing Radiation and CNS Tumors

Therapeutic ionizing radiation may be the strongest potentially modifiable CNS tumor risk factor [7,38]. Ionizing radiation used to treat tinea capitis and skin hemangioma in children or infants has been associated with relative risks of 18 for nerve sheath tumors, 10 for meningioma, and 3 for glioma [7,38]. Another report suggests that children irradiated for treatment of tinea capitis also have a greater risk of pituitary adenoma [39]. Exposure to non-dental X-rays of the head and neck did not increase glioma risk in one case-control study [40]; but both radiation therapy of the head and neck and diagnostic X-rays were found to increase brain tumor risk in another case-control study [41]. A study in the Finnish population showed that second primary brain tumors occur more frequently than expected, based on national incidence, in patients previously treated for brain tumors, especially among those treated with radiation therapy [42]. Results from one case-control study suggest that only exposure to full-mouth X-rays performed 15 to 40 years preceding diagnosis - and not to bitewing, lateral cephalometric, or panoramic X-rays - increase meningioma risk [43]. These results are supported by another study suggesting that meningioma risk among men is more strongly associated with exposures from dental X-rays taken before the age of 20 years or taken before 1945 [44].

A study of survivors of the atomic bombing of Hiroshima showed a high incidence of meningioma correlating with the dose of radiation to their brain [45]. Several studies have found that atomic bomb survivors also have higher incidences of neuroepithelial tissue tumors, schwannoma and pituitary tumors. Japanese studies of survivors of the atomic bomb have not shown an increased risk of brain tumors among those who were exposed *in utero* [38].

On the whole, results from studies of the association between exposure to ionizing radiation and CNS tumor risk are homogenous and suggest a causal association. However, few people are exposed to high doses of ionizing radiation, so such exposures probably account for only a small percentage of brain tumors.

Epilepsy and Seizures and Glioma (But Probably Not Causal)

Seizures commonly precede brain tumor diagnoses [46]. Results from studies concerning epilepsy or seizure disorders and glioma risk are relatively strong. Results from four case-control studies and three cohort studies indicate an increase in glioma risk from a history of epilepsy or seizure. Lamminpaa et al. [47] found an increase in both meningioma and glioma risk associated with history of prescribed antiepileptic medication. Schlehofer et al. [48] found an increased glioma risk associated with a history of epilepsy (RR = 6.55, 95% CI: 3.40-12.63), but the relative risk diminished when only those patients with epilepsy lasting at least 20 years were included. It is important to note that for glioma, risk has been shown to increase with the proximity of epilepsy to brain tumor diagnosis, and to decrease with duration of epilepsy, suggesting that epilepsy is not a cause but rather a result, an early effect, of glioma [49].

Allergies and Immune-Related Conditions and Glioma

Several recent reports have suggested that a history of allergies and immune-related conditions, such as asthma, eczema, and rheumatoid arthritis decrease risk of glioma. Although the mechanism governing such potential protection has not been identified, there is speculation that it may arise from the anti-inflammatory effects of cytokines involved in allergic and autoimmune disease. Five case-control studies have reported decreased odds ratios for GBM, glioma, or astrocytoma in relation to allergies and immune-related conditions, whereas results from one case-control study suggest no difference in glioma risk.

A problem with a case-control association between reported allergy status and glioma is that, due to the low survival probability from GBM, investigators have used many proxy respondents to ascertain information concerning allergic conditions. Confirming the suggestion that proxy reports may not be reliable, Schwartzbaum et al. [50] found a correlation between whether a proxy respondent was used and the presence or absence of allergic conditions. Specifically, proxy respondents reported fewer allergic conditions for index subjects than did self-reporting respondents. However, in a cohort study where information on allergic conditions was obtained on the average at least 19 years before diagnosis of a brain tumor, Schwartzbaum et al. [50] report results from the first series of cohort studies, consistent with an inverse association between allergies and glioma risk (HR = 0.45, 95% CI: 0.19-1.07) - excluding low-grade glioma - and between immune-related hospital discharges and glioma risk (HR = 0.46, 95% CI: 0.14-1.49). Moreover, Schwartzbaum et al. [51] found that germline polymorphisms associated with increased susceptibility to asthma and other allergic conditions decrease GBM risk. This result is important because it suggests that associations between allergic conditions and GBM risk are not merely reporting artifacts; however, their findings do not exclude an indirect relationship between allergic conditions and GBM [51]. The majority of the evidence, therefore, supports an inverse association between allergies and immune-related conditions and glioma - and especially GBM - risk.

RISK FACTORS WITH MODERATE EVIDENCE OF ASSOCIATION WITH CNS TUMORS

Familial Aggregation and Meningioma

Only a few epidemiologic studies have addressed the potential familial aggregation of meningioma [52-54]. Among patients with meningioma, the standardized incidence ratio (SIR) was 2.5 for having a parent with any nervous system cancer [54], and was 3.1 for having a parent with meningioma [53]. In another study, among families with an adult onset glioma, risk of meningioma was over five times that of the reference population [52]. Familial aggregation of meningioma has not been demonstrated consistently and should be validated through additional studies; however, there is some evidence for the presence of familial aggregation of meningioma.

Epilepsy and Seizures and Meningioma

There is relative consistency in the findings from case-control studies that epilepsy or seizure disorders are associated with increased meningioma risk, although not all findings have been statistically significant. Moreover, the findings concerning meningioma are not as strong as those pertaining to glioma risk. Meningioma risk does not appear to increase steadily with the proximity of epilepsy to meningioma diagnosis, and meningioma risk does not decrease steadily with the duration of epilepsy [49]. Meningioma are characteristically slow-growing, and early systemic effects from meningioma may result in epilepsy and seizures.

Estrogen and Reproductive and Menstrual Factors and Astrocytic Tumors and Meningioma

Epidemiologic research indicates that the sex hormone estrogen may be associated with decreased astrocytic tumor risk. Astrocytic tumors are approximately 40 percent more common among males than females [7]. A study of the incidence of astrocytoma subtypes occurring in the State of New York suggests that, for GBM, the protective effect of being female occurs between the approximate ages of menarche and menopause, and that this protection decreases in postmenopausal age groups [9]. Schlehofer et al. [10] report that postmenopausal women whose menopause was not surgically induced are at greater risk of glioma and acoustic neuroma, although the finding was not statistically significant. However, like the association with meningioma (described below), the association between estrogen and astrocytoma risk may not be straightforward. For example, results from two case-control studies suggest that risks of astrocytic tumors may be lower among parous women [55,56]. Schlehofer et al. [10] report no association between parity and glioma risk.

Meningioma is approximately twice as common in females as in males. In addition, some meningiomas express progesterone receptors, and this expression occurs to a greater degree among females [11]. Studies of meningioma risk and menopausal status, age at menarche, and parity have produced some results supporting the notion that greater exposure to endogenous estrogen increases meningioma risk, and some results supporting the notion that lesser exposure increases meningioma risk. Concerning age at menarche, Jhawar et al. (OR = 1.97, 95% CI: 1.06 - 3.66) [8] found that onset of menarche at a later age - after age 14 years - increased meningioma risk. Moreover, there was an increased risk of meningioma among parous women, as compared to nulliparous women (RR = 2.39, 95% CI: 0.76 - 7.53). However, findings from two case-control studies suggest no association between parity and meningioma risk. Results from a cohort study suggest that, as compared to premenopausal women, postmenopausal women who have never used estrogen replacement therapy are at greater meningioma risk (RR = 2.48, 95% CI: 1.29 - 4.77), and the risk diminishes - but remains significantly greater - when postmenopausal women who have used estrogen replacement therapy are compared to premenopausal women (RR = 1.86, 95% CI: 1.07 - 3.24) [8]. These results are supported by those of Schlehofer et al. [10], who found that, as compared to premenopausal women, postmenopausal women had a reduced risk of meningioma (RR = 0.58, 95% CI: 0.18 - 1.90).

On the whole, there is consistency among results concerning increased meningioma risk among premenopausal women; that is, among women of the same age, those who are still premenopausal are at higher risk than are those who are postmenopausal, suggesting that increased exposure to menstrual hormones might increase risk. However, results concerning parity and age at menarche suggest that estrogen or other reproductive or menstrual hormones might decrease meningioma risk. One would expect parous women and women who started menarche relatively late to have lower meningioma risk, if estrogen increases risk, because parous women and women who are older when they begin menarche are exposed to endogenous estrogen for a shorter time. Further study is required to understand hormone-related factors, especially because the findings presented here are statistically significant and opposite to those expected under the hypothesis that endogenous estrogen exposure increases meningioma risk. It is also possible that menstrual and reproductive factors alone are not sufficient to accurately classify lifetime estrogen or other hormonal exposure.

Estrogen and perhaps other hormones and menstrual and reproductive factors may alter risks of both meningioma and astrocytic tumors. Other than sex differences in incidence, there is no known evidence that estrogen, reproductive or menstrual factors alter risk of tumors of cranial and spinal nerves, CNS lymphomas, germ cell tumors, and tumors of sellar region. The relationships between brain tumor risks and endogenous and exogenous estrogen exposures appear to be complex and should be studied further. Cohort studies of brain tumor risk among women who have and have not taken estrogen replacement therapy should be conducted.

Head Injury and Trauma and Intravascular Brain Tumors

Head injury and trauma have been examined as potential brain tumor risk factors in several epidemiologic studies. Inskip et al. [57] found that, after excluding injuries occurring within the year preceding diagnosis - which could have caused a search which resulted in earlier tumor detection – intravascular tumor risk remained elevated, while risks of other brain tumor types diminished.

Cellular Telephone Use and Acoustic Neuroma

Because of public concern over possible health effects associated with cellular telephone use, several studies have addressed the potential association between use of cellular telephones and brain tumor risk. A relatively strong association (OR = 3.9, 95% CI: 1.6 – 9.5) was recently reported between a long duration (at least 10 years) of regular ipsilateral cellular telephone use and acoustic neuroma risk, but a long duration of contralateral use did not increase risk (OR = 0.9, 95% CI: 0.2 – 3.1) [58]. However, it is also possible that exposure to noise associated with cellular telephone use could have resulted in the increased acoustic neuroma risk among those reporting a long duration of use. Recently, habitual exposure to loud noise was found to increase the risk of acoustic neuroma [59]. Although potentially habitual, noise resulting from cellular telephones is not usually loud.

Calcium Intake and Glioma

Dietary calcium may decrease glioma risk through increasing apoptosis, promoting DNA repair, and decreasing the production of parathyroid hormone [60]. Tedeschi-Blok et al. [60] found that greater levels of calcium intake protect against glioma, but only among females. The results of another case-control study also suggest that calcium intake may be protective for all brain tumors combined [61].

Maternal N-nitroso Compound and Antioxidant Intakes and Childhood Brain Tumors

N-nitroso compounds - especially nitrosamides - are potent neurocarcinogens. Assessing exposure to N-nitroso compounds is difficult because they are common in both endogenous and exogenous sources, including food. Cured meats contain nitrites, which are precursors of N-nitroso compounds. Because it is possible for nitrosamides to cross the placenta, maternal exposures to N-nitroso compounds (either resulting from diet or medications, such as antihistamines) have been examined as potential risk factors for childhood brain tumors. These studies have produced mixed results [7,62]. Several studies have shown increased childhood brain tumor risk among children whose mothers either used N-nitroso-containing medications or consumed more cured meats. Although results are not homogenous, there is more evidence in support of an association between maternal N-nitroso consumption and childhood brain tumor risk. Maternal and early life consumption of antioxidants may decrease childhood brain tumor risk, perhaps through the inhibition of nitrosation. Results from several studies have suggested that childhood brain tumor risk from high maternal consumption of cured meats was reduced by use of prenatal vitamins (which contain antioxidants) and a high dietary intake of vegetables and fruits.

Maternal Folate Supplementation and Primitive Neuroectodermal Tumors

Folate protects against neural tube defects. Maternal folate supplementation has resulted in a decreased risk of primitive neuroectodermal tumors [63], and may be responsible for a decrease in the incidence of medulloblastoma [62].

Paternal Preconceptional Smoking and Childhood Brain Tumors

Several laboratory findings and two epidemiologic studies provide evidence that preconceptional paternal tobacco smoking increases childhood brain tumor risk, although the increase may be slight. However, Yang et al. found no such association for childhood neuroblastoma risk [64]. Paternal smoking should be evaluated in additional studies.

RISK FACTORS WITH LOW EVIDENCE OF ASSOCIATION WITH CNS TUMORS

Genetic Polymorphisms and Glioma and Meningioma

Only a small proportion of primary CNS tumors result from effects of inherited rare mutations in highly penetrant genes. Investigators therefore have turned their attention to common polymorphisms in genes that might influence susceptibility to CNS tumors in concert with environmental exposures. Genetic alterations that affect oxidative metabolism, detoxification of carcinogens, DNA stability and repair, or immune response, are candidates that might plausibly confer genetic susceptibility to CNS tumors.

Schwartzbaum et al. [51] selected polymorphisms that increased susceptibility to an epidemiologic risk factor inversely related to glioma - history of allergic conditions. They found that interleukin (IL)-4RA ser478pro TC, CC and IL-4RA gln551arg AG, AA are positively associated with GBM (OR=1.64, 95% CI=1.05, 2.55; 1.61, 95% CI 1.05, 2.47) while IL-13 -1112 CT, TT is negatively associated with GBM (0.56, 95% CI=0.33, 0.96) [51]. Each of these polymorphism-GBM associations is in the opposite direction of a corresponding polymorphism-asthma association, consistent with previous findings that self-reported asthmatics and people with allergic conditions are less likely to have GBM than are people who do not report these conditions (see section below on allergies and immune-related conditions). Judgments on the validity of these associations cannot be made until they are replicated by additional studies.

Results of studies of polymorphisms selected because of their associations with tumors at sites other than the brain or known carcinogenic mechanisms have not been consistent. For example, studies of polymorphisms of genes that detoxify carcinogens produce mixed results. Although one case-control study found that cytochrome p450 2D6 (CYP2D6) was associated with both astrocytoma (OR = 4.17, p = 0.004) and meningioma (OR = 4.90, p = 0.01) [65], another found no associations [66]. In two additional case-control studies, there was no association between the null genotype of CYP1A1 and risk of glioma in adults, but De Roos et al. [67] found that CYP2E1 RsaI variant was possibly associated with glioma (OR = 1.4, 95% CI: 0.9 - 2.4) and acoustic neuroma (OR = 2.3, 95% CI: 1.0 - 5.3), especially among younger people.

Detoxifying glutathione-S-transferase genes have also been studied extensively, also with mixed results. Although one study supported a strong association of glutathione transferase theta (GSTT1) deletion and astrocytoma (OR = 2.67, p = 0.0005) and meningioma (OR = 4.52, p = 0.0001) [65], others have not replicated these findings. Trizna et al. [68] and De Roos et al. [67] report no associations between the null genotype of GSTT1 and glioma risk; however, other results suggest that GSTT1 null genotype increases meningioma risk and that the GSTP1 105 Val/Val genotype is associated with increased glioma, with evidence of a dose-response trend with increasing numbers of variant alleles. Most recently, Wrensch et al. [69] found little evidence for the association of glutathione-S-transferase polymorphisms with glioma histologic variants, but did show an association of GSTT1 deletion and astrocytic tumors with p53 mutations.

Several additional polymorphisms have been evaluated for their relationship with glioma. Chen et al. [70] showed that AA or AC versus CC genotype in nucleotide 8092 of ERCC1 increased oligoastrocytoma risk (OR = 4.6, 95% CI: 1.6-13.2). Caggana et al. [71] found that the AA genotype (C to A polymorphism (R156R)) of ERCC2 was more prevalent than the CC or CA genotypes in cases with GBM, astrocytoma, or oligoastrocytoma than in controls, and the association was strongest for oligoastrocytoma (OR = 3.2; 95% CI: 1.1 - 9.5). Yang et al. [72] found the ERCC2-exon-22 T allele prevalence was 35 percent among oligodendroglioma cases, compared to 18 percent for controls, and that alterations in GLTSCR1 (or a closely linked gene) were associated with oligodendroglioma. Wang et al. [73] found that the TT genotype of XRCC7 – a gene involved in nonhomologous end joining double-strand break repair – was more common among glioma cases, compared to controls (OR = 1.86, 95% CI: 1.1-3.1, comparing TT homozygotes to all others).

Inconsistencies among genetic polymorphism studies may result from false-positive associations based on inadequate sample sizes [74] and from confounding by genes with similar functions not accounted for in the analyses. Another possibility may be that study populations consist of different proportions of types of tumors, and genetic risk for certain subtypes could be masked by lack of risk among other subtypes. When these issues are addressed, the potential interaction between genetic polymorphisms with other genetic characteristics and environmental factors can be properly evaluated. Although, based on current research, there is only a low probability of association between genetic polymorphisms and CNS tumor risk, there is a high likelihood that future research will probably identify important polymorphisms that alter risk, either alone or in concert with environmental factors.

Mutagen Sensitivity and Glioma

Bondy et al. [75] found that lymphocyte mutagen sensitivity to gamma radiation appears to increase glioma risk. Lymphocytes from glioma patients, compared to those from matched controls, are more sensitive to gamma radiation [75]. Bondy et al. [75] observed a greater frequency of chromatid breaks per cell among patients with glioma as compared to controls, and found mutagen sensitivity to be associated with increased glioma risk (OR = 2.09, 95% CI: 1.43 - 3.06). Moreover, there was evidence of a statistically significant dose-response trend between frequency of chromatid breaks and glioma risk. However, because Bondy et al. [75] used the case-control design, it is not possible to determine whether chromatid breaks increased brain tumor risk or whether they represent a systemic effect of the tumors themselves. Further, there is a possibility of confounding by age, solar exposure, diet (especially carotenoids and other antioxidants) and glioma treatment [76]. To avoid this confounding and definitively establish temporality, further studies of mutagen sensitivity must be conducted on blood from patients with glioma that is collected before initiation and development of the glioma. Given the absence of reliable information on latency for glioma, results of such a study would necessarily require careful evaluation.

Infections and Glioma, Meningioma, and Childhood CNS Tumors

Infection with polyomaviruses, such as JC, BK and simian virus 40 (SV40), and herpes viruses, such as varicella zoster virus (VZV), and nonviral infectious agents, such as Toxoplasma gondii - or immunity to these agents - might influence CNS tumor risk, although the potential risk from these agents has been inadequately addressed in epidemiologic studies. Between 1955 and 1963, an unknown proportion of all inactivated and live polio vaccines distributed was contaminated with SV40 [77]. In Germany, where children were followed over a 20-year period, those inoculated with the polio vaccine contaminated with SV40 had higher occurrences of GBM, medulloblastoma, and some less common brain tumor types than had children not given the contaminated vaccine [78]. By contrast, in the US, no difference in brain tumor risk was found for major brain tumor types (glioma and meningioma) between the two groups of children [79], but one study reported that the incidence of ependymoma was 37 percent greater among the children receiving the contaminated vaccine [77]. There is mixed evidence from laboratory studies concerning the involvement of SV40, JC virus and BK virus in the development of brain tumors. Results from a nested case-control study conducted by Rollison et al. [80] indicated that infection with either JC virus or BK virus or with SV40, as measured in sera of patients between 1 and 22 years before brain tumor diagnoses, did not significantly increase subsequent brain tumor risk. Further, Rollison et al. [81] found no increased brain tumor risk among male army veterans receiving contaminated vaccines.

Limited laboratory evidence suggests that human herpes virus 6 (HHV-6) may be involved in the development of brain tumors. However, results from three case-control studies suggest that prior clinical disease associated with VZV infection and anti-VZV immunoglobulin G levels may be inversely associated with adult glioma risk [82-84].

A history of cold or influenza infection may also be associated with decreased glioma risk. In a case-control study, Schlehofer et al. [48] found a 30 to 40 percent reduction in glioma risk associated with a self-report of a history of colds or influenza infections (RR = 0.72, 95% CI: 0.61 - 0.85). In another case-control study, Fisher et al. [85] found that treatment for at least one cold or influenza infection between 2 and 5 years before diagnosis of a glioma decreased glioma risk two- to three-fold (OR = 0.39, 95% CI: 0.18 - 0.86). These results should be validated in cohort studies with serologic or symptom-based confirmation of infection.

The potential association between infection with human immunodeficiency virus (HIV) and CNS tumor risk has not been addressed in epidemiologic studies, although it is likely that the incidence of CNS tumors among people infected with HIV is greater than that among the general population. With the exception of the fact that HIV infection is known to increase CNS lymphoma risk, there is only limited information about CNS tumors related to HIV infection.

Antibodies to toxoplasma gondii have been associated with meningioma in a case-control study and to astrocytoma in another study, but not to glioma, based on the results of Ryan et al. [86].

Results from several case-control studies have suggested that children whose mothers had viral infections during pregnancy are at greater CNS tumor risk, as well as brain tumor and neuroblastoma risks. For example, Fear at el. [87] found that children whose mothers had a clinically documented viral infection during pregnancy had approximately an 11-fold increased CNS tumor risk. Further, results from one of two ecologic studies suggested that perinatal exposure to either measles or influenza increases CNS tumor risk in children. These results should be validated in cohort studies with serologic or symptom-based confirmation of infection.

The findings concerning infections and both childhood and adult brain tumor risk are limited, inconsistent, or based exclusively on results from case-control studies. The strongest epidemiologic evidence of a potential association between infection and CNS tumor risk would be submitted from a cohort study in which serologic measurement of viral or bacterial exposure was ascertained before the development of brain tumors.

Head Injury and Trauma and non-Intravascular Brain Tumors

Hu et al. [88] found an increase in glioma risk from head trauma requiring medical attention (OR = 4.1, 95% CI: 2.5-10.3), and Hochberg et al. [89] found a large increase in GBM risk from severe head injury. However, results from four additional case-control studies, and two cohort studies suggested no such association. Results from four case-control studies suggest that head injury and trauma increase meningioma risk. Among males, Preston-Martin et al. [90] found that meningioma was more common among those who reported having ever had a head injury (OR = 1.5, 95% CI: 0.9-2.6), and that, among those with a latency of 15 to 24 years, meningioma risk was much greater (OR = 5.4, 95% CI: 1.7-16.6). However, these results are in conflict with the results of three cohort studies, which suggest no increase in meningioma risk from head injury or trauma. Findings from the three cohort studies provide much stronger evidence because it is likely that there were differences between cases and controls in the reporting of previous head injury and trauma. A large Danish cohort study provides good evidence that there is little, if any, association between head injury and trauma and either meningioma or glioma risk [57]. Inskip et al. [57] found that, after excluding injuries occurring within the year preceding diagnoses, neither glioma risk (SIR = 1.0, 95% CI: 0.8-1.2) nor meningioma risk (SIR = 1.2, 95% CI = 0.8-1.7) was elevated.

Head injury and trauma during birth have been examined as potential risk factors for childhood brain tumors; however, there appears to be only a slight, if any, increase in risk [62], and it is possible that recall bias may account for the excess risk [7]. There are no known studies specifically examining head injury and trauma and specific risks of tumors of cranial and spinal nerves, CNS lymphomas, germ cell tumors, and tumors of sellar region. With the exception of risk of some less common intravascular tumors, for which there is moderate evidence of association, there appears to be a low likelihood of association with CNS tumors risk.

N-nitroso Compounds and Glioma and Meningioma

Cured meats contain nitrites, which are precursors of N-nitroso compounds. Results from epidemiologic studies concerning brain tumor risk associated with cured meat consumption are mixed. Two case-control studies report conflicting findings of the effect of cured meat consumption on glioma risk, one showing no effect [91] and one showing that male cases, but not female cases, were more likely than controls to report higher levels of cured meat consumption [92]. However, as suggested by Schwartzbaum et al. [93], it is possible that energy intake and gamma-tocopherol modify the association between cured meat consumption and glioma risk; cured meats contain high energy and low gamma-tocopherol content. In a recent meta-analysis of nine studies addressing the possible association between cured meat consumption and glioma risk, Huncharek et al. [94] report an increase in glioma risk from cured meat consumption (pooled RR = 1.48, 95% CI: 1.20 - 1.83), but they point out that individual studies failed to adjust for potential confounding by energy intake. Further, several studies have reported a higher incidence of brain tumors in areas with greater nitrate content in the drinking water. Results from a case-control study of cured meat consumption and meningioma risk suggest an increased risk, but only for females [95].

Antioxidant Intake and Glioma

Oxidative stress results from excessive accumulation of reactive oxygen species (ROS), and can be caused by inadequate dietary antioxidant intake. Antioxidants are abundant in a diet high in fruits and vegetables. Consumption of greater amounts of vitamin C was inversely associated with glioma risk in two case-control studies, although the findings were statistically significant only among males in the study conducted by Lee et al. [92]. Schwartzbaum et al. [93] found lower levels of vitamin C intake among glioma cases as compared to controls. The results reported by Chen et al. [91], however, suggest no association between vitamin C intake and glioma risk. Dietary intake of higher levels of vitamin A or pro-vitamin A has been inversely related to glioma risk in each of three case-control studies in which it was examined, although not all findings were statistically significant. Higher levels of dietary vitamin E intake were protective for glioma in one case-control study [61], but not in two other studies. Schwartzbaum et al. [93] found lower levels of vitamin E - both alpha-tocopherol and gamma-tocopherol - intake among glioma cases as compared to controls.

Tobacco Smoking and Glioma and Meningioma

Tobacco smoking has been evaluated as a potential risk factor for CNS tumors because some carcinogenic components contained in tobacco smoke, including N-nitroso compounds, penetrate the blood-brain barrier. Results from two case-control studies and one cohort study suggest that there may be a sex difference in the association between tobacco smoking and glioma risk. In one case-control study, males, but not females, who reported a history of having ever smoked were at greater risk of glioma, while results from a cohort study suggest that tobacco smoking increases risk of adult-onset glioma only among women. Lee et al. [92] found that male glioma cases were almost two times more likely to report smoking unfiltered cigarettes, but there was no association among women.

Tobacco smoking has been shown to increase meningioma risk, but only in females [96]. Results from most studies suggest that tobacco smoking does not strongly contribute to brain tumor risk, although smoking unfiltered, but not filtered, cigarettes may increase glioma risk [92]. There is no compelling evidence that maternal tobacco use, or childhood exposure to environmental tobacco smoke, increases childhood brain tumor risk [62]. Further, results from three studies suggest no increased risk in childhood germ cell tumor risk from maternal tobacco smoking, and that neither tobacco smoking nor environmental tobacco smoke increase pituitary adenoma risk. With the exception of preconceptional paternal smoking, tobacco-related results are inconsistent and the magnitudes of the effect estimates are modest, suggesting little important effect of tobacco smoking on glioma and meningioma risks.

Alcohol and Glioma, Meningioma and Childhood Brain Tumors

Results from seven case-control studies addressing alcohol consumption and brain tumor risk are inconsistent, with four studies suggesting no increase in brain tumor risk, and three suggesting increases in risk. Alcohol consumption has not been shown to affect meningioma risk; and while glioma risk was found to be increased from higher levels of alcohol consumption in two studies, in other studies there was no increase in either glioma risk, or GBM risk. Maternal alcohol consumption is associated with only a slight increase in childhood brain tumor risk [38,97]. There are no known studies of alcohol consumption and risk of tumors of cranial and spinal nerves, CNS lymphomas, germ cell tumors, and tumors of sellar region. Overall, the results concerning alcohol and CNS tumor risk are inconsistent and the magnitudes of the positive results are modest.

Cellular Telephone Use and Non-Acoustic Neuroma Brain Tumors

One mortality study, four case-control studies and one retrospective cohort study suggest that there is no association between cellular telephone use and brain tumor risk, with the possible exception of acoustic neuromas. Results from these studies, in general, suggest that there is no increase in brain tumor risk from a longer duration of cellular telephone use and that these devices affect no specific anatomic site or brain tumor histology. However, three reports provide additional important findings. Results reported by Hardell et al. [41] suggest an increase in brain tumor risk from ipsilateral (same side) use of cellular telephones for areas of the brain with the greatest potential for microwave exposure from cellular telephone use (the temporal, temporoparietal, and occipital areas). Moreover, ipsilateral radiofrequency exposure was associated with an increased malignant brain tumor risk, and for astrocytoma, risk was nearly double [98]. The association of ipsilateral radiofrequency exposure with malignant brain tumor risk was stronger for analog than for digital radiofrequency; whereas analog cellular telephone radiofrequency signals operate in the range of 800-900 MHz, newer digital phones operate in the range of 1600-2000 MHz. Similar results concerning ipsilateral cellular telephone use were reported in a case-control study, and statistically significant increases in brain tumor risk, including astrocytoma risk, were found for both analog and digital devices - although, again, the finding was stronger for analog devices [99]. Using the same set of cases and controls, Hardell et al. [100] recently reported that the effect of digital cellular phone use on brain tumor risk is over three times greater among users residing in rural areas of Sweden, and the effect was strong for malignant brain tumors. In rural areas, there is a longer distance between base stations, which causes a greater power output level in digital phones; the analog system is less affected by this adaptive power control [100]. No association has been reported between the use of cellular telephones and brain tumor risk on the side opposite the ear generally used for telephone calls. Although results are inconsistent, if there is an increase in brain tumor risk from cellular telephone use, it may be specific to ipsilateral use, which would be expected since the radiofrequency dosage to the contralateral ear would be minimal. The relatively consistent studies also suggest increased risk from analog telephones and for the histology of acoustic neuroma. Although results from most studies of cellular telephones and brain tumors, in general, suggest no increase in brain tumor risk, it is important to continue this line of study because: 1) the use of such devices is increasingly common; and 2) it is possible that adverse health effects from this exposure may result from long-term exposure. Results from reported studies may not account adequately for the possibly long lag-time between exposure and brain tumor development, especially for slow-growing brain tumors. In addition, changes in cellular telephone technology, such as the predominance of digital versus analog telephones, as well as an overall increase in the frequency and duration of usage, have not been addressed in many studies.

Allergies and Immune-related Conditions and Meningioma

Unlike results concerning allergies and immune-related conditions and glioma risk, no inverse or positive associations of meningioma with allergies or autoimmune diseases have been found.

Electromagnetic Fields and Childhood and Adult Brain Tumors

Concern over exposure to low-frequency electric and magnetic fields (EMF) has stimulated considerable public and scientific attention. This interest arises primarily from residential studies showing increased risk of brain tumors and leukemia in children whose homes had high EMF exposures. However, for CNS tumors, exposure to EMF has, for the most part, been well evaluated through occupational studies of workers presumably exposed to greater levels of EMF than residential exposure would involve. Workers exposed to greater levels of EMF have a higher incidence of, and mortality from, brain tumors. In general, results from each of 11 case-control studies addressing occupational EMF exposure and brain tumor risk suggest an increase in brain tumor risk associated with greater levels of EMF exposure, although not every increase in risk was statistically significant. However, results from nested case-control and cohort studies have yielded inconsistent results, with six suggesting no association, and five suggesting an increase in brain tumor risk from occupational exposure to EMF. It is possible that there has been insufficient measurement of EMF exposure, and that this has accounted for the discrepant findings, especially because there may be less individual variation in assessment of occupational exposure, made on the basis of occupational codes, as compared to assessment of non-occupational exposure. It is also possible that occupational exposure to EMF, on the whole, occurs at a higher dose than that obtained from non-occupational exposure, and that this has accounted for the difference between occupational and non-occupational studies. No causal relationship has been established between exposure to EMF, either occupational or residential, and brain tumor (or astrocytoma, glioma, GBM, or meningioma) risk. Further, there is no compelling evidence that greater levels of EMF exposure increase risk of childhood brain tumors [62]. There are no known studies specifically examining EMF exposure and specific risks of tumors of cranial and spinal nerves, CNS lymphomas, germ cell tumors, and tumors of sellar region.

Risk Factors, Summary

Table 3 shows each potential CNS tumor risk factor and the corresponding likelihood that the factor increases or decreases CNS tumor risk.

Specific histologic types are mentioned when there is apparent variation according to histology. Again, it is important to emphasize that some factors with relatively low likelihood given current state of knowledge may eventually be shown to be associated with CNS tumor risk. Other than genetic characteristics, there is a high likelihood that ionizing radiation increases risk for most CNS tumors. History of epilepsy and/or seizures is strongly and consistently associated with glioma, but the association is probably due to the tumor causing the seizures, rather than vice-versa. Among the associations currently being investigated, those of greatest interest include: familial aggregation with meningioma, allergies and immune-related conditions with glioma, estrogen and reproductive and menstrual factors with both astrocytic tumors and meningioma, a variety of inherited polymorphisms with glioma and meningioma, maternal dietary factors with childhood brain tumors, and focused aspects of cellular telephone use with acoustic neuroma.

RECOMMENDED MANAGEMENT STRATEGIES AND TREATMENT

Standard treatment options for selected common CNS tumor histologies are shown in Table 4 [101-103].

There is tremendous histologic variability in response to treatments and cure rates. Pilocytic astrocytoma, mostly affecting children, is rarely fatal, with a two-year survival probability of 93.9 percent. (Note that survival probabilities given in this section are for all ages combined, and differ from the age-specific probabilities shown in Figure 4.) Diffuse astrocytoma (two-year survival probability of 61.5 percent) can progress to anaplastic astrocytoma (two-year survival probability of 44.2 percent), and, eventually, GBM (two-year survival probability of 8.8 percent); the cure rate for diffuse astrocytoma is, therefore, dependent on whether there is progression. Anaplastic astrocytoma usually progresses to GBM, which is almost always fatal within five years, regardless of treatment. Compared to patients diagnosed with an astrocytoma subtype, patients with oligodendroglioma (two-year survival probability of 82.7 percent) and anaplastic oligodendroglioma (two-year survival probability of 60.1 percent) respond more favorably to radiation therapy and chemotherapy. Patients with grade I ependymal tumors (myxopapillary ependymoma and subependymoma) have good prognoses, with long durations of survival time and high cure rates, while patients with grade II ependymal tumors (ependymoma), more common in children and young adults, have slightly poorer prognoses. Anaplastic ependymoma have accelerated growth; as a result, prognosis is not as favorable as that for ependymoma. Ependymoma and anaplastic ependymoma, combined, have a two-year survival probability of 60.1 percent.

Table 4. Summaries of standard treatment options for common CNS tumor histologies based on National Cancer Institute options [101-103]

Histologic Group	Summary of Standard Treatment Options
Tumors of Neuroepithelial Tissue	
Pilocytic Astrocytoma	Surgery alone if tumor is totally resectable; Surgery followed by radiation therapy to known/suspected residual tumor.
Diffuse Astrocytoma	Surgery plus radiation therapy; Some physicians treat with surgery alone if patient is younger than 35 years and if tumor does not contrast-enhance on computed tomographic scan.
Anaplastic Astrocytoma	Surgery plus radiation therapy and chemotherapy.
Glioblastoma	Surgery plus radiation therapy and chemotherapy;
Oligodendroglioma/ Anaplastic Oligodendroglioma	Surgery plus radiation therapy; Some physicians treat with surgery alone if patient is younger than 45 years and if tumor does not contrast-enhance on computed tomographic scan.
Grade I and II Ependymal Tumors	Surgery alone if tumor is totally resectable; Surgery followed by radiation therapy to known or suspected residual tumor.
Anaplastic Ependymoma	Surgery plus radiation therapy.
Mixed Glioma	Surgery plus radiation therapy; Surgery plus radiation therapy plus chemotherapy.
Tumors of Meninges	
Grade I Meningioma	Surgery; Surgery plus radiation therapy is used in selected cases, such as with known/suspected residual disease or recurrence after previous surgery; Radiation therapy for unresectable tumors.
Grade II and III Meningioma/ Hemangiopericytoma	Surgery plus radiation therapy.
CNS Lymphomas	Variable; Unsatisfactory results of whole-brain irradiation alone, neurologic toxic effects of chemotherapy and radiation therapy, current major focus on trials with chemotherapy alone.
Germ Cell Tumors	Variable; Depends on tumor histology, tumor location, presence and amount of biological markers, and surgical resectability.
Tumors of Sellar Region	
Craniopharyngioma	Surgery alone if tumor is totally resectable; Debulking surgery plus radiation therapy if tumor is unresectable.
Pituitary Tumors	Variable; Depends on tumor type, hormonal activity, presence of vision deterioration, and presence of extension into brain around pituitary.

Grade I meningioma are benign and almost always curable with resection, while grade II and III meningioma (which comprise between six and ten percent of all meningioma) and hemangiopericytoma (now recognized, according to the NCI as "a mesenchymal, nonmeningothelial tumor histologically indistinguishable from hemangiopericytomas occurring in soft tissue") have less favorable prognoses, but still more favorable than most astrocytic tumors. Prognoses for patients with CNS lymphoma are, in general, poor, although there are wide variabilities in treatments and prognoses, based on factors shown in Table 4, as well as the potential for acquired immunodeficiency syndrome-related comorbidities. Overall, two-year survival probability for CNS lymphoma is 26.4 percent. Patients diagnosed with localized germinoma have good prognoses (due to cure as the result of radiation therapy), but patients with other germ cell tumors (embryonal carcinoma, choriocarcinoma, and teratoma) often have variable and unsuccessful treatments and poorer prognoses. Craniopharyngioma, a benign tumor occurring in children and older adults, and pituitary tumors, which are usually benign, are often curable.

Because patients diagnosed with astrocytic tumors, especially the most common subtype, GBM, have poor prognoses, many randomized clinical trials (RCT) have been conducted and are currently in progress to examine novel treatment approaches. The standard therapy for tumors of the CNS (except for lymphoma) involves surgical excision, if possible. If operative resection is deemed too risky, then stereotactic biopsies are performed to obtain histologic confirmation of tissue. Surgery can be curative for some tumors (such as meningioma), while it is palliative for others (such as grade III or IV astrocytomas). For malignant tumors, radiation and/or chemotherapy are also employed in the postoperative setting. For the malignant glial tumors, clinical trials are being used to find additional treatments. For example, results from a recent RCT show that, among patients with high-grade glioma, survival time was longer for patients who had biodegradable carmustine-impregnated polymer placed intraoperatively at the time of initial surgery, compared with a placebo-treated group (13.9 months survival in the treated group and 11.6 months in the control group) [104]. Even more recently, the addition of oral temozolomide therapy provided at the time of radiation therapy has been shown to improve the two-year survival probability of patients with malignant gliomas to 26.5 percent, compared to 10.4 percent for patients receiving radiotherapy alone [105]. In addition, MGMT silencing by promoter methylation has been associated to improved responses to chemotherapy [106]. Another treatment option for patients with oligodendroglioma and loss of heterozygosity of chromosomes 1p/19q has been to employ chemotherapy alone, since these tumor appear to be very chemosensitive [107,108].

Other current RCT for patients with unresectable tumors or tumors with very low cure rates involve hyperfractionated or accelerated-fraction irradiation, stereotactic radiosurgery, radiosensitizers, hyperthermia, interstitial brachytherapy, intraoperative radiation therapy used in conjunction with external-beam radiation therapy, gene therapies, virotherapy, immunotherapy, and boron neutron capture therapy.

CONCLUSION

The reasons for variation in CNS tumor incidence according to time, sex, age, race, ethnicity, and geography are poorly understood, as are the factors that affect prognosis. As shown in Table 3, there are few established risk factors for CNS tumors. In addition to ionizing radiation, rare mutations in highly penetrant genes associated with certain diseases and syndromes, only the unexplained observation of familial aggregation of glioma, and the inverse association of allergies and immune-related conditions with glioma have been shown consistently. Ongoing research on CNS (and especially brain) tumors is focused on classifying homogeneous groups of tumors based on molecular markers and identifying genetic polymorphisms that may increase brain tumor risk in conjunction with developmental experiences and environmental exposures. Rather than examining individual genetic polymorphisms in isolation, new research is focusing on genetic polymorphisms in pathways involved in carcinogenesis. Related pathways are also studied simultaneously so that confounding by genes with similar functions can be avoided. Large sample sizes are required for such studies, and these larger studies avoid false-positive findings and permit examination of the modifying effects of polymorphisms on environmental exposures, as well as the potential for interaction between germline mutations and sporadic tumor mutations. There has been some limited success in the advancement of treatment of CNS tumors (such as that for oligodendroglioma), but to improve the prognoses and prolong the survival of patients diagnosed with astrocytic tumors will probably require many RCT of novel treatment strategies. Our knowledge about the causes of CNS tumors, the factors that determine prognoses, and the treatments allowing the best possible outcomes, is not extensive and should be expanded by conducting large, well-designed epidemiologic and RCT studies of potential risk and prognostic factors and treatment strategies.

ACKNOWLEDGEMENTS

This work was supported by grants RO1CA52689 and P50CA097257 from the National Institutes of Health. We thank the Central Brain Tumor Registry of the United States, in particular Jennifer Propp, for providing statistical information related to central nervous system tumor incidence and survival.

REFERENCES

[1]   CBTRUS. *Statistical Report: Primary Brain Tumors in the United States*, 1995-1999. 2002.

[2]   CBTRUS. *Statistical Report: Primary Brain Tumors in the United States*, 1997-2001. 2004.

[3]   SEER. Surveillance, Epidemiology, and End Results (SEER) Program SEER*Stat Database: Incidence - SEER 9 Regs Public-Use, Nov 2003 Sub (1973-2001), National

Cancer Institute, DCCPS, Surveillance Research Program, Cancer Statistics Branch, released April 2004.

[4]   SEER. SEER*Stat Database: Incidence - SEER 11 Regs + AK Public-Use, Nov 2003 Sub for Expanded Races (1992-2001), National Cancer Institute, DCCPS, Surveillance Research Program, Cancer Statistics Branch. 2004.

[5]   Davis FG, Bruner JM, Surawicz TS. The rationale for standardized registration and reporting of brain and central nervous system tumors in population-based cancer registries. *Neuroepidemiol* 1997;16(6):308-16.

[6]   Helseth A. The incidence of primary central nervous system neoplasms before and after computerized tomography availability. *J Neurosurg* 1995;83(6):999-1003.

[7]   Wrensch M, Minn Y, Chew T, Bondy M, Berger MS. Epidemiology of primary brain tumors: current concepts and review of the literature. *Neuro-oncology* 2002;4(4):278-99.

[8]   Jhawar BS, Fuchs CS, Colditz GA, Stampfer MJ. Sex steroid hormone exposures and risk for meningioma. *J Neurosurg* 2003;99(5):848-53.

[9]   McKinley BP, Michalek AM, Fenstermaker RA, Plunkett RJ. The impact of age and sex on the incidence of glial tumors in New York State from 1976 to 1995. *J Neurosurg* 2000;93(6):932-9.

[10]   Schlehofer B, Blettner M, Wahrendorf J. Association between brain tumors and menopausal status. *J Natl Cancer Inst* 1992;84(17):1346-9.

[11]   Yu ZY, Wrange O, Haglund B, Granholm L, Gustafsson JA. Estrogen and progestin receptors in intracranial meningiomas. *J Steroid Biochemistry* 1982;16(3):451-6.

[12]   Inskip PD, Linet MS, Heineman EF. Etiology of brain tumors in adults. *Epidemiologic Reviews* 1995;17(2):382-414.

[13]   Singh GK, Siahpush M. All-cause and cause-specific mortality of immigrants and native born in the United States. *Am J Public Health* 2001;91(3):392-9.

[14]   Brower V. Large variations seen in treatment of adults with brain cancer. *J Natl Cancer Inst* 2005;97(7):478-9.

[15]   Diete S, Treuheit T, Dietzmann K, Schmidt U, Wallesch CW. Sex differences in length of survival with malignant astrocytoma, but not with glioblastoma. *J Neuro-oncol* 2001;53(1):47-9.

[16]   Sant M, van der Sanden G, Capocaccia R. Survival rates for primary malignant brain tumours in Europe. *Eur J Cancer* 1998;34(14 Spec No):2241-7.

[17]   Lacroix M, Abi-Said D, Fourney DR, et al. A multivariate analysis of 416 patients with glioblastoma multiforme: prognosis, extent of resection, and survival. *J Neurosurg* 2001;95(2):190-8.

[18]   Lutterbach J, Sauerbrei W, Guttenberger R. Multivariate analysis of prognostic factors in patients with glioblastoma. *Strahlentherapie und Onkologie: Organ der Deutschen Rontgengesellschaft* 2003;179(1):8-15.

[19]   Jeremic B, Milicic B, Grujicic D, Dagovic A, Aleksandrovic J. Multivariate analysis of clinical prognostic factors in patients with glioblastoma multiforme treated with a combined modality approach. *J Cancer Res Clin Oncol* 2003;129(8):477-84.

[20]   Schwartzbaum J, Lal P, Evanoff W, et al. Presurgical serum albumin levels predict survival time from glioblastoma multiforme. *J Neuro-oncol* 1999;43:35-41.

[21] Arrieta O, Garcia E, Guevara P, et al. Hepatocyte growth factor is associated with poor prognosis of malignant gliomas and is a predictor for recurrence of meningioma. *Cancer* 2002;94(12):3210-8.

[22] Simmons ML, Lamborn KR, Takahashi M, et al. Analysis of complex relationships between age, p53, epidermal growth factor receptor, and survival in glioblastoma patients. *Cancer Res* 2001;61(3):1122-8.

[23] Ohgaki H, Dessen P, Jourde B, et al. Genetic pathways to glioblastoma: a population-based study. *Cancer Res* 2004;64(19):6892-9.

[24] Wang L, Wang LE, El-Zein R, et al. Human telomerase genetic variation predicts survival of patients with glioblastoma multiforme (Abstract number 2823). *Proc Am Assoc Cancer Res* 2005;46.

[25] Helseth A. Incidence and survival of intracranial meningioma patients in Norway 1963-1992. *Neuroepidemiol* 1997;16(2):53-9.

[26] Sankila R, Kallio M, Jaaskelainen J, Hakulinen T. Long-term survival of 1986 patients with intracranial meningioma diagnosed from 1953 to 1984 in Finland. Comparison of the observed and expected survival rates in a population-based series. *Cancer* 1992;70(6):1568-76.

[27] McCarthy BJ, Davis FG, Freels S, et al. Factors associated with survival in patients with meningioma. *J Neurosurg* 1998;88(5):831-9.

[28] http://www.ncbi.nlm.nih.gov/entrez/query.fcgi?DB=pubmed.

[29] Wrensch M, Lee M, Miike R, et al. Familial and personal medical history of cancer and nervous system conditions among adults with glioma and controls. *Am J Epidemiol* 1997;145(7):581-93.

[30] Bondy M, Wiencke J, Wrensch M, Kyritsis AP. Genetics of primary brain tumors: a review. *J Neuro-oncol* 1994;18(1):69-81.

[31] Malmer B, Iselius L, Holmberg E, Collins A, Henriksson R, Gronberg H. Genetic epidemiology of glioma. *British J Cancer* 2001;84(3):429-34.

[32] Malmer B, Gronberg H, Bergenheim AT, Lenner P, Henriksson R. Familial aggregation of astrocytoma in northern Sweden: an epidemiological cohort study. *Intl J Cancer* 1999;81(3):366-70.

[33] Malmer B, Brannstrom T, Andersson U, Bergh K, Gronberg H, Henriksson R. Does a low frequency of P53 and Pgp expression in familial glioma compared to sporadic controls indicate biological differences? *Anticancer Res* 2002;22(6C):3949-54.

[34] de Andrade M, Barnholtz JS, Amos CI, Adatto P, Spencer C, Bondy ML. Segregation analysis of cancer in families of glioma patients. *Genetic Epidemiol* 2001;20(2):258-70.

[35] Grossman SA, Osman M, Hruban R, Piantadosi S. Central nervous system cancers in first-degree relatives and spouses. *Cancer Investigation* 1999;17(5):299-308.

[36] Malmer B, Henriksson R, Gronberg H. Familial brain tumours-genetics or environment? A nationwide cohort study of cancer risk in spouses and first-degree relatives of brain tumour patients. *Intl J Cancer* 2003;106(2):260-3.

[37] Paunu N, Lahermo P, Onkamo P, et al. A novel low-penetrance locus for familial glioma at 15q23-q26.3. *Cancer Res* 2002;62(13):3798-802.

[38] Preston-Martin S. Epidemiology of primary CNS neoplasms. *Neurologic Clinics* 1996;14(2):273-90.

[39] Juven Y, Sadetzki S. A possible association between ionizing radiation and pituitary adenoma: a descriptive study. *Cancer* 2002;95(2):397-403.

[40] Wrensch M, Miike R, Lee M, Neuhaus J. Are prior head injuries or diagnostic X-rays associated with glioma in adults? The effects of control selection bias. *Neuroepidemiol* 2000;19(5):234-44.

[41] Hardell L, Mild KH, Pahlson A, Hallquist A. Ionizing radiation, cellular telephones and the risk for brain tumours. *European J Cancer Prevention* 2001;10(6):523-9.

[42] Salminen E, Pukkala E, Teppo L. Second cancers in patients with brain tumours - impact of treatment. *Eur J Cancer* 1999;35(1):102-5.

[43] Longstreth WTJ, Phillips LE, Drangsholt M, et al. Dental X-rays and the risk of intracranial meningioma: a population-based case-control study. *Cancer* 2004;100(5):1026-34.

[44] Preston-Martin S, Yu MC, Henderson BE, Roberts C. Risk factors for meningiomas in men in Los Angeles County. *J Natl Cancer Inst* 1983;70(5):863-6.

[45] Shintani T, Hayakawa N, Hoshi M, et al. High incidence of meningioma among Hiroshima atomic bomb survivors. *J Radiation Res* 1999;40(1):49-57.

[46] Pace A, Bove L, Innocenti P, et al. Epilepsy and gliomas: incidence and treatment in 119 patients. *J Experimental Clin Cancer Res: CR* 1998;17(4):479-82.

[47] Lamminpaa A, Pukkala E, Teppo L, Neuvonen PJ. Cancer incidence among patients using antiepileptic drugs: a long-term follow-up of 28,000 patients. *Eur J Clin Pharm* 2002;58(2):137-41.

[48] Schlehofer B, Blettner M, Preston-Martin S, et al. Role of medical history in brain tumour development. Results from the international adult brain tumour study. *Intl J Cancer* 1999;82(2):155-60.

[49] Schwartzbaum J, Jonsson F, Ahlbom A, et al. Prior hospitalization for epilepsy, diabetes, and stroke and subsequent glioma and meningioma risk. *Cancer Epidemiol Biomarkers* Prev 2005;14(3)643-50.

[50] Schwartzbaum J, Jonsson F, Ahlbom A, et al. Cohort studies of association between self-reported allergic conditions, immune-related diagnoses and glioma and meningioma risk. *Intl J Cancer* 2003;106(3):423-8.

[51] Schwartzbaum J, Ahlbom A, Malmer B, et al. Polymorphisms associated with asthma are inversely related to glioblastoma multiforme. *Cancer Res (In Press)* 2005.

[52] Paunu N, Pukkala E, Laippala P, et al. Cancer incidence in families with multiple glioma patients. *Intl J Cancer* 2002;97(6):819-22.

[53] Hemminki K, Li X. Familial risks in nervous system tumors. *Cancer Epidemiol Biomarkers Prev* 2003;12(11 Pt 1):1137-42.

[54] Hemminki K, Li X, Collins VP. Parental cancer as a risk factor for brain tumors (Sweden). *Cancer Causes Control* 2001;12(3):195-9.

[55] Lambe M, Coogan P, Baron J. Reproductive factors and the risk of brain tumors: a population-based study in Sweden. *Intl J Cancer* 1997;72(3):389-93.

[56] Cantor KP, Lynch CF, Johnson D. Reproductive factors and risk of brain, colon, and other malignancies in Iowa (United States). *Cancer Causes Control* 1993;4(6):505-11.

[57] Inskip PD, Mellemkjaer L, Gridley G, Olsen JH. Incidence of intracranial tumors following hospitalization for head injuries (Denmark). *Cancer Causes Control* 1998;9(1):109-16.

[58] Lonn S, Ahlbom A, Hall P, Feychting M. Mobile phone use and the risk of acoustic neuroma. *Epidemiol* 2004;15(6):653-9.

[59] Edwards C, Schwartzbaum J, Lonn S, Alinaghizadeh H, Ahlbom A, Feychting M. Habitual exposure to loud noise and risk of acoustic neuroma. *Submitted* 2005.

[60] Tedeschi-Blok N, Schwartzbaum J, Lee M, Miike R, Wrensch M. Dietary calcium consumption and astrocytic glioma: the San Francisco Bay Area Adult Glioma Study, 1991-1995. *Nutrition Cancer* 2001;39(2):196-203.

[61] Hu J, La Vecchia C, Negri E, et al. Diet and brain cancer in adults: a case-control study in northeast China. *Intl J Cancer* 1999;81(1):20-3.

[62] Baldwin RT, Preston-Martin S. Epidemiology of brain tumors in childhood - a review. *Toxicology Applied Pharmacology* 2004;199(2):118-31.

[63] Bunin GR, Kuijten RR, Buckley JD, Rorke LB, Meadows AT. Relation between maternal diet and subsequent primitive neuroectodermal brain tumors in young children. *N Engl J Med* 1993;329(8):536-41.

[64] Yang Q, Olshan AF, Bondy ML, et al. Parental smoking and alcohol consumption and risk of neuroblastoma. *Cancer Epidemiol Biomarkers Prev* 2000;9(9):967-72.

[65] Elexpuru-Camiruaga J, Buxton N, Kandula V, et al. Susceptibility to astrocytoma and meningioma: influence of allelism at glutathione S-transferase (GSTT1 and GSTM1) and cytochrome P-450 (CYP2D6) loci. *Cancer Res* 1995;55(19):4237-9.

[66] Kelsey KT, Wrensch M, Zuo ZF, Miike R, Wiencke JK. A population-based case-control study of the CYP2D6 and GSTT1 polymorphisms and malignant brain tumors. *Pharmacogenetics* 1997;7(6):463-8.

[67] De Roos AJ, Rothman N, Inskip PD, et al. Genetic polymorphisms in GSTM1, -P1, -T1, and CYP2E1 and the risk of adult brain tumors. *Cancer Epidemiol Biomarkers Prev* 2003;12(1):14-22.

[68] Trizna Z, de Andrade M, Kyritsis AP, et al. Genetic polymorphisms in glutathione S-transferase mu and theta, N-acetyltransferase, and CYP1A1 and risk of gliomas. *Cancer Epidemiol Biomarkers Prev* 1998;7(6):553-5.

[69] Wrensch M, Kelsey KT, Liu M, et al. Glutathione-S-transferase and adult glioma. *Cancer Epidemiol Biomarkers Prev* 2004;13(3):461-7.

[70] Chen P, Wiencke J, Aldape K, et al. Association of an ERCC1 polymorphism with adult-onset glioma. *Cancer Epidemiol Biomarkers Prev* 2000;9(8):843-7.

[71] Caggana M, Kilgallen J, Conroy JM, et al. Associations between ERCC2 polymorphisms and gliomas. *Cancer Epidemiol Biomarkers Prev* 2001;10(4):355-60.

[72] Yang P, Kollmeyer TM, Buckner K, Bamlet W, Ballman KV, Jenkins RB. Polymorphisms in GLTSCR1 and ERCC2 are associated with the development of oligodendrogliomas. *Cancer* 2005;1(103):2363-72.

[73] Wang L-E, Bondy ML, Shen H, et al. Polymorphisms of DNA repair genes and risk of glioma. *Cancer Res* 2004;64(16):5560-3.

[74] Wacholder S, Chanock S, Garcia-Closas M, El Ghormli L, Rothman N. Assessing the probability that a positive report is false: an approach for molecular epidemiology studies. *J Natl Cancer Inst* 2004;96(6):434-42.

[75] Bondy ML, Kyritsis AP, Gu J, et al. Mutagen sensitivity and risk of gliomas: a case-control analysis. *Cancer Res* 1996;56(7):1484-6.

[76] Berwick M, Vineis P. Markers of DNA repair and susceptibility to cancer in humans: an epidemiologic review. *J Natl Cancer Inst* 2000;92(11):874-97.

[77] Fisher SG, Weber L, Carbone M. Cancer risk associated with simian virus 40 contaminated polio vaccine. *AntiCancer Res* 1999;19(3B):2173-80.

[78] Geissler E, Staneczek W. SV40 and human brain tumors. *Archiv fur Geschwulstforschung* 1988;58(2):129-34.

[79] Strickler HD, Rosenberg PS, Devesa SS, Hertel J, Fraumeni JFJ, Goedert JJ. Contamination of poliovirus vaccines with simian virus 40 (1955-1963) and subsequent cancer rates. *JAMA* 1998;279(4):292-5.

[80] Rollison DEM, Helzlsouer KJ, Alberg AJ, et al. Serum antibodies to JC virus, BK virus, simian virus 40, and the risk of incident adult astrocytic brain tumors. *Cancer Epidemiol Biomarkers Prev* 2003;12(5):460-3.

[81] Rollison DEM, Page WF, Crawford H, et al. Case-control study of cancer among US army veterans exposed to simian virus 40-contaminated adenovirus vaccine. *Am J Epidemiol* 2004;160(4):317-24.

[82] Wrensch M, Weinberg A, Wiencke J, et al. Does prior infection with varicella-zoster virus influence risk of adult glioma? *Am J Epidemiol* 1997;145(7):594-7.

[83] Wrensch M, Weinberg A, Wiencke J, Miike R, Barger G, Kelsey K. Prevalence of antibodies to four herpesviruses among adults with glioma and controls. *Am J Epidemiol* 2001;154(2):161-5.

[84] Wrensch M, Weinberg A, Wiencke J, et al. History of chickenpox and shingles and prevalence of antibodies to varicella-zoster virus and three other herpesviruses among adults with glioma and controls. *Am J Epidemiol* 2005;161(10):929-38.

[85] Fisher J, Schwartzbaum J, Johnson C. Cold/influenza infection, influenza vaccination, and risk of adult glioma (abstract 116). *Am J Epidemiol* 2000;151.

[86] Ryan P, Hurley SF, Johnson AM, et al. Tumours of the brain and presence of antibodies to Toxoplasma gondii. *Intl J Epidemiol* 1993;22(3):412-9.

[87] Fear NT, Roman E, Ansell P, Bull D. Malignant neoplasms of the brain during childhood: the role of prenatal and neonatal factors (United Kingdom). *Cancer Causes Control* 2001;12(5):443-9.

[88] Hu J, Johnson KC, Mao Y, et al. Risk factors for glioma in adults: a case-control study in northeast China. *Cancer Detection Prev* 1998;22(2):100-8.

[89] Hochberg F, Toniolo P, Cole P. Head trauma and seizures as risk factors of glioblastoma. *Neurology* 1984;34(11):1511-4.

[90] Preston-Martin S, Pogoda JM, Schlehofer B, et al. An international case-control study of adult glioma and meningioma: the role of head trauma. *Intl J Epidemiol* 1998;27(4):579-86.

[91] Chen H, Ward MH, Tucker KL, et al. Diet and risk of adult glioma in eastern Nebraska, United States. *Cancer Causes Control* 2002;13(7):647-55.

[92] Lee M, Wrensch M, Miike R. Dietary and tobacco risk factors for adult onset glioma in the San Francisco Bay Area (California, USA). *Cancer Causes Control* 1997;8(1):13-24.

[93] Schwartzbaum JA, Fisher JL, Goodman J, Octaviano D, Cornwell DG. Hypotheses concerning roles of dietary energy, cured meat, and serum tocopherols in adult glioma development. *Neuroepidemiol* 1999;18(3):156-66.

[94] Huncharek M, Kupelnick B, Wheeler L. Dietary cured meat and the risk of adult glioma: a meta-analysis of nine observational studies. *J Environmental Pathology Toxicology Oncol* 2003;22(2):129-37.

[95] Preston-Martin S, Henderson BE. N-nitroso compounds and human intracranial tumours. *IARC* 1984(57):887-94.

[96] Hu J, Little J, Xu T, et al. Risk factors for meningioma in adults: a case-control study in northeast China. *Intl J Cancer* 1999;83(3):299-304.

[97] Wrensch M, Bondy ML, Wiencke J, Yost M. Environmental risk factors for primary malignant brain tumors: a review. *J Neuro-oncol* 1993;17(1):47-64.

[98] Hardell L, Mild KH, Carlberg M. Case-control study on the use of cellular and cordless phones and the risk for malignant brain tumours. *Intl J Radiation Biology* 2002;78(10):931-6.

[99] Hardell L, Mild KH, Carlberg M. Further aspects on cellular and cordless telephones and brain tumours. *Intl J Oncol* 2003;22(2):399-407.

[100] Hardell L, Carlberg M, Hansson Mild K. Use of cellular telephones and brain tumour risk in urban and rural areas. *Occup Environ Med* 2005;62(6):390-4.

[101] NCI. Primary CNS lymphoma (PDQ): Treatment health professionals version. 2004.

[102] NCI. Childhood brain tumors (PDQ): Treatment health professionals version. 2004.

[103] NCI. Adult brain tumors (PDQ): Treatment health professionals version. 2005.

[104] Westphal M, Hilt DC, Bortey E, et al. A phase 3 trial of local chemotherapy with biodegradable carmustine (BCNU) wafers (Gliadel wafers) in patients with primary malignant glioma. *Neuro-oncology* 2003;5(2):79-88.

[105] Stupp R, Mason WP, van den Bent MJ, et al. Radiotherapy plus concomitant and adjuvant temozolomide for glioblastoma. *N Engl J Med* 2005;352(10):987-96.

[106] Hegi ME, Diserens A-C, Gorlia T, et al. MGMT Gene silencing and benefit from temozolomide in glioblastoma. *N Engl J Med* 2005;352(10):997-1003.

[107] Reifenberger G, Louis DN. Oligodendroglioma: toward molecular definitions in diagnostic neuro-oncology. *J Neuropathology Experimental Neurology* 2003;62(2):111-26.

[108] Cairncross JG, Ueki K, Zlatescu MC, et al. Specific genetic predictors of chemotherapeutic response and survival in patients with anaplastic oligodendrogliomas. *J Natl Cancer Inst* 1998;90(19):1473-6.

RECOMMENDED FURTHER READING

Books

1. Principles and Practice of Neuro-Oncology (Hardcover) by David Schiff. Publisher: McGraw-Hill Professional; 1 edition (June 23, 2005)
2. Brain Tumor Pathology: Current Diagnostic Hotspots and Pitfalls (Hardcover) by Davide Schiffer. Publisher: Springer; 1 edition (April 11, 2006)
3. Brain Tumors: An Encyclopedic Approach (Hardcover) by Andrew H. Kaye and Edward R. Laws (Editors). Publisher: Churchill Livingstone; 2 edition (April 5, 2001)

Articles

1. Nakamura M, Shimada K, Ishida E, Nakase H, Konishi N. Genetic analysis to complement histopathological diagnosis of brain tumors. *Histology and Histopathology.* vol. 22, no. 3 (2007 Mar): 327-35.
2. Schwartzbaum JA, Fisher JL, Aldape KD, Wrensch M. Epidemiology and molecular pathology of glioma. *Nature Clinical Practice. Neurology.* vol. 2, no. 9 (2006 Sep): 494-503; quiz 1 p following 516.
3. Goldsmith B, McDermott MW. Meningioma. *Neurosurgery Clinics of North America.* vol. 17, no. 2 (2006 Apr): 111-20, vi.
4. Ashby LS, Ryken TC. Management of malignant glioma: steady progress with multimodal approaches. *Neurosurgical Focus.* vol. 20, no. 4 (2006): E3.
5. Lee S-W, Kim WJ, Park Jae, Choi YK, Kwon Y-W, Kim K-W. Blood-brain barrier interfaces and brain tumors. *Archives of Pharmacal Research.* vol. 29, no. 4 (2006 Apr): 265-75.
6. Robertson PL. Advances in treatment of pediatric brain tumors. *NeuroRx: the Journal of the American Society for Experimental NeuroTherapeutics.* vol. 3, no. 2 (2006 Apr): 276-91.
7. Gilbert MR. Advances in the treatment of primary brain tumors: dawn of a new era? *Current Oncology Reports.* vol. 8, no. 1 (2006 Jan): 45-9.

In: Handbook of Clinical Neuroepidemiology
Editors: V. L. Feigin and D. A. Bennett, pp. 429-464
ISBN 978-1-60021-511-7
© 2007 Nova Science Publishers, Inc.

Chapter 12

CENTRAL NERVOUS SYSTEM TOXIC AND METABOLIC DISORDERS

G. Jean Harry[1], Susan H. Brunssen[2] and Donald E. Schmechel[3]

[1]Neurotoxicology Group Laboratory of Neurobiology, National Institute of Environmental Health Sciences, National Institutes of Health Research Triangle Park, NC, 27709 USA;
[2]School of Nursing and Neurodevelopmental Disorders Research Center, University of North Carolina, Chapel Hill, NC, USA;
[3]Departments of Medicine (Neurology) and Neurobiology, Integrated Toxicology Program Duke University Medical Center, Durham, NC, USA.

ABSTRACT

Normal development and functioning of the nervous system represents the proper integration of information received and acted upon in an integrated manner. Concern is raised upon disruptions of these processes whether due to structural or functional changes induced by endogenous disease process such as, genetic based metabolic disorders or from exposure to exogenous agents in the environment. These effects can be either clinically remarkable or represent very subtle alterations that, over time, can lead to adverse health effects. This chapter presents examples of known environmental neurotoxicants and metabolic disorders and briefly discusses how one might examine and evaluate toxicological data to assess potential adverse health effects and incorporate this information into a diagnostic process.

INTRODUCTION

Normal development and functioning of the nervous system represents the proper integration of various types of information received. This information is then acted upon in a fully integrated manner. Disruptions of these processes can occur at the structural or functional level. They can be induced by endogenous disease process such as, genetic based metabolic disorders or from exposure to an exogenous agent in the environment. In either case the disruptions can be detrimental to the quality of life of the individual. One usually considers major incidents or outbreaks of chemical poisonings or early onset childhood metabolic disorders as being of primary concern; however, an increasing emphasis is being placed on possible decrement in nervous system function at a more subtle level due to low levels of environmental insult or milder abnormalities of metabolism. Questions regarding identification of an environmental exposure and the increased level of risk to human health are quite prominent in more recent environment-based neuroepidemiology studies. This chapter provides background information and summarizes what is known with regards to toxic responses in the nervous system, reviews effects by classification of agent, discusses special vulnerabilities related to developmental stage, and then briefly reviews childhood metabolic disorders that show similar neurologic effects. In addition it presents considerations in evaluating evidence from neuroepidemiology studies to assess exposure related outcomes. Considerations related to evaluating patients presenting with history and signs of possible neurotoxicity are overviewed.

THE NERVOUS SYSTEM AS TARGET SITE

The nervous system has been identified as a primary target site for toxic agents with concern raised by a number of international agencies. It is estimated that millions of people are exposed to known neurotoxicants that is supported by the number of repeated outbreaks of environmentally related neurological disease. The development of a human neurotoxic condition can be considered within a contextual framework of a continuum of events initiated by exposure to a neurotoxic substance at a level sufficient for absorption of a biologically effective dose [23]. In order to study and understand neurotoxic diseases, one must understand the anatomy, physiology, and biochemistry of the nervous system. In addition, modifying factors such as developmental stage, aging process, gender, concurrent systemic toxicity, inter-current illnesses, nutritional state, and the genetically determined effectiveness of repair and regenerative processes of the nervous system must be considered in such evaluations.

NEUROTOXICITY

As defined by a number of international health and regulatory agencies, neurotoxicity is the capacity of chemical, biologic, or physical agents to cause adverse functional or structural changes in the nervous system. Adverse effects have been defined as alterations from a baseline state that diminishes an organism's ability to survive, reproduce, or adapt to the environment. It has also been suggested that induced alterations in nervous system function or structure that are unintended or unwanted effects (side-effects) can be considered adverse. Characterization of toxicity encompasses multiple levels of organization and interactions. Such characterization includes structural, biochemical, physiological, and behavioral levels of effects. Complex cognitive functions such as speech, emotion, learning, memory, neuromuscular coordination, and autonomic control depend upon an integrative capacity. Therefore, adverse effects on the nervous system can result in a wide range of signs and symptoms depending on the dose and duration of exposure, and factors such as, age and gender. Representative chemical-induced neurotoxic effects often include seizures, paralysis, dementia, incoordination, impaired reasoning ability, memory loss, decreased vigilance, or attention, affective disorders such as episodic mood disorder, psychosis or other psychiatric dysfunction, weakness, tremor, impaired performance, and laterations in sensory function. Outcome measures that may help characterize or quantify neurotoxic effects include anatomical and functional neuroimaging, neuropsychological assessment of behavior, cognition and sensorimotor function, electrophysiological testing such as, autonomic studies (e.g. heart rate regulation), electromyography/nerve conduction studies, visual, brainstem auditory or somatosensory evoked potentials, and electroencephalography, nerve or muscle biopsy, and biological monitoring or sampling of cerebrospinal fluid.

Incidence of Neurotoxicity in the Human Population

The major routes by which agents gain access to the body are via ingestion, inhalation, topical (trans-dermal or trans-mucosal), percutaneous, or other parenteral routes. As would be expected, the greatest and most rapid effects occur with direct exposure to the bloodstream. Poisonings usually occur via oral ingestion; occupational exposure most frequently involves inhalation or direct and prolonged dermal contact; and environmental exposure involves multiple routes but usually at lower exposure levels. In many cases, information on the toxic potential of chemicals is limited with an estimated 7 percent of high production chemicals (excess of 1 million pounds/year) having a complete set of publicly available studies for basic toxicity endpoints and no data available for approximately 43 percent. Even less is known about more subtle effects of chemical exposure at low levels to the long-term functioning of the nervous system. Thus, studies to assess the impact of environmental chemicals on human health are limited to the subset of chemicals with a good data-base for toxicity and to relatively short exposures at high levels.

An increasing number of reports are available examining the possible effects of exposure to neurotoxicants and adverse human health outcomes. Many of these studies are case reports or case studies involving a small number of severely affected individuals. Such reports are often the first information available on a health related incident. Much of our knowledge regarding the neurotoxicity of specific compounds has been the result of reports of human neurotoxic disease due to environmental and industrial over-exposures as a consequence of accident or ignorance. In the occupational setting, outbreaks of neurotoxic conditions have occurred as the result of exposure to both identified and unidentified chemicals including pesticides, metals, and organic solvents. Outbreaks have also occurred in the general population. In the United States, in the 1920s, ingestion of a popular drink containing cresyl phosphates resulted in the paralysis of several thousand persons. Similar types of incidents occurred due to the contamination of cooking oil with organic compounds such as, the aniline contamination in Spain that affected 20,000 persons in 1981, cresyl phosphates in Morocco, and both polychlorinated biphenyls (PCBs) and furans in the Far East. Contamination of fish with industrial mercury containing wastes resulted in two large scale outbreaks in Japan (Minimata Disease - named for the painful neurological effects); more than 7000 persons were hospitalized in Iraq from the ingestion of grain contaminated with organomecurial fungicides; and, in 1986, bread contaminated with parathion resulted in an outbreak in Sierra Leone. The human incidence of neurotoxic disease due to chemical exposure both in the general population and in the occupational setting provide compelling evidence for the potential of different classes of chemicals to affect neurological function. The transfer of the neurotoxicity to the unborn child in the incidents with methyl mercury and PCBs raised an additional level of concern for human exposure of more vulnerable individuals such as pregnant women, unborn fetus, and children of young ages.

In the case of poisoning, or high exposure from an accident or from occupational setting, exposure and dose are much easier to determine. In this case, adverse effects are seen in a relatively short time period. However, a significant lag time occurs between exposure and the eventual manifestation of clinical symptoms. A sentinel health event is the occurrence of a neurotoxic outcome in an occupational setting. Examples of such events include toxic encephalopathy due to lead exposure in foundry workers, ship repair and bridge demolition workers; Parkinsonian-like symptoms in manganese miners, steel manufacturing and welding environments; cerebellar ataxia due to organic mercury exposure in fungicide manufacturing; and peripheral neuropathy due to n-hexane, methyl n-butyl ketone, or other solvent exposure in the furniture refinishing industry, electronics industry, plastic coating industry, paint manufacture, or reprocessing and waste disposal industries [23]. Outbreaks of carbon monoxide exposure have occurred among farmers using gasoline-powered pressure washers, indoor burning of charcoal briquettes, indoor use of gasoline-powered machinery, riding in the back of pickup trucks with faulty exhaust systems, and one of the most common sources of exposure, a faulty home heating system. In the case of CO poisoning, the patient can potentially be removed in time from the source and restoration of oxygen to hemoglobin, cytochromes, and other CO-binding sites will slowly ensue with O2 supplementation. Hyperbaric oxygen has been used successfully to accelerate the displacement of CO for the treatment of acute carbon monoxide poisoning. The specificity of the clinical effects associated with these exposures (obtundation or coma, cherry red appearance, ability to measure hemoglobin-CO levels) serves as warning and diagnostic signals to a physician. CO and related exposures such as, hydrogen sulfide gas represent agents that can produce significant long-term effects without absolute correlation to clinical status. Blood hemoglobin-CO levels may clear rapidly under O2 supplementation during transport, but tissue levels still remain high. Thus, high-risk individuals such as pregnant women that present with CO poisoning and then clear their sensorium should still be considered for hyperbaric treatment or continued attention. The clearing of blood hemoglobin and restoration of apparently "intact" mental status does not mean that intracellular CO on mitochondrial cytochromes and other targets has been adequately cleared. Likewise, both CO and hydrogen sulfide (H2S) exposures can give rise to a syndrome termed delayed neurodegeneration where one or more weeks later, significant clinical decline can occur characterized by a Parkinsonian-like syndrome with basal ganglia involvement.

Quite often it is from such descriptive case reports that we have identified neurotoxic chemicals. Such reports usually rely on the clinical symptoms that show a temporal relationship with exposure, plausibility with existing knowledge on the biological effects of the chemical, and consistency with other possible case reports. However, prolonged exposure at sufficiently high levels may subsequently lead to early health effects that may not also lead to a clinical diagnosis because of time delay or lack of information, yet are early signs of neurotoxic effects. Given the limitations in our understanding of the mechanisms of toxicity, the application of epidemiological methods to address knowledge gaps in our understanding of acute poisoning has been proposed by Buckley [15]. The implementation of such an approach may allow for the further development of biomarkers of effect in addition to those of exposure. Erythrocyte acetylcholinesterase (AchE) activity is an example of a biomarker of neurotoxic effect that is used to monitor acute or cumulative exposure to organophosphate chemicals. Such chemicals are used as pesticides and chemical warfare agents. The assumption that early and reversible biochemical changes occur with a sufficiently high level of internal exposure has led to a number of studies focused on identifying early biochemical markers of exposure/effect.

Classification of Neurotoxicants

Neurotoxic agents can be classified in a number of different ways depending on the interests and needs of the classifier. These include: chemical class and structure; intended use of the chemical; source; and effects such as, morphological target, functional or cellular target, or mechanism of action. The term *toxin* generally refers to a toxic substance produced by a biological system while *toxicant* refers to substances that are produced by or are a by-produce of man-made activities or natural elements (metals). Examples of chemical exposure demonstrated to have adverse effects on the nervous system include several classes of chemicals found in the environment or occupational setting. These include metals, solvents, insecticides, and naturally occurring toxins.

Metals

Almost all metals examined have the potential to produce adverse human health effects, including effects on the nervous system. However, as expected, effects are a matter of absorbed dose. Neurotoxic effects of aluminum have been demonstrated in dialysis encephalopathy where normal intestinal barriers to aluminum absorption are bypassed and contaminated water is used for dialysis via bloodstream. Aluminum toxicity is characterized by difficulties in speech and coordination, twitching, myoclonic jerks, affect disorders, and can progress to dementia. Speculation has been made with regards to the relationship between aluminum exposure and Alzheimer's Disease (AD); however, to date the weight of evidence does not support a causal relationship. This association was based upon early studies that reported aluminum in neurofibrillary tangles. Further studies failed to replicate this observation but rather found that chelation of aluminum onto microscopic specimens during processing lead to this artifact. In addition, elemental analysis of brain tissue did not support excess aluminum in AD pathology. Arsenic appears to target mostly other organ systems such as skin and liver; serious and fatal injury of the peripheral nervous system can occur without apparent central nervous system involvement. However, more recent experimental animal data suggests that indeed the central nervous system may be involved in the toxicity of arsenic. Barium is widely used in paints and free barium can be readily absorbed from the gut or lung. If this occurs at a sufficient level, accumulation can occur in both the skeleton and the eye. In ionic form and at high dose levels, barium can be a muscle poison leading to loss of tendon reflexes and paralysis. Bismuth poisoning can produce acute encephalopathy; depending upon the severity of the effect, memory and affective disorders can persist. Manganese is used in the metal industry and poisoning can lead to an acute psychosis, impaired motor ability, and long term impaired cognitive functioning. Inorganic mercury poisoning produces impaired cognitive function and fatigue, depression, and dysphoria. For these outcomes the aged show a greater level of sensitivity. Careful long-term epidemiological studies have shown that such dramatic outcomes in heavily exposed individuals are accompanied by significant "sub-clinical" alterations in these same measures in the entire population of exposed workers. This poses the question, should threshold limit values for exposures be based on immediate clinical measures or biomarker levels or rather, on longer-term measures of exposure. For example, in workers potentially exposed to mercury, monitoring of urinary mercury excretion is used as a biomarker of acute exposure (and potential injury to kidney). Time away from exposure and natural normalization of urinary excretion is used as a measure of clearing the body burden. With regards to a concern over dental mercury amalgam, replacement of all dental amalgam or chelation therapy has been proposed. The replacement of dental amalgam has risks for additional mercury exposure and chelation therapy can have potentially serious sideeffects due to non-specific chelation of other metals. There is no evidence-based literature to speak to the effect of long-term exposures to low levels of mercury or episodic releases (e.g. inflammatory disease of teeth and gums).

The form of the metal influences toxicity, as well as, the route of exposure. For example, methyl mercury is much more toxic than inorganic mercury. During gestation, methylmercury passes through the placenta resulting in fetal concentrations equal to or exceeding the maternal concentrations High exposure levels during development can result in sensory deficits, mental deficiency, cerebral palsy, seizures, and spasticity. At slightly lower doses (3-11ppm) the effects are characterized by mental deficiency, reflex and muscle tone abnormalities, and delayed motor development. At even lower doses (0.1-3ppm), a delay in psychomotor development can be evident. In infants with Minamata disease (methylmercury poisoning), brain gliosis and cytoarchitectural abnormalities such as, ectopic cell masses and disorganization of the cortical layers are evident. Disturbances in neuronal migration, defective lamination of the cerebral cortex, changes in the pattern of the cerebral gyri, and either gliosis or neuroglial heterotopias can also occur. In the massive epidemic of methylmercury poisoning in Iraq during 1971-72 as a result of eating bread made from contaminated grain, the threshold for minimally abnormal neurological signs in children was between 68 and 180 ppm methylmercury in maternal hair. Severe neurologic impairment was seen in children when maternal peak hair mercury values were above 165 ppm. Symptoms of poisoning included seizures and motor, speech, and mental retardation.

Lead as a Prototypic Metal Neurotoxicant

In the case of inorganic lead, epidemics of lead poisoning were recognized as early as the eighteenth century. In more modern times, there has been widespread exposure from industrial emissions, lead-based paints, food, beverages, and the use of lead-based gasoline. Occupational sources of lead exposure include mining, smelting, storage batteries, pigments, ink, ceramics, automobile radiator repair, welding, and firing ranges. With the acknowledgement of the neurotoxic properties of lead, the availability of sufficient manufacturing substitutes, and government-mandated removal of lead from gasoline, paints, and domestic cans, blood lead levels within North America began to decline [40]. More recent data is being obtained from other areas of the world with regard to the impact of lead removal from gasoline.

Blood is the vehicle of transport and distribution for lead. While blood lead levels are a good indicator for recent exposure they are reflective of only approximately 2% of the body burden. Absorbed lead is excreted primarily via the kidneys and unabsorbed lead via the feces. The half-life of lead varies for the different pools; decades for bone, 4-5 weeks for soft tissue, and in blood it is the half-life of the erythrocyte (35 days). Given the binding of lead to the erythrocyte, it is not unexpected that lead intoxication can adversely affect the hematological system. Lead inhibits gamma-aminolevulinic acid dehydratase (ALA-D) at blood levels of approximately 20 – 40 mg/dl and the activity of this enzyme is a useful biochemical indicator of early lead intoxication. A good indicator of chronic lead intoxication is the measurement of blood zinc protoporphyrin due to the elevation in free erythrocyte protoporphyrin.

Most cases of human toxicity to lead are the result of chronic exposures lasting weeks to months. Given that lead is excreted by the kidneys, one would expect this organ to be a major primary target site for toxicity. Indeed, chronic lead toxicity in the adult can produce an irreversible chronic interstitial nephropathy. In children, lead containing intranuclear inclusion bodies can be evident in proximal renal tubule epithelial cells. This condition is reversible depending on the level of damage and removal of the person from exposure. With regards to the nervous system, encephalopathy of various degrees occurs primarily in children. The incidence of lead poisoning is highest between the ages of 12 and 36 months. During this age, the hand to mouth activities of the child are most pronounced and Pica can be determined by a good history of activities. Clinical signs include gastrointestinal distress, behavioral abnormalities, and increased intracranial pressure. These signs are accompanied by gross and microscopic changes in the brain structure that have been well described in the neuropathology literature [19]. Chronic changes can be seen in the cerebellum and include focal atrophy and gliosis with loss of Purkinje cells and internal granular layer neurons. As would be expected, anemia usually accompanies neurological symptoms. This being said, lead encephalopathy can also occur in various levels of severity such that these pathological alterations may not be easily recognized.

In adults, clinical outcome of lead exposures is primarily neuropathic. In the peripheral motor neuropathy, upper limbs are involved more than the lower limbs. When a peripheral neuropathy does occur in children, it tends to involve the lower limbs with signs of foot drop. In each case, the neuropathy is motor in nature and commonly devoid of sensory signs or symptoms. In typical cases of radial nerve involvement with wrist drop, there is a progressive involvement of the extensors radiating from the middle and ring fingers to include the wrist. Based on these clinical outcomes in very high exposures, electrophysiological studies have been conducted in the occupational setting with lesser exposures to determine the relationship between blood lead levels and peripheral neuropathy. While such studies suggested minor abnormalities in nerve conduction, the measurement techniques differed thus, making comparisons across studies difficult. For example, in a small cohort of subjects with significant lead exposure (7 of 14 with lead levels > 120 mg/dl) no difference was found in the maximal motor or sensory nerve conduction velocity. However, a decrease was seen in the ratio of the amplitude of the compound muscle action potential suggestive of a minor degree of conduction block between the knee and the ankle [16]. Other occupationally related confounders were not addressed in the study. Seppalainen et al. [49] examined a group of 26 storage battery factory workers with blood lead levels <70 mg/dl and reported a slight but significant slowing of maximal motor conduction velocity for the ulnar and median nerves. Conduction velocity of the slower motor fibers was also reported as decreased. While the study showed a relative reduction as compared with the control group, the sample size was small and the values fell within the normal range of the general population. A similar problem arose in a study examining 20 workers with maximal blood lead levels of 70 – 140 mg/dl [14]. Motor conduction velocity in the median nerve was reduced by a mean 5.5 m/sec that was found to be statistically significant but all subjects remained within the laboratory's normal range. Thus, while statistical significance has been reported and lead intoxication can cause peripheral neuropathy, when examined more closely, most studies have not established a correlation between blood lead level and reduction of nerve conduction velocity. This situation points to a fundamental problem in most studies of clinical outcome in neurotoxic exposures. The observed wide variability of most clinical and electrophysiological measures in the general population (presumably developmentally, genetically, and environmentally modulated) is such that clinically significant changes in a given individual are not detected. The ideal case would to monitor an individual's specific clinical status and measurements by any of the outcome measures mentioned above before, during, and after exposures, instead of comparing to population means. Here, significant change would be determined by trajectory of single individual with appropriate adjustment for age-related change, regression to the mean, and other influences and variables. In individual cases, acquiring clinical measures such as neuropsychological assessment, electrophysiological studies, blood/tissue samples, neuroimaging at time of first assessment will, nevertheless, assist in assessment and long-term management of the case. While the neuropathology of human lead neuropathy is poorly characterized, segmental demyelination has not been described and the general conclusion is that the histopathological process is mainly one of Wallerian degeneration. The speculation that lead exposure may play a role in the pathogenesis of amyotrophic lateral sclerosis [11,4] is based, not on the human pathophysiology, but rather on experimental rodent studies. In adult rats, lead exposure over an extended period produces primary demyelination of the peripheral nerve with possible involvement of the spinal roots and anterior horn cells.

The evidence of clinical symptoms with lead intoxication raised the concern for subclinical lead poisoning and permanent neurological sequelae from lesser exposures. This concern was most pronounced for childhood exposure [6,20,32,43]. In fact, clinical studies have shown that children with subclinical lead poisoning have a number of neurobehavioral characteristics and problems, poor academic achievement, and intellectual and sensory-motor deficits. Following these reports, population based, cross-sectional epidemiological studies were undertaken. Changes in cognitive function were assessed by standardized intelligence and psychometric tests and related to lead exposure as determined by either blood or tooth lead. Assessment methodologies and specific potential confounders differed across studies. Many of the studies reported an inverse association between intelligence test scores and blood lead levels exceeding 25-30 mg/dl. Subsequent prospective studies shared common design elements including subject recruitment, similar test methods for outcome measures, and repeated testing including school-age years [6]. These studies demonstrated decrement in intelligence test scores with blood lead levels at or slightly less than 20 mg/dl (8). While primary attention has been paid to childhood exposure, changes in neurological function have also been related to occupational lead exposure. In adults, blood lead levels of 40 mg/dl produce a decrease in sensory-motor reaction time, mild attention impairment, deficits in verbal memory and reasoning, and linguistic processing. The work of Bleecker et al. [9] suggests that the susceptibility to chronic lead exposure is increased in the older individual and thus, identifies this population as one of greater risk comparable to the child. More recent data suggests that the current blood lead threshold limit of 10 mg/dl should be lowered to 2 mg/dl as a level of concern for childhood exposure and long-term effects. However, the weight of evidence is not yet conclusive for such an action but given the nature of the effects one can conclude that any efforts to lower exposure would be of benefit. Moreover, attaining such a low standard for lead levels may not be technically or economically feasible given the current ubiquitous nature of lead in our environment.

Organic Solvents

Most of our data regarding neurotoxicity of solvents comes from the occupational setting. As most solvents are volatile, they can be readily inhaled or dermally absorbed by the worker. In many clinical cases, proposed protective means such as suits, masks with respiratory filters, washing, etc were either not provided, defective or not utilized due to lack of workplace education or individual decision. Clinical outcomes are also affected in chronic exposures by the eventual loss of olfactory cues to exposure and even acclimatization to such cues as headaches. Often workers in these industries are inadequately informed with regard to human health and toxic agents, and have limited opportunity to distance themselves from the occupational exposure setting. It can be found that workers deal with their toxic headache syndrome by excess use of caffeine. Organic solvents are also lipid soluble and accumulate in adipose tissue and organs or tissues with "fat" such as peripheral or central myelin, liver, and can be carried as with other neurotoxic agents on clothes that then expose family members in the home place. Organic solvents have the potential of perturbing membrane stability and function, of initiating or seeding lipid peroxidation in target tissues or organs. Downstream effects on nervous system function could result from disruption of blood-brain (retina or nerve) barriers or by indirect effects on nervous tissue through derangement of homeostasis and function of other tissues such as, choroid plexus, liver, kidney, etc. Significant deep targets without blood brain barrier protection exist in the brain including the circumventricular organs such as, the median eminence, OVLT, subcommisural organ, etc. Recent studies suggest a relationship between possible organic solvent encephalopathy and pathological sleep apnea. Obstructive sleep apnea (OSAS) could result from weight increase in susceptible individuals and/or increase in mass and inflammation of retropharyngeal tissues. As such, it may represent a target syndrome for toxic exposures that alter affect (e.g., depression with weight gain) and/or inflammation and allergic reaction. Subsequent case control studies with occupational solvent exposure have yet to clearly demonstrate an association with the pathogenesis of obstructive sleep apnea syndrome (OSAS), the most common organic disorder related to the symptom of excessive daytime somnolence. In cross-sectional studies, the minimum prevalence of OSAS among adult men is about 1% with the highest, 8.5%, among men aged 40-65 years. For example, carbon disulfide exposure in workers can increase the frequency of depression and other measures of affective disturbance. Repeated exposures have been suspected to contribute to chronic encephalopathy. The dye solvent and cleaning agent, methyl-n-butyl ketone can cause a peripheral nervous system neuropathy with the degeneration of nerve fibers. Abuse of organic solvents, such as those in glues, can lead to permanent neurological effects. Glue-sniffing and inhalation of other organic solvents and aerosols points out that acute exposures to many liquid or gaseous substances can produce "pleasurable" intoxication or narcosis of the sensorium and contribute to recurrent substance abuse.

Pesticides

Under this classification, one finds insecticides, fungicides, rodenticides, and herbicides. Active ingredients are combined with inert substances to make numerous pesticide formulations. While these formulations are the most commonly encountered class of neurotoxic substances, obvious signs of poisoning are most common in a subset of persons with chronic heavy exposures, namely, farm workers. Other occupations and pastimes at risk include amateur and professional gardeners, landscape personnel, and pest-control personnel. Signs and symptoms of pesticide toxicity include tremors, weakness, ataxia, visual disturbances, and short-term memory loss. The organophosphorous insecticides act by covalent modification of the serine esterase protein, neuropathy target esterase, and the inhibition of acetylcholinesterase. These compounds include parathion and currently account for a large percentage of the registered pesticides in the United States. The are also be used as additives in plastics and petroleum products such as, the gasoline additive, tri-o-cresylphosphate (TOCP). With certain forms of these compounds, not only can acute symptoms of poisoning occur, but delayed neurotoxicity also can be seen with irreversible loss of motor function and associated neuropathology. With TOCP consumption, a peripheral neuropathy can develop in the absence of cholinergic poisoning. This was demonstrated by the severe central peripheral distal axonopathy occurring in humans with the outbreak following consumption of the Ginger Jake drink contaminated with TOCP and in the Morocco outbreak from olive oil contaminated with TOCP. The herbicides and cotton defoliants O-ethyl O-4-nitrophenyl phenylphosphonothionate (EPN) and O-(4-bromo-2,5-dichlorophenyl) O-methyl phenylphosphonothionate (leptophos) have also been reported to produce peripheral neuropathies.

Polyhalogenated Biphenyls (PHBs)

The PHBs are found in all environments and populations throughout the world. They are stored primarily in adipose tissue and bioaccumulate in mammals due to long half-lives of approximately 12 years. The PHBs are transplacentally transferred and in the adult female are preferentially stored and excreted in the breast milk lipids raising concern for post-natal exposure. Human milk is usually 1-4% fat and is in equilibrium with the other fat stores of the body. Highly lipid soluble chemicals like PCBs, DDT, dieldrin have been shown to appear in the fat of a high percentage of human milk samples. The amounts are generally in the milligram per kilogram of fat range, thus in parts per billion of whole milk. While no disease has been associated with exposure at these levels, our knowledge and ability to detect subtle neurological and clinical alterations limits our ability to discount this route of exposure as safe for the infant. However, a metabolite of DDT, DDE, has been demonstrated to produce hyporeflexia in human infants. Intrauterine growth retardation has been reported in the Yu-cheng and Yusho populations in China and the PCB Michigan fish eater population. The ingestion of polychlorinated biphenyl-contaminated rice oil during pregnancy and lactation resulted in low-birth-weight infants, growth retardation, abnormal skin pigmentation, bone and tooth defects, and functional neurological deficits, including decreased scores on neurological tests and decreased motor tone and reflexes. Despite these observations, a dose-response relationship was difficult to identify, as often the dose levels within the breast milk were within range of the normal levels in the general population.

Toxins

Mycotoxins, or fungal toxins, occur in field crops and grains used for livestock and can incorporate into grain based products for human consumption. As many of these fungal toxins produce ergot alkaloids they can have adverse effects on the nervous and vascular system if consumed in large quantities. Ergotism or St. Vitus Dance was described during Middle Ages when ergot-contaminated wheat was consumed. Constriction of peripheral and central blood vessels occurred with painful, encephalopathic and potentially fatal consequences. In modern times, rare clinical cases occur when ergot-like substances for control of migraines or headaches are consumed. As another example of interplay between toxic exposure and clinical response of exposed person (illustrated above in abnormal behavioral decisions and responses of solvent-exposed individuals), persons with subclinical ergotism and damage to deep gray and white matter (small penetrator arteriolar vessels are most at risk) can then lose common-sense and continue exposure and behavior without insight or assessment of their decline. Ergot alkaloids are also produced by morning glories and thus, can be incorporated inadvertently into various crops during harvest. Numerous other classes of marine toxins can be produced in dinoflagellates and accumulate in fish or shellfish, such as mussels containing domoic acid, that are excitotoxins to the nervous system. Such events are often first discovered during large-scale outbreaks which occurred in the Prince Edward Island poisoning with domoic-acid contaminated mussels. As for ciguatera-poisoning with reef-fish (groupers, barracuda), the neurotoxin is not poisonous to the host or concentrating organism, is concentrated in the food chain and is not detectable to the human palate. The relatively large amounts of some toxins can permit relatively rapid discovery of the substances and mechanisms, such as occurred for domoic acid with rough isolation of the proposed toxin, exposure of a rodent model, and then characterization of substance and pathobiology. Other biotoxins and marine toxins may be more potent and therefore less easy to characterize or study. Many of the proposed potent marine toxins are small molecular weight polyethers or other unusual compounds. Pfisteria toxin(s) can be produced by certain members of Pfisteria family and are apparently used to stun or predate on other organisms. There is some evidence that emergence of this marine toxin was related to algal blooms secondary to human contamination of the estuarine environment by both agricultural and metropolitan contribution of inorganic phosphate and other contaminants. The first apparent clinical case of neurotoxicity was in a scientist studying and characterizing the organisms during experimental laboratory fish kills. The significance in the natural environment remains controversial, although several laboratory workers have presumptive neurological syndromes after exposure.

CLASSIFICATION BY TARGET ORGAN

Myelin Disruption

Myelin is another target site within the nervous system for chemical-induced damage. Isoniazid targets the peripheral nervous system in man with peripheral neuritis as the major effect. Triethyltin is highly toxic to oligodendroglia and causes severe damage to white matter throughout the CNS. Hexachlorophene (2,2'-methylenebis(3,4,6-trichlorophenol) is an antimicrobial agent that produces similar morphological changes to that seen with triethyltin. These findings were clearly manifested in infants or in patients with extensive epidermal damage due to burns or ichthyosis bathed with antibacterial soaps and antiseptic solutions containing the substance. In some infants, application of 3 to 6% HCP to normal skin in the diaper area resulted in excoriation which facilitated the absorption of HCP leading to fatal intoxication. While neuropathological changes in the white matter of the brain can be seen in adults with epidermal damage, the brains of low birth weight, premature infants of less than 1440 gm birth weight are highly susceptible to the effects of HCP at less than 1400 gram body weight.

Lead exposure in adults causes a primary disruption to myelin of the peripheral nervous system. In contrast, childhood exposure to lead results in neurotoxic damage to the central nervous system resulting in cognitive defects with a possible involvement of central myelin. Poisoning with thallium salts causes damage to myelin sheaths similar to that seen with lead exposure yet, damage also occurs to ventral horn cells and dorsal root ganglion cells. Neurological signs include ataxia and painful paresthesias, weakness, and diminished sensation. Tellurium exposure to manufacturing workers results in mild neurological effects. However, neurotoxicity of tellurium in animals is characterized by a peripheral neuropathy due to segmental demyelination occurring from damage to Schwann cells.

Peripheral Axonopathies (Dying-back Axonopathies)

While Schwann cells and the myelin sheath comprise one general target site of chemicals inducing peripheral neuropathies, the neuron and its axon represent the other component of the peripheral nerve targeted in neurotoxic injuries. Usually, an extended period of time is required for the clinical manifestation of such damage. However, nerve damage can be evident within a time period as short as one week. An example is severe arsenic poisoning with ascending paralysis occurring within the first week. Chronic ethyl alcohol intake can result in axonal degeneration of motor neurons within the distal nerve segments. Acrylamide is a vinyl monomer that can be dermally absorbed, inhaled, or ingested. Chronic exposure to the monomer form of acrylamide results in a primary sensory neuropathy in the limbs accompanied by weakness and ataxia. Experimental animal models have shown that both the sensory and motor fibers are damaged by p-bromophenylacetylurea exposure. Carbon disulfide exposure causes psychosis, tremor, and polyneuritis in man. The accumulation of neurofilaments within the axon has been correlated with the neuropathy possibly due to a cross-linking of filaments. n-hexane and methyl n-butyl ketone are metabolized to 2,5-

hexanedione and the primary neurotoxic effect is the formation of large swellings in motor and sensory fiber axons and in the long fiber pathways in the spinal cord caused by cross-linking of neurofilaments. Experimental animal studies have shown damage to axons in the spinal cord and brainstem with 3,3'-iminodipropionitrile (IDPN) exposure. While the "waltzing syndrome" is likely due to degeneration of the vestibular sensory hair cells, massive neurofilament-filled swellings also occur in the proximal axons of peripheral nerves. With the organophosphorus compounds, delayed neuropathy has been shown for triorthocresyl phosphate (TOCP), cresyldiphenyl phosphate, o-isopropylphenyldiphenyl phosphate, diisopropyl fluorophosphates, leptofos, and mipafox.

Neuronopathies

In classifications of toxic chemicals by their primary target site, the neuronal cell body can also be the site of the initial events. Neuronopathies can be more easily identified and measured in the peripheral nervous system but similar changes can likely be found in comparable sets of vulnerable central nervous system neurons. For example, organomercuricals produce one of their earliest pathological changes in the sensory cell bodies of the dorsal root ganglia with the dispersion of the rough endoplasmic reticulum. Specific populations of neurons within the central nervous system are also affected, e.g., granule cell neurons within the cerebellum. While mercury causes a variety of aberrations in cellular function it is likely that numerous mechanisms come into play for the selective neuronal loss. It has also been proposed that all structural components of the neuron are concurrently affected rather than and one distinct primary target sites. Doxorubicin is an anthracycline antibiotic derivative that is known to damage dorsal root ganglion and autonomic ganglion neurons in the peripheral nervous system. Studies with acrylamide suggest that the earliest morphological event is within the neuronal cell body; however, this is often considered to be as a retrograde reaction to the axonal changes. A similar pattern of morphological change is observed in the large neurons of the cerebellum. In this case, whether they correlate with axonal change is more difficult to determine morphologically.

Based upon their anti-mitotic actions targeted to microtubules, vincristine and vinblastine are used therapeutically for the treatment of leukemia. Colchicine is also a microtubule inhibitor and is used primarily in the treatment of gout. However, the use of each of these agents can result in polyneuropathy with sensory and motor nerve disruption along with muscle atrophy. Filamentous aggregates are also found in the neurons of the brainstem, spinal cord, and dorsal root ganglia. Paclitaxel (Taxol) also targets microtubules; however, rather than disrupting microtubules there is a stabilization of the polymerization form. This type of disruption also results in sensorimotor or autonomic axonopathy in patients receiving large chemotherapeutic doses.

Neuromuscular Junction

A number of pharmacological agents have been designed to target the neuromuscular junction. However, certain biologically derived toxic substances can also have effects on the terminals of motor neurons. Botulinum toxin (clostridium botulinum) has an LD 50 of approximately 0.00001 mg/kg and interferes with the release of acetylcholine from the axon terminal; the muscle responds as if denervated and the neuron responds as if the axon had been severed. Tetrodotoxin has an LD50 of 0.10 mg/kg and death results from skeletal muscle paralysis with effects on the sensory nerves due to a blockage of the axonal sodium channel. The actions of saxitoxin actions are similar to tetrodotoxin. Batrachotoxin depolarizes nerve membrane by increasing the permeability of the resting membrane to sodium ions. Chemical substances can also disrupt the function of the neuromuscular junction. DDT or dichlorodiphenyltrichloroethane and allethrin cause repeated depolarization of the presynaptic nerve terminal. Lead causes a presynaptic block and depresses the end-plate potential.

Central Nervous System

Similar functional distinctions can be made for the central nervous system with white matter or gray matter as the initial demarcating principle for targets of neurotoxic substances. Quite often, specific anatomical regions and even distinct neuronal populations or subsets show differential vulnerabilities to different compounds as well as regional effects upon the different glia populations of the brain. Specifically in the CNS, 1-methyl-4-phenyl-1,2,3,6-tetrahydropyridine (MPTP) produces marked progressive degeneration of dopaminergic neurons in the substantia nigra [35]. MPTP is converted to MPP+ by a two-electron oxidation step primarily in the astrocyte. Upon release from the astrocyte, MPP+ enters dopaminergic neurons via the dopamine uptake system where it acts as a general mitochondrial toxin blocking respiration at complex I which results in cell death. Repeated MPTP ingestion results in the recruitment of the pigmented noradrenergic neurons of the locus ceruleus to the injury.

Anoxic Brain Injury

The brain is critically dependent upon an uninterrupted supply of oxygen. For this reason, any disruption in blood flow, oxygen capacity, or related processes can lead to brain damage. This effect is clearly evident in stroke patients. There are a number of toxic disease processes that produce neuropathological changes consistent with loss of oxygen supply. For example, while recovery from a barbiturate coma usually occurs without a neurological deficit, the anoxia produced from a coma lasting a number of days can result in laminar cortical cell death, specific neuronal death in the hippocampus CA1 region, and loss of cerebellar Purkinje cells. Carbon monoxide combines with hemoglobin to form carboxyhemoglobin and with cytochrome oxidase in mitochondria, resulting in both direct and indirect cellular level anoxia or disturbance of oxidative metabolism. With prolonged CO or H2S exposure, ischemic anoxic damage occurs within the basal ganglia and deep thalamic neurons. Leukencephalopathy can occur as a consequence of carbon monoxide coma. A delayed neurotoxicity or relapse can occur, as well as, a delayed neurotoxicity following repeated exposures. CO neurotoxicity is characterized by a sudden onset of behavioral confusion, disorientation, ataxia, rigidity, incoordination, and muscle weakness. These symptoms can progress over a few weeks leading to death. The neuropathological changes following CO delayed toxicity are classified as severe status spongiosus with demyelination. Short fibers connecting the cortical columns and axons are often spared. With cyanide poisoning, inhibition of cytochrome oxidase, cytotoxic anoxia, and hypotension are thought to be the mediators of damage in the cortical gray matter, hippocampus CA1 pyramidal cell region, corpus striatum, substantia nigra, and corpus callosum. Azide poisoning shows a strong resemblance to the outcomes of cyanide poisoning. The level of detail needed to discuss focal toxicities within the brain is not within the scope of the current chapter but is available in the published literature.

NEUROMETABOLIC DISORDERS

X-linked Adrenoleukodystrophy

X-linked adrenoleukodystrophy (ALD) is a progressive disorder with multiple phenotypic variations often characterized by Addison disease, childhood dementia, and progressive neurologic deterioration. The most common clinical phenotypes are: 1) childhood cerebral ALD with presentation between 4 and 8 years of age with rapidly progressive and diffuse demyelination usually leading to death within less than 5 years and; 2) adrenomyeloneuropathy beginning after 10 years of age and is characterized as a slowly progressive distal axonopathy. A report of differing clinical characteristics in monozygotic twins suggests a role for environmental factors influencing the phenotypic expression of this disease. Primary treatment has been related to symptomatic targets; however, other treatments include stabilization of the neurological progression by hematopoietic stem cell transplantation (HSCT). This treatment is indicated only in the childhood form of the disease after early onset of symptoms, primarily in boys with early cerebral ALD as confirmed by neurological examination, MRI-visible lesions, and neuropsychological testing. It is counter-indicated once significant neurologic deterioration becomes evident. Adrenal insufficiency occurs in about 10% of patients with elevated plasma VLCFA levels. VLCFAs accumulate primarily in the brain and adrenal cortex thus, producing the neuropathological changes. The source of VLCFA is dietary, as well as, endogenous production by microsomes. Thus, both to limit intake and to decrease synthesis of C26:0 fatty acids, a dietary therapy is being developed in addition to the steroid treatment. Magnetic resonance spectroscopy (MRS) examinations over time, following increases in choline/creatine and myo-inositol/creatine ratios and decreases in N-acetyl aspartate/creatine can be used as indicators of disease progression.

Lysosomal Diseases

The lysosome is an organelle containing acid hydrolases necessary for the digestion of cellular constituents. This intracellular digestive process is blocked by the defective catabolic activity of any of these related enzymes. This then results in the accumulation of undigested substrate within the lysosome forming inclusion bodies. In the CNS there are autosomal recessive disorders and the two X-linked recessive disorders, Fabry's disease and Hunter's disease. The lysosomal storage diseases are classified by the type of undigested substrate accumulated. As to be expected, they show multiple clinical phenotypes. The sphingolipidoses are a group of lysosomal storage diseases caused by a deficit in the lysosomal enzymes necessary for the degradation of sphingolipids. This results in a blockage and excessive storage of the substrate. Included in this group of diseases are gangliosidoses (defective degradation of gangliosides in the CNS and are comprised of the GM1 and GM2 groups), Niemann-Pick disease types A and B (acid sphingomyelinase deficient), Gaucher's disease (glucosylceramide), Farber's disease (ceramidase deficiency), Fabry's disease (deficient alpha-galactosidas A), metachromatic leukodystrophy (deficiency in arylsulfatase A), multiple sulfatase deficiency, Krabbe's disease (deficent galactosylceramidase), and sphingolipid activator protein deficiency (deficit in small non-enzymatic glycoprotein cofactors). The mucopolysaccharidoses are diseases due to inborn errors of lysosomal glycosaminoglycan metabolism. Dermatan sulfate is accumulated in Hurler, Hunter, Maroteaux-Lamy and Sly syndromes with severe skeletal abnormalities. Heparan sulfate accumulates in Hurler, Hunter, and Sanfilippo syndromes and is associated with mental retardation. Gangliosides are the major neuronal storage materials in mucopolysaccharidoses.

Organic Acid Disorders

Organic acid disorders include glutaryl-CoA dehydrogenase deficiency (glutaric aciduria type l), mevalonic aciduria, L-2-hydroxyglutaric aciduria, and N-acetylaspartic aciduria (Canavan disease) can result in CNS neurodegeneration. Clinical findings include ataxia, myoclonus, extrapyramidal symptoms, metabolic stroke, and megalencephaly. For Canavan's disease, a rare genetic disorder that results in white matter changes, gene therapy is now available and magnetic resonance spectroscopy (MRS) imaging can monitor the treatment related reduction of increased signal of N-acetyl aspartate in the brain associated with progressive disease. Creatine deficiency is the result of a rare genetic disorder and, on MRS, presents a brain spectrum with the striking absence of a creatine peak. Therapy with oral creatine can replenish this peak and provide a partial reversal of neurological deficit when the gene deletion directly affects creatine biosynthesis. However, oral replacement is ineffective when the gene deletion targets the creatine-transporter.

Molecular defects have been identified in disorders of peroxisome biogenesis and function. Of 11 complementation groups, groups 1-10 are associated with the phenotypes of Zellweger syndrome, neonatal adrenoleukodystrophy, or infantile Refsum disease, and Group 11 is associated with the rhizomelic chondrodysplasia punctata phenotype (RCDP). Refsum disease is a genetic peroxisomal disorder with a defect in the enzyme phytanoyl-coenzyme A hydroxylase and impaired capacity to degrade phytanic acid. The clinical signs include retinitis pigmentosa, hearing deficits, progressive neuropathy, ataxia and ichthyosis. For infantile Refsum's disease, presentation usually occurs after the neonatal period. For the adult disease, presentation usually occurs prior to 20 years of age with symptoms of decreased visual acuity, peripheral neuropathy, cerebellar ataxia, sensorineural hearing deficits, cardiac disorders, and ichthyosis. Two forms exist, Batten disease or the infantile NCL-1 form of the disease caused by a defect in the lysosomal enzyme, palmitoyl-protein thioesterase and a second NCL-2 associated with a lysosomal peptidase defect. These diseases are pathologically characterized by an accumulation of autofluorescent ceroid lipofuscin materials in the cytoplasm of neurons and other cell types. In Niemann-Pick C (NPC) disease there is an excessive accumulation of unesterified cholesterol resulting in progressive ataxia, eye movement disturbances, dementia and hepatosplenomegaly. Smith-Lemli-Opitz syndrome is due to a defect in cholesterol biosynthesis with symptoms of facial abnormalities, syndactyly, cataracts, cryptorchidism, and mental retardation. Leukoencephalopathy is a chronic-progressive disorder characterized by episodes of deterioration and loss of white matter in the cerebral hemispheres and pontine tegmentum. Cerebral folate deficiency is characterized by low cerebrospinal fluid levels of the active folate metabolite, 5-methyltetrahydrofolate. Clinical symptoms display as sleep disturbances, psychomotor retardation, cerebellar ataxia, spastic paraplegia, and dyskinesia. Autoimmune disorders with antibodies targeting the folic acid receptor may present with cerebral degeneration and can only be reversed with leucovorin.

Mitochondrial Disorders

Mitochondrial dysfunction, mitochondrial DNA function, oxidative phosphorylation, and disorders of fatty acid oxidation can lead to neurological disease often termed mitochondrial encephalomyopathies. Mitochondrial disorders are characterized according to the genomic site of the molecular lesions. Correlation of this classification system with the biochemical abnormalities is not clear-cut. Diagnosis is based initially on the clinical presentation with laboratory confirmatory data. With regards to nervous system involvement, mitochondrial disorders can affect both the central and peripheral nervous systems and can both grey and white matter. Grey matter involvement varies from rarefaction and spongy change accompanying neuronal loss and astrogliosis to a more pronounced ischemic-like neuronal necrosis. White matter changes ranges from spongy myelinopathy to cystic necrosis. Medium chain 3-ketoacyl coenzyme A thiolase deficiency and 3-hydroxy-3-methylglutaryl-coenzyme A synthase deficiency are associated with coma and ketosis in infancy or early childhood. Serine deficiency disorders are inborn errors of metabolism diagnosed by the detection of low concentrations of both serine and glycine in plasma and cerebrospinal fluid. Neurological symptoms include congenital microcephaly, seizures, psychomotor retardation, and polyneuropathy. Leukotriene C4 synthesis occurs in brain tissue and a biological deficiency is characterized by severe muscular hypotonia, psychomotor retardation, microcephaly, and absence of cysteinyl leukotrienes in blood cells.

AGE RELATED DIFFERENTIAL SUSCEPTIBILITY

While much of this chapter has focused on adult exposure in which there is a relative homeostatic stability in the nervous system with regards to structure and function the susceptibility of the developing child and the aging nervous system with limited reserve capacity is of major concern within the area of neurotoxicology.

The Developing Nervous System

Neurobehavioral assessment of chemical exposure and toxicity is complicated by having to measure functional impairment within a changing and maturing organ system of emergence of capabilities, maturation of these skills, and the later gradual decline in capabilities [34]. Neurobehavioral functions emerge according to a rather well defined developmental schedule of phases from the neonatal stage through to adolescence, continuing into adulthood. Temporal and spatial organization of nervous system development is a precise and complex process with the basic framework laid down in a stepwise fashion in which each step is dependent upon the proper completion of the previous one. Thus, a relatively minor disturbance resulting in a perturbation of developmental interactions between selected cell groups for a limited time period may result in a major deleterious outcome. An insult occurring at any of these vulnerable time windows may be reflected only in the impairment of the functions emerging at that time; however, they may also ultimately appear as delays in the appearance of new functions. Neurotoxic effects may be either due to the specific target site susceptible to damage at that time window or rather dependent upon the complicated interdependent and progressive nature of development and functional maturation of the nervous system. Major differences in sensitivity to insult are related to changing cell structure and morphology, the degree of development of the blood-brain barrier, the degree of myelination of tracts, the degree of arborization of dendritic and axonal processes, and the extent of development of the cerebral vascular bed and capillary endothelium. In any case, there are critical periods of development occurring during gestation and post-natally in which the nervous system may be differentially sensitive to chemical exposure. While an insult occurring at the time of a developmental event may result in a given malformation, it may also result in an alteration in the developmental program thus affecting any or all events that are subsequent to the insult. In addition, early episodes of exposure may result in damage that will not be manifest behaviorally for several months or years thus forming the framework for the hypothesis of a fetal basis of adult disease.

The developing human can be adversely affected by body burdens of environmental chemicals that do not affect the adult. The toxic effects seen in the developing human can be more varied, more severe, and more debilitating than those seen in the adult. In the human infant, several studies have provided evidence supporting the concept of a critical period from birth to about 2 years of age during which the nervous system is most vulnerable to malnutrition and not responsive to nutritional therapy. Children can have exposure to chemicals by direct contact or indirectly through the parents. This exposure can occur during gestation, lactation, and even from the clothing and body surfaces of parents exposed in an occupational setting. The fetus can be exposed to both nutrients and xenobiotics via the maternal circulation. The main route of exposure is trans-placental. The placenta is metabolically active toward xenobiotics and the nature of the compounds reaching the fetal circulation may depend on multiple placental biotransformation reactions. Chemical exposure *in utero* can be manifested as altered newborn growth and abnormal functional development. It needs to be noted that exposure to a chemical during pregnancy may not necessarily result in any observable alteration within a short time period after birth but may instead take years before the toxicity becomes overt. Some of the best examples available are those related to hormonal changes during development; the use of diethylstilbestrol during pregnancy to prevent miscarriage. It was found that female fetuses exposed to diethylstilbestrol are at an increased risk for adenocarcinoma of the vagina. This type of malignancy is not discovered until after puberty [39]. Additional clinical findings indicate that male offspring were not spared from the effects of the drug and also demonstrate later abnormalities of the reproductive system [52].

It is well established that many drugs are excreted into the breast milk and are bioavailable to the infant. In much the same fashion, environmental chemicals can be transferred to the nursing infant. Exposure during lactation has also been known to result in persistent toxicity. While breast-feeding offers many positive features to the newborn, it also can serve as a source of infant exposure to drugs and chemicals even thought the amount of drug present in maternal milk is only a small fraction of the adult intake. Environmental exposure via breast-feeding may be chronic and consequently more toxic, unlike therapeutic agents that can be voluntarily terminated. The amount of drug that is available for transfer to milk is dependent on certain maternal factors such as dosage, frequency, and route of administration and all other relevant pharmacokinetic principles of absorption, distribution, metabolism and excretion. In addition to the pharmacokinetic factors of the mother, the flow and pH of blood to the breast, the composition and pH of milk, and the rate of milk production and resorption of the drug from milk into the maternal circulation are factors that affect the amount of actual drug delivery to the child. General factors that may influence breast milk concentrations include maternal age, parity, maternal body weight, and fat content of the breast milk. Human milk is a suspension of fat and protein in a carbohydrate-mineral solution. Milk proteins are fully synthesized from substrate delivered from the maternal circulation with the major proteins identified as casein and lactalbumin. Drug excretion into milk may be accomplished by binding to the proteins, lipids, or onto the surface of the milk fat globule.

The physiochemical features of the compound are the most important factors influencing drug excretion into the breast milk. Such things as degree of ionization, molecular weight, lipid solubility, and protein binding capacity, will affect the ability of the chemical to traverse the mammary gland epithelium. The mechanisms that determine the concentration of a drug in breast milk are similar to those existing elsewhere within the organism. Drugs traverse membranes primarily by passive diffusion and the concentration achieved is dependent upon the concentration gradient and on the intrinsic lipid solubility of the drug and its degree of ionization, as well as binding to protein and other cellular constituents. In general, drugs and chemicals bind more readily to plasma proteins than to milk proteins; thus, the dosage to the infant is dependent upon the degree of plasma protein binding of the drug. For drugs that bind to milk proteins, accumulation and delayed response must be considered. For example, exposure via breast milk to the fungicide, hexachlorobenzene, resulted in persistent manifestations of hexachlorobenzene-induced porphyria cutanea tarda including, hyperpigmentation and severe scarring of the face and hands continuing for 25 years [25]. The human maternal ingestion of hexachlorobenzene via treated wheat in Turkey resulted in chemical accumulation of the fungicide in breast milk and infants showing symptoms of a disease called pembe yara and the condition drug-induced porphyria cutanea tarda. The evaluation of potential risk of toxicity on the child must consider all exposure routes both during pregnancy and after birth.

Assessment of Neurotoxicity in Children

The actual assessment of children for neurobehavioral outcomes brings with it an additional set of problems related to attention span and dependence on parental and environmental supports. With age comes increasing complexity of functional capabilities and any test evaluation must be appropriate for the age at which it is to be administered. If there is a delay in maturation, unless the test is repeatedly administered, the outcome may be erroneously viewed as a deficit rather than a delay. While this may not compromise the identification of an exposure related effect it would indeed have a significant impact on the parent and on any course of action outlined by the physician. Childhood assessment brings with it additional covariates that need to be considered in their influence on human cognitive development. Two of the most prominent covariates are parental intelligence and quality of the home environment. These variables have been clearly demonstrated to impact associations between lead exposure and intelligence [7]. Although progress has been made in the development of assessment techniques in children, more research is needed to establish normative data for use in different populations and cultures. Other confounders due to socioeconomic status such as, nutritional status, might further change threshold limits to be very context specific.

Heightened Vulnerability in the Aged

In addition to adverse developmental responses in the young, there is concern that neurotoxic exposure may be a contributory factor in neurodegenerative processes related to aging. The aged population may represent a susceptible group due to various metabolic and reserve capacity changes occurring during the aging process. Neurotoxic exposure and effects occurring during development, adolescence, or young adult period may be latent and not manifest in clinical signs until much later in life. While this potential area of latent developmental effects is appreciated it has not received the research attention necessary to determine particulars of relevance to human health and disease. For example, animal and human data support very early and measurable effects of presence of the susceptibility gene for AD, apolipoprotein E, in 'adverse' (i.e., Western) dietary conditions, well before the onset of AD neuropathology or clinical presentation.

EVALUATING EVIDENCE FOR NEUROTOXICITY

Epidemiologic Studies

Descriptive case reports have identified neurotoxic agents based upon clinical symptoms displayed by individuals that show a temporal relationship with exposure, plausibility with existing knowledge on the biological effects of the chemical, and consistency with other possible reports. As a next step in exploring causality and exploring potential mechanisms of injury, epidemiological studies have demonstrated that neurotoxicity may be occurring in humans at levels considerably lower than those necessary to produce frank manifestations of neurological illness. Many different study designs are available to examine the relationship between exposure and adverse human health outcome. Specific study designs have been applied to detailed analysis of dose-response relationships and route of exposure in the occupational setting that allows for a more defined description of exposure. Other approaches have focused on the study of larger populations. These populations can be based on analysis of subjects either defined as clinically asymptomatic or with a confirmed diagnosis depending upon the study design. Epidemiologic studies vary widely in terms of study population and sampling, timing and intensity of sampling, study design, outcome measures, the study question, and the inferences possible from the data generated. For example, documentation of actual overt poisonings and associated clinical symptoms and therapeutic intervention are often some of the initial questions. In the occupational setting, initial studies were designed to identify and to detect adverse outcomes in the worker population in order to set exposure limits (threshold limit values) and to establish surveillance and monitoring programs for health effects. The results of such occupational studies and the follow-up data with long term human exposure have formed the basis for many of the recent study designs examining possible exposure related health effects in the general population. These attempts then led to studies to detect and to characterize potentially more subtle neurotoxic effects from specific environmental exposures such as metals, pesticides, or solvents.

In the examples of childhood lead and mercury exposure, epidemiological studies have been conducted from which the resultant data have then been used in risk assessment analysis to set threshold standards for human exposure. More recently, analysis of high dose effects, experimental animal studies, and neuropathological similarities between experimental animal models and fatal human exposure, have formed a basis for epidemiologic studies of associations between exposure and classical neurodegenerative diseases in the population. Epidemiological studies have been undertaken to determine if chemical exposure increases not only the risk for immediate adverse human health outcomes but also increased long-term risk for specific human diseases such as, Parkinson's Disease (PD), Alzheimer's Disease (AD), Multiple Sclerosis (MS), and amyotrophic lateral sclerosis (ALS; Lou Gehrig Disease).

Issues of Outcome Measurement in Population Assessments

In a clinical neurology setting, establishing a differential diagnosis requires sampling through history and physical examination of a comprehensive array of cognitive, affective, sensorimotor, and neurobehavioral functions. Traditional full neuropsychological assessment, electrophysiological studies, and neuroimaging can be applied as in general clinical neurology. However, more specific test methods have been developed or modified for the study of targeted exposed populations. These are usually shortened test batteries of clinical neuropsychological tests that focus on those effects most commonly seen in CNS toxic disorders. The World Health Organization (WHO) proposed the standardization of test methods in the field of human neurotoxicity with a Neurobehavioral Core Test Battery (NCTB) that can be used on an international scale. This test battery is relatively inexpensive and easy to administer, has a large control database [1] and consists of tests that have most consistently identified neurotoxic effects in occupational settings [2]. A number of computerized test batteries have also been developed [27,31]. However, they do not allow for detection of different aspects of fine and gross motor abilities, language use, constructional disorders, and stereoagnosis. A common characteristic of psychological test instruments is their sensitivity to many subject variables that need to be considered in both the design and interpretation of neurotoxicity studies [51]. Different tests and test methods show sensitivity to a variety of factors and have led to the publication of criteria for the evaluation of human neurobehavioral studies of neurotoxicity by the European Community (1996).

Psychiatric inventory and symptom questionnaires often are included in individual assessment of neurotoxicity and are used in epidemiologic studies of exposed populations based upon changes in affect in severe neurotoxic exposures to mercury, arsenic, manganese, and carbon disulfide [10,37,54] and solvent exposure or painter's syndrome. A number of questionnaires and rating scales have been developed to obtain similar information in a standardized manner. However, these instruments each rely on self-report and thus are subject to reporting bias. Within the occupational setting these measures include the Q16 questionnaire [29,50], the Neurotoxic Symptom Checklist-60 (NSC-60) [30], and an analogue rating scale developed in Germany [33]. More recently, the symptom questionnaire EUROQUEST (EQ) has been developed with the goal of simplifying the evaluation of health effects associated with long-term solvent exposure.

Due to the demonstrated involvement of sensory and motor components in a neurotoxicologic response to chemical exposure, these endpoints have been included in neurological examination and symptom questionnaires. Quantitative measures have been developed to assess visual, somatosensory and olfactory function, and to assess gait, postural balance, and tremor for use in health surveillance in field studies of exposed workers. Most of these test measures were developed following exposure incidents and are now intended to be used as indications of involvement in exposure. For example, following the initial reports of color vision loss in n-hexane-exposed workers [42] color arrangement tests have been incorporated into the monitoring of workers exposed to a number of different solvents including carbon disulfide [45], styrene [24], toluene [56], and mixed organic solvents [45,30,13]. Similar tests have been developed to assess changes in the somatosensory system, olfactory perception, and postural stability of exposed workers.

Based upon solvent and acrylamide exposure, electrophysiological evaluations of the peripheral nerve have been included in assessing neurotoxicity in exposed workers. Nerve conduction velocity can be obtained with surface electrodes and thus are suitable for use in epidemiological studies [3,47,46]. Electrophysiological techniques can be used to evaluate CNS dysfunction and include electroencephalography (EEG) and different types of evoked potentials (EPs) such as, somatosensory, visual, and brainstem auditory system. The use of EEGs for differential diagnosis and in assessing exposed populations is limited [38,48,46] while sensory evoked potential testing has been used in a number of studies to examine the effects of solvents, metals, and pesticides in exposed populations. In most studies, abnormalities of evoked potentials usually dominate over abnormalities of cortical encephalographic rhythms probably reflecting the greater involvement of subcortical white matter involvement. The usual caveat applies to the assessment of these tests for individuals in that there is a large and normal population variance of event times in evoked potentials and the relevant pre- and post-exposure data for a given individual are rarely available.

Even considering differences in study measures, if well designed and conducted, each is capable of contributing to the risk assessment for particular exposures. Significant progress has been made in the last decade to develop and validate methods for detecting neurotoxicity in humans as well as an increased understanding of the factors that impact on the validity and reliability of such measures. Standardized neuropsychological tests, computer-assisted test batteries, neurophysiologic and biochemical tests, and imaging techniques have been refined for use in both clinical and research applications. While standardized and validated methods are available for outcome measures, the existing literature continues to be limited due to the variability of the chosen testing methods used thus, making it still quite difficult to compare results across studies.

ISSUES OF EXPOSURE ASSESSMENT

Any study, in any form, is only as good as the tools employed. A great deal of effort has been spent over the years to develop and validate test methods and batteries to assess human nervous system function. Whether standardized tests for intelligence, cognitive function, motor or sensory function, outcome measures can be accurately assessed. Similarly, advancements have been made in exposure assessment tools. Yet, often there is scarce data on individual or population exposure. Rarely do we find the best of both exposure assessment and outcome assessments in any one study.

In order to interpret findings of exposure studies, it is necessary to understand the inherent advantages and limitations in methods and approaches both concerning subject selection and outcome measurements and the inferences that can be made with regard to a causal relationship between exposure to a particular agent and an adverse health outcome. Since the determination of exposure-response/effect is a prerequisite for inferring a causal relationship between a chemical and a particular health effect, reliable and valid methods to accurately determine exposure are of critical importance. Exposure determination becomes of immensely greater difficulty when the population under study is not one identified at high exposure or one identified with acute clinical symptoms but rather is identified a population at low level exposures and one with sub-acute clinical outcomes with long latency. With continued environmental mediation and identification of potential neurotoxic agents, it is precisely this numerous population of low exposures and long latency that is most critical. The cost of expensive and debilitating developmental abnormalities or neurodegenerative illnesses must be balanced appropriately against the costs to society of remediation of identified causes. Reviews of the different types of epidemiological studies in neurotoxicology are available [36,17,44] as well as guidelines for conducting environmental epidemiology studies [55].

In epidemiological studies, the majority of approaches to assess exposure are subjective in nature (5). While the personal interview is the most commonly used method in general epidemiology, with increased sample sizes the time involved in this part of the study is significantly increased and has quite often been replaced by self-administered questionnaire. When exposure is related to occupation, often employment data is collected and used to classify individuals on the basis of their degree of exposure. A related approach has been the job exposure matrix (JEM) method, working from a database regarding the degree and type of exposure associated with different job titles in different industries. This information is then used to help estimate the degree of specific exposures [e.g., 41]. Errors arise due to the fact that exposures may vary widely between workers with the same job title in the same industry or even plant. As with any other measure dependent upon self-report, accuracy comes into question. However, when compared to actual biological monitoring, data obtained from detailed job-specific questionnaires agreed better with analytical measures of internal exposure than did data obtained with the more traditional questionnaire methods [53].

Individual exposure assessments can be conducted by personal monitors, monitoring of an occupational or residential setting, or actual testing of air, water, or foods consumed. Yet, determining the actual body burden of a chemical or peak level of a compound at the target organ, in this case the nervous system, under specific conditions of age and general health status is not possible. Instead, measurements in biological tissues such as, blood or urine are typically used to provide an estimate of exposure. Alternatively, chemical levels can be determined from other biological samples such as fat tissue or breast milk for highly lipid-soluble compounds like PCBs, teeth for lead, hair for mercury. In all cases, the measurement of internal levels of the parent compound or its metabolites in exposed individuals provides a more direct assessment of exposure and dose than measurements of external levels for exposure.

The minimal standard in occupational studies includes intensity of exposure reported by the study participants as provided by checklists, questionnaires, and other self-report measurement tools coupled with actual exposure measurements in the workplace. Yet, misclassification of exposure can challenge the validity of epidemiologic studies [e.g., 22]. Quite often, the exposure assessment for neuroepidemiological studies is limited to self-report, questionnaires, diaries, employment histories, and, in very detailed studies, possible environmental exposure levels in air, water, food, or soil, which may, or may not, be an accurate reflection of the individual exposure. The quality of exposure data reported in epidemiologic neurotoxicology studies has been criticized for the quality of exposure data reported [51]. Without direct evidence of dose-effect relationships, it is impossible to infer a causal link between exposure and effect. Thus, increasing sample size may actually heighten the concern for generalizability of results if the increased size and sampling burden leads to more abbreviated methods of collecting exposure data with increase in sample size. In addition, hypotheses are often developed for specific single agent exposures such as, particular pesticides, mercury, lead, and PCBs. Human exposure is comprised not of individual chemicals in isolation but rather as mixtures. Thus, when one examines exposure related effects on health outcome all components of the exposure need to be considered. For example, while PCB body burdens have been measured in a majority of epidemiological studies, PCBs may simply reflect exposure to other fish-born contaminants such as methylmercury, p,p'lDDE, and pesticides given the multi-contaminant nature of exposure. In solvent studies, the role of adjuvant compounds such as methyl-ethyl ketone is rarely considered, or the multiple ingredients in mixed solvent exposures. Moreover, exposure outcomes may be also affected by nutritional status, intercurrent illness such as chronic pulmonary disease or acute illness such as viral syndromes with diminished host responses such as glutathione status.

INTERPRETATION OF TOXICOLOGICAL DATA

Interpretation of data from neurotoxicity studies can be considered judgments of the adversity and neurotoxicity of an exposure. Adversity depends in part on psychological perceptions, framing of the questions, social values, and the population affected. Neuropathologic effects are the easiest to interpret as adverse outcomes although the actual functional consequences may be unclear. Neurophysiologic and neurochemical effects are generally considered to be adverse outcomes but their adversity depends more on their empirical and presumptive functional consequences. Changes in behavior such as organic affective syndrome (one of the most common clinical outcomes of many neurotoxic occupational exposures) are considered adverse and are thought to represent the integration of a number of processes within the nervous system yet, their representation of actual neurotoxicity are the most difficult to assess and to determine and usually depend on a variety of constructs and other measures. Several decision points could be used in a stepwise fashion to guide interpretation of data from toxicology studies. First, it should be considered whether a putative chemical-induced neurobiological change has not occurred merely on the basis of chance and normal variance and that while the change is an unwanted or unintended effect it is unrelated to the exposure. The possibility that a chemical-induced change in the structure or function of the nervous system is due to confounding non-specific alterations must then be considered. Well-designed studies incorporate a range of exposures and exposure conditions to permit the assessment of the nervous system at all relevant dose levels. Chemical-induced neurobiological alterations that appear to be nervous system specific can then be evaluated for persistence, relationship to a known neurotoxic mechanism, covariance with a known neurotoxic effect or possibility as a significant health hazard.

It is possible that changes in the structure and function of the nervous system might be produced by indirect or secondary mechanisms. For example, in animal studies or in defined human populations, dietary restriction and loss of body weight or lack of body weight gain during development as a result of chemical-induced systemic toxicity could result in changes in neurobehavioral endpoints indirectly and could lead to the erroneous labeling of a chemical as a primary neurotoxicant. The presence of systemic toxicity might complicate the interpretations of functional changes in toxicological studies but does not preclude their use in defining neurotoxicity. Functional changes in the nervous system that are dose or exposure-dependent, related to neuroanatomical or other functional measures and that occur in the absence of observed systemic toxicity or any clear pathway for the systemic toxicity to produce CNS damage are indicative of neurotoxicity of the particular substance. It is likely, however, that many substances (for example, volatile organic compounds or arsenic) have both direct systemic and direct nervous system toxicity. Likewise, substances that perturb liver function or intestinal absorption may produce CNS damage in a somewhat indirect fashion. For example, severed thiamine or vitamin E deficiencies are known to produce CNS damage.

Another issue, relative to direct versus indirect sites of toxicity, is related to irritation due to direct contact of chemicals on sense organs or respiratory epithelia. An example would be significant functional changes, including behavioral changes, following contact with an irritating agent such as ammonia. Such an effect would be adverse; however, would it be neurotoxic? Toxicity may depend upon the dose level and duration of exposure and the potential damage to the sensory organ involved. Obviously, ototoxicity, vestibular toxicity, retinal damage can be become very defined examples of neurotoxicity to sensory organs, epithelia or primary sensory pathways. With pulmonary and respiratory epithelial damage, there may be production of upper airway allergic responses or inflammation conducive to obstructive sleep apnea syndromes.

Another component in the evaluation of data is to determine if the effect is irreversible or reversible. If the effect is reversible the data should be examined in the context of four criteria 1) environmentally relevant exposure conditions, 2) known mechanisms for effect; 3) biomarker of effect, and 4) evidence of latent effect. These criteria would then serve to direct consideration toward a neurotoxic effect. For example solvents or anesthetics may produce functional changes in the nervous system by acting at specific cellular level; however, if the effects are short lived are they neurotoxic? Again, this may depend upon the dose level, the number of exposures and the length of exposure. Progressive damage may occur with repeated exposures. If a chemical produces reversible effects by a known neurotoxicological mechanism of action it could be considered potentially neurotoxic. For example cholinesterase inhibiting insecticides produce signs of neurotoxicity by inhibiting the breakdown of the neurotransmitter acetylcholine (Ach). This neurotoxicologic effect increases Ach at the synaptic cleft, stimulates cholinergic receptors, and leads to overactivity of cholinergic pathways. Overstimulation of the parasympathetic nervous system leads to a syndrome of neurotoxicity characterized by muscular weakness, fasciculations, respiratory difficulties, increased bronchial secretions, salivation and lacrimation, sweating, increased gastrointestinal tone, and peristalsis. Although these effects are transient in nature, they represent a neurotoxic event. Other examples of reversible effects caused by a known neurotoxicologic mechanism of action are DDT-induced tremor and behavioral hyperexcitability and domoic acid-induced seizures. Reversible effects should be evaluated cautiously due to the ability of the nervous system to compensate for damage. However, there is a limited capacity for such repair. Apparent reversibility of effects may mask residual effects or loss of reserve that persist beyond a recovery period or become evident only after a challenge such as stress, increased workload, pharmacological manipulation, disease, or aging. Subsequent exposure to the same or similar chemical could result in additional cell death and diminish the function and ability to compensate. This becomes important when one starts to examine the cumulative effects of either multiple exposures or exposures to different chemicals acting via a common mode of action. Perhaps the best example of this phenomenon is destruction of dopaminergic neurons by small exposures to 1-methyl-4-phenyl-1,2,3,6-tetrahydrophrindine (MPTP) in humans where transient Parkinsonian syndromes occurred, but then disappeared with re-establishment of homeostasis of the striatal-nigral system. However, these exposures result in actual dopaminergic cell loss in a system that can take up to 80-95% cell loss without obvious clinical consequence. Extensive injury to white matter and CNS myelin or members of diffuse projections such as, hypothalamus-cortex or ascending reticular activating system (dopaminergic, serotoninergic, noradrenergic, and groups CH5-9 of cholinergic systems) with non-specific or even no clinical signs and symptoms. Such injuries to non-primary motor/sensory/cerebellar systems may result in depression, sleep disorders, organic affective disorders, fatigue, neurasthenia, difficulties in attention and learning. These disturbances that can be the result of neurotoxic exposures, nevertheless, can overlap or be mimicked by the normal and variable degree of psychological distress in persons who know that they may have been exposed to toxic substances.

Assumptions for Interpretation of Experimental Animal Data

Given the inability to conduct experimental studies on humans, an assessment of what is know about the neurotoxicity of a chemical requires the inclusion of data from animal studies. Several assumptions are required in categorizing of a neurotoxic effect and in the extrapolation from experimental animals to humans. First, it is assumed that if a chemical produces an effect in animal studies, it is likely that humans will also be affected. A good database should be available in support of this assumption. Second, it is assumed that qualitative and quantitative differences may exist between animals and humans due to species differences in the organization and maturation of the nervous system. No obvious animal model exists for effects seen in humans on verbal behavior or speech, due to the lack of an analogous response that can be measured in animals. As an example, there are essentially no gabaergic interneurons in thalamic gray matter in rodents (with the exception of thalamic reticular nucleus) in striking contrast to primates and humans. Third, it has been assumed that a neurotoxicant must exceed a threshold level to induce toxicity. The threshold level is based on the known capacity of the nervous system to compensate for and/or repair a certain amount of damage at the cellular, tissue, or organ level. However, more recent data suggests that the concept of a threshold dose may not be appropriate for neurotoxicants especially with regards to populations at higher risk. For example, the Parkinsonian-like syndrome of progressive supranuclear palsy (PSP) is probably environmentally mediated in some persons by prolonged exposures to agricultural chemicals and pesticides, but susceptibility may further depend on the presence of common polymorphisms in the non-coding promoter region of the tau gene coding neurofilament protein. Likewise, many of the relatively common polymorphisms in apolipoprotein E, hemochromatosis gene, mitochondrial proteins (glutathione S-transferase) may confer susceptibility for onset of neurodegenerative disorders such as AD and PD. Many of these genes are environmentally modulated or are genes that respond to acute phase reaction. Since the carrier populations for these polymorphisms range from 10-30% or more, it is hard to imagine that formulating a *single* threshold limit unless it is the limit for the most susceptible individuals makes sense. This brings up the further question of protecting persons with greater genetic susceptibility (e.g, polymorphisms or mutations with 1% or less prevalence) or at risk populations such as the very young or old.

In addition, pharmacokinetic, pharmacogenomic, metabolic differences, or other factors can play a critical role in the manifestation of neurotoxicity and comparison to the human may require the identification of the most relevant experimental animal model.

CONSIDERATIONS FOR INDIVIDUAL CLINICAL ASSESSMENT

The clinical assessment of potential neurotoxicity in an individual patient known or reported to have environmental exposure is carefully conducted to establish a differential diagnosis not only to identify a potential neurotoxic insult(s) but also to rule out other possible etiologies and to identify other contributing factors or illnesses. In the normal clinical setting, the reverse is also true in that a differential diagnosis is conducted to identify a disease but should also consider and rule out other possible etiologies like an exposure-related insult. The neurological examination has been well defined and characterized for the use in neurotoxicology over the years [12]. Depending on the presentation of signs and symptoms and the nature of the exposure, more specialized evaluations may be indicated including an assessment of exposure [18]. Possible confounding, contributing or independent factors need to be carefully sought such as pre-existing or current substance use/abuse, sleep disorders (commonly underdiagnosed), pre-existing or current neurological or psychiatric illness, effects of prescribed medications or OTC preparations (particularly herbals, supplements) are the major considerations.

For human neurotoxic disease, causation criteria have been proposed [46]. These include 1) independent from subject confirmation of exposure to the suspected agent 2) severity and temporal onset of the clinical symptoms are commensurate with level and duration of exposure 3) the condition is self-limiting and either clinical improvement or lack of progression follows with cessation of exposure 4) the clinical features are consistent with patterns presented by previous cases; 5) support of adverse effects by experimental models. There are examples of progression after cessation of exposure (item 3) so the criteria must be weighed against clinical or experimental experience with the particular exposure. An example would be CO or H2S exposures with delayed neurodegeneration, some mixed volatile organic solvent injuries with significant white matter damage, and the reasonable concept that damage to CNS may accelerate the eventual onset of neurodegenerative disorders (e.g., low doses of MPTP with eventual clinical Parkinsonism). In a given case with progression after cessation of injury, a long list of possibilities emerges including modeling, factitious behavior or malingering for secondary gain, primary effects of the initial exposure with progression of injury, or increased susceptibility to 'normal' aging, normal environmental factors such as diet, or other common-place environmental exposures. A relatively unexplored mechanism is immunological mediation of damage through either cell and/or humoral mediated mechanisms after priming or exposure of CNS-related antigens during the initial exposure or the injury/repair process.

The single most useful information and often the most difficult to obtain is an accurate history of exposure. Aside from the standard modifying factors, if the exposure level and duration is sufficient to produce structural damage in the nervous system, any single chemical will likely produce similar dysfunctions in most individuals. Quite often, similar patterns of neuropathological changes will also occur in experimental animal models. Like all clinical evaluations, a detailed medical history and standard clinical neurological examination are conducted. Secondary informants, although not always independent and impartial, are vital if available. However, the history includes environment related questions such as occupation, activities prior to onset of clinical symptoms, possible exposures e.g., source of heating within a home, hobbies, dietary practices or other questions that may identify exposure to known neurotoxicants including metals, pesticides, solvents, gaseous agents. Secondary sources such as previous employment histories or evaluations, school records and performance, previous medical examinations can be invaluable sources for evaluating change after exposure and for evaluating possible influence of previous illnesses or exposures. Information obtained from such expanded histories can serve as a guide for examination of specific endpoints. In cases where there is an indication of cognitive or affective changes, neuropsychological testing is often carried out and can help to rule out other etiologies [21,46]. While the choice of tests vary, they are aimed at assessing a wide range of functions.

The ability to make appropriate diagnoses and outline a therapeutic course of action for the patient is the strongest argument to be made for the practicing physician to maintain an informed knowledge base with regards to neurological outcomes as the result of environmental, chemical, or drug exposure. Many potential environmentally mediated diagnoses (such as agricultural chemical exposure in cases of PSP, chronic CO exposure with Parkinsonism) are overlooked for lack of directed history taking and inventory of all present and past exposures. For neurotoxicology, the challenge for the clinician can come in many forms; managing the care of a patient following acute exposure to a neurotoxicant including prompt and urgent referral where indicated (e.g., consideration for hyperbaric treatment for CO or H2S exposures); providing medical care and advice to patients employed in occupations in which there is exposure to neurotoxic agents; determining the etiology of a disease process; addressing the concerns of patients with regards to exposure related issues; addressing questions with regards to safety of therapeutics such as vaccines; and addressing questions with regards to expensive and/or invasive and/or potentially harmful interventions for removal of chemicals from the body e.g., chelation therapy, dental amalgam removal, use of multiple nutritional supplements. These and other issues support the need for evidence-based- medicine and for this approach to be inclusive of all data available to make an informed clinical decision. The process is similar to the steps required to conduct an adequate risk assessment using a weight of evidence approach.

Even with the multi-dimensional nature of the nervous system, common manifestations of effects often occur across chemical classes. This is particularly true for substances that damage myelin or interfere/injure the deep white matter. The best clinical model for considering this possible presentation is multiple sclerosis or demyelinating disease where clinical presentation can be multiple, mimic primary psychiatric illness, and be state-dependent (variation with fatigue, illness, body temperature). Thus, it is often difficult to identify a specific culprit unless there is a confirmed exposure assessment and exposure limited to a specific chemical. In addition, the exposure needs to be at a dose and for sufficient time to produce an adverse effect. Epidemiological studies offer little practical help in setting practice guidelines to assist physicians in clinical decision-making; however, they can offer information on the types of clinical outcome measures to incorporate into their clinical assessment and a framework in which to compare similar measures. Population based studies really do not address the concerns of the individual with regards to neurotoxicant exposure. More recent studies are examining the interactions between the genetic background of the individual and exposure to environmental agents in the attempt to identify polymorphisms and susceptible populations. As this field of research advances, data from human studies may provide relevant information in identifying genetic risk factors that can be used in setting practice guidelines as they apply to a particular susceptible population.

From a clinical standpoint, persons presenting with new or existing neurological or psychiatric illness should be considered as possible examples of past and/or present environmental exposures. Depending on the anatomical localization of the illness (peripheral nerve, muscle, white matter), minimally an appropriate list of possible exposures that could produce or exacerbate the syndrome should be considered. Conversely, the person presenting with putative exposure should be carefully considered for non-environmental causes of the same syndrome. In both cases, a careful clinical approach and transaction with the actual patient is of great benefit. A single diagnosis is rare, and multiple diagnoses common for presence of independent or contributing conditions. Where multiple anatomical systems are involved (CNS and peripheral nerve), it may be of benefit to list out separate diagnoses and to pursue their normal work-up, rather than to assume or fall into one unitary, neurotoxic causation. Where exposure is suspected or clinical condition is significant, the early use of ancillary measurements for staging is crucial: neuropsychological testing (with MMPI and neuropsychiatric scales for depression, psychosis, etc), neuroimaging, and electrophysiological studies. Overnight polysomnography is generally underutilized. Use of other specialists or studies for concurrent illness or dysfunction of other organ systems (liver, kidney) is essential. A major omission in many cases is collection of relevant tissue samples at the time of exposure in seriously injured cases. These might include cerebrospinal fluid, blood, fat biopsy, and peripheral nerve or muscle biopsy; however, the normal clinical venue is ill equipped for cataloging and storing such samples for eventual analysis. Another major omission in many cases with significant persistent illness or deficit is consistent monitoring or follow-up with ancillary testing. Informal practice guidelines or guidelines adapted from other illnesses (e.g., multiple sclerosis) can be employed (e.g., monitoring of neuropsychological status every 18-24 months, neuroimaging status every year if significant abnormality was present). This monitoring can be very useful for cases with unremitting symptoms or progression. At all times, such testing and monitoring must be indexed to the actual clinical status of the person with appropriate education and guidance of the person and their relatives or support system. A commonly unrecognized or under-appreciated clinical occurrence is primary and/or secondary psychiatric disorder from the initial injury and/or the reaction to the injury with the possibility of adverse long-term outcomes (episodic mood disorder, unemployability, depression, divorce, suicide, etc). Likewise, the exposure may directly or indirectly contribute to onset of other significant secondary conditions or illness such as substance abuse, dietary indiscretion, obesity, coronary artery disease, etc. The goal of the physician faced with caring for persons with actual or potential neurotoxic exposures should be optimal clinical care and management, and provision of sufficient information at the onset and during follow-up to allow the eventual analysis of such cases by other clinicians or researchers for integration with the data bases from large-scale epidemiological studies.

CONCLUSION

Evaluation of environmentally induced or metabolically determined neurotoxicity, the identification of risk factors for human health, and the impact of therapeutic intervention require an understanding not only of the biological processes underlying the perturbation but also details of exposure and impact of confounders. While numerous epidemiology studies are available on a limited number of specific diseases or environmental exposures, the focus of these studies limit the ability to make a more broad generalization. In addition, the requirement of non-invasive procedures for the majority of existing epidemiology studies results in an inability to collect data on more clinically relevant endpoints.

REFERENCES

[1]   Anger, W.K., Cassito, M.G., Liang, Y-X., et al. (1993). Comparison of performance from three continents on the WHO-recommended Neurobehavioral Core Test Battery (NCTB). *Environmental Research 62*, 125-147.

[2]   Anger, W., Liang, Y-X., Nell, V., et al. (2000). Lessons learned – 15 years of the SHO-NCTB: A review. *Neurotoxicology 21*, 837-846.

[3]   Araki, S., Yokoyama, K., Murata, K. (1997). Neurophysiological methods in occupational and environmental health: methodology and recent findings. *Environmental Research 73*, 42-51.

[4]   Armon, C. (2003). An evidence-based medicine approach to the evaluation of the role of exogenous risk factors in sporadic amyotrophic lateral sclerosis. *Neuroepidemiology 22*, 217-228.

[5]   Armstrong, B.K., White, E., Saracci, R. (eds.) (1992). *Principles of exposure measurement in epidemiology*. New York, NY: Oxford University Press.

[6]   Baghurst, P.A., McMichael, A.J., Wigg, N. (1992). Environmental exposure to lead and children's intelligence at the age of seven years. The Port Pirie Cohort Study. *New England Journal of Medicine 327*, 1279-1284.

[7] Bellinger, D.C. (1995). Interpreting the literature on lead and child development: The negelected role of the "experimental system." *Neurotoxicology and Teratology 17*, 201-212.

[8] Bellinger, D., Sloman, J., Leviton, A., et al. (1991). Low level lead exposure and children's cognitive function in the pre-school years. *Pediatrics 87*, 219-227.

[9] Bleecker, M.L., Lindgren, K.N., Ford, D.P. (1997). Differential contribution of current and cumulative indices of lead dose to neuropsychological performance by age. *Neurology 48*, 639-645.

[10] Bolla, K.L., & Roca, R.P. (1994). Neuropsychiatric sequelae of occupational exposure to neurotoxins. In Bleeker, M. (ed.) *Occupational Neurology and Clinical Neutotoxicology*. Baltimore, MD: Williams and Wilkins, 148-158.

[11] Boothby, J.A., DeJesus, P.V., Rowland, L.P. (1974). Reversible forms of motor neuron disease. Lead "neuritis". *Archives of Neurology 31*, 18-23.

[12] Bradley,W.G., Daroff, R.B., Feniehel, G.M., Marsden, C.D. (eds.) (1996). *Neurology in clinical practice*. Boston, MA: Butterworth-Heinemann.

[13] Broadwell, D.K. Darcey, D.J. Hudnell, H.K. et al. (1995). Work-site clinical and neurobehavioral assessment of solvent-exposed microelectronics workers. *American Journal of Industrial Medicine 27*, 677-698.

[14] Buchthal, F. & Behse, F. (1979). Electrophysiology and nerve biopsy in men exposed to lead. *British Journal of Industrial Medicine 36*, 135 -147.

[15] Buckley, N.A. (1998). Poisoning and epidemiology: 'toxicoepidemiology'. *Clinical Experimental Pharmacology Physiology 25*, 195-203.

[16] Catton, M.J. Harrison, M.J.G. Fullerton, P.M. et al. (1970). Subclinical neuropathy in lead workers. *British Medical Journal 2*, 80-82.

[17] Checkoway, H., & Cullen, M.R. (1998). Epidemiological methods in occupational neurotoxicology. In Costa, L.G. & Manzo, L. (eds.) *Occupational Neurotoxicology* Boca Raton, Florida: CRC Press.

[18] Chern, C.M., Proctor, S.P., Feldman, R.G. (1995). Exposure assessment in clinical neurotoxicology. Exvironmental monitoring and biologic markers. In Chang, L.W. & Slikker, W. (eds.). *Neurotoxicology: Approaches and methods*. New York, NY: Academic Press. 695-709.

[19] Cory-Schlecta, D.A., & Schaumburg, H.H. (2000). Lead, Inorganic In Spencer, P.S. & Schaumburg H.H. (eds). *Experimental and Clinical Neurotoxicology* (2nd edn.). New York, NY: Oxford University Press. 708-725.

[20] Dietrich, K.N., Succop, P.A., Berger, O.G., et al. (1993). Lead exposure and the central auditory processing abilities and cognitive development of urban children: The Cincinnati lead study cohort at 5 years of age. *Neurotoxicology and Teratology 14*, 51-56.

[21] Feldman, R.G. (1999). *Occupational and environmental neurotoxicology*. Philadelphia, PA: Lippincott-Raven.

[22] Flegal, K.M., Keyl, P.M., Nieto, F.J. (1991). Differential misclassification arising from nondifferential errors in exposure measurement. *American Journal of Epidemiology 134*, 1233-1244.

[23] Ford, D.P., Schwartz, B.S., Rothman, N. (1994). Assessment of exposure and dose in neurotoxicology: Clinical and epidemiologic applications. In Bleeker ML & Hansen JA (eds.), *Occupational Neurology and Clinical Neurotoxicology*. Baltimore, Maryland: Williams and Wilkins, 23-42.

[24] Gobba, F. Galassi, C. Imbiani, M. et al. (1991) Acquired dyschromatopsia among stryrene-exposed workers. *Journal of Occupational Medicine 33*, 761-765.

[25] Gocmen, A. Peters, H.A. Cripps D.J. et al. (1989). Hexachlorobenzene episode in Turkey. *Biomedical Environmental Science 2*, 36-43.

[26] Guzelian, P.S. Victoroff, M.S., Haimes, N.C. et al. (2005). Evidence-based toxicology: a comprehensive framework for causation. *Human Experimental Toxicology 24*, 161-201.

[27] Hartman, D.E. (ed.) (1995). *Neuropsychological toxicology: Identification and assessment of human neurotoxic syndromes*. (2nd edn.) New York, NY: Plenum Press.

[28] Hill, A.B. (1965). The environment and disease: Association or causation? *Proceedings of the Royal Society of Medicine 58*, 295-300.

[29] Hogstedt, C. Andersson, K. Hane, M. (1984). A questionnaire approach to themonitoring of early disturbances in central nervous function. In Aito, A, Rihimaki, V. & Vainio, H. (eds.) *The biological monitoring of exposure to industrial chemicals*. Washington DC: Hemispheres. 275-287.

[30] Hooisma, J. Hanninen, H. Emmen, H.H. et al. (1994). Symptoms indicative of the effects of organic solvent exposure in Dutch painters. *Neurotoxicology and Teratology 16*, 613-622.

[31] Iregren, A. 1998 computer- assisted testing. In: Costa LG and Manzo L ed. *Occupational neurotoxicology*. Boca Raton, Florida, CRC Press pp 213-233.

[32] Johnson M.V., & Goldstein G.W. (1998). Selective vulnerability of the developing brain to lead. *Current Opinions in Neurology 11*, 689-693.

[33] Kieswetter, E., Stetmann, B., Seeber, A. (1997). Standardization of a questionnaire for neurotoxic symptoms. *Environ Res 73*: 73-80.

[34] Landrigan, P.J., Weiss, B., Goldman, L.R. (2000). The developing brain and the environment. *Environmental Health Perspectives 108*, 373-595.

[35] Langston, J.W., Forno, L.S., Tetrud J., et al. (1999). Evidence of active nerve cell degeneration in the substantia nigra of humans years after 1-methyl-4-phenyl-1,2,3,6-tetrahydropyridine exposure. *Annuals of Neurology 46*, 598-605.

[36] Longstreth, W.T., Koepsell, T.D., Van Belle, G. (1994). Neuroepidemiology as it applies to occupational neurology. In Bleeker, M.L. & Hansen, A.A. (eds.) *Occupational neurology and clinical neurotoxicology*. Baltimore, Maryland: Williams and Wilkins. 1-21.

[37] Mikkelsen, S. (1995). Solvent encephalopathy: disability pension studies and other case studies. In Chang, L.W. & Dyer, R.S. (eds.) *Handbook of Neurotoxicology*. New York, NY: Marcel Dekker, 323-338.

[38] Nuwer, M. (1997). Assessment of digital EEG, quantitative EEG, and EEG brain mapping: Report of the American Academy of Neurology and the American Clinical Neurophysiology Society. *Neurology 49*, 277-292.

[39] Palmer, J.R., Anderson, D., Helmrich, S.P., et al. (2000). Risk factors for diethylstilbestrol-associated clear cell adenocarcinoma. *Obstetrics and Gynecology 95*, 814-820.

[40] Pirkle, J.L., Brody, D.J., Gunter, E.W., et al. (1994). The decline in blood lead levels in the United States. The National Health and Nutrition Examination Surveys (NHANES). *Journal of the American Medical Association 272*, 284-291.

[41] Plato, N., & Steineck, G. (1993). Methodology and utility of a job-exposure matrix. *American Journal of Industrial Medicine 23*, 491-502.

[42] Raitta, C., Seppalainen, A.M., Huuskonen, M.S. (1978). n-Hexane maculopathy in industrial workers. *Albrecht Von Graefes Archives Klin Experimental Ophthalmology. 209*, 99-110.

[43] Ris, M.D., Dietrich, K.N., Succop, P.A., et al. (2004). Early exposure to lead and neuropsychological outcome in adolescence. *Journal of International Neuropsychology Society 10*, 261-270.

[44] Rothman, K.J., & Greenland, S. (eds.) (1998). *Modern Epidemiology.* (2nd edn.). New York, NY: Lippincott Williams and Wilkins.

[45] Ruijten, M.W.M.M., Salle, H.J.A., Verberk, M.M. (1990). Special nerve functions and color discrimination in workers with long-term low level exposure to xylene and mixed organic solvents in shipyard spray painters. *Neurotoxicology 15*, 613-620.

[46] Schaumburg, H.H. (2000). Human Neurotoxic Disease In Spencer, P.S. & Schaumburg, H.H. (eds.). *Experimental and Clinical Neurotoxicology* (2nd edn.). New York, NY: Oxford University Press. 55-82.

[47] Seppalainen, A.M. (1988). Neurophysiological approaches to the detection of early neurotoxicity in humans. *CRC Critical Reviews in Toxicology 18*, 245-298.

[48] Seppalainen, A.M. (1998). Electrophysiological approaches to occupational neurotoxicology. In Costa, L.G. & Manxo, L. (eds.) *Occupational Neurotoxicology.* Boca Raton, Florida: CRC Press. 185-197.

[49] Seppalainen, A.M., Tola, S., Hernberg, S., et al. (1975). Subclinical neuropathy at "safe" levels of lead exposure. *Archives of Environmental Health 30*, 180-183.

[50] Smargiassi, A., Bergamaschi, E., Mutti, A., et al. (1998). Predictive validity of the Q16 questionnaire: A comparison between reported symptoms and neurobehavioral tests. *Neurotoxicology 19*, 703-708.

[51] Stephens, R., & Barker, P. (1998). Role of human neurobehavioral tests in regulatory activity on chemicals. *Occupational and Environmental Medicine 55*, 210-214.

[52] Strohsnitter, W.C., Noller, K.L., Hoover, R.N. (2001). Cancer risk in men exposed in utero to diethylstilbestrol. *Journal of the National Cancer Institute 93*, 545-551.

[53] Tielemans, E., Heederik, D., Burdorf, A., et al. (1999). Assessment of occupational exposures in a general population: Comparisons of different methods. *Occupational Environmental Medicine 56*, 145-151.

[54] White, R.F., & Proctor, S.P. (1995). Clinico-neuropsychological assessment methods in behavioural neurotoxicology. In Chang, L.W. & Slikker, W. (eds.). *Neurotoxicology: Approaches and methods.* New York, NY: Academic Press 711-726.

[55] WHO (2000). Guideline document – Evaluation and use of epidemiological evidence for environmental health risk assessment. Copenhagen, *World Health Organization Regional Office for Europe.*

[56] Zavalic, M., Mandic, Z., Bogadi-Sare, A., et al. (1998). Quantitative assessment of color vision impairment in workers exposed to toluene. *American Journal of Industrial Medicine 33*, 297-304.

RECOMMENDED FURTHER READING

1. Bellinger DC. What is an adverse effect? A possible resolution of clinical and epidemiological perspectives on neurobehavioral toxicity. *Environmental Research* 2004;95:394-405.

2. Berlin CM, LaKind JS, Fenton SE, et al. Conclusions and recommendations of the expert panel: technical workshop on human milk surveillance and biomonitoring for environmental chemicals in the United States. *Journal of Toxicological and Environmental Health* 2005; *A 68*, 1825-1831.

3. Crump KS & Rousseau P. Results from eleven years of neurological health surveillance at a manganese oxide and salt producing plant. *Neurotoxicology* 1999; 20, 273-86.

4. Gerr F & Letz R. Epidemiological case definitions of peripheral neuropathy: experience from two neurotoxicity studies. *Neurotoxicology* 2000; 21, 761-768.

5. Jin CF, Haut M, Ducatman A. Industrial solvents and psychological effects. *Clinical and Occupational Environmental Medicine* 2004; 4, 597-620.

6. Klaassen CD. (Editor). *Casarett and Doull's Toxicology: The basic science of poisons.* 6th Edition, New York, NY: McGraw-Hill, 2001

7. Needham LL, Barr DB, Caudill SP, et al. Concentrations of environmental chemicals associated with neurodevelopmental effects in U.S. population. *Neurotoxicology* 2005; 26, 531-545.

8. Spencer PS, Schaumburg HH, & Ludolph AC. *Experimental and Clinical Neurotoxicology*, 2nd Edition. New York, NY: Oxford University Press, 2000.

In: Handbook of Clinical Neuroepidemiology
Editors: V. L. Feigin and D. A. Bennett, pp. 465-502
ISBN 978-1-60021-511-7
© 2007 Nova Science Publishers, Inc.

Chapter 13

NEUROLOGICAL ASPECTS OF AGING

Jeffrey C.L. Looi[1,2], *Julian N. Trollor*[3,4] *and Perminder S. Sachdev*[3,4]

[1]Research Centre for the Neurosciences of Ageing, Academic Unit of Psychological
Medicine, Australian National University Medical School,
Canberra, Australia;
[2]Laboratory of Neuro Imaging, Department of Neurology, David Geffen School of
Medicine, University of California, Los Angeles, USA;
[3]School of Psychiatry, Faculty of Medicine University of New South Wales, Australia;
[4]Neuropsychiatric Institute, Prince of Wales Hospital, Sydney, Australia.

ABSTRACT

This chapter outlines brain and nervous system aging from structural, molecular, neurochemical and functional viewpoints. There is evidence of generalised cerebral atrophy with aging. At the microstructural level, there are changes in neuronal structure and function. Neuronal loss increases with age, but neuronal plasticity is preserved. Functional imaging of the brain demonstrates age-related declines in cerebral activation. There are age-related declines in neurotransmitter levels, particularly in acetylcholine and dopamine. There is considerable variation in the trajectory of cognitive performance with aging. Whilst aging of the nervous system is inevitable, function is usually preserved. Nonetheless, impact may be assessed via systematic history and examination.

INTRODUCTION

Inside every 75 year old is a 25 year old wondering what the hell happened!

Norwegian Proverb.

The aging brain must be considered as a special case within the domain of aging. While age-related changes in the brain in general parallel those of the body, there are some important exceptions. It is not uncommon to see a very active mind in a frail body. Brain diseases that are usually regarded as concomitants of old age, such as Alzheimer's disease (AD) and Parkinson's disease, are sometimes seen in the young, and most elderly individuals manage to evade them. The popular conceptualization is that of an elderly person as being forgetful, incapable of change, and slow in thinking, but cognitive decline is not a uniform occurrence with aging. Our examination of the aging brain must therefore occur in the context of a neurobiological understanding and sound empirical evidence. In this chapter, we review the major changes that occur in the brain with aging, and how these might impact on the interpretation of clinical data, especially when a clinician attempts to distinguish age-related brain disease from aging-related brain change. There are limitations to the data being reviewed, which are highlighted in table 1.

Table 1: Limitations of the data on healthy brain ageing

- Brain changes in the elderly are a combination of aging-related changes and age-related diseases, and it is difficult to separate the two.
- Cross-sectional comparisons of young and old individuals are compromised by cohort differences (e.g. education, nutrition, cultural factors, socioeconomic status).
- Even in longitudinal studies, arguably the best methodology, survivor effect results in an over-representation of the very healthy.
- Most samples have an ascertainment bias toward health, which is more marked when demands on subjects are high, as in neuroimaging studies.
- Assessments of change are bedevilled by methodological issues and limitations of power.

It should be remembered that the definition of the elderly as being over 65 is an administrative demarcation introduced by Otto Van Bismarck during the 19th Century Prussian Empire. Demographically, there is a distinction between the younger old (60-75) and the older old (75 years plus). This distinction has been variously defined [1], with some studies characterizing a further category of 'oldest old' (age 84 and above). The latter may represent a true cleavage point in survival, with only the young old commonly graduating to the next category. They certainly represent different age cohorts and, by far the largest increase in the developing world in the coming decades will be in the younger old from the 'baby boomer' generation (those born in the 1950s).

BRAIN MORPHOLOGICAL CHANGES WITH AGE

Gross Brain Structure

A clear understanding of structural brain changes associated with normal aging is of importance as it allows the clinician the opportunity to evaluate a CT or MRI scan of a patient's brain in the context of their age. As age is a key risk factor for many neurodegenerative conditions, a fundamental issue for structural studies of normal brain aging is whether to exclude those with or at risk of an age-related neurodegenerative disorder. The study of 'supernormals' (ie those carefully screened for the absence of such disorders) has the advantage of allowing an appreciation of changes distinct to the aging process per se, but the ability of the data to inform regarding age-related changes representative of the general population is diminished. In this section, we will examine both pathological studies and structural neuroimaging studies, to ascertain key elements of structural changes on the brain during the aging process.

Cerebral Atrophy

Postmortem pathological studies [2] reveal small but distinct declines in brain volume in normal subjects with age. This decline is apparent for both cortical and white matter volumes, but may be more pronounced in the latter. Cross-sectional CT and volumetric MRI studies also provided support for a general reduction in brain volume and increase in CSF volume with age [3,4]. Interpretation is complicated by methodological issues such as controlling for cranial size, sociodemographic background and cohort effects. The demonstration of a gradual increase in brain weight in the general population from the mid-19th to the 20th century [5], is thought to be due to improved nutrition and general health status. This may have contributed to an apparent reduction in brain size in some cross-sectional studies of brain aging.

Longitudinal analysis allows each subject to act as his or her control, thus eliminating a number of biases including the cohort effect. Longitudinal analysis of whole brain volume has revealed an increase in lateral ventricular size (central atrophy) and an increase in sulcal volume (cortical atrophy) that are relatively independent of one another [6]. The pathological basis for these atrophic changes is the subject of a lively debate (see below). Significant advances have been made in computational methods which allow the registering of serial brain images from the same individual. This has allowed the longitudinal assessment of brain volumes in a semiautomated fashion, together with estimates of percentage volume loss per year. Although such longitudinal studies are invariably short and as yet span only a few years, results do suggest that rates of generalised atrophy increase progressively with age, even in healthy individuals. This volume loss appears steady in midlife, but is slightly elevated in older individuals [7] at approximately 0.3-0.5% per year. This acceleration of age-related volume loss appears most obvious in the subcortical regions [7].

Changes observed with normal aging appear quantitatively distinct from those observed in early Alzheimer's disease (AD) or its precursor, Mild Cognitive Impairment (MCI). For example, subjects with AD demonstrate an accelerated annual global atrophy rate of 2 - 3% compared with age matched controls [8]. Furthermore, accelerated global atrophy has been identified in individuals at risk of later cognitive decline [8], and may be predictive of transition from normal aging to cognitive decline.

Regional Brain Atrophy

The frontal lobes of normal individuals show preferential atrophy [9] at a rate of about twice that found in the temporal or parietal neocortex [10]. This loss of volume may be greater in the grey matter than white matter [4]. It has been proposed that a decrease in frontal white matter volume does not start until late life but that grey matter volume loss takes place gradually over the full span of adult years [11]. The disproportionate loss of volume in the frontal lobes supports a role for this area in cognitive aging.

Some studies show preferential age-related decline in volume of the dorsolateral [9] and orbitofrontal cortex [9], whilst other studies demonstrate the greatest age-related decreases in the anterior cingulate and dorsolateral prefrontal cortex and preservation of the orbitofrontal cortex [12,13]. Discrepancies between results from the various studies are in part determined by disparate methodology and image analysis. Longitudinal studies suggest that accelerated temporal lobe volume decline is a better predictor of early AD than prefrontal atrophy [14,15]. The dissociation between physiological brain shrinkage in the frontal lobe and accelerated pathological change in the temporal lobe is likely to be a focus of study over the next few years.

The temporal lobes also show definitive evidence of reduction in volume with age [16]. Age-related effects are apparent in the hippocampus [4], with some studies suggesting preferential age-related atrophy in the head of the hippocampus [17]. The age-effects in the hippocampus have been implicated in decline in declarative memory, new learning and spatial navigation skills [18]. Accelerated hippocampal volume loss is a feature of transition from MCI to AD [19] and from normal to cognitive decline [20]. The effect of APOE on the status of hippocampal volume in normal older persons has been variable [21,22]. Volume loss in the entorhinal cortex is an early feature in MCI [23] and AD [14], whereas studies of normal aging show little if any change [24].

Age effects in other regions have received some attention. Structures such as locus coeruleus and substantia nigra show marked sensitivity to age-related volume losses [25]. Age related reductions in volume are apparent in the caudate and putamen nuclei [26] whereas globus pallidus and thalamus appear minimally affected [4]. Studies of the cerebellum suggest a moderate decline in volume [4].

White Matter Changes

Periventricular hyperintensities and deep white matter hyperintensities become increasingly common with advancing age [16]. The presence of deep white matter lesions appears to correlate with presence of cerebrovascular risk factors and MRI infarction [16]. Furthermore, MRI infarction appears to correlate with reduction in brain volume in many brain regions [16]. WMH are most often found in the subcortical frontal regions, periventricular area and internal capsule. Changes in these regions are inversely correlated to performance on tasks of executive function [27,28] and speed of information processing [28]. A summary of brain morphological changes as revealed on neuroimaging is presented in table 2.

Microscopic Brain Structure

Demylineation

Post-mortem analyses indicate a greater loss of white than grey matter [29]. Although correlates of reduction in white matter of volume with age are not entirely clear, it is probably associated with leukoariosis on CT scan, WMHs seen on MRI [30] and histological changes such as myelin pallor, gliosis and axonal loss. Granular degeneration of myelinated axons is observed with increasing frequency from midlife, and is a ubiquitous finding in brains of older individuals [31]. The resultant reduction in axonal conductance may be a correlate of motor and cognitive slowing that is a core component of age-related cognitive decline [32].

Table 2: Neuroimaging of Normal Aging (Looi & Sachdev, 2003)

Atrophy and ventricular enlargement
Both CT and MRI studies demonstrate ventricular enlargement with increasing age. This process begins in the 30s in men and 40s in women.

Gross brain volumes
These decrease with age, with consistent findings of regional decreases in frontal and temporo-parietal volumes.

Cortex
This area is advancing very rapidly but measurement/analytic error remains a problem. Age-related decreases in the hippocampal and parahippocampal volumes have been characterized at 5-10% per decade.

Subcortical & Deep White Matter Regions
White matter hyperintensities in the periventricular regions reach a prevalence of almost 100% in the elderly. Whilst mostly mild, there is evidence of lesion progression. In the subcortical regions, the prevalence is of the order of 20%.

Cerebellum, Midline, Midbrain & Basal Ganglia
There is evidence of volume loss, but the inconsistency of findings and low numbers make firm conclusions difficult.

Senile Plaques

Senile plaques (SPs) are heterogenous structures that contain a variety of components including amyloid, degenerating neuronal components and reactive glial cells [31]. Several types of plaques can be identified depending on the nature of the amyloid and neuronal content within the plaques [31]. Their features may help to distinguish senile plaques of aging from those associated with AD. There are two main competing theories regarding formation of senile plaques. The first theory is that synaptic and axonal injury is primary and followed by deposition of amyloid. The second theory is that deposition of amyloid is the primary event, leading to neural cell death. Cell death is thought to arise from excitotoxic activity mediated by immunological activation of microglia that also inhabit the SP region [33].

Diffuse plaques are those with poorly circumscribed deposits of beta-amyloid with few or no degenerating neural components and few or no reactive glial cells. Neuritic or classical plaques are those containing a more compact core of beta-amyloid and contain prominent degenerative neuronal components, surrounded by reactive microglia and astrocytes. Diffuse plaques can be abundant in older people showing no signs of dementia. Diffuse plaques are thought to be generated by a separate biological process involving cleavage of amyloid precursor protein into shorter amyloid subunits resulting in deposits that are less neurotoxic than dense SPs [34]. When SPs do occur in the normal aged, they tend to accumulate in the association cortices, are moderately dense in the visual and auditory cortex and seem to spare the primary sensory and motor cortices [35]. Dense plaques in which neuronal processes or neurites contain paired helical filaments and neurofibrillary tangles are characterised by tau immunoreactivity and are characteristic of AD.

Neurofibrillary Tangles

Neurofibrillary tangles represent intraneuronal accumulation of fibrous protein comprised of paired helical filaments consisting predominantly of phosphorylated tau, a micro tubule associated protein. Tau promotes stabilisation of cellular microtubles, an ability that decreases when it is phosphorylated. Hyperphosphorylated tau spontaneously self assembles to form PHFs [36]. There is some contrast in the distribution of neurofibrillary tangles in normal aging and in neurodegenerative conditions such as AD. Neurofibrillary tangles are almost always found in the elderly brain but are generally restricted to a select few brain regions [31], including the entorhinal cortex, basal nucleus of Meynert and locus ceruleus. Hippocampal involvement is unpredictable [31]. In non-demented people, NFTs do not progress to inhabit cortical neurons. By contrast, NFTs and abnormally phosphorylated tau are widespread throughout almost all cortical areas in AD individuals [31]. At the cellular level, NFTs are often found in the neural processes (neuropil threads) in AD but almost never in the normal elderly [34].

Cerebrovascular Change

Changes in the cerebral vasculature with age are of importance, as the high energy demands of the brain require delivery of blood, together with energy and nutrients to function normally. Common changes occurring with age include reduced capillary density, increased microvessel deformity, intimal thickening and amyloid angiography in cerebral arteries. Capillary density is reduced in most parts of the brain with age [37]. Microvessel abnormalities increase progressively from midlife [38], and appear to be more prevalent in those with dementia than in age-matched controls [39]. Tortuosity of vessels is related to increased basement membrane thickening in capillaries, which can leave vessels susceptible to endothelial and luminal compression, brain-barrier leakage and endothelial-mitochondrial depletion [40]. Such changes may lead to neuronal dysfunction as a result of disruption of delivery of glucose and oxygen across the capillary wall [41]. Within larger vessels, change begins mostly in the intima. In the fourth decade, about 50% of vessels show intimal thickening and by the eighth decade it is seen in about 80% of all vessels studied [42]. The distribution of these changes is not uniform, with the middle cerebral artery territories being particularly affected and cerebellar and brainstem arteries relatively spared. These changes are often the precursors to arteriosclerosis which increases vascular resistance and decreases perfusion pressure, thereby ultimately compromising neurocognitive function. Amyloid is found in small arteries and arterioles of approximately 30% of cognitively intact individuals, and is a more common finding in those with AD. The distribution is widespread in AD but in healthy aging is most often encountered in the occipital lobes [43].

Does Neuronal Loss Occur with Age?

Reduction in neuronal number was long assumed to underlie age-related reduction in brain volume. Furthermore, the presumption of neuronal loss provided a convenient explanation for cognitive decline with age. Neuronal loss is also pivotal to theories of brain aging that invoke neuronal apoptosis as a central causal mechanism [44]. However, the results of studies examining neuronal loss with aging have varied depending on the region being studied and the technique used to assess neuronal populations. Stereological methods of neuron counting avoid biases inherent in earlier techniques [45,46] and suggest that these assumptions may have been inaccurate [47]. It is probable that much of the apparent neuronal loss previously reported can be attributable to a reduction in neuronal size with age rather than actual reduction of cell number. For a detailed review of stereological studies, the reader is referred to the publication by Long and colleagues [48]. An important finding from this review is the lack of definitive evidence of widespread neuronal loss with age. However, some regions within the hippocampus e.g. regions CA4 and the subiculum appear particularly susceptible to neuronal loss [49] . While the studies of neuronal numbers are numerous, fewer studies have examined the morphology and integrity of the aging neurons. There is suggestion of reduced synaptic density [50] with age, but little is known about age effects on axons [51] and glial cells [52]. The demonstration of neurogenesis in the mouse hippocampus in response to cognitive stimulation in both young [53] and old [54] animals as well as the demonstration of the capacity of hippocampal neurons to replicate in humans [55] has challenged the long-held view that neurogenesis was absent in mature animals.

Changes in Neuronal Plasticity

There are small regionally discrete changes in neuronal dendritic branching and spine density with aging, in contrast to previous observations of profound neuronal loss with aging [56]. In particular, carefully controlled studies have demonstrated that increased dendritic branching occurs in the dentate and parahippocampal gyri of aged individuals compared with younger middle-aged individuals. Animal studies also show that modifications to the neuronal ensemble subserving cognition occur with age, such as the ensemble characteristics of dentate gyrus granule cells may, with loss of long-term potentiation, contribute to failures of spatial representation networks [56]. In summary, most aging related behavioral impairments result from regionally specific changes in cellular connectivity, calcium dysregulation, gene expression and dendritic morphology, thus altering plasticity and the network function of neural ensembles supporting cognition [56].

Brain Function

Studies of Cerebral Blood Flow (CBF) and Metabolism in Healthy Aging

The work of Kety and Schmidt [57] formed the basis for early conclusions that cerebral blood flow and oxygen consumption reduced progressively from puberty. These early studies were, by today's methodological standards, seriously flawed. Subsequent studies using the xenon inhalation technique reinforced the idea of reduction in global CBF with age [58-60], but this was by no means a universal finding [61]. Some of these studies noted an emphasis in reduction in regional CBF (rCBF) in the anterior or middle cerebral artery territories with age [58,60]. A subsequent flurry of single photon emission computed tomography (SPECT) studies using technetium 99m hexamethylpropylamine oxime (^{99m}Tc-HMPAO) has challenged the notion of age-dependent decline in global CBF somewhat, returning a number of negative studies [62,63]. Using SPECT, some regionally specific reduction in rCBF is noted with age particularly in frontal regions CBF [62], with a less dramatic effect being apparent in the temporal regions [62,63].

A modest decline in global CBF has been observed in some positron emission tomography (PET) studies [64,65], but not others [66]. A non-linear decline in CBF which slows in later decades has been proposed [67]. A number of studies document a small global decline in cerebral metabolic rate of oxygen ($CMRO_2$) with age, ranging from 0.3% -0.6% per annum [64,65]. Some studies demonstrate a discrepancy between age effects on global $CMRO_2$ and CBF [68,69], raising the possibility of an uncoupling between CBF and $CMRO_2$ as a factor of age [69]. However, it remains unclear whether under this uncoupling is artefactual [68]. Studies remain divided on whether there are changes in oxygen extraction ratio (OER) with age [64,68], with overall results suggesting that the increase in OER may simply be a reflection of reciprocal decreases in CBF.

A number of studies have attempted to evaluate the effects of aging on global cerebral metabolic rate of glucose (CMRglu), with conflicting results [70-72]. Typically, studies reporting decline in global CMRglu have produced rates of between 0.21% and 0.6% per year [71,73,74], owing to a number of methodological limitations.

The disparate methodology of PET studies which evaluate regional changes in $CMRO_2$ or CMRglu with age provides a challenge to the reviewer. However, regional specificity of age-related changes in $CMRO_2$ and CBF have been examined in a number of studies with the most obvious finding being a discrepancy between white matter regions (largely unaffected by age) and grey matter regions (showing modest reduction with age) [75,76]. Within cortical grey matter there is some regional specificity to decline in CBF and CMRO2, with the most common finding being a bilateral reduction in selected frontal and temporal regions [65,75] although some studies have noted a left-sided [69,77] or right-sided emphasis [76] for particular regions. Consistent with these effects are the regional patterns of reduction in CMRglu observed with age. Findings have included frontal reduction [65,71] in CMRglu, including the anterior cingulate [71,78], reductions in specific anterior, posterior and lateral temporal regions [71] and in parietal cortex [74]. The effect of aging on CMRglu in the deep grey matter nuclei is occasionally reported as a reduction, and in the study by Bentourkia et al [65], this was maximal in the right striatum. The effect of aging on CMRglu in the cerebellum, occipital cortex and white matter appears to be minimal.

Effect of Cerebrovascular Risk Factors

Very early studies [79] failed to demonstrate an effect of hypertension alone on CBF or $CMRO_2$. More recent studies have suggested a significant impact of untreated hypertension on cerebral parameters. Neurologically asymptomatic hypertensives have shown focal and diffuse hypometabolism in a cross-sectional study [80]. The presence of hypertension may specifically affect areas such as the perforating vessels and watershed regions. A significant reduction in CMRglu was demonstrated in regions supplied by basal ganglia perforating arteries and at the middle cerebral/anterior cerebral artery watershed [81] in elderly hypertensives compared with non-hypertensive controls. The short-term beneficial effect of treatment of hypertension on CBF was demonstrated using ^{133}Xe inhalation in a 36-month prospective study [82]. Overall, it appears that the presence of hypertension alone has a modest but appreciable influence on CBF and CMRglu. The impact of the presence of other risk factors for cerebrovascular disease and stroke is less clear. While early studies indicated that CBF and $CMRO_2$ declines in the presence of systemic arteriosclerosis or frank cerebrovascular disease [79], the presence of risk factors per se may not substantially influence CBF [83] or CMRglu [84]. The functional significance of white matter hyperintensities appears related to their volume, with one PET study [85] showing that when WMHs comprise >0.5% of intracranial volume, they are associated with cognitive deficits and reduced frontal CBF. One study suggests that in the neurologically normal subjects there is a stronger relationship between CMRglu and periventricular hyperintensities than for deep white matter or basal ganglia hyperintensities [86].

Activation Studies in Aging

There is a growing literature is examining age-related differences in activation patterns in response to a variety of tasks using fMRI, SPECT and PET. Activation procedures are of interest as they may allow an unmasking of changes not appreciable at rest, may allow a better understanding of the functional effect of the aging process, and provide a means by which the functional integrity of brain networks in older individuals may be assessed. Such an approach may allow a broader appreciation of the effect of the aging process on cognitive, motor and sensory processing. Activation experiments of most relevance to the aging brain can be divided into three key areas: motor and sensory, complex tasks and memory tasks.

Motor and Sensory Stimulation

A number of simple motor and visual stimulation studies have investigated the relationship between the blood oxygen level-dependent (BOLD) haemodynamic response and aging. While some studies have found a relative decrease in amplitude of the haemodynamic response in the visual cortex in the elderly, others have found no difference compared with young subjects. These somewhat contrasting results underscore the complexity the influences on the BOLD signal [87]. In a simple reaction time task which compared to young and elderly subjects, D'Esposito et al [88] found a reduced number of suprathreshold voxels and lower signal-to-noise ratio (SNR) in the elderly, but no significant group differences in the shape of the haemodynamic response. In a BOLD contrast fMRI experiment using photic stimulation [89], mean BOLD signal response to photic stimulation in the visual cortex was significantly reduced in aged compared with young subjects. Huettel et al, [90] used checkerboard stimuli and noted an earlier peak in the haemodynamic response, smaller spatial extent of activation and lower SNR in the elderly compared with subjects. A subsequent study [87] with a simple visual and motor task demonstrated similar peaks in the HDR in elderly and young subjects but a more sustained bold response for the elderly, and a higher percentage of a negative voxels in the elderly group in the visual region. A number of possible explanations underlie changes in the BOLD signal and HDR with age. These include alterations in responsiveness of the cerebral vasculature, local steal phenomena in the aged or differences in unrestrained cognitive processing between elderly and younger groups within the scanner. Pre-existing cerebrovascular disease may also influence the shape and reduced the amplitude of the bold haemodynamic response [91].

More complex visual processing experiments seem to indicate that the elderly brain has a less efficient way of processing sensory information. For example, in facial and spatial matching ^{15}O PET experiments Grady et al [92] demonstrated less distinct functional separation of dorsal (occipitoparietal) versus ventral (occipitotemporal) pathways in aged compared with young subjects. In addition the latter study demonstrated greater and more bilateral activation by older adults in a number of regions, suggesting reduction in processing efficiency and compensatory recruitment of additional networks. Similar results have also been noted in tasks of selective and divided attention in elderly individuals [93]. In an experiment in which subjects discriminated between pairs of vertical sinusoidal gratings of differing spatial frequency [94], additional distinct regions were activated by older individuals in a manner that correlated with task performance, suggesting that additional recruitment of networks was important in maintenance of performance.

Complex Tasks

The effect of age on activation induced by complex cognitive tasks (for example card sorting, progressive matricies, word identification) has been examined in a number of studies. These studies suggest reduction in rCMRO$_2$ activation effects with age [95,96]. In addition, aged subjects activate areas which are normally suppressed in younger individuals. Reduced activation in key areas normally subserving these more complex neuropsychological functions appears linked with decrements on task performance. However, it remains unclear whether enhanced activation in regions normally suppressed by younger individuals represents use of alternative cognitive strategies or inefficiency networks subserving these cognitive tasks [96].

Memory Tasks

The encoding of visual and verbal information has been the subject of a series of studies. The often conflicting results must be understood in the context of major methodological differences between the studies including the wide variety of tasks employed. Although some studies have shown a reduced ability of aged subjects to activate typical networks involved in encoding verbal or visual information [97,98] using ^{15}O PET , other studies [99] have not shown an age effect, or have shown the opposite effect [93]. The variability of these findings raise the possibility that age related differences in rCBF during encoding may vary across tasks rather than as a function of age *per se*. A number of studies have examined the effects of age on functional imaging correlates of retrieval from verbal memory. Although the comparability of results is limited by the widely differing paradigms, there is some support for loss of the normal retrieval asymmetry and activation of more extensive bilateral frontal networks in aged subjects compared with younger controls [98,100].

In summary, there is evidence, from studies employing simple motor and sensory paradigms, of an age-related decline in cerebral activation, an effect that may have its basis in dysfunction in pathways subserving sensory and motor functions. For cognitive processes, a unifying observation is that during many cognitive tasks, elderly subjects activate brain networks that are similar to those activated by young subjects. However, the extent of this activation is reduced in elderly subjects and for encoding and recall tasks, a more bilateral pattern of prefrontal activation has generally been observed. Together with data suggesting subtle reduction in frontal rCBF and CMRglu with age, the enhanced activation in response to cognitive tasks could be viewed simplistically as an attempt to compensate for reduced functionality of this brain region with age.

Brain Neurochemistry and Aging:

Acetylcholine

Foremost in the neurotransmitter theories of aging and neuropsychiatric disease is the cholinergic hypothesis. The relevance of the cholinergic hypothesis to memory function has been demonstrated by a series of animal and human experiments, in which administration of a cholinergic antagonists such as atropine [101] or scopolamine [102] disrupted learning and memory. Furthermore, the observation that young primates given scopolamine performed like old monkeys on cognitive tasks [102] suggested a role for cholinergic dysfunction in age related memory decline. The demonstration that aged rodents had reduced acetylcholine synthesising capacity [103] and reduced responsiveness of their hippocampal pyramidal cells to acetylcholine [104] provided more direct evidence of an age-related alteration of cholinergic neurotransmission. The cholinergic hypothesis of human memory function has played a pivotal role in understanding the early and preferential failure of episodic memory function in AD and has been an important key in the development of treatments for AD. Alterations to cholinergic neurotransmission observed in AD include a decrease in choline acetyltransferase (CAT) [105]; reduced levels of acetyl cholinesterase [106] and reduced capacity for acetylcholine synthesis [107]. Some post-mortem studies are at odds with the above studies. For example, Davis et al found no evidence of reduction in acetylcholinesterase activity or choline acetyltransferase in early AD [108]. In another study [109], choline acetyltransferase activity was actually upregulated in MCI subjects. However, as these enzymes are not rate limiting steps for cholinergic transmission, a negative finding does not necessarily point to intact cholinergic function in these abnormal populations.

Of major importance is whether such alterations in cholinergic neurotransmission play a role in normal aging. With age a number of alterations to cholinergic neurotransmission have been documented including a minimal change in acetylcholine synthesis, minimal alteration to acetylcholinesterase activity, modest reduction in choline acetyltransferase, reduced acetylcholine release following neural stimulation and reduced sensitivity of autoreceptors [110]. PET studies using muscarinic ligands have also indicated an age associated reduction in muscarinic receptors [111]. Overall, the modest alteration in cholinergic neurotransmission observed with age stands in some contrast to the significant reduction in cholinergic integrity seen in AD. In isolation, alterations to cholinergic function do not appear to adequately explain loss of cognitive function in normal aging.

Dopamine

The changes that occur to the dopaminergic system with age have received considerable attention. Reported alterations include the loss of dopaminergic cell bodies in the substantia nigra, decrease in tyrosine hydroxylase activity, decrease in activity of dopamine decarboxylase, reduction in the dopamine transporter and increase in monoamine oxidase B enzyme activity [112]. Studies of dopamine receptor density suggest a possible but inconsistent reduction in D1 receptor density in the striatum and a more consistent reduction in D2 receptor density [112]. Dopaminergic changes have been suggested as the most reliable age-related change in the human brain [113]. PET studies have pointed to significant alteration in dopamine neurotransmission with age, including reduction in density of striatal D_2 receptors [114], decreased striatal D_1 receptors [115] and reductions in striatal dopamine transporters [116]. Reduction in D_2 binding has been shown to correlate with age-related decrements in motor tasks (e.g. finger tapping) and neuropsychological tests of frontal lobe function [117]. Correlations with other neuropsychological domains have been less impressive. A correlation has been demonstrated between the age-related reduction in striatal D_2 binding and reduction of metabolism in frontal and anterior cingulate regions [118].

Other Neurotransmitters

A number of other neurotransmitter abnormalities have been associated with the aging process. A detailed review is beyond the scope of this chapter. However, a number of post-mortem, PET and SPECT studies have indicated reduction in 5-HT_{2A} binding sites in both aging and AD [119]. Serotonin transporter binding is also reduced as a function of age, but these reductions are less dramatic than reduction in dopamine transporter binding in the striatum [120]. Reductions have been noted with age for 5HT_{1A} receptor binding [121]. Age-related changes in serotonergic function have been hypothesised to underlie a variety of psychobiological changes including alterations in mood, sleep and eating [122].

Cognitive Changes with Aging

While there is debate about the specific types of changes in cognitive and intellectual functioning with age, there is agreement that cognitive change is not unitary [123,124]. Three distinctive patterns have been described:

Life-long Decline

Some cognitive abilities, often considered basics to cognitive processing, tend to decline through the life span: information processing speed, working memory, and encoding of information into episodic memory. Cross-sectional studies suggest that information processing speed declines by about 20% at age 40 and by 40-60% at age 80 compared to a 20 year old [125]. Longitudinal data, especially from the influential Seattle Longitudinal Study [126], support this, with small changes between 20% and 60% but an accelerated decline thereafter.

Late-life Decline

Well-practiced tasks and crystallized intelligence (vocabulary, information, similarities, etc.) show little or no decline until very late in life. Short-term or working memory is characterized by small declines through life but an increased decline after age 70 years. Longitudinal studies suggest slight declines in vocabulary after age 60. There is an acceleration of decline in information processing speed and working memory 3-6 years prior to death, presumably related to neuropathology. Cognitive decline is therefore a predictor of mortality even after accounting for demographic and health variables [127].

Life-long Stability

Abilities that appear to be stable into late life are autobiographical memory, semantic memory, emotional processing and automatic memories. It may be the preservation of autobiographical and semantic memories that account for the 'wisdom' generally attributed to old age. It would appear that elderly individuals rely on preserved knowledge and experiences whereas younger people rely on processing ability to perform tasks [124].

Inter- and Intra-Individual Differences

Most studies suggest that individual differences in speed and memory increase with age [123]. Education, absence of Apolipoprotein E ε4, and good health protect against decline. Older individuals also show greater intra-individual variability in test performance, and this may be a marker of subtle neurological impairment [128].

MOLECULAR THEORIES OF BRAIN AGING

Oxidation, Free Radicals and Mitochondrial DNA

The free radical theory of aging proposes that reactive oxygen and nitrogen species cause damage to critical lipid, protein and DNA components of cells. These highly reactive molecules contain an unpaired electron which can react with cellular components, generating further reactive oxygen species, resulting in a cumulative burden of oxidative damage with age which leads to neuronal dysfunction and cell death. The production of reactive oxygen species and is enhanced by the presence of transition metals such as Cu^+ and Fe^{2+}. Free radicals are produced throughout life and there are endogenous antioxidant mechanisms in place which assist in the maintenance of homoeostasis. The role and impact of reactive oxygen and nitrogen species has been debated as under certain circumstances they may themselves exert neuroprotective effects [129]. A number of observations support a role of reactive oxygen and nitrogen species in the aging process and have been summarised in a recent publication [130]. Briefly stated, the evidence includes observations that the rate of reactive oxygen species production of mitochondria in post mitotic tissues is lower in long-lived than short-lived species and that the level of endogenous antioxidants correlate inversely with longevity in vertebrates. Decline in mitochondrial function as a consequence of oxidative damage has been proposed as a key factor in the aging process and neurological disease [131]. Advancing age and reduction in the mitochondrial process of oxidative phosphorylation are thought to promote mutations in the mitochondrial genome [132]. In turn, mutations in mitochondrial DNA may result in depressed cell respiration, enhanced free radical formation and increase susceptibility to apoptosis. This process is thought to result in accelerated generation of reactive oxygen species, promoting further damage [132]. Results from human studies of mitochondrial function in human brain are now being reported and suggest that reduction in mitochondrial respiratory enzyme activity is associated with increasing age [133]. For a detailed review of the impact of oxidative stress and age mitochondrial function, the reader is referred to a recent publication by Harper et al [134]. There is accumulating evidence implicating the role of oxidative stress in the pathology of diseases such as Alzheimer's disease and other age related neuropsychiatric diseases such as Parkinson's disease [130].

A number of compounds with antioxidant activity have demonstrable neuroprotective effects in vitro and in animal models, including vitamins [such as Vitamin E (alpha-tochopherol), Vitamin C (Ascorbic Acid), Beta Carotene], enzymes (e.g. superoxide dismutase, glutathione peroxidase), hormones (e.g. melatonin) and other neuroprotective agents (e.g. monoamine oxidase inhibitors). The possible neuroprotective and antiaging effects of some of these antioxidants have been explored in a number of studies. Administration of exogenous vitamin E has no demonstrable effect in Parkinson's disease [135], is of equivocal benefit in treatment of tardive dyskinesia [136], and has only limited efficacy in AD [137]. Higher consumption of dietary and supplemental antioxidants in community samples has not benefited cognitive function in middle age [138] or elderly samples [139]. The monoamine oxidase inhibitor selegiline has shown some ability to slow progression of AD [137], and may delay onset of disability in early Parkinson's disease [135]. Overall, administration of exogenous antioxidants has not been an effective strategy to reduce aging or all age related neuropsychiatric disease. There remains a possibility however, that exogenous antioxidants may have some role in protecting against increased oxidative stress of an exogenous origin [130].

Ion Homoeostasis

A related theory of brain aging proposes that changes in ion homoeostasis with age lead to sustained changes in intracellular ion levels which threaten cellular integrity. Although one of the most prominent ions implicated is Ca^{2+}, there is also considerable interest in the effect of aging on other ion channels such as Na^+ and K^+ [129]. Alterations in calcium regulation occur with age at a variety of levels [140]. These may include: changes in calcium influx via membrane based calcium channels; dysregulation of intracellular stores via malfunction of intracellular calcium channels in the endoplasmic reticulum and alteration in intracellular cytosolic buffers; inefficiency of calcium clearance as a result of impaired extrusion into extracellular space, and reduced reaccumulation into endoplasmic reticulum. Alterations to calcium homoeostasis may also have a bearing on mitochondrial function [129]. Key markers of calcium dyshomoeostasis in brain aging include an increase in calcium dependent afterhyperpolarisation in the hippocampus, an increase in specific subtypes of voltage gated calcium channels in hippocampus CA1 region and the appearance of larger calcium transients in response to stimuli including toxic challenge [141]. Although disturbance in calcium homoeostasis produces significant alterations in neuronal physiology, synaptic function and neuronal plasticity [142], its direct role in the aging process is a matter for continuing debate. Thus, significant questions remain unanswered concerning the primacy of calcium dysregulation in both healthy aging and pathological processes [140].

Gene Expression

The cloning of the human genome and the advent of microarray techniques has made it feasible to study the effect of age on gene expression in animal and human brains with relative ease. Preliminary evidence suggests a significant alteration to genetic expression with age in both animals and humans. Such alteration may play an important role in modulating vulnerability to oxidative stress, inflammatory response and regulation of DNA repair. Illustrative work in mice indicates that with age, gene expression in the neocortex and cerebellum is increased [143] for those genes involved in inflammatory and stress responses and reduced for those genes linked to neuronal plasticity and central nervous system development. In humans, age effects on RNA expression in prefrontal cortex show significant reduction in expression in those genes the play a role in synaptic function and plasticity, including some genes that mediate synaptic vesicle release and recycling [144]. RNA expression was also reduced for signal transduction systems that mediate long-term potentiation. Age-related increase in expression of RNA was seen in genes that mediate stress response and repair. Such studies suggest that genetic expression will be significantly altered as a function of age in a manner that has a direct bearing on synaptic plasticity and vulnerability to oxidative stress.

Gene-diet interactions have become a recent focus of aging research. The ability of caloric restriction to extend maximum lifespan of rats is well known. However, the molecular mechanisms of this phenomenon are only just beginning to be understood. Recent microarray analysis of aging rodents undergoing dietary restriction indicate significant modification of expression of genes involved in stress and immune mediated responses as well as genes involved in neural growth and plasticity [143]. It remains unclear to what extent these alterations are responsible for the beneficial effects of dietary restriction. However, dietary restriction in rats has been shown to increase the resistance of hippocampal neurons to toxic insult [145], suggesting a direct protective effect. Of interest is whether a protective effect against age-related neurodegenerative disease is observable in humans undertaking dietary restriction. Preliminary studies suggest that low calorie and low-fat diets reduce relative risk for Alzheimer's disease and Parkinson's disease [146,147].

Table 3: What is the role of genes in brain ageing?

1. Multiple genes contribute to ageing. These genes may be particular to the individual ('Private') or be shared across populations and species ('public').
2. Ageing results from an accumulation of somatic damage because of limited or deficient maintenance and repair.
3. It is likely that the longevity genes influence the ability to repair DNA or provide antioxidant defence.
4. There may additionally be some genes that exert an adverse effect at old age. These genes either escape natural selection or trade beneficial effect at an early age with harm later.
5. It is unlikely that specific genes exist that promote brain ageing with large effects.

Ref. Kirkwood TBL, Austad SN. Why do we age? Nature 2000; 408: 233-238.

Glucocorticoids

Converging evidence suggests that glucocorticoids have a bimodal effect on cognition, with transient glucocorticoid increases improving performance in spatial memory tasks but long-term elevations producing performance decrements [148]. In addition to the effect on learning, glucocorticoids are implicated in aging. The hippocampus has been the central focus of research on the effect of glucocorticoids on the brain. Hippocampal-dependent learning and memory is mediated by a process of strengthening synaptic communications, known as long-term potentiation (LTP). The effect of glucocorticoid has on this process is represented by an inverted 'U', with glucocorticoid insufficiency and excess both inhibiting LTP. Studies of the effects of glucocorticoids have indicated adverse effects on memory in endogenous excess states [149] and with administered glucocorticoids [150]. Progressive elevations of serum cortisol are observed with age and are associated with higher risk of cognitive impairment [148]. Aging subjects with elevated and increasing basal cortisol levels over a four year period have been shown to demonstrate reduction in hippocampal volumes and memory deficits [151]. Another study that followed up elderly women with elevated cortisol at baseline found that further increases in urinary cortisol secretion over a 2.5 year follow-up were associated with declines in memory performance, whereas women with decreases in urinary cortisol secretion demonstrated improvements in memory performance [142]. Various cellular mechanisms have been proposed to explain the detrimental effect of chronic elevations of cortisol on cognition [148]. Whilst short-term elevation of cortisol may help protect hippocampal neurons against excitotoxic damage, long-term elevation of cortisol is associated with increased vulnerability to excitotoxic damage. A variety of mechanisms have been proposed including reduced neurogenesis, attenuation of glucose uptake, accumulation of extracellular glutamate and elevation of Ca^{2+}.

Homocysteine

Elevated levels of the plasma based amino acid homocysteine have been shown to be a risk factor for vascular disease and age associated neuropsychiatric diseases. A strong association has been noted between elevated homocysteine levels and risk of stroke in large prospective studies [153]. Precursors of stroke such as carotid artery stenosis, intimal thickening and plaque formation [154] also appear to be increased in those with elevated homocysteine levels. The results of the Framingham heart study suggest that people with elevated homocysteine levels are at increased risk for Alzheimer' s disease [155]. Studies of cognition and homocysteine levels in the elderly suggest an association between elevated homocysteine and reduced cognitive performance [156], but this finding is by no means a universal one [157]. Early studies suggest a relationship between elevated homocysteine levels and various neuroanatomical markers such as ventricular dilation in normal healthy elderly [158]. As vitamins B12, B6 and folate are cofactors in homocysteine metabolic pathways, their deficiency is associated with elevated levels of homocysteine [159]. Animal models of diseases such as Alzheimer's disease and Parkinson's disease suggest that folate deficiency and the resultant increase in homocysteine levels may increase the risk for these disorders by rendering neurons vulnerable to age-related oxidative stress [160]. However, the mechanisms by which elevated homocysteine mediates its effect on the aging brain requires further evaluation.

NEUROLOGICAL EXAMINATION OF AN ELDERLY INDIVIDUAL

When the map differs from the terrain, believe the terrain

Norwegian Proverb

Interviewing Style

A more formal and patient interviewing style is often helpful in working with older patients. As Sir William Osler observed, *'Listen to the patient and he will tell you the diagnosis'*. This is not to be construed, however, as encouragement to be too directive. Indeed, open-ended questioning and a polite preamble will help in building rapport. Often, a patient's spouse will be in attendance, and may serve as a useful source of information, as may other family members, within the bounds of the patient's wishes for confidentiality.

Whilst observing for unusual delays, some allowance must be made for the decreased motor/cognitive-processing speed of elderly especially when asking them to participate in the physical examination or provide a history. A further source of misunderstanding may be deafness, or significant language difficulties (especially in the older generations of immigrants from impoverished or countries lacking in basic educational infrastructure).

It is helpful to send out a letter or request that patients bring in relevant investigations prior to an office consultation, such as brain scans, blood test results among other investigations.

History-Taking

Particularly with older people, a life-course history of illnesses is useful in determining the context of symptoms, possible aetiological factors and precipitants. Indeed, the contribution of stroke, diabetes, hypertension, ischaemic heart disease and cerebrovascular disease among other systemic processes to age-related neurologic disease has been remarked upon in the dementias [161].

A comprehensive accounting of all medication and herbal remedies prescribed and being taken should be performed. This may necessitate a staff-member visiting the patient's home, with permission to locate all available medicaments. Similarly, a comprehensive overview of the other physicians and services being consulted by the patient is mandatory to avoid miscommunication and iatrogenic complications. Accurate information regarding alcohol and other drug intake should be obtained, especially in the still-working young-old group. Occupational commitments and voluntary work should be assessed, as should the impact of any symptoms on such work. Social and instrumental supports should be ascertained. For example, the level of contact with family members and, the community services (financial support, meals etc.) accessed.

NEUROLOGICAL EXAMINATION

Considerations from Findings in Normal Aging

Disturbances of Gait & Balance

The development of an extraordinarily cautious gait characterised by slowed walking, increased unsteadiness (secondary to extrapyramidal, frontal-lobe and postural control disturbances) and fear of falling has been described [162]. It has been suggested that this may be due to a disorder of frontal subcortical white matter. Furthermore, this disorder was significantly associated with higher levels of depression (Geriatric Depression Scale [GDS]), anxiety (Spielberger State-Trait Anxiety Inventory [STAI]) and lower scores on the Mini-Mental State Examination (MMSE). A large US epidemiological study assessed gait speed, chair standing, standing balance, cognition with a modified MMSE and digit symbol substitution test (DSST) [163]. A statistically significant association was found between physical and cognitive function in otherwise healthy elderly. Their conclusion was that slow gait speed can be an indicator of impaired executive cognitive function.

Similarly, previous research showed that membership of the oldest old subgroup was best predicted by poor performance in clinical tests of balance (heel-toe walking and one-leg balancing with eyes closed) [164]. Other studies have also demonstrated statistically significant decline in gait disturbance with age [165].

Assessing Parkinsonism

Mild, clinically detectable tremor was found in 96% of a 103 normal control subjects 65 years and older [166]. Of these, 28% had a clearly oscillatory tremor of moderate amplitude present during maintenance of posture or task performance [166]. Other studies have shown the prevalence of mild Parkinsonism (as defined by the presence of two or more of the signs bradykinesia, gait disturbance, rigidity or tremor) to be 14.9% for those 65-74, 29.5% for those 75 to 84 rising to 52.4% in the age range 85 and above [167]. Furthermore, the presence of Parkinsonism, thus defined, was associated with a two-fold increased risk of death. There is also evidence that those who meet criteria for essential tremor have a mildly reduced body mass index, presumably due to the physiological effects of the tremor on metabolism [168].

The Unified Parkinson's Disease Rating Scale (UPDRS) has been demonstrated to provide an empirical basis for summarizing the main components of Parkinsonism and is used widely in clinical and research practice. Hoehn-Yahr staging is useful for assessing the staging of the disease. Nonetheless, the differential diagnosis of Parkinson's disease remains difficult, with misdiagnosis rates approximating 25%, with the most common misdiagnoses being progressive supranuclear palsy, corticobasal degeneration, or multiple system atrophy. Unfortunately, diagnosis remains primarily a clinical process, with the cost-effectiveness and availability of specialised tests such as SPECT, PET and specialised MRI still to be determined [169].

The Peripheral Nervous System

A recent study of chronic idiopathic axonal polyneuropathy conducted by Vrancken et al. [170] has informed us about the aging of the peripheral nervous system [171]. Whilst defined as a successfully aging group, the controls were primarily characterized by the absence of neurological or other diseases. Vrancken et al. [170] found that 65% of the 108 controls had sensory signs such as reduced light touch or vibration sense, and absent tendon reflexes. Controls 65 years and older had significantly lower sensory score of the legs. Other studies have also demonstrated age-related decreases in vibration sense [171]. A larger population-based study of women showed that perceived vibration threshold declined most, with the lowest decrement in light touch discrimination [172]. However, all domains assessed, muscle strength, balance, gait, somatosensory discrimination and reaction time declined with increasing age [172]. Another population-based study showed rare absence of deep tendon reflexes and impaired proprioceptive sensation [173].

Nerve conduction studies show an age-related decline in normal aging [171]. In the absence of other electrodiagnostic abnormalities, the consensus has been to discount a finding of the absence of a sural response [171]. In electrodiagnostically confirmed peripheral neuropathy for persons aged 50-80, two of three signs: Achilles' reflex (absent despite facilitation), vibration (128 Hz tuning fork for <10 s) and position sense (<8/10 1-cm trials), identified peripheral neuropathy [174]. Re-emergence of primitive reflexes may also be associated with increased age [165].

Intra-epidermal nerve fiber density has been described as the most sensitive test for detecting small fiber neuropathy, but the results have been conflicting as to whether there is a trend for change with aging. Sural biopsy is a rather invasive and uncomfortable procedure [171].

Central Nervous System

Cranial Nerve Function

The oldest old subgroup (those greater than 84 years) perform poorly relative to young old (65-74 years) cohorts on tests of smell and visual pursuit [164]. Limitation of upward gaze and convergence have also been described as being common, especially with advanced age [173].

Cognitive Assessment

Whilst a decline in cognitive performance occurs with aging, there is now evidence of considerable variability in the degree and rate of decline. There is evidence, that within the healthy elderly without major illness aged 65-94, cognition is relatively stable over short epochs such as four years, albeit in a highly select group as the authors admitted [1].

How a clinician should screen for cognitive decline is somewhat controversial as most of the short screening scales are incomplete and not intended for assessing normal aging. The Folstein MMSE has been translated into several languages (including ideographic languages such as Chinese) and has the advantage of being relatively quick to administer. It also correlates well with other cognitive assessment batteries [175].

The Folstein MMSE has been shown to have effectiveness in separating those with mild Alzheimer's disease from healthy elderly, mild cognitive impairment and depression [175]. However, the separation of the other categories from each other is more problematic and additional history is required. Alternatives are the Mental Status Questionnaire or the Abbreviated Mental Test Scale, but these are disadvantaged by not being as rigorously evaluated as the MMSE. The cutoff for AD was at or equal to 24. However, lower educational levels, illiteracy and non-native language administration may also result in unusually low scores not reflective of cognitive function. The score must be supplemented by an assessment of the person's functional abilities related to cognition (eg. reading, writing, paying bills, shopping).

This can be supplemented by a clock-drawing task to assess executive cognitive function. The caveats to the above assessments are that the MMSE be administered in a first language, educational level be ascertained and visual/auditory deficits be noted.

The Addenbrookes Cognitive Examination (ACE), which incorporates the MMSE, has been demonstrated to be sensitive to early dementia and useful in clinical practice in determining a cutoff score above which dementia is unlikely, 83 (moderate likeliehood ratio - LR) – 88 (large LR) [177].

Assessment of Motor Vehicle Driving Capacity

The independence of many older people, particularly in first world countries is highly dependent on reliable transport. For many, the main mode of transport is the motor vehicle. Driving is a complex neurocognitive task and because of the potential of impairment to impact upon others, any assessment of capacity must be made judiciously.

However, the emotional response and consequences of restriction of driving can be considerable and place great strain on the physician-patient relationship.

Recent research has demonstrated that a comprehensive history, physical examination, neuropsychological and laboratory tests are significantly helpful for the prediction of on-road driving performance by neurologists. In a study of early Alzheimer's dementia and on-road driving performance as assessed by a driving instructor, personal and informant ratings of performance were not significantly related to actual performance [178]. However, a neurologist's assessment, based upon a comprehensive neurological examination was predictive of performance on a formal driving instructor's assessment.

SUGGESTED PROTOCOL FOR NEUROLOGICAL HISTORY & EXAMINATION

Medical History

- Presenting Symptoms
- History of Presenting Illness (especially localizing signs, evolution, remissions)
- Current Medications
- Allergies (Including Medications)
- Past Medical History (previous major illnesses, surgery)
- Family Medical History (heritable diseases)
- Social history (living circumstances, occupation, family & social supports)
- Ability in daily function (activities of daily living: washing, cleaning, cooking, & functional abilities: reading, writing etc.

Neurological Examination

Mental Status Examination
- Attention: Level of attentiveness, note any fluctuations in attention
- Orientation: Time, place, person
- Speech: Speed, clarity,
- Comprehension: Ability to comprehend questions and simple commands in order to undertake the examination
- Mood: Prevailing reported emotional state eg. Happy, sad, angry
- Affect: Observation of patient's emotional state, including fluctuations
- Thought form: Logical sequence of thoughts, eg. Flight of ideas (rapid progression from topic to topic faster than is usual); Knight's move thinking (progression of ideas in which the intervening steps can no longer be discerned); concreteness (literality of thought without regard for contextual, complexity of meaning)
- Thought content: Prevailing thoughts, presence of delusions (fixed false beliefs), presence of hallucinations (sensory percepts without objective stimulus eg. Hearing voices in an otherwise empty room)

Cognitive Assessment

(Suggest Folstein MMSE, Mental Status Questionnaire, Addenbrookes Cognitive Examination [177].

Cognitive assessement can be supplemented by a clock-drawing task: eg. 'Please draw a clock-face with all the numbers on it, and then draw the hands of the clock at ten minutes past eleven'.

Cranial Nerve Examination

First cranial nerve (olfactory): whilst smell is not ordinarily assessed in younger patients, it may be worthwhile assessing persons suspected of having cognitive impairment as there have been findings of deficits in mild cognitive impairment and Alzheimer's disease. However, assessment is somewhat problematic due to the lack of odoriferous materials in most physicians' practices apart from a decomposing uneaten breakfast/lunch/dinner. Alcohol and other irritants test nociceptive receptors of the 5th cranial nerve (trigeminal) [179].

The cranial nerves subserving the visual system (2nd optic, 3rd oculomotor, 4th trochlear and 6th abducens) are usually assessed together. Visual acuity (corrected) can be assessed with a Snellen card. Visual fields are assessed and pupillary shape, size and accommodation to ascertain integrity of the optic nerve and visual pathways. Extraocular eye movements are explored to assess the 3rd, 4th (inversion) and 6th (abduction) nerves.

The 5th cranial nerve (trigeminal) has three sensory divisions. A disposable neurological lancet is used to assess facial sensation in the ophthalmic, maxillary and mandibular divisions, whilst a cotton ball wisp is used to assess the corneal reflex. The motor function of the trigeminal is tested by palpating the masseter muscles whilst the patient clenches his/her teeth.

The 7th cranial nerve is assessed by observation for hemifacial weakness. If the ability to frown and close the eye is preserved, the facial motor weakness is likely due to an upper motor neuron lesion. The sensory component is rarely assessed as this involves taste in the anterior two-thirds of the tongue.

The 8th cranial nerve has auditory and vestibular components. The auditory component may be assessed by whispering a number in each ear whilst the other is covered. Vestibular function is assessed by tests of gait and balance (see below).

The 9th (glossopharyngeal) and 10th (vagus) cranial nerves are usually assessed together. This is tested by eliciting the gag reflex.

The 11th (spinal accessory nerve) is tested by having the patient turn their head against resistance provided by the examiner's hand and assessing the elevation of the shoulders by the trapezius.

The 12th (hypoglossal) nerve is assessed by examining tongue protrusion.

Peripheral Nervous System & Motor Function

An inspection should be conducted for atrophy, abnormal movements (fasciculations, tremor, myoclonus, chorea, Parkinsonism).

Muscle strength can be graded conventionally on a scale of 0 to 5. No movement can be scored as 0, trace movement as 1, able to move with the assistance of gravity 2, movement against gravity but not resistance 3, movement against resistance from the examiner 4, and normal strength 5.

Assessment of rising from a sitting position, standing, getting off a bed (or examination couch) are good functional assessments of motor system function. Similarly, testing of gait can also be performed, by observation of unassisted walking, heel-toe walking. Postural sense (Romberg test) can be carefully assessed by asking the patient to stand with eyes closed and then the examiner gently attempting to unbalance via a push. Observation of arm swing should also should be noted for evidence of Parkinsonism [180].

Sensory Examination

Screening can be performed using a disposable neurological lancet (which has a dull tip and the sharper non-penetrating lancet end). This applied to the face, neck, torso and all limbs. A wisp from a cotton ball is used to assess light touch. Proprioceptive loss as noted above may occur with aging and is assessed by moving terminal phalanges up or down and asking the patient to describe the direction of movement with their eyes closed.

Stereognosis is tested by asking the patient to identify an object placed in their hand, whilst ability to discern numbers written on hands is graphesthesia.

Vibration sense can be assessed with a tuning fork (125 Hz) placed over bony prominences in the extremities.

Reflex Examination

As noted above, with advancing age, there may be some loss of deep tendon reflexes and re-emergence of primitive reflexes. The DTR (and their innervation) assessed are:

- Biceps (C-5)
- Radial (C-6)
- Triceps (C-7)
- Quadriceps knee jerk (L-4)
- Ankle jerk (L-5, S-1)

The lateral aspect of the sole of the foot is stroked to elicit the plantar response, of which the Babinski sign indicates a spinal upper motor neuron lesion.

Neurologic Investigations

Computed Tomography (CT)

This is available in most centres and suffices for investigation of most brain, spine and gross spinal cord lesions (although MRI confers particular advantages for imaging the spinal cord). It has the disadvantages of difficulty in visualizing structures in the posterior fossa, radiation exposure and lower resolution. Iodinated contrast can be used to visualize the cerebral vasculature, although there is a low risk of stroke in carotid angiography. It has advantages of availability and speed.

Magnetic Resonance Imaging (MRI)

This method is generally superior for visualization of neural structures, and spinal abnormalities impinging upon the cord. It also has the advantage that different protocols (image scanning sequences differing on strength, duration and type of the magnetic field applied) can be used to distinguish particular pathologies. Diffusion-weighted imaging can be used to detect areas of reduced vascular perfusion. T2 and Fluid Attenuation Inversion Recovery (FLAIR) methods can be used to detect areas of inflammation and/or demyelination. Gadolinium contrast can be used to visualize demyelination, inflammation and neoplastic lesions. The disadvantages of MRI are lack of availability in all centres and contraindication for those with cardiac pacemakers, aneurysm clips and movable metallic prostheses.

PET & SPECT

Both PET (Positron Emission Tomography) and SPECT (Single Photon Emission Computed Tomography) remain largely research tools, although they are occasionally used for adjunctive information when a particular pathology such as a dementia or an encephalopathy is suspected.

Cerebral Angiography

Using contrast dye, X-ray images can delineate arterial and venous circulation in the brain. Digital subtraction angiography has improved the quality of images obtained. In this way, information regarding the vasculature can be found complementing the information from CT and MRI.

EEG

Electroencephalography is useful for assessment of suspected epilepsy. Slow wave changes from focal cerebral lesions such as tumors, or generalized as in the case of delirium or encephalopathy. It can be useful in assessing episodic altered consciousness.

Evoked Responses

Visual, auditory, or tactile stimuli can be used. The computerized analysis of the electrical activity in the cortex reflects the integrity of the neuroanatomic pathway.

Electromyography & Nerve Conduction Studies

Electromyography can be used to establish which nerves or muscles are affected by a lesion. This involves insertion of a needle to record the electrical activity of the muscle, which is displayed via a monitor and heard via loudspeaker.

The time to initiate a contraction after a series of stimulations is used to assess nerve conduction velocity. This method can be useful in the evaluation of a demyelinating or neuromuscular disease.

**Table 4: Neurological signs attributable to ageing,
and not suggestive of a disease process.**

1. <u>Hearing</u>: Progressive loss (presbycusis), esp. for high tones.
2. <u>Vision</u>: impairment of accommodation (presbyopia); small pupils with sluggish reaction to light and accommodation; restricted convergence and upward conjugate gaze,;loss of bells' phenomenon.
3. <u>Smell and taste</u>: Reduction in sense (smell > taste).
4. <u>Motor system</u>: slowed reaction time; decreased fine coordination and agility, reduced muscle power (legs > arms, proximal > distal); loss of muscle mass (esp. anterior tibial, thenar and dorsal interossei muscles).
5. <u>Sensory system</u>: Vibratory sense reduced or lost in feet and ankles; slight increase in threshold for touch sensation; proprioception largely unchanged.
6. <u>Reflexes</u>: Achilles reflexes reduced or absent. Some primitive reflexes appear (snout, palmomental or glabellar), but grasp or sucking reflex generally indicate pathology.
7. <u>Posture, stance and gait</u>: Reduced agility; slightly stooped posture; slowness and stiffness of walking; shortening and broadening of the stride (senile gait); reduced gracefulness and adaptability of gait.

Refs: Critchley M. Neurologic changes in the aged. J Chronic Dis 1956; 3:459.

Jenkyn LR, Reeves AG. Neurologic signs in uncomplicated aging (senescence). Semin Neurol 1981; 1:21.

Benassi G, D'Allesandro R, Gallasi R et al. Neurological examination in subjects over 65 years: an epidemiological survey. Neuroepidemiology 1990; 9:27.

Lumbar Puncture

This is performed in special circumstances, after exclusion of a bleeding diathesis, raised intracranial pressure, obstruction to CSF flow (Arnold Chiari) and skin infection at the puncture site. A CT or MRI is performed to rule out a mass lesion in the presence of papilledema or localizing neurological signs. The CSF is examined for intracranial pressure and composition. Cell count, glucose and protein levels are determined [181].

Table 4 summarises some neurological changes that may be regarded as normal aspects of the aging process and are not uncommon in the octo- and nonagenarians.

CONCLUSION

In this chapter, we have reviewed the brain morphological and functional changes associated with aging, the majority of which paint a negative picture. We wish to end the chapter with a positive view of the aging brain. As noted previously, autobiographical and semantic memory are preserved into old age. The aging brain therefore accumulates a lifetime of experiences which commonly translates into worldly wisdom. Older individuals also have a more positive emotional bias in information processing than younger people. There is some evidence from imaging studies that the elderly show less amygdala activation to negative emotional pictures, but there is no difference in subjective response or brain activation to positive images [182]. Older people have been noted to pay more attention to their emotional lives. Beliefs that creativity and productivity decline greatly with age and beginning to be challenged, and it is time that we begin to challenge some of the stereotypes related to the aging brain.

ACKNOWLEDGEMENTS

Angie Russell for assistance with final editing and referencing.

A/Prof Looi acknowledges: Dr Arthur Toga, Professor of Neurology, and Director of the Laboratory of Neuro Imaging, David Geffen School of Medicine for hosting A/Prof Looi as a Fulbright Visiting Scholar; and the Australian-American Fulbright Commission for academic and financial support in the preparation of his section of the chapter (January-June 2005) - http://www.loni.ucla.edu/About_Loni/people/Indiv_Detail.jsp?people_id=154

REFERENCES

[1]   Hickman, S. E., Howieson, D. B., Dame, A., Sexton, G., Kaye,J. Longitudinal analysis of the effects of the ageing process on neuropsychological test performance in health young-old and oldest-old. *Develop Neuropsychol* 2000;17:323-337.

[2]   Miller, A. K., Alston, R. L., Corsellis, J.A. Variation with age in the volumes of grey and white matter in the cerebral hemispheres of man: measurements with an image analyser. *Neuropathol & Applied Neurobiology* 1980;6:119-132.

[3]   Coffey, C. E., Wilkinson, W. E., Parashos, I.A., Soady, S.A., Sullivan, R.J., Patterson, L.J., et al. Quantitative cerebral anatomy of the aging human brain: a cross-sectional study using magnetic resonance imaging. *Neurology* 1992;42:527-536.

[4]   Raz, N., Craik, F., Salthouse, T. "Aging of the brain and its impact on cognitive performance: Integration of structural and functional findings". *The Handbook of Aging and Cognition*. New Jersey: Lawrence Erlbaum Associates; 2000:1-90

[5]   Miller, A.K., Corsellis, J.A. Evidence for a secular increase in human brain weight during the past century. *Ann Human Biol* 1977;4:253-7.

[6]   Forstl, H., Zerfab, R., Geiger-Kabisch, C., Sattel, H., Besthorn, C., Hentschel, F. Brain atrophy in normal ageing and Alzheimer's disease: Volumetric discrimination and clinical correlations. *Br J Psychiatry* 1995;167:739-746.

[7]   Scahill, R.I., Frost, C., Jenkins, R., Whitwell, J.L., Rossor, M.N., Fox, N.C. A longitudinal study of brain volume changes in normal aging using serial registered magnetic resonance imaging. *Arch Neurol* 2003;60:989-994.

[8]   Fox NC, Scahill RI, Crum WR, Rossor MN. Correlation between rates of brain atrophy and cognitive decline in AD. *Neurology* 1999;52:1687-1689.

[9]   Raz N, Gunning F, Head D, Dupuis J, McQuain J, Briggs S, et al. Selective aging of human cerebral cortex observed in vivo: Differential vulnerability of the prefrontal gray matter. *Cerebral Cortex* 1997;7:268-282.

[10] Murphy, D., DeCarli, C., McIntosh, A., Daly, E., Mentis, M., Pietrini, P., et al. Age-related differences in volumes of subcortical nuclei, brain matter, and cerebro-spinal

fluid in healthy men as measured with magnetic resonance imaging (MRI). *Arch Gen Psychiatry* 1996;53:585-94

[11] Tisserand, D.J., Pruessner, J.C., Sanz Arigita, E.J., van Boxtel, M.P., Evans, A.C., Jolles J, et al. Regional frontal cortical volumes decrease differentially in aging: an MRI study to compare volumetric approaches and voxel-based morphometry. *Neuroimage* 2002;17:657-669.

[12] Salat, D.H., Kaye, J.A., Janowsky, J.S. Selective preservation and degeneration within the prefrontal cortex in aging and Alzheimer disease. *Arch Neurol* 2001;58:1403-1408.

[13] Tisserand, D.J., Bosma, H., van Boxtel, M.P., Jolles, J. Head size and cognitive ability in nondemented older adults are related. *Neurology* 2001;56:969-971.

[14] Bobinski, M., De Leon, M., Convit, A., De Santi, S., Wegiel, J., Tarshish, C., et al. MRI of entorhinal cortex in mild Alzheimer's disease. *Lancet* 1999;353:38-40.

[15] Convit, A., De Leon, M., Tarshish, C., De Santi, S., Tsui, W., Rusinek, H., et al. Specific hippocampal volume reductions in individuals at risk for Alzheimer's disease. *Neurobiol Aging* 1997;18:131-138.

[16] DeCarli, C., Massaro, J., Harvey, D., Hald, J., Tullberg, M., Au, R., et al. Measures of brain morphology and infarction in the Framingham heart study: establishing what is normal. *Neurobiol Aging* 2005;26:491-510.

[17] Jack, C.R., Jr., Petersen, R.C., Xu, Y., O'Brien, P.C., Smith, G.E., Ivnik, R.J., et al. Rate of medial temporal lobe atrophy in typical aging and Alzheimer's disease. *Neurology* 1998;51:993-999.

[18] Stern, C., Hasselmo, M. Bridging the gap: integrating cellular and functional magnetic resonance imaging studies of the hippocampus. *Hippocampus* 1999;9:45-53.

[19] Jack, C.R., Jr., Petersen, R.C., Xu, Y., O'Brien, P.C., Smith, G.E., Ivnik, R.J., et al. Rates of hippocampal atrophy correlate with change in clinical status in aging and AD. *Neurology* 2000;55:484-489.

[20] Rusinek, H., De, S.S., Frid, D., Tsui, W.H., Tarshish, C.Y., Convit, A., et al. Regional brain atrophy rate predicts future cognitive decline: 6-year longitudinal MR imaging study of normal aging. *Radiology* 2003;229:691-696.

[21] Reiman, E., Caselli, R., Yun, L., Chen, K., Bandy, D., Minoshima, S., et al. Preclinical evidence of Alzheimer's disease in persons homozygous for the E4 allele for apolipoprotein E. *New Engl J Med* 1996;334:752-758.

[22] Plassman, B., Welsh-Bohmer, K., Bigler, E., Johnson, S., Anderson, C., Helms, M., et al. Apolipoprotein E epsilon 4 allele and hippocampal volume in twins with normal cognition. *Neurology* 1997;48:985-999.

[23] Shah, Y., Tangalos, E., Petersen, R. Mild Cognitive Impairment: When is it a precursor to Alzheimer's disease? *Geriatrics* 2000;55:62-68.

[24] Insausti, R., Jouttonen, K., Soininen, H., Insausti, A., Partanen, K., Vainio, P., et al. MR volumetric analysis of the human entorhinal, perirhinal, and temporopolar cortices. *Am J Neuroradiol* 1998;19:659-671.

[25] Doraiswamy, P., Na, C., Husain, M., Figiel, G., McDonald, W., Ellinwood, E., et al. Morphometric changes in the human midbrain with normal aging: MR and stereologic findings. *Am J Neuroradiol* 1992;13:383-386.

[26] Raz, N., Torres, I., Acker, J. Age, gender, and hemispheric differences in human striatum: a quantitative review and new data from in vivo MRI morphometry. *Psychobiology* 1995;21:151-160

[27] Valenzuela, M., Sachdev, P., Wen, W., Shnier, R., Brodaty, H., Gillies, D. Dual voxel proton magnetic resonance spectroscopy in the healthy elderly: Subcortico-frontal axonal N-acetylaspartate levels are correlated with fluid cognitive abilities independent of structural brain changes. *Neuroimage.* 2000;12:747-756.

[28] Ylikoski, R., Ylikoski, A., Erkinjuntti, T., Sulkava, R., Raininko, R., Tilvis, R. White matter changes in healthy elderly persons correlate with attention and speed of mental processing. *Arch Neurol* 1993;50:818-824.

[29] Double, K., Halliday, G., Kril, J., Harastay, J., Cullen, K., Brooks, W., et al. Topography of brain atrophy during normal ageing and Alzheimer's disease. *Neurobiol Aging* 1996;17:513-521.

[30] Pantoni, L., Garcia, J. Pathogenesis of leukoaraiosis: A review. *Stroke* 1997;28:652-659.

[31] Dickson, D., Timiras, P., Bittar, E. Structural changes in the aged brain. *Advances in Cell Aging and Gerontology.* Jai Press: Greenwich, 1997:51-76.

[32] Salthouse, T. The processing-speed theory of adult age differences in cognition. *Psychol Rev* 1996;103:403-428.

[33] McGeer, P., McGeer, E. Autotoxicity and Alzheimer's Disease. *Arch Neurol* 2000;57:789-790.

[34] Dickson, D., Crystal, H., Mattiace, L., Masur, D., Blau, A., Davies, P., et al. Identification of normal and pathological aging in prospectively studied non-demented elderly humans. *Neurobiol Aging* 1992;13:1-11.

[35] Guillozet, A., Smiley, J., Mash, D., Mesulam, M. The amyloid burden of the cerebral cortex in non-demented old age. *Soc Neurosci Ab.* 1995;21:1478.

[36] Yen, S., Liu, W., Hall, F., Yan, S., Stern, D., Dickson, D. Alzheimer neurofibrillary lesions: molecular nature and potential roles of different components. *Neurobiol Aging* 1995;16:381-387.

[37] Jucker, M., Battig, K., Meier-Ruge, W. Effects of aging and vincamine derivatives on pericapillary environment: stereological characterization of the cerebral capillary network. *Neurobiol Aging* 1990;11:39-46.

[38] Fang, H., Terry, R., Gershon, S. Observations on aging characteristics of cerebral blood vessels, macroscopic and microscopic features. *Neurobiology of Aging.* New York: Raven Press, 1976:155-66.

[39] Hassler, O. Vascular changes in senile brains. *Acta Pathologica (Berl)* 1965;5:40-53.

[40] de la Torre, M., Timiras, P., Bittar, E. Cerebrovascular changes in the aging brain. *Advances in Cell Aging and Gerontology.* Greenwich: JAI Press; 1997:77-107.

[41] Mooradian, A. Effect of aging on the blood-brain barrier. *Neurobiol Aging* 1988;9:31-39.

[42] Klassen, A., Sung, J., Stadlan, E. Histological changes in cerebral arteries with increasing age. *J Neuropath Exp Neurol* 1968;27:607-623.

[43] Schochet, S.S., Jr. Neuropathology of aging. *Neurologic Clinics* 1998;16:569-580.

[44] Zakeri, Z., Locksin, R. Physiological cell death during development and its relationship to aging. *Ann NY Acad Sci* 1994;719:212-229.

[45] Sterio, D. The unbiased estimation of number and sizes of arbitrary particles using the disector. *J Microscopy* 1984;134:127-136.

[46] West, M. Stereological methods for estimating the total number of neurons and synapses: Issues of precision and bias. *Trends Neurosci* 1999;22:51-61.

[47] Wickelgren, I. Is hippocampal cell death a myth? *Science* 1999;271:1229-1230.

[48] Long, J., Mouton, P., Jucker, M., Ingram, D. What counts in Brain Aging? Design-based stereological analysis of cell number. *J Gerontol: Biol Sci* 1999;54A:B407-B17.

[49] West, M.J., Coleman, P.D., Flood, D.G., Troncoso, J.C. Differences in the pattern of hippocampal neuronal loss in normal ageing and Alzheimer's disease. *Lancet* 1994;344:769-772.

[50] Hamrick, J., Sullivan, P., Scheff, S. Estimation of possible age-related changes in synaptic density in the hippocampal CA1 stratum radiatum. *Soc Neurosci Ab* 1998;24:783.

[51] Wickett, J., Vernon, P. Peripheral Nerve Conduction Velocity, Reaction Time, and Intelligence: An Attempt to Replicate Vernon and Mori. *Intelligence* 1994;18:127-31.

[52] Laming, P., Sykova, E., Reichenbach, A., Hatton, G., Bauer, H., Laming, P., et al. *Glial Cells: Their role in Behaviour.* Cambridge: Cambridge University Press, 1998.

[53] Kempermann, G., Kuhn, G., Gage, F. More hippocampal neurons in adult mice living in an enriched environment. *Nature* 1997;386:493-5.

[54] Kempermann, G., Kuhn, G., Gage, F. Experience-induced neurogenesis in the senescent dentate gyrus. *J Neurosci* 1998;18:3206-3212.

[55] Eriksson, P., Bjork-Eriksson, T., Alborn, A., Nordborg, C., Peterson, D., Gage, F. Neurogenesis in the adult human hippocampus. *Nat Med* 1998;4:1313-1317.

[56] Burke, S.N., Barnes, C.A. Neural plasticity in the ageing brain. *Nat Rev Neurosci* 2006;7:30-40.

[57] Kety, S.S., Schmidt, C.F. Nitrous oxide method for the quantitative determination of cerebral blood flow in man: theory, procedure and normal values. *J Clin Invest* 1948;27:476-483.

[58] Matsuda, H., Maeda, T., Yamada, M., Gui, L.X., Tonami, N., Hisada, K. Age-matched normal values and topographic maps for regional cerebral blood flow measurements by Xe-133 inhalation. *Stroke* 1984;15:336-342.

[59] Takeda, S., Matsuzawa, T., Matsui, H. Age-related changes in regional cerebral blood flow and brain volume in healthy subjects. *J Am Geriatr Soc* 1988;36:293-297.

[60] Tsuda, Y., Hartmann, A. Changes in hyperfrontality of cerebral blood flow and carbon dioxide reactivity with age. *Stroke* 1989;20:1667-1673.

[61] Iwata, K., Harano, H. Regional cerebral blood flow changes in aging. *Acta Radiologica - Supplementum.* 1986;369:440-443.

[62] Waldemar, G., Hasselbalch, S.G., Andersen, A.R., Delecluse, F., Petersen, P., Johnsen, A., et al. 99mTc-d,l-HMPAO and SPECT of the brain in normal aging. *J Cereb Blood Flow & Metabolism* 1991;11508-521.

[63] Swartz, J.R., Lesser, I.M., Boone, K.B., Miller, B.L., Mena, I. Cerebral blood flow changes in normal aging - SPECT measurements. *Intl J Geriatr Psychiatry* 1995;10:437-446.

[64] Leenders, K.L., Perani, D., Lammertsma, A.A., Heather, J.D., Buckingham, P., Healy, M.J., et al. Cerebral blood flow, blood volume and oxygen utilization. Normal values and effect of age. *Brain* 1990;113:27-47.

[65] Bentourkia, M., Bol, A., Ivanoiu, A., Labar, D., Sibomana, M., Coppens, A., et al. Comparison of regional cerebral blood flow and glucose metabolism in the normal brain: effect of aging. *J Neurol Sci* 2000;181:19-28.

[66] Itoh, M., Hatazawa, J., Miyazawa, H., Matsui, H., Meguro, K., Yanai, K., et al. Stability of cerebral blood flow and oxygen metabolism during normal aging. *Gerontology* 1990;36:43-48.

[67] Mozley, P.D., Sadek, A.M., Alavi, A., Gur, R.C., Muenz, L.R., Bunow, B.J., et al. Effects of aging on the cerebral distribution of technetium-99m hexamethylpropylene amine oxime in healthy humans. *E J Nuclr Med* 1997;24:754-761.

[68] Yamaguchi, T., Kanno, I., Uemura, K., Shishido, F., Inugami, A., Ogawa, T., et al. Reduction in regional cerebral metabolic rate of oxygen during human aging. *Stroke* 1986;17:1220-1228.

[69] Takada, H., Nagata, K., Hirata, Y., Satoh, Y., Watahiki, Y., Sugawara, J., et al. Age-related decline of cerebral oxygen metabolism in normal population detected with positron emission tomography. *Neurological Research* 1992;14:S128-131.

[70] Duara, R., Grady, C., Haxby, J., Ingvar, D., Sokoloff, L., Margolin, R.A., et al. Human brain glucose utilization and cognitive function in relation to age. *Ann Neurol* 1984;16:703-713.

[71] Petit-Taboue, M.C., Landeau, B., Desson, J., Desranges, B., Baron, J. Effects of healthy aging on the regional cerebral metabolic rate of glucose assessed with statistical parametric mapping. *Neuroimage* 1998;7:176-184.

[72] Ibanez, V., Pietrini, P., Furey, M.L., Alexander, G.E., Millet, P., Bokde, A.L., et al. Resting state brain glucose metabolism is not reduced in normotensive healthy men during aging, after correction for brain atrophy. *Brain Res Bull* 2004;63:147-154.

[73] Kuhl, D.E., Metter, E.J., Riege, W.H., Phelps, M.E. Effects of human aging on patterns of local cerebral glucose utilization determined by the [18F]fluorodeoxyglucose method. *J Cerebral Blood Flow & Metabolism* 1982;2:163-171.

[74] Moeller, J., Ishikawa, T., Dhawan, V., Spetsieris, P., Mandel, F., Alexander, G., et al. The metabolic topography of normal aging. *J Cerebral Blood Flow & Metabolism* 1996;16:385-398.

[75] Pantano, P., Baron, J.C., Lebrun-Grandie, P., Duquesnoy, N., Bousser, M.G., Comar, D. Regional cerebral blood flow and oxygen consumption in human aging. *Stroke* 1984;15:635-641.

[76] Marchal, G., Rioux, P., Petit-Taboue, M.C., Sette, G., Travere, J.M., Le, P.C., et al. Regional cerebral oxygen consumption, blood flow, and blood volume in healthy human aging. *Arch Neurol* 1992;49:1013-1020.

[77] Martin, A.J., Friston, K.J., Colebatch, J.G., Frackowiak, R.S. Decreases in regional cerebral blood flow with normal aging. *J Cerebral Blood Flow & Metabolism* 1991;11:684-689.

[78] Garraux, G., Salmon, E., Degueldre, C., Laureys, S., Franck, G. Comparison of impaired subcortico-frontal metabolic networks in normal aging, subcortico-frontal dementia, and cortical frontal dementia. *Neuroimage* 1999;10:149-162.

[79] Shenkin, H.A., Novak, P., Goluboff, B., Soffe, A.M., Bortin, L. The effects of aging, arteriosclerosis, and hypertension upon the cerebral circulation. *J Clin Investigation* 1953;32:459-465.

[80] Nobili, F., Taddei, G., Vitali, P., Bazzano, L., Catsafados, E., Mariani, G., et al. Relationships between tc-99m-hmpao ceraspect and quantitative eeg observations in alzheimers disease. *Arch Gerontol Geriatr* 1998;S6:363-368.

[81] Salerno, J.A., Waltenbaugh, C., Cianciotto, N.P. Ethanol consumption and the susceptibility of mice to Listeria monocytogenes infection. *Alcoholism: Clin Expl Res* 2001;25:464-472.

[82] Meyer, J.S., Rogers, R.L., Mortel, K.F. Prospective analysis of long term control of mild hypertension on cerebral blood flow. *Stroke* 1985;16:985-990.

[83] Claus, J.J., Breteler, M.B., Hasan, D., Krenning, E.P., Bots, M.L., Grobbee, D.E., et al. Regional cerebral blood flow and cerebrovascular risk factors in the elderly population. *Neurobiol Aging* 1998;19:57-64

[84] Yoshii, F., Barker, W.W., Chang, J.Y., Loewenstein, D., Apicella, A., Smith, D., et al. Sensitivity of cerebral glucose metabolism to age, gender, brain volume, brain atrophy, and cerebrovascular risk factors. *J Cerebral Blood Flow & Metabolism* 1988;8:654-661.

[85] DeCarli, C,, Murphy, D.G., Tranh, M., Grady, C.L., Haxby, J.V., Gillette, J.A., et al. The effect of white matter hyperintensity volume on brain structure, cognitive performance, and cerebral metabolism of glucose in 51 healthy adults. *Neurology* 1995;45:2077-2084.

[86] Takahashi, W., Takagi, S., Ide, M., Shohtsu, A., Shinohara, Y. Reduced cerebral glucose metabolism in subjects with incidental hyperintensities on magnetic resonance imaging. *J Neurol Sci* 2000;176:21-27.

[87] Aizenstein, H.J., Clark, K.A., Butters, M.A., Cochran, J., Stenger, V.A., Meltzer, C.C., et al. The BOLD hemodynamic response in healthy aging. *J CogNeurosci* 2004;16:786-793.

[88] D'Esposito, M., Zarahn, E., Aguirre, G.K., Rypma, B. The effect of normal aging on the coupling of neural activity to the bold hemodynamic response. *Neuroimage* 1999;10:6-14

[89] Ross, M.H., Yurgelun-Todd, D.A., Renshaw, P.F., Maas, L.C., Mendelson, J.H., Mello, N.K., et al. Age-related reduction in functional MRI response to photic stimulation. *Neurology* 1997;48:173-176.

[90] Huettel, S.A., Singerman, J.D., McCarthy, G. The effects of aging upon the hemodynamic response measured by functional MRI. *Neuroimage* 2001;13:161-175.

[91] Pineiro, R., Pendlebury, S., Johansen-Berg, H., Matthews, P.M. Altered hemodynamic responses in patients after subcortical stroke measured by functional MRI. *Stroke* 2002;33:103-109.

[92] Grady, C.L., Maisog, J.M., Horwitz, B., Ungerleider, L.G., Mentis, M.J., Salerno, J.A., et al. Age-related changes in cortical blood flow activation during visual processing of faces and location. *J Neurosci* 1994;14:1450-1462.

[93] Madden, D.J., Turkington, T.G., Provenzale, J.M., Hawk, T.C., Hoffman, J.M. Selective and divided visual attention - age-related changes in regional cerebral blood flow measured by (h2o)-o-15 pet. *Human Brain Mapping* 1997;5:389-409.

[94] McIntosh, A.R., Sekuler, A.B., Penpeci, C., Rajah, M.N., Grady, C.L., Sekuler, R., et al. Recruitment of unique neural systems to support visual memory in normal aging. *Current Biology* 1999;9:1275-1278.

[95] Madden, D.J., Turkington, T.G., Coleman, R.E., Provenzale, J.M., DeGrado, T.R., Hoffman, J.M. Adult age differences in regional cerebral blood flow during visual world identification: evidence from H215O PET. *Neuroimage* 1996;3:127-142.

[96] Esposito, G., Kirkby, B.S., Van Horn, J.D., Ellmore, T.M., Berman, K.F. Context-dependent, neural system-specific neurophysiological concomitants of ageing: mapping PET correlates during cognitive activation. *Brain* 1999;122:963-979.

[97] Grady, C.L., McIntosh, A.R., Horwitz, B., Maisog, J.M., Ungerleider, L.G., Mentis, M.J., et al. Age-related reductions in human recognition memory due to impaired encoding. *Science* 1995;269:218-221.

[98] Cabeza, R., Grady, C.L., Nyberg, L., McIntosh, A.R., Tulving, E., Kapur, S., et al. Age-related differences in neural activity during memory encoding and retrieval: a positron emission tomography study. *J Neurosci* 1997;17:391-400.

[99] Herholz, K., Ehlen, P., Kessler, J., Strotmann, T., Kalbe, E., Markowitsch, H.J. Learning face-name associations and the effect of age and performance: a PET activation study. *Neuropsychologia* 2001;39:643-50.

[100] Cabeza, R., Anderson, N.D., Houle, S., Mangels, J.A., Nyberg, L. Age-related differences in neural activity during item and temporal-order memory retrieval: a positron emission tomography study. *J Cog Neurosci* 2000;12:197-206.

[101] Whitehouse, J.M. Effects of atropine on discrimination learning in the rat. *J Comparative and Physiological Psychology* 1964;57:13-15.

[102] Bartus, R.T. Short term memory in the rhesus monkey: disruption from the anticholinergic scopalamine. *Pharmacol Biochem Behav* 1976;5:39-46.

[103] Sastry, B.V., Janson, V.E., Jaiswal, N., Tayeb, O.S. Changes in enzymes of the cholinergic system and acetylcholine release in the cerebra of aging male Fischer rats. *Pharmacology* 1983;26:61-72.

[104] Lippa, A.S., Pelham, R.N., Beer, B., Critchett, D.J., Dean, R.L., Bartus, R.T. Brain cholinergic dysfunction and memory in aged rats. *Neurobiology of Aging* 1980;1:13-9.

[105] Bowen, D.M., Smith, C.B., White, P., Davison, A.M. Neurotransmitter-related enzymes and indicies of hypoxia in senile dementia and other abiotrophies. *Brain* 1976;99:459-496.

[106] Op, D.V. Some cerebral proteins and enzyme systems in Alzheimer's presenile and senile dementia. *J Am Geriatr Soc* 1976;24:12-16.

[107] Sims, N.R., Bowen, D.M., Smith, C.C. Glucose metabolism and acetylcholine synthesis in relation to neuronal activity in Alzheimer's disease. *Lancet* 1980;1:333-336.

[108] Davis, K.L., Mohs, R.C., Marin, D., Purohit, D.P., Perl, D.P., Lantz, M, et al. Cholinergic markers in elderly patients with early signs of Alzheimer disease. *JAMA* 1999;281:1401-1406.

[109] DeKosky, S.T., Ikonomovic, M.D., Styren, S.D., Beckett, L., Wisniewski, S., Bennett, D.A., et al. Upregulation of choline acetyltransferase activity in hippocampus and frontal cortex of elderly subjects with mild cognitive impairment. *Ann Neurol* 2002;51:145-155.

[110] Muller, W.E. Central cholinergic function and aging. *Acta Psychiatrica Scandinavica.* 1991;366:S34-S39.

[111] Suhara, T., Inoue, O., Kobayashi, K., Suzuki, K., Takeno, Y. Age-related changes in human muscarinic acetylcholine receptors measured by positron emission tomography. *Neuroscience Letters* 1993;149:225-228.

[112] Reeves S, Bench C, Howard R. Ageing and the nigrostriatal dopaminergic system. *Intl J Geriatr Psychiatry* 2002;17:359-370.

[113] Kelly, J., Roth, G., Timiras, P., Bittar, E. Changes in Neurotransmitter Signal Transduction Pathways in the Aging Brain. *Advances in Cell Aging and Gerontology.* Greenwich, CT: Jai Press; 1997:243-278.

[114] Volkow, N.D. Measuring age-related changes in DA D2 receptors with [11C]raclopride and with [18F]N-methylspiroperidol. *Psychiatry Res* 1996;67:11-16.

[115] Suhara, T. Age-related changes in human D1 dopamine receptors measured by positron emission tomography. *Psychopharmacology* 1991;103:41-45.

[116] Volkow, N.D., Ding, Y.S., Fowler, J.S., Wang, G.J., Logan, J., Gatley, S.J., et al. Dopamine transporters decrease with age. *J Nucl Med* 1996;37:554-559.

[117] Volkow, N.D., Gur, R.C., Wang, G.J. Association between decline in brain dopamine activity with age and cognitive and motor impairment in healthy individuals. *Am J Psychiatry* 1998;155:344-349

[118] Volkow, N.D., Logan, J., Fowler, J.S., Wang, G.J., Gur, R.C., Wong, C., et al. Association between age-related decline in brain dopamine activity and impairment in frontal and cingulate metabolism. *Am J Psychiatry* 2000;157:75-80.

[119] Meltzer, C.C., Smith, G., DeKosky, S.T., Pollock, B.G., Mathis, C.A., Moore, R.Y., et al. Serotonin in aging, late-life depression, and Alzheimer's disease: the emerging role of functional imaging. *Neuropsychopharmacology* 1998;18:407-430.

[120] Kuikka, J.T., Raitakari, O.T., Gould, K.L. Imaging of the endothelial dysfunction in coronary atherosclerosis. *E J Nucl Med* 2001;28:1567-1578.

[121] Tauscher, J., Verhoeff, N.P., Christensen, B.K., Hussey, D., Meyer, J.H., Kecojevic, A., et al. Serotonin 5-HT1A receptor binding potential declines with age as measured by [11C]WAY-100635 and PET. *Neuropsychopharmacology* 2001;24:522-530.

[122] Cidis, M.C., Drevets, W.C., Price, J.C., Mathis, C.A., Lopresti, B., Greer, P.J., et al. Gender-specific aging effects on the serotonin 1A receptor. *Brain Research* 2001;895:9-17.

[123] Christensen, H., Kumar, R. Cognitive changes and the ageing brain. In Sachdev, P. (ed) *The Ageing Brain.* Lisse: Swets & Zeitlinger, 2003:75-95.

[124] Hedden, T., Gabrieli, J.D.E. Insights into the ageing mind: A view from cognitive neuroscience. *Nature Rev Neurosci* 2004;5:87-96.

[125] Salthouse, T.A. *Adult Cognition.* New York: Springer Verlag, 1982.

[126] Schaie, K.W.. Intellectual development in adulthood. *The Seattle Longitudinal Study.* Cambridge UK: Cambridge University Press, 1996.

[127] Small, B.J., Blackman, L. Cognitive correlates of mortality: evidence from a population based study of very old adults. *Psychol Aging* 1997;12:309-313.

[128] Hultsch, D.F., MacDonald, S.W.S., Hunter, M.A., Levy-Bencheton, J., Strauss, E. Intraindividual variability in cognitive performance in the elderly: Comparison of adults with dementia, adults with arthritis and healthy adults. *Neuropsychology* 2000;15:588-598.

[129] Annunziato, L., Pannaccione, A., Cataldi, M., Secondo, A., Castaldo, P., Di, R.G., et al. Modulation of ion channels by reactive oxygen and nitrogen species: a pathophysiological role in brain aging. *Neurobiol Aging* 2002;23:819-834.

[130] Barja, G. Free radicals and aging. *Trends Neurosci* 2004;27:595-600.

[131] Beal, F., Hyman, B., Koroshetz, W. Do defects in mitochondrial energy metabolism underlie the pathology of neurodegenerative diseases? *Trends Neurosci* 1993;16:125-131.

[132] Brewer, G.J. Neuronal plasticity and stressor toxicity during aging. *Experimental Gerontology* 2000;35:1165-1183.

[133] Ojaimi, J. Mitochondrial respiratory chain activity in the human brain as a function of age. *Mechanism Ageing Develop.* 1999;111:39-47.

[134] Harper, M.E., Bevilacqua, L., Hagopian, K., Weindruch, R., Ramsey, J.J. Ageing, oxidative stress, and mitochondrial uncoupling. *Acta Physiologica Scandinavica* 2004;182:321-331.

[135] The Parkinson Study G. Effects of tocopherol and deprenyl on the progression of disability in early Parkinson's disease. *New England J Medicine* 1993;328:176-183.

[136] Lohr, J.B. A double-blind placebo-controlled study of vitamin E treatment of Tardive Dyskinesia. *J Clin Psychiatry* 1996;57:167-173.

[137] Sano, M. A controlled trial of selegiline, alpha-tocopherol, or both as a treatment for Alzheimer's disease. *New England J Medicine* 1997;336:1216-1222.

[138] Peacock, J.M., Folsom, A.R., Knopman, D.S., Mosley, T.H., Goff, D.C., Szklo, M. Dietary antioxidant intake and cognitive performance in middle-age adults. *Public Health Nutrition* 2000;3:337-343.

[139] Mendelsohn, A.B., Beele, S.H., Stoehr, G.P., Ganguli, M. Use of antioxidants and its association with cognitive function in a rural elderly cohort-the movies project. *Am J Epidemiology* 1998;148:38-44.

[140] Verkhratsky, A. Calcium and neuronal ageing. *Trends Neurosci* 1998;21:2-7.

[141] Toescu, E.C., Verkhratsky, A., Landfield, P.W. Ca2+ regulation and gene expression in normal brain aging. *Trends Neurosci* 2004;27:614-620.

[142] Gareri, P. Role of calcium in brain aging. *General Pharmacology* 1995;26:1651-1657.

[143] Lee, C.K., Weindruch, R., Prolla, T.A. Gene-expression profile of the ageing brain in mice. *Nature Genetics* 2000;25:294-297.

[144] Lu, T., Pan, Y., Kao, S.Y., Li, C., Kohane, I., Chan, J., et al. Gene regulation and DNA damage in the ageing human brain. *Nature* 2004;429:883-891.

[145] Zhu, H., Guo, Q., Mattson, M.P. Dietary restriction protects hippocampal neurons against the death-promoting action of a presenilin-1 mutation. *Brain Research* 1999;842:224-229.

[146] Logroscino, G., Marder, K., Cote, L., Tang, M.X., Shea, S., Mayeux, R. Dietary lipids and antioxidants in Parkinson's disease: a population-based, case-control study. *Ann Neurol* 1996;39:89-94.

[147] Luchsinger, J.A., Tang, M.X., Shea, S., Mayeux, R. Caloric intake and the risk of Alzheimer disease. *Arch Neurol* 2002;59:1258-1263.

[148] Patel, N.V., Finch, C.E. The glucocorticoid paradox of caloric restriction in slowing brain aging. *Neurobiol Aging* 2002;23:707-717.

[149] Starkman, M.N., Gebarski, S.S., Berent, S., Schteingart, D.E. Hippocampal formation volume, memory dysfunction, and cortisol levels in patients with Cushing's syndrome. *Biological Psychiatry* 1992;32:756-765.

[150] McEwen, B.S., Sapolsky, R.M. Stress and cognitive function. *Current Oppinion in Neurobiology* 1995;5:205-216.

[151] Lupien, S., De Leon, M., De Santi, S., Convit, A., Tarshish, C., Nair, N., et al. Cortisol levels during human aging predict hippocampal atrophy and memory deficits. *Nature Neurosci* 1998;1:69-73.

[152] Seeman, T.E., McEwen, B.S., Singer, B.H., Albert, M.S., Rowe, J.W. Increase in urinary cortisol excretion and memory declines: MacArthur studies of successful aging. *J Clin Endocrinol Metab* 1997;82:2458-2465.

[153] Perry, I.J. Prospective study of serum total homocysteine concentration and risk of stroke in middle aged British men. *Lancet* 1995;346:1395-1398.

[154] McQuillan, B.M., Beilby, J.P., Nidorf, M., Thompson, P.L., Hung, J. The risk of carotid atherosclerosis with hyperhomocysteinemia and the C677T mutation of the methylenetetrahydrofolate reductase. The Perth Carotid Ultrasound Assessment Study (CUDAS). *Circulation* 1999;99:2383-2388.

[155] Seshadri S, Beiser A, Selhub J, Jacques PF, Rosenberg IH, D'Agostino RB, et al. Plasma homocysteine as a risk factor for dementia and Alzheimer's disease.[see comment]. *New England Journal of Medicine 346(7)*:476-83. 2002.

[156] Selhub, J., Bagley, L.C., Miller, J., Rosenberg, I.H. B vitamins, homocysteine, and neurocognitive function in the elderly. *Am J Clini Nutr* 2000;71:614S-20S.

[157] Ravaglia, G. Elevated plasma homocysteine levels in centenarians are not associated with cognitive impairment. *Mechanisms of Ageing and Development* 2000;121:SI251-261.

[158] Sachdev, P.S., Valenzuela, M., Wang, X.L., Looi, J.C., Brodaty, H. Relationship between plasma homocysteine levels and brain atrophy in healthy elderly individuals. *Neurology* 2002;58:1539-1541.

[159] Beilby, J. Homocysteine and disease. *Pathology* 2000;32:262-273.

[160] Mattson MP. Gene-diet interactions in brain aging and neurodegenerative disorders. *Ann Internal Med* 2003;139:441-444.

[161] Whalley, L.J., Dick, F.D., McNeill, G. A life-course approach to the aetiology of late-onset dementias. *Lancet Neurology* 2006;5:87-96.

[162] Giladi, N., Herman, T., Reier-Groswasser, I.I., Gurevich, T., Huasdorff, J.M. Clinical characteristics of elderly patients with a cautious gait of unknown origin. *J Neurol* 2005;252:300-306.

[163] Rosano, C., Simonsick, E.M., Kritchevsky, S.B., Brach, J., Visser, M., Yaffe, K., et al. Association between physical and cognitive function in health elderly: the health aging and body composition study. *Neuroepidemiology* 2005;24:8-14.

[164] Kaye, J.A., Oken, B.S., Howieson, D.B., Howieson, J., Holm, L.A., Dennison, K. Neurologic evaluation of the optimally healthy oldest old. *Arch Neurol* 1994;51:1205-1221.

[165] Odenheimer, G., Funkenstein, H.H., Beckett, L., Chown, M., Pilgrim, D., Evans, D., et al. Comparison of neurologic changes in "successfully aging" persons versus the total aging population. *Arch Neurol* 1994;51:573-580.

[166] Louis, E.D., Ford, B., Pullman, S.L., Baron, K. How normal is normal? Mild tremor in a multiethnic cohort of normal subjects. *Arch Neurol* 1998; 55:222-227.

[167] Bennett, D.A., Beckett, L.A., Murray, A.M., Shannon, K.M., Goetz, C.G., Pilgrim, D.M., et al. Prevalence of Parkinsonian signs and associated mortality in a community population of older people. *New England J Medicine* 1996;334:71-76.

[168] Dogu, O., Sevim, S., Louis, E.D., Kaleagasi, H., Aral, M. Reduced body mass index in patients with essential tremor. *Arch Neurol* 2004;61:386-389.

[169] Tolosa, E., Wenning, G., Poewe, W. The diagnosis of Parkinson's disease. *Lancet Neurology* 2006;5:75-86.

[170] Vrancken, A.F.J.E, Franssen, H., Wokke, J.H.J,. Teunissen, L.L., Notermans, N.C. Cnronic idiopathic axonal polyneuropathy and successful aging of the peripheral nervous system in elderly people. *Arch Neurol* 2002;59:533-540.

[171] Wolfe, G.I. Chronic idiopathic axonal polyneuropathy and successful aging of the peripheral nervous system in elderly people. *Arch Neurol* 2002;59:520-522.

[172] Sands, M.L., Schwartz, A.V., Brown, B.W., Nevitt, M.C., Seeley, D.G., Kelsey, J.L. Relationship of neurological function and age in older women. *Neuroepidemiology* 1998;17:318-329.

[173] Benassi, G., D'Allessandro, R., Gallassi, R., Morreale, A., Lugaresi, E. Neurological examination in subjects over 65 years: an epidemiological survey. *Neuroepidemiology* 1990;9:27-38.

[174] Richardson, J.K. The clinical identification of peripheral neuropathy among older persons. *Arch Physical Med Rehab* 2002;83:1553-1558.

[175] Benson, A.D.S., M.J., Tran, T.T., Petrella, J.R., Doraiswamy, P.M. Screening for early Alzheimer's disease: is there still a role for the Mini-Mental State Examination? *Primary Care Companion Journal of Clinical Psychiatry* 2005;7:62-67.

[176] Mahuranath, P.S., Nestor, P.J., Berrios, G.E., Racowicz, W., Hodges, J.R. A brief cognitive test battery to differentiate Alzheimer's disease and frontotemporal dementia. *Neurology* 2000;55:1613-1620.

[177] Larner, A.J. An audit of the Addenbrookes Cognitive Examination (ACE) in clinical practice. *Intl J Geriatr Psychiatry* 2005;20:593-594.

[178] Brown, L.R., Ott, B.R., Papandonatos, G.D., Sui, Y., Ready, R.E., Morris, J.C. Prediction of on-road driving performance in patients with early Alzheimer's disease. *J Am Geriatr Soc* 2005;53:94-98.

[179] Merck Manual. Available from: http://www.merck.com/mrkshared/mmanual/section14/chapter165/165c/165d.jsp

[180] Clinical Neurological Examination. Available from: http://www.dundee.ac.uk/medther/StrokeSSM/ClinExamNeuro.htm

[181] Aminoff, M.J., Simon, R.R., Greenberg, D. *Clinical Neurology.* 6th ed. San Francisco: McGraw-Hill, 2004.

[182] Mather, M., Canli, T., English, T., Whitfield, S., Wais, P., Ochsner, K., Gabrielli, J.D.E., et al. Amygdala responses to emotionally valenced stimuli in older and younger adults. *Psychol Sci* 2004;15:259-263.

RECOMMENDED FURTHER READING

1. Aminoff MJ, Simon RR, Greenberg D. Clinical Neurology 6th ed. San Francisco: McGraw-Hill Medical, 2004. *For a description of a detailed neurological examination for the non-specialist.*

2. Burke SN, Barnes CA. Neural plasticity in the aging brain. *Nature Reviews Neuroscience* 2006;7:30-40.

3. DeCarli C, Massaro J, Harvey D, Hald J, Tullberg M, Au R, et al. Measures of brain morphology and infarction in the framingham heart study: establishing what is normal. *Neurobiology of Aging.* 26(4):491-510 2005.

4. Hedden T, Gabrieli JDE. Insights into the aging mind: A view from cognitive neuroscience. *Nature Rev Neurosci* 2004; 5:87-96.

5. Hodges, JR Cognitive Assessment for Clinicians. Oxford: Oxford University Press, 1994. *For descriptions of a detailed neuropsychological examination for the non-specialist.*

6. Jack CR, Jr., Petersen RC, Xu Y, O'Brien PC, Smith GE, Ivnik RJ, et al. Rates of hippocampal atrophy correlate with change in clinical status in aging and AD. *Neurology* 2000;55(4):484-489.

7. Kirkwood TBL, Austad SN. Why do we age? *Nature* 2000; 408: 233-238.

8. Long J, Mouton P, Jucker M, Ingram D. What counts in Brain Aging? Design-Based Stereological Analysis of Cell Number. Journal of Gerontology: *Biological Sciences* 1999;54A(10):B407-B417.

9. Mahuranath PS, Nestor PJ, Berrios GE, Racowicz W, Hodges JR. A brief cognitive test battery to differentiate Alzaheimer's disease and frontotemporal dementia. Neurology 2000;55:1613-1620. *For the Addenbrooke's Cognitive Examination screening test.*

10. Raz N, Craik F, Salthouse T. Aging of the Brain and its Impact on Cognitive Performance: Integration of Structural and Functional Findings. In: *The Handbook of Aging and Cognition.* New Jersey: Lawrence Erlbaum Associates; 2000. p. 1-90.

11. Rusinek H, De SS, Frid D, Tsui WH, Tarshish CY, Convit A, et al. Regional brain atrophy rate predicts future cognitive decline: 6-year longitudinal MR imaging study of normal aging. *Radiology.* 229(3):691-6 2003.

12. Sachdev P (ed.) *The Ageing brain: the neurobiology and neuropsychiatry of ageing.* Lisse: Swets & Zeitlinger, 2003.

13. Schaie KW. *Intellectual development in adulthood. The Seattle Longitudinal Study.* Cambridge UK: Cambridge University Press, 1996.

In: Handbook of Clinical Neuroepidemiology   ISBN 978-1-60021-511-7
Editors: V. L. Feigin and D. A. Bennett, pp. 503-526   © 2007 Nova Science Publishers, Inc.

Chapter 14

NEUROPSYCHIATRIC DISORDERS

Perminder Sachdev

School of Psychiatry, University of New South Wales, and Neuropsychiatric Institute,
Prince of Wales Hospital, Sydney, Australia.

ABSTRACT

Neuropsychiatry pertains to the application of the neurological or neuroscientific paradigm to psychiatric and behavioural syndromes. The scope of the discipline has seen many ebbs and flows since its origin in the 19th century. Its epidemiology has been influenced by developments in psychiatric epidemiology in general, but continues to be challenged by problems in definition and ascertainment. In this chapter, these challenges are highlighted by three examples of neuropsychiatric disorders par excellence - schizophrenia-like psychosis associated with epilepsy, tardive dyskinesia and Tourette syndrome - and demonstrate various solutions to these problems. Further systematic epidemiological studies are needed to signal the maturity of the discipline.

INTRODUCTION

What is Neuropsychiatry?

Neuropsychiatry or 'Organic Psychiatry' can trace its origins to the mid-19th century, or even earlier to the 17th century, much before modern psychiatry was born. It pertains to the application of the neurological or neuroscientific paradigm to psychiatric and behavioural syndromes. In its current form, it is regarded not merely as a borderland between Psychiatry and Neurology but as a discipline with a distinctive approach and a clinical territory. It brings together the descriptive, nosological and therapeutic strengths of psychiatry, the empirical foundations of neurology and the assessment skills of neuropsychology to deal with these disorders. Its sister discipline within Neurology is Behavioral Neurology, which covers the same territory but with a neurological bias in training and clinical emphasis [1].

The Emergence of Neuropsychiatric Epidemiology

The European clinician-scientists took an exceptional interest in the interface between the specialties of Neurology and Psychiatry in the 19th century. Linking case studies with neuropathology, they described conditions such as schizophrenia, Alzheimer's disease, and the spectrum of neuropsychiatric disorders in epilepsy. For much of the 19th and 20th centuries this work remained institution and hospital based, with clinicians expressing little interest (or indeed awareness) about the need for representative population based data.

Psychiatric epidemiology was the earlier to emerge, with the evolution of what have been described as the first-generation studies [2]. Interestingly, some of these were neuropsychiatric, for example that done in the 1920's by Goldberger [3] wherein the role of nutritional deficiencies in the development of psychosis due to Pellagra was examined. The second-generation studies followed World War II as in this period psychiatric illness was the leading cause for men being rejected for or discharged from military service. The main improvement in the second-generation studies was that subjects were directly interviewed. Further, this period witnessed clinical and reliability studies, and the use of the first edition of the Diagnostic and Statistical Manual (DSM-I) of the American Psychiatric Association [4] for classification. The development of the Feighner criteria [5] followed. Well-conceived, designed and executed third generation studies have followed these early efforts and in the past two or three decades have brought an element of sophistication to psychiatric epidemiology, tremendously advancing our understanding of mental health.

While the interface between the specialties is not new, the study of epidemiology in neuropsychiatry is, and has evolved only over the last three or four decades. Much of this development has come from the study of comorbidity or associations, rather than from well-designed population based research aimed at addressing this interface. As a consequence, a number of methodological considerations continue to plague this interface.

METHODOLOGICAL ISSUES IN NEUROPSYCHIATRIC EPIDEMIOLOGY

Neuropsychiatric Territory v Approach

For a borderland discipline, one of the challenges has been to categorize 'neuropsychiatric disorders' so as to delineate a 'neuropsychiatric territory'. Here, one can distinguish between neuropsychiatric 'territory' and 'approach', although the need for the latter influences the former. As an example, the management of Tourette syndrome requires familiarity with movement disorders as well as obsessive-compulsive disorder, attention deficit disorder, conduct disorder, mood disorders, specific developmental disabilities, and sleep disorder. It requires skills in pharmacotherapy, behavior therapy, family therapy, genetic counseling and rehabilitation. The neuropsychiatrist brings together the basic skills of psychiatry and neurology, and combines them with expertise in neuroimaging, neuropsychology and neurophysiology to bear upon the condition, thereby demonstrating the neuropsychiatric approach. This would appear to be the essence of neuropsychiatry. By its application, however, some disorders can be identified that are best dealt with the neuropsychiatric approach, thereby delineating the 'territory' of the discipline.

Defining 'Organic' Etiology

The term 'organic' in reference to psychiatric disorders is the topic of much contemporary debate [6]. Its origins are rooted in the late 19th century move to distinguish 'functional' (or psychological) disorders from 'structural' brain diseases in the spirit of Cartesian dualism. In modern neurobiology, there is an understanding of an interaction of structure and function whereby no disorder of the brain (or mind) can be based solely on disturbance of structure or function alone. In addition to its philosophical baggage, 'organic' presents practical problems. According to ICD-10 [7] organic mental disorders are "a range of mental disorders grouped together on the basis of their having in common a demonstrable etiology in cerebral disease, brain injury, or other insult leading to brain dysfunction". It goes on to say that 'organic' means no more and no less than that the syndrome so classified can be attributed to an independently diagnosable cerebral or systemic disease or disorder. The working hypothesis is that the cerebral or systemic dysfunction is directly responsible for the disorder, and is not a fortuitous association with such a disease or dysfunction, or a psychological reaction to its symptoms.

In practice, however, there are no infallible guidelines to establish a direct association, and the following considerations are generally given: i) A temporal association between the onset, exacerbation, or remission of the medical condition and the mental disorder. However, there are many exceptions to this; ii) The presence of features that are atypical of the primary mental disorder; iii) Evidence from the literature of a well-established or frequently encountered association between the general medical condition and the phenomenology of a specific mental disorder. The situation is often not ambiguous. We recognise that psychiatric illnesses have multiple etiological factors (e.g. genetics, coarse brain disease, personality, stress), some of which would be recognized as being 'organic' in most cases. The approach taken by DSM-IV to address the problems associated with 'organic' was to retire the term and replace it with 'secondary' (or 'symptomatic'). It is not being argued that primary psychiatric disorders do not have a basis in brain dysfunction, but that their etiology is poorly understood and they are therefore 'idiopathic', akin to the primary-secondary dichotomy used in medicine. While this does not make the process of etiological determination any easier, it is a philosophically more comfortable position.

Problems with Ascertainment

Neuropsychiatric disorders present special problems in their ascertainment. To take the example of epilepsy, incidence and prevalence figures have varied considerably in different studies because of this [8]. Not all patients with epilepsy are aware of their attacks. There is significant under-reporting due to the transient nature of the illness, with attacks often going unwitnessed. Medical professionals in primary care have a small number of patients in their register and limited expertise. Therefore, patients with epilepsy often do not consult a physician for their seizures, especially if they are in remission [8]. There are also problems in making an epilepsy diagnosis even in specialist settings, with 5-20% of all subjects with epilepsy diagnosis being identified as having a non-epileptic attack disorder. Comorbid psychiatric disorder in epilepsy poses other problems as these episodes (both psychotic and affective somatoform) are intimately linked to seizures, are often transient, and are characterised by features that resemble those of epileptic seizures. Further, these disturbances often do not match conventional descriptions or psychiatric criteria, even when this is clinically applied. Ascertainment of comorbid psychiatric disorder can therefore be as difficult as the ascertainment of epilepsy.

Problems with Psychiatric Instruments and Criteria

Generic tools used in psychiatric research have been applied in a number of epilepsy studies. The semi-structured clinical examination relies upon the skill and experience of the clinician to reduce measurement error. A degree of structure is introduced to increase reliability. However, the validity of the semi-structured examination has not been the subject of extensive investigation and they have been assumed to bring their credentials with them, from their development with psychiatric patients and their use in clinical research [9]. The use of such instruments in the epilepsy setting does confer certain advantages, provided of course the clinician concerned has expertise in the neuropsychiatry of epilepsy. A variant of this approach is the structured measure, for example the Structured Clinical Interview for DSM (SCID), the Composite International Diagnostic Interview (CIDI), the Diagnostic Interview Schedule (DIS), and the Clinical Interview Schedule-Revised (CIS-R). All of these rely on trained interviewers - in some cases with mental health backgrounds, as opposed to clinical psychiatrists. While these tend to have good psychometric properties they do not allow, unlike their semi-structured peers, the luxury of expert clinical interpretation. Further, these generic instruments do not ask questions relevant to epilepsy, and rely on computer programs and operational rules to generate diagnosis based on standard ICD and DSM criteria, which again do not take into account the psychopathologies specific to epilepsy [10].

Other psychometric measures include the General Health Questionnaire (GHQ), Hospital Anxiety and Depression Scale (HADS), Beck Depression Inventory (BDI), Hamilton Anxiety and Depression Ratings Scales (HARS/HDRS), Minnesota Multiphasic Personality Inventory (MMPI), Schedule for Affective Disorders and Schizophrenia (SADS) etc. In general, all these instruments have demonstrated good psychometric properties in relevant populations, both normal individuals and those with psychiatric disorder. Further, the ability of these instruments to identify "cases" with relevant psychiatric disorders is not in question. However, that these are in most cases screening and not diagnostic tools is rather conveniently ignored and several papers are published each year with "psychiatric diagnosis" having been made in epilepsy patients using one of these instruments. The identification of "caseness" without re-confirmation using accepted diagnostic instruments is potentially flawed, and must be approached with caution.

The other potential problem in many studies is the use of criteria such as ICD and DSM. While this results in the identification of "cases" as described in psychiatric literature, it is suspected to exclude many cases with disabling clinical psychiatric problems linked to epilepsy, as they fail to meet temporal or other diagnostic criteria. Thus, while a depressive episode needs to last as along as two weeks in ICD-10 [7], interictal dysphoric disorder of epilepsy (IDD) is often punctuated by severe but brief bouts of depression, anxiety and other somatic symptoms, which do not last longer than hours to days in many cases. The other problem alluded to elsewhere in this review is the tendency of these systems to label all psychiatric disorders in someone with epilepsy as organic, thus presuming a direct link. In both clinical and research terms, this is unhelpful.

The Range of Neuropsychiatric Disorders

There is no general consensus on what comprises the territory of neuropsychiatry. The approach in the Diagnostic and Statistical Manual, 4th edition (DSM-IV) of the American Psychiatric Association [11] is to include disorders characterized by the presence of mental symptoms that are judged to be the direct physiological consequence of a general medical condition. These disorders were previously categorised as 'organic mental disorders'. DSM-IV distinguishes those mental disorders that are due to a general medical condition from those that are substance induced and those that have no specified etiology. The latter are, as a short hand, called *primary mental disorders*, and the former two are *secondary mental disorders*. There are situations in which psychosocial factors produce an exacerbation of a disorder with a primary 'organic' etiology. It is therefore important in any psychiatric disorder to consider the biological, psychological and social factors, even when the primacy of one or the other factor may be apparent. The DSM-IV categorization of secondary mental disorders is presented in Table 1.

Another approach to the territory of neuropsychiatry is to examine which disorders are treated by neuropsychiatrists. Table 2 is a list of disorders commonly seen in the neuropsychiatric clinic. The management of these disorders is not exclusively within the domain of neuropsychiatry, but these disorders may be regarded as prototypically neuropsychiatric. Since it is not possible to examine the epidemiology of all these disorders, we will consider three representative disorders to highlight issues pertaining to neuropsychiatric epidemiology: epilepsy and chronic schizophrenia-like psychosis, tardive dyskinesia and Tourette's syndrome.

Table 1. Classification of organic mental syndrome according to DSM-IV[1]

Cognitive disorders
1. Delirium due to a general medical condition or substance
2. Dementia due to a general medical condition or substance
3. Amnestic disorder due to a general medical condition or substance
Non-cognitive disorders
4. Psychotic disorder due to a general medical condition or substance
     4a. With delusions; 4b. With hallucinations
5. Mood disorder due to a general medical condition or substance
     5a. With depressive features; 5b. With major depressive-like episode
     5c. With manic features; 5d. With mixed features
*6. Catatonic disorder due to a general medical condition
7. Anxiety disorder due to a general medical condition or substance
     7a. With generalized anxiety; 7b. With panic attacks
     7c. With obsessive-compulsive features; 7d. With phobic symptoms
*8. Personality disorder due to a general medical condition
9. Sexual dysfunction due to a general medical condition or substance
10. Sleep disorder due to a general medical condition or substance

[1]Diagnostic and Statistical Manual of Mental Disorders, 4th edition.
*These syndromes are not generally diagnosed as substance-induced. All other syndromes can be caused by general medical conditions or substances.

EXAMPLE 1

Epilepsy and Chronic Schizophrenic-like Psychosis (SLP)

The association between epilepsy and schizophrenia has attracted the attention of psychiatrists since the 19th century. This clinically observed association was seen as a starting point for exploration of the brain basis of mental illness, with epilepsy-related psychosis as a possible model of schizophrenia. Epilepsy has been linked with both brief (ictal, postictal and interictal) and chronic psychosis. The investigation of the relationship with chronic SLP was brought into the modern era by Slater et al [12]. Despite a great deal of further work, many aspects of this relationship remain controversial, and the promised insights have been slow to arrive.

Table 2. Disorders commonly seen in neuropsychiatric practice

- Dementia, mild cognitive impairment and other neurocognitive disorders
- Delirium
- Drug-induced movement disorders
    - Tardive dyskinesia
    - Akathisia
    - Tardive dystonia and other tardive syndromes
    - Neuroleptic malignant syndrome
    - Other drug-induced movement disorders
- Tourette syndrome
- Attention deficit hyperactivity disorder
- Chronic fatigue syndrome
- Cognitive, behavioral or affective disturbance associated with
    - Parkinson's disease, dystonia and other movement disorders
    - Epilepsy
    - Cerebrovascular disease
    - Head injury
    - Alcohol and substance abuse.
- Neurodevelopmental disorders, including mental retardation.

Evidence for Association

The evidence that there is indeed an affinity between schizophrenia and epilepsy must come from epidemiological data. The epidemiological evidence for this association is summarized in Table 3. The rates must be interpreted in light of the general prevalence of psychosis, schizophrenia, and epilepsy in the general population. Schizophrenia is estimated to have a prevalence of 0.5%-1% in the general population, but if we use a broad concept of psychosis, the prevalence is likely to be much higher [13]. Epilepsy has a point prevalence of 0.4%-1% in the general population, and the lifetime risk of having at least one unprovoked seizure is 2%-5% [14]. The prevalence is low in the first decade of life, increases to a plateau in the adult years, and increases further in the elderly [15]. Methodological difficulties in the studies should also be taken into account in the interpretation of the prevalence data. For example, the classic study by Slater et al. [12] drew its subjects from tertiary centres in two major London hospitals. The overall evidence suggests that schizophrenia-like psychosis is many times higher in epileptic patients than in the general population. A recent study based on the Danish longitudinal registers is particularly noteworthy for its comprehensive coverage of a population of 2.7 million [16]. The relative risk of schizophrenia in patients with epilepsy was 2.48 (95% CI 2.20-2.8) and of schizophrenia-like psychosis 2.93 (95% CI 2.69-3.20). The risk was the same in men and women, and increased with age and with family history of schizophrenia or epilepsy.

Table 3. Epidemiological evidence for the association between epilepsy and schizophrenia-like psychosis (SLP)

Measure and Authors	N	%	Comment
Prevalence of SLP in epilepsy clinic groups: Gibbs and Gibbs (1952) [17]	11,612	2.8	Reliability of psychiatric diagnosis uncertain; majority of subjects young
Currie et al (1971) [18]	666	1.8	No criteria described; only patients with temporal lobe epilepsy included
Standage and Fenton (1975) [19]	37	8.0	Temporal lobe epilepsy not different from other epilepsies
Mendez et al (1993) [20]	1,611	9.25	1.06% of migraine (comparison) subjects had schizophrenia-like psychosis; comprehensive assessment used DSM-III-R criteria
Schmitz and Wolf (1995) [21]	697	4.0	Both generalized and focal epilepsies represented
Onuma et al (1995) [22]	1,285	9.1	Point prevalence 4.0%
Prevalence of SLP in epileptic patients in community-based studies: Krohn (1961) [23]	-	2.0	Additional 9% had incapacitating behavioral disorder
Gudmundsson (1996) [24]	987	8.1	Entire epileptic population of Iceland studied
Qin et al (2005) [16]	2.27x106	RR2.93 (2.6-2.20)	Danish longitudinal register. Risk increased with age and family history of schizophrenia and epilepsy.
Prevalence of epilepsy in psychotic patients: Kat (1937) [25] Davison & Bagley (1969) [26] Betts (1981) [(27]	50,000 1,950	0.33 1-10 2.1	Estimates from published data Hospitalised patients
Annual incidence of psychosis in epileptic patients: Lindsay et al (1979) [28]	87	10	Temporal lobe epilepsy subjects followed up for 39 years
Onuma et al (1995) [22]	1,285	0.3	

Risk Factors of Chronic SLP with Epilepsy

While a number of studies have examined the risk factors, the literature remains contentious, without a clear consensus emerging on many variables. The putative risk factors are summarized in Table 4.

Table 4. Putative risk factors for chronic schizophrenia-like psychosis of epilepsy

1. Age: Early age of onset, but evidence conflicting
2. Sex: A female bias reported by one group but not others
3. Family history of psychosis or epilepsy
4. Characteristics of epilepsy:
    a. Many years (usually 10-14) between onset of epilepsy and onset of psychosis
    b. Severe epilepsy: multiple seizure types, history of status epilepticus, multiple hospital admissions, resistance to drugs
    c. Partial complex epilepsy, especially of mediobasal temporal lobe origin
    d. History of secondary generalization
    e. Left sided focus
5. Neuropathology:
    f. Presence of neuroembryodysplastic lesions, e.g. gangliogliomas, hamartomas.
    g. Bilateral pathology
6. Neurological examination: sinistrality

1. Age at Onset, Duration, and Severity of Epilepsy

Epilepsy beginning at an early age and enduring through puberty [29] has been associated with schizophrenia-like psychosis. Other studies have found no relationship to age of onset [30] or have associated psychosis with later age of onset of epilepsy [16,20]. In the large Danish study [16], for every five year increase in the age at diagnosis of epilepsy, there was an increased relative risk of 1.2 (1.14 – 1.26, p<0.0001) of schizophrenia-like psychosis. Many years (usually 10-14) are said to intervene between the onsets of epilepsy and schizophrenia-like psychosis [13,31,32], but this period is highly variable and patients who develop epilepsy after the psychosis are usually excluded from such analyses. Moreover, the peak age at onset for epilepsy is in any case earlier than that for schizophrenia [33], thus making the relevance of this observation somewhat ambiguous.

It is often noted that the patients who develop psychosis have a severe form of epilepsy involving multiple seizure types, a history of status epilepticus [12], and resistance to drug treatment. The risk was higher in epileptics with multiple admissions in the Danish study [16]. The frequency of seizures at the time of development of the psychosis is variable; some authors report an improvement [34], whereas others report a worsening [20]. Most often, it is not possible in the case of chronic psychosis to relate the onset of the psychosis to any change in seizure frequency [12].

2. Is Greater Risk of Psychosis Particular to Temporal Lobe Epilepsy (TLE)?

Suggestions that psychosis in epilepsy might be exclusively or preferentially associated with temporal lobe epilepsy are supported by a majority of case series [12,31,35]. Mendez et al. [20] reported a higher rate of partial complex seizures, but not temporal lobe foci, in their group with schizophrenia-like psychosis plus epilepsy than in their nonschizophrenic epilepsy comparison subjects. In the large Danish study, the relative risk associated with complex partial epilepsy was slightly but non-significantly higher than other types of epilepsy [16] (relative risk, after adjustment for complex partial epilepsy 3.38, for other partial epilepsy 3.18, for generalized epilepsy 2.81). Another argument has been that the proportion of temporal lobe epilepsy in epilepsy-psychosis patients is no different from that in the adult epileptic population in general [13], the latter being estimated to be about 60% [14,33]. This debate, therefore, has not resolved but continues to be in favor of a special but not exclusive relationship between schizophrenia-like psychosis and temporal lobe epilepsy. Additionally, there are neuroimaging and neuropathological data linking the temporal lobe with psychosis (discussed in later sections).

There is also a suggestion that the phenomenology of the psychosis associated with TLE is somewhat different from that associated with generalized epilepsy. The latter are reportedly relatively mild, shorter in duration, often associated with confusion in the early stages, and lacking in Schneiderian first-rank symptoms.

3. Mediobasal or Neocortical Temporal Lobe Epilepsy?

Kristensen and Sindrup [30] reported that psychotic patients had a substantial preponderance of temporal mediobasal spike foci, recorded on sphenoidal electrodes, and an excess of epigastric auras. Hermann et al. [36] reported a higher frequency of schizophrenia and other psychopathology in patients with an aura of fear. Mendez et al. [20] reported more psychic and autonomic auras in the psychotic patients. The neuropathological literature (see later section) has supported a predominant abnormality in the medial temporal structures, although more widespread damage has also been reported [37]. The majority of the evidence, therefore, points to a mediobasal rather than neocortical temporal lobe abnormality underpinning psychosis when the focus is in the temporal lobes.

4. Laterality of Epileptic Focus?

Since the suggestion by Flor-Henry [38] of a preponderance of left-sided pathology in patients with schizophrenia-like psychosis, many studies have examined this issue. In the EEG studies, the majority opinion favors an excess of left temporal foci in the patients with temporal lobe epilepsy and schizreniform psychosis [35], although there have been some negative laterality studies [30,39]. There are many problems with the available data. First, the rigor with which laterality was established differs across studies, and the use of surface EEG recordings to establish laterality is open to question. Second, the presence of an epileptic focus on one side does not mean that pathology is restricted to that side. Third, left-sided preponderance of temporal lobe foci may not be restricted to psychotic individuals, as the evidence supports a left-sided bias for temporal lobe epilepsy in general [40]. Fourth, there is emerging evidence that epilepsy patients with schizophrenia have generalized seizures even when they have a temporal focus [31,41]. Fifth, the instruments and diagnostic criteria used for psychosis are language dependent, thus introducing a left-side bias [13].

The neuroimaging studies that examined laterality were inconclusive. The CT [31,32] and MRI [42] studies failed to demonstrate lateralized lesions, although the patients with hallucinations had higher T1 values in the left temporal lobe. Two small functional imaging studies [43,44] provided preliminary evidence of greater left medial temporal lobe dysfunction in schizophrenia-like psychosis with epilepsy. The neuropathological studies [37,45] have not supported lateralization of pathology.

The laterality issue therefore remains undecided, but the importance of a left-sided focus is not striking. It is possible that the structural abnormality in epileptic psychosis is not lateralized, and is possibly bilateral, but that the functional abnormality is predominantly left-sided. However, right-sided abnormality seems to be sufficient, and generalization of the epileptic disturbance is commonly present.

5. Sex

A female sex bias was reported by one group [29] but is not generally supported [12,16,31,32].

6. Family History

Patients who have schizophrenia-like psychosis with epilepsy generally have been reported not to have a greater than normal familial aggregation of schizophreniform disorders [12,31,32]. In the Danish longitudinal registers study [16], family history of psychosis was associated with a relative risk of 3.12 (2.83 – 3.43) of schizophrenia-like psychosis associated with epilepsy. Interestingly, a family history of epilepsy also increased the risk of schizophrenia or schizophrenia-like psychosis, even after adjusting for the effects of personal history of epilepsy and other confounding factors. This familiar aggregation of epilepsy and schizophrenia-like psychosis suggests shared genetic and/or environmental factors.

7. Premorbid Personality

Since patients with primary schizophrenic illness often have abnormalities in their premorbid personalities, their assessment has been considered a measure of vulnerability. Slater et al. [12] argued that the premorbid personalities of subjects with psychosis related to epilepsy were normal, suggesting that they were different from primary schizophrenics. However, assessments of premorbid personalities are notoriously unreliable, and other studies have not commented on this aspect.

8. Temporal Lobectomy and Post-lobectomy Psychosis

Schizophrenia-like psychosis may develop de novo many months or years after temporal lobectomy for the treatment of intractable epilepsy. Rates from 3% to 28% have been reported [46]. Shaw et al. [46] recently summarized the literature on post-lobectomy psychosis, noting reports of 50 cases of de novo psychosis following temporal lobectomy, and added 11 of their own. They reiterate the excess of congenital lesions such as dysembryoblastic neuroepithelial tumours in the excised lobes rather than the typical mesial temporal sclerosis. They also emphasise bilateral temporal lobe abnormalities, reporting bilateral EEG abnormalities preoperatively and a small amygdala on the unoperated side, but right-sided lobectomy did not emerge as a significant risk factor in their series. There are some reports of improvement of schizophrenic symptoms with temporal lobectomy; it is interesting that these cases were associated with left-sided surgery [45].

EXAMPLE 2

Tardive Dyskinesia

The term 'tardive dyskinesia' (TD) refers to the delayed or tardive onset of dyskinetic movements secondary to neuroleptic drug use. The term dyskinesia (literally 'abnormal movement') is a generic term that refers to a range of movement abnormalities. In the case of TD the movements are either choreiform (rapid, jerky and nonrepetitive, involving particularly the proximal muscles), athetoid (slow, sinuous or writhing, and involving distal muscles), dystonic (slow and sustained muscle contractions) or stereotypic (rhythmic and repetitive) or a combination of these. The movements in TD most commonly involve the oro-buccal, lingual and facial muscles, especially in older individuals.

While there is an extensive literature on the epidemiology of TD, the findings are varied, even though consensus has emerged on many aspects. The diversity of the epidemiological findings calls for an explanation, and many possible reasons can be suggested. Importantly, the very definition of TD has been the subject of much debate. While the movements that are characteristic of TD are usually choreoathetoid, neuroleptic-induced tardive movements may also be dystonic, akathisic, tic-like, myoclonic or tremorous in their manifestation. This has led to a debate between the 'lumpers' and 'splitters', i.e. those who include all these different movements within the rubric of TD, and those who make a distinction between TD and other tardive syndromes such as tardive dystonia, tardive akathisia, or tardive tics. Another issue is the time factor of the condition as implied by the term "tardive" which is derived from the French word "tardif" meaning "late". Until the widely accepted criteria proposed by Schooler and Kane [47] in 1982 which specified a time criteria for persistent TD (3 months) and chronic TD (6 months), there had been a lack of standardization which made comparisons among studies problematic. These criteria also specify that a definite research diagnosis of TD be made only if movements of moderate severity are present in one or more body parts, or of mild severity in two or more body parts. This would exclude cases with mild movement in one body area which Jeste and Wyatt [15] have proposed to be sufficient to diagnose TD.

Other factors that may confound any epidemiological study include the following: temporal aspect of TD (fluctuating course of the condition); differences in assessment (nominal vs. ordinal criteria, use of different rating instruments, single or multiple assessments); differences in treatment practices (type, dosage and duration of neuroleptic treatment, concurrent medication, e.g. anticholinergic drugs, whether patients are currently on neuroleptics at time of assessment, etc.); and the heterogeneity of the patient population (age, sex, ethnicity, duration of illness, exposure to medications, diagnosis, the presence of pseudoparkinsonism masking the disorder). In a critical examination of the literature, all these factors need to be taken into consideration.

Prevalence

In two key review articles [48,49] that examined the prevalence rates of TD in the diverse studies, the authors used the retrospective "pooled data" method where frequency figures from selected primary studies were pooled and a mean was calculated. In a review of 56 studies which spanned from 1959 to 1979, Kane and Smith [48] reported point prevalence rates ranging from 0.5% to 65%, with an average point prevalence of 20%. In a later review of 76 published studies, Yassa and Jeste [49] reported an overall prevalence of 24% among a total of 39,187 patients. The clinical significance of these figures is limited as they were derived from studies that differed in assessment criteria, methodology and population characteristics.

The study by Woerner et al. [50] attempted to address some of the previous methodological issues. The overall prevalence of TD in neuroleptic-treated individuals in this study was 23.4%, of which 3.8% had another neuromedical illness that might have had an etiological role, thus giving a conservative prevalence rate of 19.6%. The rate varied with the setting, being 13.3% at a voluntary hospital with a young population, 23% in a Veterans Administration hospital and 36% in a state hospital. In the same study, when a group of patients with no evidence of TD was withdrawn from neuroleptic drugs and examined weekly for 3 weeks, 34% developed emergent dyskinesia.

Another large-scale study by Muscettola et al. [51] reported a prevalence rate of 19.1% among 1651 psychiatric patients. However, the samples of these two studies were different: the study by Woerner et al. [50] was on normal subjects as well as those with a range of psychiatric disorders while the study by Muscettola et al. [51] was on mixed psychiatric disorders. While both studies used the operationalized criteria of Schooler and Kane [47], it also meant that those with mild dyskinetic movements were excluded.

Spontaneous Dyskinesia

Hyperkinetic involuntary movement also occurs in some individuals without any known causes. Prevalence rates of 0.8%, 6.0% and 7.8% for spontaneous dyskinesia have been reported in the 6th, 7th and 8th decades of life respectively in otherwise healthy subjects [52]. Kane et al. [53] reported a rate of 4.0% in healthy elderly (mean age 73 years) subjects. Prevalence is higher in psychogeriatric patients, especially in those with dementia [54]. Most of the studies were performed in elderly populations, owing to the observation that spontaneous dyskinesias are more common in the elderly. However, one study [55] found that 12.6% of neuroleptic-naive young subjects (aged 3 – 7 years) had at least a rating of "mild" on the Abnormal Involuntary Movement Scale (AIMS), and 4.1% fulfilled the Schooler and Kane [47] criteria for TD.

The presence of spontaneous dyskinesias in psychiatric populations confounds the true prevalence rate of neuroleptic-induced TD. Studies have reported that the prevalence of these spontaneous movements is higher among neuroleptic-naïve patients with schizophrenia than that found among older non-psychiatric patients and patients with other psychiatric diagnoses [56]. Age is a risk factor as well. Reviewing 14 studies which reported prevalence rates of spontaneous dyskinesia among neuroleptic-naïve schizophrenic patients, Fenton [57] found a positive correlation with age: 12% among schizophrenic patients with mean age of 30 years or younger, 25% among those between 31 to 50 years, and 42% among those over 60 years.

The pathophysiology of such spontaneous dyskinesia is unknown. The evidence though not very robust, suggests that these spontaneous movements are found more significantly among neuroleptic-naive schizophrenic patients than neuroleptic-naïve patients with other diagnoses [57]. It has been suggested that this abnormality of movement is intrinsic to the pathophysiology of schizophrenia and Waddington and Crow [54] have suggested it may be a manifestation of brain damage. Whether the presence of spontaneous dyskinesia will worsen or accentuate neuroleptic-induced TD remains to be elucidated, as there is no study to date that has prospectively examined this relationship.

Incidence

Given the difficulties inherent in prevalence estimates, it has been much more rewarding to examine the incidence of TD, the salient studies having been summarized in Table 5. The varying rates probably reflect differences in methodologies and samples as discussed previously. Notwithstanding the difficulties, these studies suggest that the cumulative incidence of TD increases with increasing duration of neuroleptic treatment at the rate of about 3-5% per year for the first several years, to reach a plateau at about 20-25%, but new cases continue to occur many years after drug initiation. It is difficult to identify a point in time after which the risk decreases. The plateau is accounted for by cases that remit while new cases are being added. The two largest prospective studies from Yale [58] and Hillside Hospital, New York [59] provided sizable patient populations that were followed up for 5 and 7 years respectively. However, both studies examined patients who had been psychiatrically unwell and treated with neuroleptics for some time prior to onset of study, with the implication that any past history of TD could not have been excluded.

Of great clinical interest is the incidence of TD in drug-naïve patients with a first episode psychosis. Such studies have the advantages of a "cleaner" cohort without the likelihood of past history of TD. The prospective medication and clinical data also enable a more robust examination of the relationship of TD with other factors. In a prospective study [60] of 118 patients with first episode schizophrenia (mean age 25.2 years), the cumulative incidence of TD was 4.8% in the first year, 7.2% in year 2, and 15.6% after 4 years. The incidence is many times higher in elderly individuals with reported cumulative annual incidence of TD of more than 25% [61,62]. Jeste et al. [63] reported that among older patients (mean age of 66.2 years), the risk of TD is high even after a short duration of typical neuroleptic treatment, with a mean cumulative incidence of TD of 3.4% and 5.9% after 1 and 3 months of treatment respectively.

The advent of atypical neuroleptics is likely to have an impact on the future incidence of TD. The preliminary data with the atypical neuroleptics indicate a lower risk for TD with an expectant fall in the incidence of TD. However, most of the studies to date are of relatively short follow-up periods that do not allow any confident predictions for the development of TD [64].

Table 5. Summary of longitudinal studies of incidence of tardive dyskinesia in schizophrenia patients

Authors	N	Years	Risk/year	5-year risk
Gibson, 1981 [65]	343	3	5.6%	24.4%
Kane et al., 1984 [66]	554	7	3.9%	17.8%
Yassa & Nair, 1984 [67]	108	2	3.9%	17.8%
Chouinard et al., 1986 [68]	131	5	8.7%	35.1%
Morgenstern & Glazer, 1993 [69]	398	5	8.7%	35.1%
[1]Jeste et al., 1995 [61]	266	3	20%	>60%
[2]Chakos et al., 1996 [70]	118	4	5.2%	19.5%
[3]Caligiuri et al., 1997 [71]	378	3	7.6%	22.9%
[1]Woerner et al., 1998 [72]	261	3	17.6%	53%

[1]Elderly neuropsychiatric patients; [2]First-onset schizophrenic patients followed-up; [3]Severe tardive dyskinesia only

Risk Factors

A large number of risk factors for TD have been identified, although in the individual patient it is still not possible to predict the onset of this side effect. The more salient risk factors are listed in Table 6. Advancing *age* is the most consistently established risk factor for TD, and there appears to be a linear correlation between age and both the prevalence and severity of TD [73]. TD in the elderly is also more likely to affect the oro-buccal-facial-lingual musculature, develop early in the course of neuroleptic treatment and be irreversible. The elderly also show a higher frequency of abnormal movements from other causes [74]. While TD has been reported in children and adolescents, it is considered to be uncommon [75], but adequate epidemiological studies are few. Rates of withdrawal-emergent dyskinesia of 8% [76] and 51% [77] have been reported in two studies of children on long-term neuroleptics. A number of studies have indicated a higher risk for women to develop TD, but other studies have either failed to find an association or have conversely reported a higher risk for men [78].

Of the other risk factors, the dose, type and duration of neuroleptic drug use deserve special mention. Recent longitudinal studies have provided that empirical support for higher dose increasing the risk [71,79]. There is no convincing evidence that once drug dosage has been accounted for, any of the conventional neuroleptics presents a differentially smaller risk; nor is there empirical evidence that depot neuroleptics are more likely to cause TD [80]. However, atypical neuroleptics as a class have much lower propensity for causing TD. While there are anecdotal reports of TD with risperidone, olanzapine and quetiapine, there is no convincing report of TD with clozapine monotherapy and this may indeed be the safest drug [81].

Table 6. Risk factors for tardive dyskinesia

1. Increasing age
2. Women in older age group
3. Race: higher in African Americans; possibly lower in Asians
4. Neuroleptic drugs:
    a. Higher dose
    b. Longer duration
    c. Type of drug (Atypical > Typical)
    d. Later age of initiation of treatment
    e. Drug holidays (nil or increased risk)
    f. History of early extrapyramidal side effects
5. Other drugs:
    g. Lithium: no increased risk or protective?
    h. Anticholinergic drugs: worsen manifestation but not increased risk
    i. Tricyclics or SSRIs: can rarely cause TD
6. Diagnosis:
    j. Negative schizophrenia with cognitive deficits
    k. Affective disorder
    l. Brain damage (dementia, trauma, epilepsy etc.)
    m. Mental retardation
7. Genetic factors: poorly understood
    n. Poor metabolisers (low CYP2D6 activity)
    o. Certain DRD2 and D3 polymorphisms
8. Other risk factors:
    p. Diabetes mellitus
    q. Alcohol abuse
    r. Smoking
    s. Dental status – ill-fitting dentures, edentulous status

EXAMPLE 3

Tourette Syndrome

Tourette Syndrome (TS), named after the French neurologist Gilles de la Tourette, is a neuropsychiatric disorder par excellence. It is currently recognised as a childhood onset disorder with a strong genetic basis and characterized by the presence of multiple motor and at least one vocal tic which are present for at least one year (DSM-IV) [11]. The disorder was once considered to be quite rare. The earlier prevalence rates were based on large registries of patients, and an often quoted figure was 1 per 2000 individuals [82]. More systematic studies performed recently have subsequently shown that this was an under-estimate.

An early population-based study was conducted in the Israeli army in which all young recruits were assessed for TS, and a prevalence of 4.28 per 10,000 was reported [83]. A study performed in south-eastern USA interviewed 4,500 children aged 9, 11 and 13 years and reported a prevalence rate of 0.1% [84].

More recent prevalence studies have been conducted in schools, and a summary of these is presented in Table 7. Four of these studies have been in large representative populations and have used multiple sources of information. The studies generally use a two-stage procedure - an initial screening followed by direct interview of the subject. The screening procedures may vary, and include questionnaires filled by the children and/or their parents and teachers, as well as direct observation of children in the classroom. The variations in rates may be explained to some extent by these methodological differences. The suggested prevalence from these studies is between 0.6% and 1% of children aged 5-17 years. The total prevalence of tic disorders, of which TS is the more sever form, was much higher – 6.6% in the Swedish study [85] and 2.9% in the Italian study [86].

The prevalence of tic disorders and TS is even higher in certain select populations. In a study in a Californian school district, of 3034 pupils referred for psycho-educational assessments, 28% were reported to have a history of tics and 12% met criteria for TS [69]. In a study from West Essex, UK [88], students with behavioural and emotional problems were noted to have tics in 65% cases, whereas those with learning difficulties had a prevalence of 24%, with other problems 6%, compared to no tics in children with any problems. TS does not, however, appear to be over-represented in adult psychiatric inpatients [88].

Table 7. Prevalence of TS in mainstream school populations (after Lanzi et al)

Author	Country	Age (yrs)	Sample Size	Procedure	Prevalence (%)
Kurlan et al (1994) [89]	USA	7-14	35	Observation + interview	3.0
Mason et al (1998) [90]	UK	13-14	166	Self-report, parents' Q, teachers' Q, and observation	2.9
	Sweden	11	435	Clinical examination	0.15-1.1
Kadesjo and Gillberg (2000) [85]	UK	13-14	918	Self-report, parents' Q, teachers' Q, and two interviews	0.76-1.85
Hornsey et al (2001) [91]	USA	8.5-17.5	1255	Interviews	3.8
	Italy	6-11	2347	Classroom and observation	0.68
Kurlan et al (2001) [92]					
Lanzi et al (2004) [86]					

CONCLUSION

The three examples above represent the challenges to neuropsychiatric epidemiology and how different solutions have emerged, depending upon the nature of the disorder being addressed. In the case of epilepsy and psychosis, epidemiological studies have the promise of informing the pathophysiology of schizophrenia. In tardive dyskinesia, there are clear implications for the treatment of psychiatric patients, and in the epidemiology of Tourette Syndrome, we see the relevance to service planning. Many other neuropsychiatric disorders could similarly benefit from informed epidemiology. Problems with definition continue to confound the epidemiology of many neuropsychiatric disorders, such as attention deficit hyperactivity disorder, chronic fatigue syndrome, etc. Other syndromes, such as delirium, are very common but under-recognised, and epidemiological studies can further emphasize their importance, and suggest pathophysiological mechanisms. Some disorders, such as early-onset dementia, are uncommon but their public health impact is out of proportion to their prevalence. Further systematic epidemiological studies can signal the maturity of the discipline of neuropsychiatry.

ACKNOWLEDGEMENTS

I would like to thank Dr ES Krishnamoorthy for his contribution to this chapter and Ms Angie Russell for manuscript preparation.

REFERENCES

[1]   Sachdev, P. S. Whither Neuropsychiatry? *J Neuropsychiatry Clin Neurosci* 2005;17:140-144.

[2]   Dohrenwend, B. P., & Dohrenwend, B.S. Perspectives on the past and future of psychiatric epidemiology. The 1981 Rema Lapouse lecture. *Am J Pub Health* 1982;72:1271-1279.

[3]   Terris M. (ed). *Goldberger on Pellagra*. Baton Rouge: Louisiana State University Press, 1964.

[4]   American Psychiatric Association. *Diagnostic and Statistical Manual of Mental Disorders* (1st edn). (DSM-I). Washington, DC: American Psychiatric Association, 1952.

[5]   Feighner, J. P., Robins, E., Guze, S. B., et al. Diagnostic criteria for use in psychiatric research. *Arch Gen Psychiatry* 1972;26:57-63.

[6]   Sachdev, P. A critique of 'organic' and its proposed alternatives. *Aust N Z J Psychiatry*1996; 30:165-170.

[7]   World Health Organisation. *International classification of diseases and health related problems* (10th edn). Geneva: World Health Organisation, 2000.

[8]   Sander, J. W. & Shorvon, S. D. Epidemiology of the epilepsies. *J Neurol, Neurosurg Psychiatry* 1996;61:433-443.

[9]   Spitzer, R. L., Williams, J. B. W., Gibbon, M., et al. The Structured Clinical Interview for DSM-III-R (SCID). I: History, rationale and description. *Arch Gen Psychiatry* 1992;49:624-629.

[10] Krishnamoorthy, E. S. (2000). An approach to classifying neuropsychiatric disorders in epilepsy. *Epilep Behav* 2000;1:373-377.

[11] American Psychiatric Association. *Diagnostic and statistical manual of mental disorders* (4th edn). Text revision (DSM-IV-TR). Washington, DC: American Psychiatric Association, 2000.

[12] Slater, E., Beard, A., Gilthero, E. The schizophrenia-like psychoses of epilepsy. *British Journal of Psychiatry* 1963;109:95-150.

[13] Stevens, J. R. "Psychosis and the temporal lobe" In Smith, D., Treiman, D., Trimble, M. (eds). *Neurobehavioral problem in Epilepsy: Advances in Neurology*. New York: Raven Press.1991:79-96.

[14] Hauser, W. A., Annegess, J. F., Rocca, W. A. Descriptive epidemiology of epilepsy – contributions of population-based studies from Rochester, Minnesota. *Mayo Clinical Proceedings* 1996;71:576-586.

[15] Jeste, D.V. & Wyatt, R.J. *Understanding and treating tardive dyskinesia*. New York: Guildford Press, 1982.

[16] Qin, P., Xu, H., Laursen, T. M., et al. Risk for schizophrenia and schizophrenia-like psychosis among patients with epilepsy: population based cohort study. *Br Med J* doi:10.1136/bmj.38488.462037.8F, 2005.

[17] Gibbs, F. A., Gibbs, E. L. Atlas of Electroencephalography, Vol. 11: Epilepsy. Cambridge, Mass: Addison-Wesley, 1952.

[18] Currie, S., Heathfield, K. W. G., Henson, R. A., et al. Clinical course and prognosis of temporal lobe epilepsy. *Brain* 1971;94:173-190.

[19] Standage, K. F., & Fenton, G. W. Psychiatric profiles of patients with epilepsy: a controlled investigation. *Psychol Med* 1975;5:152-160.

[20] Mendez, M. F., Grau, R., Doss, R. C. et al. Schizophrenia in epilepsy: seizure and psychosis variables. *Neurology* 1993;43;1073-1077.

[21] Schmitz, B., & Wolf, P. Psychosis in epilepsy: frequency and risk factors. *J Epilepsy* 1995;8:295-305.

[22] Onuma, T., Adachi, N., Ishida, S., et al. Prevalence and annual incidence of psychoses in patients with epilepsy. *Epilepsia* 1995;32 (Suppl 3):S218.

[23] Krohn, W. (1961). A study of epilepsy in Northern Norway: its frequency and character. *Acta Psychiatr Scand* 1961;150:215-225.

[24] Gudmundsson, G. Epilepsy in Iceland – a clinical and epidemiological investigation. *Acta Neurol Scand* 1966;25:1-124.

[25] Kat, W. Uber den Gegensatz Epilepsie-Schizophrenie und das kombinieerte Vorkommen dieser Krankheiten (Antagonism between epilepsy and schizophrenia and simultaneous occurrence of these diseases). *Psychiatr en Eurol Bl* 1937;41:733-745.

[26] Davison, K., & Bagley, C. R. Schizophrenia-like psychosis associated with organic disorder of the central nervous system: a review of the literature. In Herrington, R. N.

(ed). *Current Problems in Neuropsychiatry: British Journal of Psychiatry Special Publication 4*. Ashford, Kent, England: Headley Brothers, 1969:1-45.

[27] Betts, T. A. Epilepsy and the mental hospital. In Reynolds, E. H., Trimble, M. R. (eds). *Epilepsy and Psychiatry*. Edinburgh: Churchill Livingstone, 1981:175-184.

[28] Lindsay, J., Ounstead, C., Richards, P. Long term outcome in children with temporal lobe seizures. III: psychiatric aspects in childhoold and adult life. *Develop Med Child Neurol* 1979;21:630-636.

[29] Taylor, D. C. Factors influencing the occurrence of schizophrenia-like psychosis in patients with temporal lobe epilepsy. *Psychol Med* 1975;5:249-254.

[30] Kristensen, O. & Sindrup, H. H. (1987). Psychomotor epilepsy and psychosis. *Acta Neurol Scand* 1987;57:361-379.

[31] Toone, B. K., Garralda, M. E., Ron, M. A. The psychoses of epilepsy and the functional psychoses. *Br J Psychiatry* 1982;141;256-261.

[32] Perez, M. M., Trimble, M. R., Murray, N. M. F. et al. Epileptic psychosis: an evaluation of PSE profiles. *Br J Psychiatry* 1985:146;155-163.

[33] Shorvon, S. D. Epidemiology, classification, natural history, and genetics of epilepsy. *Lancet* 1990;336:93-96.

[34] Lindsay, J., Ounstead, C., Richards, P. Long term outcome in children with temporal lobe seizures. III: Psychiatric aspects in childhood and adult life. *Develop Med Child Neurol* 1979;21:630-636.

[35] Perez, M. M., Trimble, M. R. Epileptic psychosis-diagnostic comparison with process schizophrenia. *Br J Psychiatry* 1980;137:245-249.

[36] Hermann B. P., Dikmen, S., Schwartz, M. S. et al. Interictal psychopathology in patients with ictal fear: a quantitative investigation. *Neurology* 1982;32:7-11.

[37] Bruton, C. J., Stevens, J. R., Frith, C. D. Epilepsy, psychosis, and schizophrenia: clinical and neuropathologic correlations. *Neurology* 1994;44:34-42.

[38] Flor-Henry, P. Psychosis and temporal lobe epilepsy. *Epilepsia* 1969;10:363-395.

[39] Shukla, G. D., Srivastava, O. N., Katiyar, B. C., et al. Psychiatric manifestations of temporal lobe epilepsy: a control study. *Br J Psychiatry* 1979;135:411-417.

[40] Currie, S., Heathfield, K. W. G., Henson, R. A. et al. Clinical course and prognosis of temporal lobe epilepsy. *Brain* 1971;94:173-190.

[41] Wolf, P. "Acute behavioural symptomatology at disappearance of epileptiform EEG abnormality: paradoxical or "forced" normalization" In Smith, D., Treiman, D., Trimble M. (eds). *Neurobehavioral Problems in Epilepsy: Advances in Neurology* Vol.55. New York: Raven Press, 1991:127-142.

[42] Conlon, P., Trimble, M. R., Rogers, D. A study of spileptic psychosis using magnetic resonance imaging. *Br J Psychiatry* 1990;156:231-235.

[43] Gallhofer, B., Trimble, M. R., Frackowiak, R. et al A study of cerebral blood flow and metabolism in epileptic psychosis using positron emission tomography and oxygen. *J Neurol, Neurosurg Psychiatry* 1985;48:201-206.

[44] Marshall, J. E., Syed, G. M. B., Fenwick, P. B. C. et al A pilot study of schizophrenia-like psychosis in epilepsy using single-photo emission computerised tomography. *Br J Psychiatry* 1993;163:32-36.

[45] Roberts, G. W., Done, D. J., Bruton, C., et al. A "mock up" of schizophrenia: temporal lobe epilepsy and schizophrenia-like psychosis. *Biological Psychiatry* 1990;28:127-154.

[46] Shaw, P., Mellers, J., Henderson, M., et al. Schizophrenia-like psychosis arising de novo following a temporal lobectomy: timing and factors. *J Neurol Neurosurg Psychiatry* 2004;75:1003-1008.

[47] Schooler, N.R. & Kane, J.M. Research diagnosis for tardiv dyskineasia. *Archif Gen Psychiatry* 1982;39:486-487.

[48] Kane, J.M. & Smith, J. Tardive dyskinesia: prevalence of risk factors 1959-1979. *Arch Gen Psychiatry* 1982;39:473-481.

[49] Yassa, R. & Jeste, D.V. Gender differences in tardive dyskinesia: a critical review of the literature. *Schizophr Bull* 1992;18:701-715.

[50] Woerner, M.G., Kane, J.M., Lieberman, J.A., et al. The prevalence of tardive dyskinesia. *J Clin Psychopharm* 1991;11:34-42.

[51] Muscettola, G., Pampallona, S., Barbato, G., et al Persistent tardive dyskinesia: demographic and pharmacological risk factors. *Acta Psychiatr Scand* 1993;87:29-36.

[52] Klawans, H. L., Barr, A. Prevalence of spontaneous lingual-facial-buccal dyskinesias in the elderly. *Neurology* 1982;32:558-559.

[53] Kane, J. M., Weinhold, P., Kinon, B., et al. Prevalence of abnormal involuntary movements ("spontaneous dyskinesias") in the normal elderly. *Psychopharm* 1982;77:105-108.

[54] Waddington, J. L., Crow, T. J. "Abnormal involuntary movements and psychosis in the preneuroleptic era and in unmedicated patients: Implications for the concept of tardive dyskinesia" In Wolf, M. E., Mosnaim, A. D (eds.). *Tardive dyskinesia: Biological mechanisms and clinical aspects.* Washington DC: American Psychiatric Press, 1988:49-66.

[55] Magulac, M., Landsverk, J., Golahan, S., et al. Abnormal involuntary movements in neuroleptic-naive children and adolescents. *Canadian J Psychiatry* 1999;44:368-373.

[56] Chong, S-A., Sachdev, P. S. "The epidemiology of tardive dyskinesia." In Sethi, K. D. (ed.). *Drug-induced movement disorders.* New York: Marcel Dekker, 2994:37-60.

[57] Fenton, W.S. Prevalence of spontaneous dyskinesia in schizophrenia. *J Clin Psychiatry* 2000;61(Suppl 4):10-14.

[58] Morgenstern, H., Glazer, W. M. Identifying risk factors of tardive dyskinesia among long-term outpatients maintained with neuroleptic medications. Results of the Yale Tardive Dyskinesia Study. *Arch Gen Psychiatry* 1993;50:723-733.

[59] Kane, J. M., Woerner, M., Weihold, P., et al. Incidence of tardive dyskinesia: five-year data from a prospective study. *Psychopharm Bull* 1984;20:387-389.

[60] Chakos, M. H., Alvir, J. M. J, Woerner, M. G., et al. Incidence and correlates of tardive dyskinesia in first episode of schizophrenia. *Arch Gen Psychiatry* 1996;53:313-319.

[61] Jeste, D. V., Caliguiri, M. P., Paulsen, J.S., et al Risk of tardive dyskinesia in older patients: A prospective longitudinal study of 266 patients. *Arch Gen Psychiatry* 1995;52:756-765.

[62] Saltz, B. L., Woerner, M. G., Kane, J.M. et al. Prospective study of tardive dyskinesia incidence in the elderly. *JAMA* 1991;266:2402-2406.

[63] Jeste, D. V., Lacro, J. P., Palmer, B., et al. Incidence of Tardive Dyskinesia in early stages of low-dose treatment with typical neuroleptics in older patients. *Am J Psychiatry* 1999;156:309-311.

[64] Barnes, T. R., McPhillips, M. A. Critical analysis and comparison of the side-effect and safety profiles of the new antipsychotics. *Br J Psychiatry* 1999;174(Suppl. 38), 34-43.

[65] Gibson, A. C. Incidence of tardive dyskinesia in patients receiving depot neuroleptic inujection. *Acta Psychiatr Scand* 1981;297:111-116.

[66] Kane, J. M., Woerner, M., Weihold, P., et al. Incidence of tardive dyskinesia: Five-year data from a prospective study. *Psychophar Bull* 1984;20:387-389.

[67] Yassa, R., Nair, V., Schwartz, G. Tardive dyskinesia: A two-year follow-up study. *Psychosomatics* 1984;25:852-855.

[68] Chouinard, G., Annable, L., Mercier, P., et al. A five-year follow-up study of tardive dyskinesia. *Psychopharm Bull* 1986;22:259-263.

[69] Morgenstern, H., Glazer, W. M. (1993). Identifying risk factors of tardive dyskinesia among long-term outpatients maintained with neuroleptic medications. Results of the Yale Tardive Dyskinesia Study. *Arch Gen Psychiatry* 1993;31:723-733.

[70] Chakos, M. H., Alvir, J. M. J., Woerner, M. G., et al. Incidence and correlates of tardive dyskinesia in first episode of schizophrenia. *Arch Gen Psychiatry* 1996;53:313-319.

[71] Caligiuri, M. P., Lacro, J. P., Rockwell, E., et al. Incidence and risk factors for severe tardiv dyskinesia in older patients. *Br J Psychiatry* 1997;171:148-153.

[72] Woener, M. G., Alvir, J. M. J., Saltz, B. L., et al. Prospective study of tardive dyskinesia in the elderly: Rates and risk factors. *Am J Psychiatry* 1998;155:1521-1528.

[73] Smith, J. M., Baldessarini, R.J. (1980). Changes in prevalence, severity and recovery in tardive dyskinesia with age. *Arch GenPsychiatry* 1980;37:1368-1373.

[74] Khot, V., Wyatt, R.J. Not all that moves is tardive dyskinesia. *Am J Psychiatry* 148, 661-666. YEAR

[75] Silverstein, F. S., Johnston, M. V. Risks of neuroleptic in children. *J Child Neurology* 1987;2;41-43.

[76] McDermid, S. A., Hood, J., Bockus, S., et al. Adolescents on neuroleptic medication - is this population at risk of tardive dyskinesia? *Ca J Psychiatry* 1998;43:629-631.

[77] McAndrew, J. B., Case, Q., Treffert, D.A. Effects of prolonged phenothiazine intake on psychotic and other hospitalized children. *J Autism Child Schizophr* 1972;2:75-91.

[78] Van Os, J., Walsh, E., Van Horn, E., et al. on behalf of the UK700 Group. Tardive dyskinesia in psychosis: are women really more at risk? *Acta Psychiatr Scand* 1999;99:288-293.

[79] Waddington, J. L. Schizophrenia, affective psychoses and other disorders treated with neuroleptic drugs: the engima of tardive dyskinesia, its neurological determinants and the conflict of paradigms. *Intl Rev Neurobiol* 1989;31:297-353.

[80] Kane, J. M., Jeste, D. V., Barnes, T. R. E, et al (eds). *Tardive dyskinesia: A task force report of the American Psychaitric Association.* Washington DC: American Psychiatric Press, 1992.

[81] Spivak, B., Mester, R., Abesgaus, J. Clozapine treatment for neuroleptic induced tardive dyskinesia, parkinsonism, and chronic akathisia in schizophrenic patients. *Journal of Clinical Psychiatry* 1997;58:318-322.

[82] Brunn, R. D. Gilles de la Toureete's syndrome: an overview of clinical experience. *J Am Acad Child Psychiatry* 1984;23:126-133.

[83] Apter, A., Pauls, D. L., Bleich, A., et al. (1992). A population-based epidemiological study of Tourette syndrome among adolescents in Israel. *Advan Neurology* 1992;58:61-65.

[84] Costello, E. J., Angold, A., Burns, B. J., et al. The Great Smoky Mountains Study of Youth. Goals, design, methods, and the prevalence of DSM-III-R disorders. *Arch Gen Psychiatry* 1996;53:129-1136.

[85] Kadesjo, B., & Gillberg, C. Tourette's disorder: epidemiology and comorbidity in primary school children. *J Am Acad Child Adoles Psychiatry* 2000;39:548-555.

[86] Lanzi, G., Zambrina, C. A., Termine C., et al. Prevalence of tic disorders among primary school students in the city of Pavia, Italy. *Arch Dis Child* 2004;89:45-47.

[87] Comings, D. E., Hines, J. A., Comings, B. G. An epidemiologic study of Tourette's syndrome in a single school district. *J Clin Psychiatry* 1990;51:563-569.

[88] Eapen, V., Robertson, M. M., Zeitlin, H. et al. Gilles de la Tourette's syndrome in special education schools: a United Kingdom study. *J Neurol* 1997;244:378-382.

[89] Kurlan, R., Whitmore, D., Irvine, C., et al. Tourette's syndrome in a special education population: a pilot study involving a single school district. *Neurology* 1994;44:699-702.

[90] Mason, A., Banerjee, S., Eapen, V., et al. (1998). The prevalence of Tourette syndrome in a mainstream school population. *Develop Med Child Neurol* 1998;40:292-296.

[91] Hornsey, H., Banerjee, S., Zeitlin, H., et al. The prevalence of Tourette syndrome in 13-14 year old in mainstream schools. *J Child Psychol Psychiatry* 2001;42:1035-1039.

[92] Kurlan, R., McDermott, M. P., Deeley, C., et al. Prevalence of tics in school children and association with placement in special education. *Neurology* 2001;57:1381-1388.

RECOMMENDED FURTHER READING

1. Yudofsky, S. C., Hales, R.E. (eds). *American Psychiatric Publishing Textbook of Neuropsychiatry and Clinical Neurosciences*, 4th edition. Washington DC: American Psychiatric Association Publishing, 2002.

2. Lishman, W. A. *Organic Psychiatry*, ed 3 Oxford: Blackwell Scientific, 1998.

3. Foge, B. S., Schiffer RB, Rao SM (eds.). *Neuropsychiatry: A comprehensive textbook*, 2nd edition. Baltimore: Lippincott Williams and Wilkins, 2003.

4. Coffey, C. E., Cumming, J. L. (eds.) *The American Psychiatric Press Textbook of Geriatric Neuropsychiatry*. Washington, DC: American psychiatric Publishing, 2000.

5. Trimble, M. R., Schmitz, B. (eds.) *The Neuropsychiatry of Epilepsy*. Cambridge, UK: Cambridge University Press, 2000.

6. Robinson, R.G. *The Clinical Neuropsychiatry of Stroke: Cognitive, Behavioral and Emotional Disorders Following Vascular Brain Injury.* Cambridge, UK: Cambridge University Press, 1998.

7. Mesulam, M-M. (ed.) *Principles of Behavioral and Cognitive Neurology.* New York: Oxford University Press, 2000.

8. Lezak, M. D., Howieson, D. B., Loring, D. W., Hannay, H. J., Fischer, J. S. *Neuropsychological assessment.* New York: Oxford University Press, 2004.

9. Heilman, K. M., Valenstein, E. (eds.) Clinical Neuropsychology, 4th edition. New York: Oxford University Press, 2003.

10. Sachdev, P. S. (ed.) *The Ageing Brain.* Lisse, Netherlands: Swets & Zeitlinger, 2003.

In: Handbook of Clinical Neuroepidemiology   ISBN 978-1-60021-511-7
Editors: V. L. Feigin and D. A. Bennett, pp. 527-556   © 2007 Nova Science Publishers, Inc.

Chapter 15

PARKINSON'S DISEASE

Yacov Balash[1] and Amos D. Korczyn[2]

[1]Movement Disorders Unit, Department of Neurology, Tel-Aviv Sourasky Medical
Center, Tel-Aviv, Israel;
[2]Sieratzki Chair of Neurology, Tel-Aviv University Medical School, Ramat-Aviv, Israel.

ABSTRACT

The etiology and pathogenesis of Parkinson's disease (PD) are remain unclear and calls for intensive researches, especially with the growing proportion of elderly people and related rising of PD incidence worldwide. In this chapter we considere a modern descriptive and analytic studies in epidemiology of PD. Marked methodological differences in the descriptive studies with absence of unified epidemiological approach should be underlined. These studies have substantial differences in numbers of prevalence and incidence of PD, and did not expose neither endemic nor racial predominance of PD around the world. Despite the fact that the twin studies stated that the major factors in the etiology of PD are probably non-genetic, the genetic component in the PD pathogenesis is suggested to be an important. Indeed the statistically significant associations were found between PD and some of genetic factors like alpha–synuclein, parkin, LARRK2, glucocerebrosidase, protein Tau H1 haplotype, debrisoquine hydroxlase in cytochrome P450D6 (CYP2D6) and apolipoprotein E. However, these studies did not examine family members and failed to reveal family aggregation for the typical (late onset) PD. From another side, numerous environmental factors like exposure to pesticides, herbicides, insecticides, fungicides, farm residence, and/or farming, welding; solvents are considered a probable cause of PD. However, the results of the above mentioned analytic studies are contradictory and cannot be considered as evidence based. To our knowledge the main reason explaining this complex situation is a lack of biological marker of PD suitable for epidemiologic studies, which could distinguish PD from other various kinds of parkinsonism and improve quality of epidemiological studies and its significance. Further fundamental studies are warranted to elucidate the causes of PD and its relationships to neurobiology of ageing.

INTRODUCTION

Epidemiological studies in Parkinson's disease (PD) have a great potential as tools for exploring PD etiology as well as for the identification of risk factors, and may lead to the development of rational preventative approaches for the disease. They are also important in the planning and development of services for affected individuals.

Currently PD is conceived as a slowly progressive neurodegenerative disease of unknown etiology. The symptoms result from the death of selected populations of neurons, first in the dorsal vagal nuclei and the olfactory bulb, later in some other catecholaminergic and serotoninergic brain-stem nuclei and subsequently in the neuromelanin-containing dopaminergic neurons of the pars compacta of the substantia nigra (SN), the cholinergic nucleus basalis of Meynert, hypothalamic neurons, and small cortical neurons (particularly in the cingulate gyrus and entorhinal cortex) [1]. Alpha-synuclein immunoreactive inclusions are found in the gastric myenteric and submucosal (Meissner's and Auerbach's) plexuses, whose axons project into the gastric mucosa [2]. Sympathetic ganglia and parasympathetic neurons in the gut are also affected [3].

There is no adequate (sensitive, specific, inexpensive and repeatable) biological marker for PD, which can be used for epidemiological studies. Such markers are important to exclude people presenting with parkinsonian symptoms due to causes other the PD, and to identify presymptomatic cases or those in an early stage in whom the disease can be suspected although they still do not fulfill clinical criteria (such as monosymptomatic cases). Methods of early, pre-motor diagnosis of PD such us smell tests, ultrasonography of brain parenchyma, or brain PET or SPECT are either not sufficiently sensitive or specific, or are too complex and expensive to be used in epidemiological studies.

The diagnosis of PD in clinical practice is based on a combination of cardinal signs - bradykinesia, extrapyramidal rigidity, 4-6 Hz rest tremor, impairment of postural reflexes and good response to levodopa. The accuracy and validity of this method was determined by clinico-pathological correlations, performed in the UK by PD society Brain Bank investigators [4]. The presence of three cardinal features except for postural instability has a sensitivity of 0.65 and a specificity of 0.71. Asymmetrical onset with absence of atypical features improved both sensitivity and specificity to 0.75. In another series, 20 percent of patients diagnosed in life as having PD had some other diagnoses, usually some form of atypical parkinsonism, at autopsy [5]. However, the clinical diagnosis can only be made late in the course of the disease and it is critically dependent on the professionalism of the neurological examination. For community studies of PD the sensitivity can be increased by reducing the number of required criteria to two (or even one), obviously at the cost of reduced specificity, as shown by de Rijk et al [6].

These results highlight the possibility that some cases of atypical parkinsonism (multiple system atrophy, vascular parkinsonism, progressive supranuclear palsy etc.) may be erroneously diagnosed as PD. Inclusion of these cases in risk factor studies lessen the likelihood that a variable associated with PD can be identified. Their inclusion in genetic studies may lead to erroneous conclusions about the contribution of heredity.

At present, an increasing number of genetic causes of parkinsonism are being recognized [7], and a conservative estimate suggests that about 10 per cent of cases are genetically determined. Obviously, inclusion of such cases in studies exploring possible environmental factors of PD might introduce noise, while it is justified to include them in studies related to health expenditures and planning.

The existence of a long presymptomatic phase of PD proven by Braak [1] also complicates the identification of environmental risk factors. For example, if the presymptomatic stage is 10 years or longer as many investigators believe, then inclusion of this decade in the period in which exposure is being studied (as done e.g. by Przuntek et al, [8]) is inappropriate, while recollection of earlier exposures may be biased and lead to mistakes. Similarly, the identification of familial patterns of disease is made difficult when pathologically affected family members die before clinical signs become apparent. The late onset of PD also complicates genetic investigations, because few families will include living ancestors and data on abnormalities in previous generations, if available, may not be accurate. For example, if a parent is said to have had tremor, it will be almost impossible to know whether this was parkinsonian or essential tremor (the latter being more common than PD in the general population). As a result, clinical information and diagnostic accuracy are limited for ancestors.

Nevertheless, the findings of studies on the epidemiology of PD are supported when examining the ageing of the populations in industrialized and developing countries, which show an increasing PD prevalence, and economic and social burden of the disease. A report prepared for the US PD Foundation in 1998 indicated that in 1997 the averaged annual individual costs related to PD were about $24,000. Only one third of this sum was related to direct medical expenditures such as clinic visits, hospitalizations, physical therapy, assisted living and nursing home care. Drug costs accounted for $2137, and the remainder, $15,169 per patient per year, came from indirect costs such as loss of productivity [9]. In Europe in 1994-2005, the total direct costs per year were € 4710-8160 and indirect ones were € 5810-6590 [10].

PREVALENCE

Prevalence is the total number of cases in a population at a given time. Roughly, 0.3% of the population, or near a million persons, suffers with PD in the USA alone. The prevalence of PD increases with age (Figure 1). In individuals over 65 years of age the prevalence rises to as high as 3%, and in individuals 80 years and older, the prevalence may be as high as 10% [11]. The increasing of PD prevalence with ageing is a general common feature.

Comparison of prevalence of PD around the world gives variable results, which do not lead to simple conclusions about endemic foci of PD and do not establish obvious racial, social or cultural differences. For example, crude prevalence rates of PD as high as 786.8 and 1507.5/100000 for population aged ≥ 55 years were reported in prospective population–based cohort studies conducted in Spain and the Netherlands [13,14].

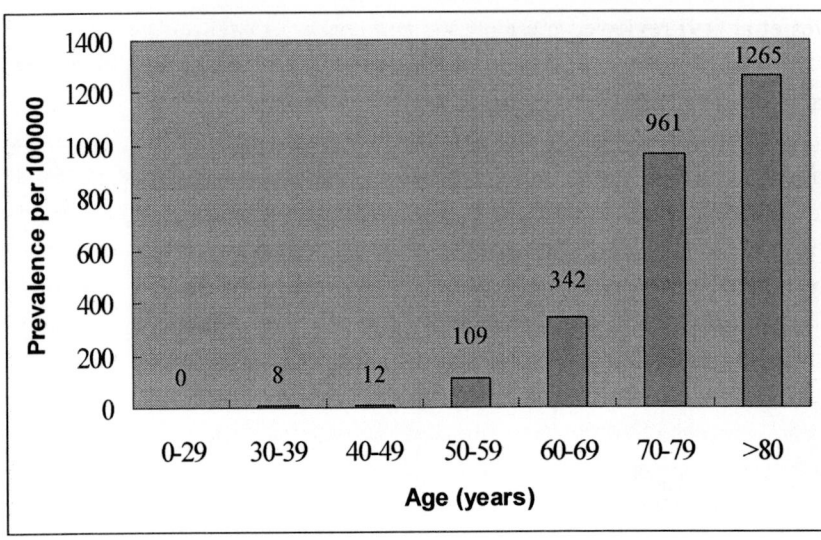

Figure 1. Age and prevalence for PD (Schrag et al, 2005 [12])

While comparison of prevalence may theoretically provide useful clues to the etiology, the accuracy of prevalence estimation needs to be considered. Prevalence can be affected by the incidence of the disease and survival after diagnosis, but confounding factors and methodological issues such as difference in study design and diagnostic criteria, as well as the experience of the examiners, affect the results [15].

Considerably high degree of geographical variability, various methods of screening and diagnostic criteria, more or less intensive methods of case-finding, absence of standardized international questionnaires, different age distribution etc. gives these heterogeneous results only modest value.

An example for this statement is a comparison between two careful studies of PD prevalence in China, performed in 1993 [16] and 2005 [17] by the same investigators. The latter study used trained neurologists and revealed considerably higher prevalence rates of PD [17].

INCIDENCE

Incidence is a more relevant estimate of disease frequency when attempting to identify risk factors, as it is the measure of the number of new cases occurring in a given time period for a specific location, and it is relatively unaffected by survival. The incidence rates for PD range from 4.5-21 new cases for 100,000 people per year, reflecting variations in study design, ascertainment methods, case definition, and age distribution [18]. It is estimated that 50,000 to 60,000 new cases of PD are diagnosed each year in the United States alone [11].

Incidence of PD is harder to establish then prevalence because it requires repeated screenings of larger populations, and attempts to identify missing cases as these could bias the results. In addition, diagnostic accuracy is lower early in the disease. Case ascertainment methods, such as review of hospital records, tend to underestimate the true number of cases.

Twelves et al [19] reviewed the methods and results of twenty-five incidence studies of PD. Each of them used different methods to identify PD patients, although most screened both primary care and hospital records. Only eight studies were prospective, and only two of them had a follow-up evaluation. The diagnostic criteria for PD varied (11 studies used two or more cardinal motor features, four used the UK Brain Bank criteria), as did the exclusion criteria and the definition of an incident case. Only 16 studies included a movement disorders specialist as part of the study team to support the clinical diagnosis. Five studies were sufficiently similar to merit comparison. Four of these gave a similar incidence (16-19/100000/year), but one from Italy had a much lower incidence (8.4/100000), the reason for which was unclear. This review highlighted the difficulties in performing good quality studies of incidence of PD and recommended a set of criteria, which would improve the consistency of such studies (size of screened population - 250,000 to 500,000 people, prospective study; screening of parkinsonian symptoms with validated questionnaires, participation of movement disorder specialist for the confirmation of the diagnosis, using the UK Brain Bank diagnostic criteria, follow up study for providing information on levodopa efficacy, unified age stratification).

Mayeux et al. [20] developed a registry of PD patients drawing on a diverse group of sources ranging from hospital and administrative billing records to private practitioner office records and rosters from senior centers in the geographical area of Northern Manhattan, New York. Using this registry, this group found an overall incidence of PD of 13 new cases per 100,000 persons per year. This figure is probably an underestimation since many cases remain undiagnosed particularly among the elderly.

MORTALITY

In theory, mortality data should provide figures similar to incidence data. However, this assumption depends on the source of information. Death certificates are relatively inaccurate, particularly if death occurred because of an unrelated illness (e.g. myocardial infarction, where cardiovascular disorders such as hypertension are mentioned as underlying causes rather than PD, particularly if the latter was not severe). If autopsy data are used, the differences between clinical and pathological diagnoses will also complicate the analysis.

Increased number of deaths resulting from PD from 16959 to 17898 was registered in the USA in 2002 and 2003, respectively, corresponding to age-adjusted death rates of 5.9 to 6.1 per 100,000 populations [21]. Therefore, the increased number of deaths could be accounted for the ageing of the population. PD individuals, compared with reference subjects, showed a 1.5 – 2 increased risk of death [14,22,23]. In Chinese population of the Ilan county, Taiwan, the relative risk of death for PD cases versus non-PD cases was 3.38 (95% CI: 2.05-4.34) [24]. Pneumonia and cachexia were the most common causes of death among PD patients [23]. PD patients have also an increased risk of dementia (hazard ratio 2.8; 95% CI: 1.8-4.4) and in turn increased mortality risk [25], although this is not always seen [26]. In absence of dementia the hazard risk was modest and depended on the duration of PD (HR increase per year = 1.03; 95% CI, 0.99-1.07 [25]. Depression was another independent predictor of mortality in PD with risk rate as high as 2.66 (95% CI: 1.59-4.44) [27,28].

AGE AND PD

PD is rare before age 40, and becomes increasingly common through subsequent decades. The peaks of incidence and prevalence are between 70-79 years of age. Although some studies have found lower PD prevalence in the very elderly, this is possibly because of the difficulties to identify parkinsonism in very old patients. In addition, the accuracy of the diagnosis may be limited in old age because of the common existence of co-morbidities, particularly vascular brain disease and dementia and the difficulty to differentiate bradykinesia because the slowness that occurs commonly in older people, as well as postural instability which in old people is frequently multicausal. Low neuron density in the ventro-lateral quadrant of the substantia nigra was revealed on autopsy in elderly persons aged 74-97 years even without a diagnosis PD in life, but with certain signs of extrapyramidal disease [29]. This finding may be the basis for parkinsonian signs in the elderly, but again raises the question of the diagnostic criteria and the accuracy of PD diagnosis in the absence of biological criteria. For example, should we give bradykinesia or postural instability the same weight in an octogenarian as we do in a 50 year old person? Nevertheless, the question of whether incidence increases in the ninth or tenth decade of life has important implications to the understanding of the disease pathogenic mechanisms, as well as to the planning of services in a world in which the population of that age increases in absolute numbers and even more proportionately.

GENDER

Some gender differences in the prevalence of PD have been reported previously in epidemiological studies in Europe and the USA, which have established that the prevalence of PD is higher among men than women [12,14,30].

A meta-analysis of published articles was performed to recognize the differences in incidence of PD between men and women. Seven selected studies that met six stringent inclusion criteria (publication after 1980 to rule out progressive supranuclear palsy, multiple system atrophy, post-encephalitic parkinsonism etc.; exclusion of secondary parkinsonism; at least 50 cases of PD; provision of data on the sex of the probands; inclusion of age groups; based on general population). As a result significantly higher incidence rate of PD was found among men (relative risk =1.49, 95% CI: 1.24-1.95) [31].

The reasons for the increased risk in men are not known, but factors such as toxicant exposure and head trauma in men or neuroprotection by estrogens in women can be considered. However, in Yamagata Prefecture, Japan, (population 1,244.040) the prevalence of PD was 61.3/100,000 for men and 91.0/100,000 for women, showing that women were significantly more affected by PD (p<0.001) [32]. This difference theoretically reflects differential referral to medical services in Japan, although no differences were observed in the men-to-women ratio (which was 1.00:1.04) of all patients in 2 of 12 of randomly selected hospitals in Japan [33]. Another and more interesting option is that Japanese women with PD lived longer than men. However, the male-to-female ratio of the incidence of PD was reported to be 1.0:1.3 in Wakayama, Japan [33]. Therefore, it was concluded that, differently from the prevailing situation in Europe and the USA, PD more frequently affected women than men in Japan.

Early, similar results were obtained in study of Kusumi et al [34] in Yonago City, Japan where prevalence of PD per 100,000 populations was 117.9 (72.8 in males and 159.1 in females), and Morioka et al [33] in Wakayama, where incidence was 16.9 per 100,000 and male to female ratio was 1:1.4.

Japanese observations not withstanding, these data suggest that female hormones might affect PD risks. Indeed, several lines of evidence from human and animal studies suggest a protective role for estrogens in PD. Among women estrogen users with PD were less cognitively impaired and more independent in their activities of daily living. However, more estrogen users were depressed and used antidepressants than non-users [35], and these differences were independent of age. It is assumed that estrogen may have dopamine-sparing properties resulting from inhibition of catechol-O-methyltransferase (COMT) gene expression as well as interaction of the estrogen metabolite, catecholestrogen with the COMT enzyme [36].

On the other hand there are anecdotal observations reporting worsening of PD symptoms during pregnancy and especially in the postpartum period, which possibly may have a long-term adverse effect on the course of the disease [37]. The mechanism underlying the deterioration of PD symptoms and the marked increase in the requirement for levodopa both during pregnancy and in the postpartum period is unknown. The dramatic increase in levodopa dosage in the early postpartum period was suggested to reflect the decline in estrogen levels [38].

Although estrogen therapy has been associated with some positive clinical effects [39], whether estrogen therapy affects the risk of PD is still questionable. In a case-control study, which compared postmenopausal women with PD and control subjects with regard to estrogen exposure, more women were found in the control group who took estrogen than women in the PD group 36 [50%] of 72 women vs. 17 [25%] of 68 women; P<0.003), and those who had taken postmenopausal estrogen were less likely to develop PD than those who had not (OR=0.40; 95% CI: 0.19-0.84, P<0.02). Among PD cases only, postmenopausal estrogen use was not associated with age of onset [40].

The association of postmenopausal hormone use with PD risk was shown to depend on the type of menopause. As opposed to the previous results, among women with a history of hysterectomy with or without an oophorectomy, estrogen use alone was associated with a 2.6-fold increased risk of PD (OR=2.6, 95% CI: 1.1-6.1). In contrast, among women with natural menopause, no increased risk of PD, or a protective effect were observed with hormone use [41].

The conflicting findings suggest that several variables, including age, estrogen dose and formulation, progesterone addition, and timing and length of dosing period, may determine the risks or benefits and their nature. Further investigation is therefore needed to understand the relationship between estrogen and the nigrostriatal dopaminergic system.

RACE/ETHNICITY

Several previous studies have suggested that the prevalence of PD is lower in African Africans and, in addition, that this rate is also lower in African Americans as compared to Caucasians [16,42,43,44]. Critical analysis of this assumption showed that a difference in the prevalence of PD between black and other populations is unproven and requires comprehensive well-designed new studies [45]. In a recent study, the incidence rates by race/ethnicity and gender were studied [46] in the multiracial population of Northern California. The age- and gender-adjusted incidence rates were highest among Hispanics, followed by non-Hispanic Whites, Asians, and Blacks. However, no comparisons of age- and gender-adjusted incidence rates between individual groups were statistically significant (i.e., non-Hispanic White vs. Asian, 13.6 vs. 11.3 per 100,000, p = 0.07; Hispanic vs. Asian, 16.6 vs. 11.3 per 100,000, p = 0.10; non-Hispanic White vs. Black, 13.6 vs.10.2 per 100,000, p = 0.11) (Figure 2, see page 51).

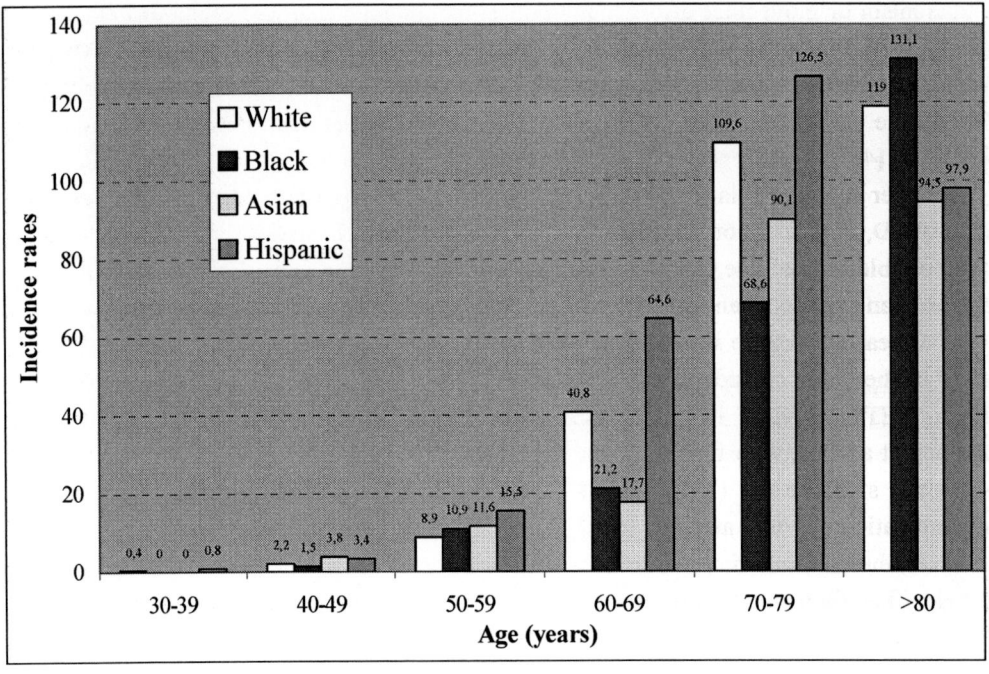

Figure 2. Age-specific and annual incidence rates of PD by gender and race/ethnicity (Van den Eden et al, 2003 [46])

HEREDITY FACTORS

Twin studies are a classic tool for assessing the influence of hereditary factors in diseases. They estimate the relative contribution of genes and environment to PD. If genetics are important, monozygotic (MZ) twins, who are genetically identical, will be concordant considerably more often than dizygotic (DZ) twins [47]. In 1983, the first series of twin studies was published [48]. This study failed to demonstrate differences in concordance between MZ and DZ twins (the latter are expected to show the same frequency of disease as would other siblings, no more than 50% for an autosomal dominant disorder). In the largest twin study Tanner et al. [47] studied 71 MZ and 90 DZ twin pairs. They found no difference in concordance for PD between MZ and DZ co-twins with typical age at onset of the disease, which was 64.5±9.1 years (range: 25-79 years), where pair wise concordance was similar (0.155 MZ and 0.111 DZ; RR=1.39; CI: 0.63-3.1). However, exception was for 16 pairs of PD patients with onset of the disease before age 51 years at least in one of them, where MZ concordance significantly exceeded that of DZ (1.0 MZ and 0.167 DZ; RR=6.0; CI: 1.69-21.26). No evidence for heritability of PD was shown in the recent Swedish twin study, where 247 twins with PD diagnosis in the Inpatient Discharge Register (called "possible PD") and 517 twins who reported parkinsonian symptoms or use of antiparkinsonian medication ("suspected parkinsonism or movement disorder") were identified [49]. For possible PD, there were only two concordant pairs. Similarly, concordances were low in all zygosity groups when the definition of affected was expanded to include twins with suspected parkinsonism or movement disorder in addition to possible PD. The authors found that MZ and DZ twin concordance rates were low (MZ=11%, DZ=8%). The correlations between twins, measured by tetrachoric correlation coefficients were also low (MZ=0.39, DZ=0.28). None of the differences between MZ and DZ concordances or correlations were statistically significant [49].

Another problem relates to the age factor. Even if two siblings are equally genetically prone to PD, they will not necessarily develop clinical manifestations at the same age. So, it is impossible to exclude the possibility that even those co-twins who have no manifest parkinsonian symptoms and signs at the time of a cross-sectional study may develop PD later.

If a mean difference in age of onset of 10 years is hypothesized, this will decrease the power of the study considerably. This can be partially corrected by using ancillary markers such as PET or SPECT imaging of the dopaminergic system. This approach was used by Laihinen et al [50], who found that in the parkinsonian co-twins, the accumulation of [18F] 6-FD was significantly (P < 0.01) decreased in the putamen when compared with the asymptomatic co-twins, and this difference was most pronounced in the posterior putamen. However, the accumulation of [18F] 6-FD in the putamen of the asymptomatic co-twins was also significantly lower than that in normal subjects. The MZ and DZ non-affected subgroups did not differ significantly from each other.

These findings are consistent with possible predominant environmental causes of PD, although cannot exclude all-important genetic contributions including gene-by-environment interactions. However, smaller longitudinal studies do not support the above-mentioned data. The combined concordance levels for subclinical dopaminergic dysfunction diagnosed with [18F] 6-FD PET and clinical PD were 75% in the 12 MZ and 22% in the 9 DZ twin pairs evaluated twice [51]. These contradictory results may reflect differences in the populations studied.

Several other observations have suggested that heredity may be important. Large kindreds with PD in multiple generations were described [52]. Each had clinically atypical features - younger age at onset and more rapid progression - but autopsies in one or two members showed changes resembling in appearance typical PD.

In a case-control study with 722 alive and dead PD patients diagnosed over the last 50 years in Iceland, a grand digital database was used, which contained the genealogy of 610 920 Icelanders over the last 11 centuries. The patients had in-between family relations significantly higher than their control groups. These family relations extended far from the nuclear family. It was concluded that PD should have a genetic component together with an environmental one, which could affect patients in the same family [53].

Family history of PD was shown to be consistently associated with an increased PD risk in a case-control study and in a sample of siblings with the disease [53,54]. One obvious limitation of such studies is the fact that evaluation of cases is usually unblinded. The evaluators are thus aware that the subject they are examining is related to an index PD case.

These thorough studies probably reflect a genetic predisposition to PD. Although other studies have reported that relatives of persons with PD appear to have higher risk for the disorder than do members of the general population, few reported familial cases were evaluated by neurological examination. In some series, subjects were selected by positive family history, raising the question of their representativeness to the entire population [55]. Moreover, families also typically share common living and/or working environments, diets, hobbies and religious habits, any of which might alter exposure to an environmental cause of disease. The Mayo Clinic Family Study of PD [56] investigated the incidence of PD and other neurodegenerative diseases among 1,001 first-degree relatives of 162 patients with PD and 851 relatives of 147 controls representative of the population of Olmsted County, Minnesota, USA. In addition, authors studied 2,713 first-degree relatives of 411 patients with PD referred to the Mayo Clinic as well as a group of 625 spouses of either cases or controls. Using the family study method this work failed to reveal any substantial family PD aggregation. Earlier this group confirmed previous reports suggesting an increased risk of PD among first-degree relatives of probands with younger onset of PD (risk ratio, 2.62; 95% CI, 1.66–4.15), but not among relatives of probands with later onset of PD [57].

These data confirm previous findings of Tanner et al [47] that genetic factor do not play a major in causing PD, but are probably important when the disease begins before age 50 years [58].

Thus, epidemiologic role of genetic factors in PD reported in some studies was not replicated in others and the results concerning heredity of PD in a majority of cases remain indefinite, conflicting, and unclear.

One of the main problems in the genetic studies mentioned so far is that they failed to include molecular genetic analyses. Since several mutations have recently been identified which contribute to dominantly or recessively inherited PD [7,59], these could possibly have been included among some of the familial cases. Inclusion of such families will trivialize the results and would prevent them from being generalizable to "sporadic" PD, although they nay of course indicate common molecular mechanisms.

GENETIC RISK FACTORS RELATED TO SPORADIC PD

The epidemiological "weight" of familial PD is unknown, but no more than 10 % of sporadic patients with PD have affected relatives [60]. Totally, the known and still unknown Mendelian PD genes (either autosomal-dominant or autosomal-recessive) are likely to explain no more than 5–10% of the overall PD population [60] (Table below).

Genes possibly associated with PD

Gene	Inheritance	Pathology	Location	Protein
PARK1	Dominant	Nigral degeneration with Lewy bodies	4q21	Alpha synuclein
PARK2	Recessive	Nigral degeneration without Lewy bodies,	6q25	Parkin
PARK8	Dominant	Variable: alpha synuclein and tau pathology, also Lewy bodies	12cen	LRRK2 (dardarin)
Glucocerebrosidase gene	Recessive	Nigral degeneration with Lewy bodies	1q21	Glucocerebrosidase
Tau gene	Recessive	Neuronal loss and gliosis	17q21	Tau
Debrisoquine hydroxylase gene	Recessive	Degeneration with Lewy bodies	22	Debrisoquine hydroxlase in cytochrome P450 D6 (CYP2D6)

Alpha Synuclein

A new era in PD research emerged in 1997 when a mutation in the α-synuclein gene was shown to cause an autosomal-dominant form of familial PD in a large Greek-Italian family [61]. This family had clinical and pathological features that were similar to typical PD and responded to levodopa. Since then additional mutations have been discovered, providing conclusive evidence that qualitative changes in this protein cause a form of PD that clinicians and pathologists would otherwise recognize as the "idiopathic" form described by Parkinson [62,63]. Further, whole-gene duplications and triplications have also been found in autosomal-dominant PD families and gene dosage may reflect on the amount of Lewy bodies seen at autopsy [64,65]. Both major quantitative and qualitative changes in α-synuclein may cause PD, but whether minor variations in either gene expression or protein function itself are a risk factor in the more common forms of PD remains unclear as is whether α-synuclein inclusions are directly toxic or if the α-synuclein proto-fibrils are the pathogenic species.

This finding led to the discovery that α-synuclein was a major component of Lewy bodies in sporadic PD [66], and enabled Braak et al [1] to trace the development of synucleopathy in specific regions of the nervous system in PD patients, revealing the beginning of the process in the medulla oblongata/pontine tegmentum and olfactory bulb/anterior olfactory nucleus, but not the SN compacta as the single target area in PD. This region suffers later but makes the problem clinically visible.

Now the theory of PD pathogenesis as a growing accumulation of α–synuclein in the CNS seems to be most promising and efforts are directed to study causes and/or triggers, which result in changing of native properties of this protein to become misfolded and enhance its propensity to aggregate.

Parkin

At present parkin mutations are considered the commonest genetic cause identified in familial parkinsonism. Various reports for parkin mutations suggest a prevalence of up to 50% of familial autosomal-recessive early onset parkinsonism cases. Parkin-associated parkinsonism should be considered in all early-onset (<45 years) hypokinetic movement disorders, and especially in patients with a symmetrical slowly progressive disease course, early-onset dystonia and responsiveness to levodopa [67].

LRRK2

An autosomal dominant inheritance has been proposed in each case. LRRK2 gene mutations, identified in 2002 [68] were shown to cause an autosomal dominant disease with typical late onset PD cases responsive to levodopa with Lewy bodies demonstrated in autopsy. Other cases, however, had different neurological and pathologic changes, ranging from nigral degeneration without α-synulein positive inclusions to τ-positive inclusions and β-amyloid deposits and/or anterior horn cell loss as in amyotrophic lateral sclerosis [69,70]. The LRRK2 gene encodes a protein, dardarin, related to kinases, which being mutated, increase other proteins phosphate-adding activity [71]. However, still there are no proofs that LRRK2 overactivity results in neuronal death.

Glucocerebrosidase

If homozygous mutations in the glucocerebrosidase gene have long been known to cause Gaucher's disease, non-neuronopathic type-1 of the disease has occasionally been associated with parkinsonian symptoms. An association between Gaucher disease and parkinsonian signs has been demonstrated by the concurrence of Gaucher disease and parkinsonism in some patients [72,73] and the identification of glucocerebrosidase mutations in probands with sporadic PD [72]. The hallmark of this atypical parkinsonism was appearance of extrapyramidal signs in 40-60 years, rapid aggressive progression of the signs and no response to levodopa [72]. Such patients have a common "non-neuronopathic" N370S mutation, including some N370S homozygotes. While brain glucosylsphingosine levels were not elevated, Lewy bodies were seen post mortem. The glucocerebrosidase deficiency can contribute to a vulnerability of the patients to parkinsonism [74]. Screening the glucocerebrosidase gene for common gene mutations in 99 Ashkenazi Jewish patients with PD and 1543 controls revealed that 31% of the PD group carried heterozygous mutations compared with 6% of controls. Aharon-Peretz et al. concluded that heterozygous mutations in this gene predisposed to "idiopathic" PD in Ashkenazi Jews [75], and postulated that this might result from aberrant protein degradation due to reduced cellular glucocerebrosidase activity and/or the accumulation of glucocerebroside. Alternatively, these may act by reducing lipid affinity for alpha-synuclein, leading to the accumulation of cytoplasmic α-synuclein and aggregate formation [76].

Protein Tau H1 Haplotype

Linkage analysis in families with late onset PD showed strong evidence for linkage with a region on chromosome 17 encompassing the large τ-gene with 16 coding exons [77]. This gene encodes a microtubule-associated protein that is expressed in the brain and forms paired helical filaments in Alzheimer disease, fronto-temporal dementia with parkinsonism, and progressive supranuclear palsy [77]. The association between the τ-H1 haplotype and risk of PD in a family based study included a sample of 1056 individuals from 235 families selected from 13 clinical centers in the United States and Australia [78]. Significantly increased risk of PD among persons with the τ-H1 haplotype (OR=5.52; 95% CI: 2.64-11.10) was found in case–control studies both in a Norwegians [79] and in a southeast England population (OR=1.34; 95% CI: 1.04–1.72) [80]. The latter study included a sample of 580 patients with PD, and found that homozygosity for the τ-H1 genotype (H1H1) increased PD risk by 57% (95% CI, 33 - 85%; p< 0.00001) compared with H2 haplotype carriers (H1H2 and H2H2) [80].

In a meta-analysis of results of 14 independent case-control studies included 2,093 PD cases and 2,258 controls pooled odds ratios were 1.42 (95% CI, 1.23–1.65) for those with H1/H1 genotype compared with all others and confirmed the statistical linking between PD gene τ-H1 genotype [81].

However, the pathogenic mechanism of the τ-protein in PD remains unknown. Possibly τ-protein dysfunction or deposition accelerates dopaminergic neuronal degeneration, with co-aggregation [82] or independently of α-synuclein [83].

Apolipoprotein E

A polymorphic gene located on chromosome 19 encodes apolipoprotein E (APOE). The association of one of the polymorphic forms, APOE ε4, with Alzheimer's disease has been demonstrated in 1993 [84] and confirmed by several groups [85]. The mechanism underlying this connection is unclear, but may be related to the fact that APOE serves as a trophic factor in the brain. Its association with other neurodegenerative diseases is therefore possible [86,87]. According to Li et al [88] APOE ε4 was significantly associated with risk of developing PD and reduced the age at onset of the disease by approximately three years. Moreover family-based association stratified analysis revealed that APOE was associated with families with a positive PD family history [88].

Analysis of the APOE genotype in sib pairs with PD showed the APOE ε4 allele was over-represented in those who shared adjacent chromosome 19 markers. This may suggest that APOE ε4 is responsible for the linkage peak in this region and that it is a modest risk factor for PD [89]. However, systematic review and meta-analysis of results from 22 case-control studies for PD and that reported APOE genotype frequencies showed the APOE ε2 allele, but not APOE ε4 allele was slightly positively associated with PD (OR = 1.20; 95% CI, 1.02-1.42) [90] Huang et al, 2004). PD patients had an increased risk of dementia (HR=2.8; 95% CI: 1.8-4.4), which was especially pronounced in carriers at least one APOE gene ε2 allele (RR=13.5; CI: 4.5-40.6) [25]. These data were confirmed in a prospective, population-based cohort study in 107 PD patients with and without dementia, where the presence of at least one ε2 allele significantly increased the risk of PD (OR = 1.7; 95% CI: 1.0-2.8) [91].

Mitochondrial Mutations in PD

PD is characterized by a systemic loss of activity of complex I of the respiratory chain (NADH: ubiquinone oxidoreductase), which is the target enzyme of the parkinsonism producing neurotoxin, methyl-phenyl-tetrahydropyridine (MPTP). Experiments with cybrid cells, in which mitochondria from platelets obtained from PD patient or control donors transferred into mitochondrial DNA-depleted recipient neuron-based cells, suggest that the loss of complex I activity arises from mitochondrial DNA (mt-DNA) [92]. Heteroplasmic mutations in the ND5 region of the mt-DNA, which is a mitochondrial gene encoding a complex I subunit in brain tissue, segregated PD from controls [93]. Several reports have shown that mitochondrial dysfunction associated with oxidative stress can trigger α-synuclein aggregation and accumulation, although the exact mechanisms remain unclear [94]. Accumulation of mitochondrial DNA mutations accelerate with normal aging, leading to oxidative damage to nuclear DNA, and impairs gene transcription [95]. In turn, accumulation through life of amino acid-changing mutations leading to systemic loss of activity of complex I of the mitochondrial electron transport chain may be a key factor explaining the increase of PD prevalence with ageing [96]. However, until now, no mitochondrial mutations have been identified as being responsible for PD, and maternal transmission has not been confirmed.

ENVIRONMENTAL RISK FACTORS FOR PD

Lifestyle Factors

Smoking

Smoking was first observed to have an inverse association with PD in a study of US military veterans in the late 1960s [97] and this observation was repeatedly confirmed in a number of case-control and cohort studies [98-100]. Contradictory results where no association between smoking and PD (OR= 1.1; p= 0.6) are also known [101]. However, systematic review of prospective studies showed an obvious protective effect of current smoking in the pooled estimate (RR=0.35; 95% CI, 0.26-0.47), and former smokers had lower risk compared with never smokers (RR=0.66; 95% CI: 0.49-0.88) [102]. The risk for PD was shown to be dose dependent - it was lowest in current smokers, increasing slightly in those who quit recently and rising to a risk nearly as high as that of nonsmokers in those who quit smoking several years previously [103]. This dose-response relationship suggests a pharmacologic action of some compound in cigarette smoke to lower the risk of PD. Inverse associations were reported also between PD and tobacco chewing and snuff use, in a case–control study conducted with data from the Rochester Epidemiology Project [104]. Smokeless tobacco use was found inversely associated with age-adjusted risk of PD (RR=0.22; CI: 0.07-0.67), and PD mortality in current users compared to never users [105]. These reports suggest that it is nicotine, rather than some other component in cigarette smoke, to be responsible factor. Risk of PD inversely correlated with the dose of tobacco smoking. In 33 discordant MZ pairs and 39 discordant DZ pairs, the twins without PD smoked more than their affected sibs (32.5 vs. 22.7 pack-years, p=0.026). Because MZ twins are genetically identical and are similar behaviorally, this difference is unlikely to result from genetic factors, and suggests a true biologic protective effect of cigarette smoking [106]. These statistical associations probably represent a real protective effect of tobacco, although a result of personality characteristics and behavioral reactions of PD patients have been discussed [106].

Dietary Factors

Dietary fats. Anderson et al. [107] found that high intake of animal fats estimated according to self-reported past food intake is associated with a more than threefold increased risk of PD (OR =3.30; 95% CI: 1.43–7.61) in a case-control study. This association was confirmed in the population-based case-control study in Detroit where high intake of total fat, saturated fats and cholesterol was associated with enhanced risk of PD (OR=1.94, 95% CI: 1.05-3.58 and OR= 2.11, 95% CI: 1.14-3.90, respectively) [108]. On the contrary, in the Rotterdam prospective population-based cohort study, no associations were found for dietary saturated fat and cholesterol. Moreover, intakes of total fat, monounsaturated fatty acids and polyunsaturated fatty acids were significantly associated with a lower risk of PD, with an adjusted hazard ratio per SD increase of energy-adjusted intake of 0.69 (95%; CI: 0.52 - 0.91) for total fat, of 0.68 (95% CI 0.50-0.94) for monounsaturated acids, and 0.66 (95%; CI: 0.46-0.96) for polyunsaturated ones [109].

Milk. Findings based on dietary intake in 7,504 men in the Honolulu Heart Program suggest that milk intake is associated with an increased risk of PD. There was a 2.3-fold excess of PD (95% CI: 1.3 - 4.1) in the highest intake group (>16 oz/day) vs. those who consumed no milk. The effect of milk consumption on PD was independent of the intake of calcium. Calcium from dairy and nondairy sources had no relation with the risk of PD [110]. The effect of milk on the risk of PD was strongest in the first 15 years of follow-up (p < 0.01) [110].

Caffeine (coffee, tea, cola). Detailed analyses of coffee consumption and risk of PD were conducted in a number of case-control studies. Hellenbrand et al [111] compared the dietary habits of 342 patients with PD and found that coffee consumption was neuroprotective (OR=0.27, 95% CI: 0.14-0.52). This ratio was not significant, however, for tea. Fall et al. [112] reported a significantly reduced risk among both coffee (OR = 0.14, 95% CI: 0.03-0.44) and tea (OR = 0.31, 95% CI: 0.10-0.87) drinkers. However, reduced risks were observed for consumption of 2 cups/day or more of tea (OR = 0.4, 95% CI: 0.2-0.9) and two or more cola drinks/day (OR = 0.6, 95% CI: 0.3- 1.4) [113].

A prospective study based on 30 years of follow-up in 8,006 Japanese-American men, showed that coffee non-drinkers experienced a 5-fold excess in the risk of PD as compared to men who consumed 28 oz (approximately 800 cc) per day or more (10.4 versus 1.9/10,000 person years, respectively). The study participants completed 24-hour diet recall in 1965 – 1968 at enrollment and were repeatedly examined thereafter. In this study the effect of coffee was dose-dependent and the risk of PD declined according to increasing in amount of coffee consumed (p<0.001) [114]. In the Health Professionals' Follow-Up Study, which included 47,351 men and 88,565 women, an inverse association between the risk of PD and caffeine consumption was observed 0.42 (95% CI: 0.23–0.78). This association was recognized with consumption of coffee, caffeine from non-coffee sources, tea but not decaffeinated coffee. Among women, the relationship between caffeine or coffee intake and risk of PD was significant only in a group with moderate intakes (1–3 cups of coffee/day) [115]. Thus, caffeine consumption was associated with a reduced risk of PD in men but not in women. This gender difference may be due to an interaction between caffeine and use of postmenopausal estrogens [116].

Infections and Inflammation

Inflammation is a typical feature of neurodegenerative diseases of aging. In 1988, McGeer et al [117] observed an activation of the microglia (HLA-DR-positive macrophages) in the SN and striatum of brains from all patients with PD. Langston et al [118] described gliosis and clustering of microglia around nerve cells in the SN in autopsy of three patients exposed to MPTP several years before death. In turn, an inflammatory process in the SN, with activated microglia, was shown to initiate or aggravate nigral degeneration in PD [119]. Indicators of inflammation such as increased levels of pro-inflammatory cytokines (tumor necrosis factor (TNF)-alpha, interleukin-1beta, and interleukin-6) and decreased levels of neurotrophins (brain-derived neurotrophic factor (BDNF)) were found in the nigrostriatal region of postmortem brains and in the CSF from patients with PD, and in animal PD models [120].

Chen et al. [121] repeatedly reported that regular use of ibuprofen lowers risk of the developing PD. This effect had begun from a dosage of two tablets (400mg totally) per week and was dose dependent, whereas duration of ibuprofen use was not related to PD risk. Unlike ibuprofen, the use of aspirin, other non-steroid anti-inflammatory drugs, or acetaminophen was not associated with PD risk. The causes of this selective effect of ibuprofen among other cyclooxygenase inhibitors are unclear.

A retrospective case-control study (172 cases, 343 age- and sex-matched controls) of a possible relationship between environmental factors encountered during fetal life and infancy and the later risk of developing PD revealed that neither birth weight, weight at 1 year of age, nor any aspect of the childhood domestic environment were associated with risk of PD. However, subjects who later developed PD were more likely to have suffered croup (OR = 4.1; 95%: CI: 1.1–16.1) or diphtheria (OR = 2.3; 95% CI: 1.1–3.6) [122]. Another retrospective case-control analysis of PD showed a significant negative association for a history of measles before college entrance (OR=0.53; 95% CI: 0.31-0.93) [123]. The results of these studies suggest that infections in childhood possibly contribute to development of PD, whereas unfavorable conditions of early growing are probably not. However the retrospective nature of these studies must be acknowledged, as well as their marginal statistical significance. The hypothesis that PD could be a late complication of intrauterine influenza (or other viral) infection that affects the fetal SN was also suggested [124,125].

Thus, epidemiologic data on the relationship between infections in early life period and risk of PD remain unclear.

Occupational Risk Factors

Pesticides, Herbicides, Insecticides, Fungicides

In one case-control study, Baldi et al. [126] found positive association between PD and exposure to pesticides (OR = 2.2, 95%; CI: 1.1-4.3). Other studies failed to confirm this dependence. In a recent prospective population-based case-control study comparing 250 PD patients with 338 age- and sex-matched healthy control subjects odds ratios for occupational exposures were non significant (pesticide worker: OR= 2.07; CI: 0.67-6.38; crop farmer: OR=1.65; CI: 0.84-3.27; animal and crop farmer: OR= 1.10; CI: 0.60-2.00; and dairy farmer: OR=0.88; CI: 0.46-1.70) [127]. No evidence of risk from home-based pesticide exposures was found [127]. Earlier, significant association of occupational exposure to herbicides was found in a population-based case-control study consisting of 144 PD patients older than 50 years and 464 control subjects. For herbicides OR=4.10; 95% CI: 1.37-12.24) and insecticides (OR= 3.55; CI: 1.75-7.18) but no relation was found with fungicide exposure [128].

The above-mentioned epidemiologic studies are limited by a lack of detailed and validated pesticide exposure assessment. In animal studies, no pesticide has yet demonstrated the selective set of clinical and pathologic signs that characterize human PD, particularly at levels relevant to human exposure. Thus, the association between pesticide exposure and PD remains tenuous [129].

Farm Residence and Farming

Gorell et al. [128] found that farming as an occupation is significantly associated with PD (OR= 2.79; CI: 1.03- 7.55), however no increased risk of the disease with rural or farm residence or well water use was established. Hertzman et al. [129] revealed a statistically significant increased risk for working in orchards (OR = 3.69; CI: 1.34-10.27). However, these data were not confirmed by other investigators [130,131].

The information about the use of well water possibly associated with contaminants in rural living or farming is controversial. For example, Koller et al. [132] found that rural living and drinking well water were significantly increased among PD patients (OR = 1.70; p=0.03) and Smargiassi et al. [133] had confirmed that well water drinking is associated with PD (OR=2.78; CI: 1.46-5.28). However, again others failed to confirm this association [128,134].

Welding

Welders had a younger age at onset (46 years) of PD compared with sequentially ascertained controls (63 years; p < 0.0001) [135]. No other differences in clinical features, family history, depression, dementia, or drug-induced psychosis were detected between the welders and the two control groups. All treated welders responded to levodopa like controls [135]. Other studies showed no association for occupational exposures to heavy metals in general [134,136].

Manganese

In population-based case-control study Gorell et al. [134] found that in miners occupational exposure to manganese more than 20 years is a risk factor to PD (OR=10.61, 95% CI: 1.06-105.83) but others have not found this association [137]. Heavy exposure to manganese is associated with hypokinetic- rigid syndrome with early intellectual decline, gait disorders, and poor response to levodopa treatment. Thus, this entity can be clearly distinct from PD by clinical, neuroradiological and pathological data [138,139].

Solvents

A few epidemiologic studies found a possible association between exposure to solvents and PD. One study examined exposure to organic solvents and found a statistically significant relationship to the development of PD (OR=2.78, CI: 1.23-6.26) [139]. According to Pezzoli et al. [140] exposure to hydrocarbon solvents led to an earlier appearance of signs of PD. Ohlson and Hogstedt [141] did not find evidence that occupational exposure to organic solvents (carbon disulfide) increases the risk of PD. Seidler et al. [136] in another case control study found an association between contacts only with wood preservatives (OR=1.9 CI: 1.2-3.0).

CONCLUSION

Thus, PD etiology remains an enigma without clear conceptions. The study is complicated by absence of robust biomarkers, inexact diagnosis, and contradictory epidemiological data. Possibly, this is a result of a mismatch in differentiation between "sporadic" or "idiopathic" PD with other kinds of parkinsonisms (vascular, infective, toxic, parkinsonism plus syndromes, hereditary etc.) with different pathogeneses. PD is an idiopathic progressive neurodegeneration, which manifests by intraneuronal accumulation of α-synuclein in selected populations of neurons – first in the dorsal motor vagus, intermediate reticular zone, and in specific nerve cell types of the gain setting system (coeruleus-subcoeruleus complex, caudal raphe nuclei, gigantocellular reticular nucleus). In contrast, many other pathological processes could result from a direct lesion of the SN (for example, methyl-phenyl-tetrahydropyridine, brain stem vascular lesions). However, these diseases have only phenotypic resemblance with PD, but a different pathogenesis, progression and outcome.

Thus, epidemiological data of PD so far fail to elucidate the etiology of PD. While ageing remains the only significant and clear risk factor (beyond genetics), the reason that only a minority of older individuals is affected is unclear. In the level of present knowledge with absence of a reliable biological marker of PD suitable for field studies make it impossible to reach definitive epidemiological conclusions.

REFERENCES

[1]   Braak H, de Vos RA, Bohl J, Del Tredici K. Gastric alpha-synuclein immunoreactive inclusions in Meissner's and Auerbach's plexuses in cases staged for Parkinson's disease-related brain pathology. *Neurosci Lett*. 2005 Dec 2; [Epub ahead of print]

[2]   Braak H, Del Tredici K, Bratzke H, Hamm-Clement J, Sandmann-Keil D, Rub U. Staging of the intracerebral inclusion body pathology associated with idiopathic Parkinson's disease (preclinical and clinical stages). J Neurol. 2002; 249 Suppl 3:III/1-5.

[3]   Korczyn AD. The gut in PD. *Neurology*. 1993; 43(3 Pt 1): 629-630.

[4]   Hughes AJ, Ben-Shlomo Y, Daniel SE, et al: What features improve the accuracy of clinical diagnosis in Parkinson's disease: A clinicopathologic study. *Neurology* 1992; 42: 1142–1146.

[5]   Siderowf A. Parkinson's disease: clinical features, epidemiology and genetics. *Neurol Clin*. 2001; 19(3): 565-578.

[6]   De Rijk MC, Rocca WA, Anderson DW, Melcon MO, Breteler MM, Maraganore DM. A population perspective on diagnostic criteria for Parkinson's disease. *Neurology*. 1997; 48(5): 1277-1281.

[7]   Jain S, Wood NW, Healy DG Molecular genetic pathways in Parkinson's disease: a review. *Clin Sci (Lond)*. 2005; 109(4): 355-364.

[8]   Przuntek H, Muller T, Riederer P. Diagnostic staging of Parkinson's disease: conceptual aspects. *J Neural Transm*. 2004; 111(2): 201-216.

[9]   *The Average Per-Patient Costs of Parkinson's Disease*. New York, NY: John Robbins Associates, 1998.

[10] Lindgren P, von Campenhausen S, Spottke E, Siebert U, Dodel R. Cost of Parkinson's disease in Europe. *Eur J Neurol*. 2005; 12 Suppl 1:68-73.

[11] Rajput ML, Rajput AH. Epidemiology of parkinsonism. In: Factor SA, Weiner WJ, eds. *Parkinson's Disease Diagnosis and Clinical Management*. New York, NY: Demos; 2002: 31-40.

[12] Schrag A, Ben-Shlomo Y, Quinn NP. Cross sectional prevalence survey of idiopathic Parkinson's disease and Parkinsonism in London. *BMJ*. 2000; 321(7252): 21-22.

[13] Benito-Leon J, Bermejo-Pareja F, Morales-Gonzalez JM, Porta-Etessam J, Trincado R, Vega S, Louis ED; Neurological Disorders in Central Spain (NEDICES) Study Group. Incidence of Parkinson disease and parkinsonism in three elderly populations of central Spain. *Neurology*. 2004; 62(5): 734-741.

[14] De Lau LM, Giesbergen PC, de Rijk MC, Hofman A, Koudstaal PJ, Breteler MM. Incidence of parkinsonism and Parkinson disease in a general population: the Rotterdam Study. *Neurology*. 2004; 63(7): 1240-1244.

[15] Von Campenhausen S, Bornschein B, Wick R, Botzel K, Sampaio C, Poewe W, Oertel W, Siebert U, Berger K, Dodel R. Prevalence and incidence of Parkinson's disease in Europe. *Eur Neuropsychopharmacol*. 2005; 15(4):473-490.

[16] Zhang ZX, Roman GC. Worldwide occurrence of Parkinson's disease: an updated review. *Neuroepidemiology*. 1993; 12(4): 195-208.

[17] Zhang ZX, Roman GC, Hong Z, Wu CB, Qu QM, Huang JB, Zhou B, Geng ZP, Wu JX, Wen HB, Zhao H, Zahner GE. Parkinson's disease in China: prevalence in Beijing, Xian, and Shanghai. *Lancet*. 2005; 365(9459): 595-597.

[18] Tanner CM, Hubble JP, Chan P. Epidemiology and genetics of parkinson's disease. In: Watts RL, Koller WC eds: *Movement Disorders. Neurologic principles and practice*. NY, USA: McGraw-Hill; 1991:124-146.

[19] Twelves D, Perkins KS, Counsell C. Systematic review of incidence studies of Parkinson's disease. *Mov Disord*. 2003; 18(1): 19-31.

[20] Mayeux R, Marder K, Cote LJ, Denaro J, Hemenegildo N, Mejia H, Tang MX, Lantigua R, Wilder D, Gurland B. The frequency of idiopathic Parkinson's disease by age, ethnic group, and sex in northern Manhattan, 1988-1993. *Am J Epidemiol*. 1995; 142(8): 820-827.

[21] Hoyert DL, Kung HC, Smith BL. Deaths: preliminary data for 2003. *Natl Vital Stat Rep*. 2005; 53 (15): 1-48.

[22] Herlofson K, Lie SA, Arsland D, Larsen JP. Mortality and Parkinson disease: A community based study. *Neurology*. 2004; 62(6): 937-942.

[23] D'Amelio M, Ragonese P, Morgante L, Reggio A, Callari G, Salemi G, Savettieri G. Long-term survival of Parkinson's disease A population-based study. *J Neurol*. 2005 Jul 18; [Epub ahead of print]

[24] Chen RC, Chang SF, Su CL, Chen TH, Yen MF, Wu HM, Chen ZY, Liou HH. Prevalence, incidence, and mortality of PD: a door-to-door survey in Ilan county, Taiwan. *Neurology*. 2001; 57(9): 1679-1686.

[25] De Lau LM, Schipper CM, Hofman A, Koudstaal PJ, Breteler MM. Prognosis of Parkinson disease: risk of dementia and mortality: the Rotterdam Study. *Arch Neurol.* 2005; 62(8): 1265-1269.

[26] Nussbaum M, Treves TA, Inzelberg R, Rabey JM, Korczyn AD. Survival in Parkinson's disease: the effect of dementia Parkinsonism Relat Disord. 1998; 4(4): 179-181.

[27] Ross HF, Hughes TA, Boyd JL, Biggins CA, Madeley P, Mindham RH, Spokes EG. The evolution and profile of dementia in Parkinson's disease. *Adv Neurol.* 1996; 69:343-347.

[28] Hughes TA, Ross HF, Mindham RH, Spokes EG. Mortality in Parkinson's disease and its association with dementia and depression. *Acta Neurol Scand.* 2004; 110(2): 118-123.

[29] Ross GW, Petrovitch H, Abbott RD, Nelson J, Markesbery W, Davis D, Hardman J, Launer L, Masaki K, Tanner CM, White LR. Parkinsonian signs and substantia nigra neuron density in decendents elders without PD. *Ann Neurol.* 2004; 56(4): 532-539.

[30] Baldereschi M, Di Carlo A, Rocca WA, Vanni P, Maggi S, Perissinotto E, Grigoletto F, Amaducci L, Inzitari D. Parkinson's disease and parkinsonism in a longitudinal study: two-fold higher incidence in men. ILSA Working Group. Italian Longitudinal Study on Aging. *Neurology.* 2000; 55(9):1358-1363.

[31] Wooten GF, Currie LJ, Bovbjerg VE, Lee JK, Patrie J. Are men at greater risk for Parkinson's disease than women? *J Neurol Neurosurg Psychiatry.* 2004; 75(4): 637-639.

[32] Kimura H, Kurimura M, Wada M, Kawanami T, Kurita K, Suzuki Y, Katagiri T, Daimon M, Kayama T, Kato T. Female preponderance of Parkinson's disease in Japan. *Neuroepidemiology.* 2002; 21(6):292-296.

[33] Morioka S, Sakata K, Yoshida S, Nakai E, Shiba M, Yoshimura N, Hashimoto T. Incidence of Parkinson disease in Wakayama, *Japan. J Epidemiol.* 2002; 12(6): 403-407.

[34] Kusumi M, Nakashima K, Harada H, Nakayama H, Takahashi K. Epidemiology of Parkinson's disease in Yonago City, Japan: comparison with a study carried out 12 years ago. *Neuroepidemiology.* 1996;15(4):201-207.

[35] Fernandez HH, Lapane KL. Estrogen use among nursing home residents with a diagnosis of Parkinson's disease. *Mov Disord.* 2000; 15(6): 1119-1124.

[36] Zhu BT. Catechol-O-Methyltransferase (COMT)-mediated methylation metabolism of endogenous bioactive catechols and modulation by endobiotics and xenobiotics: importance in pathophysiology and pathogenesis. *Curr Drug Metab.* 2002; 3(3): 321-349.

[37] Routiot T, Lurel S, Denis E, Barbarino-Monnier P. Parkinson's disease and pregnancy: case report and literature review. *J Gynecol Obstet Biol Reprod* (Paris). 2000; 29(5): 454-457.

[38] Shulman LM, Minagar A, Weiner WJ. The effect of pregnancy in Parkinson's disease. *Mov Disord.* 2000; 15(1):132-135.

[39] Tsang KL, Ho SL, Lo SK. Estrogen improves motor disability in parkinsonian postmenopausal women with motor fluctuations. *Neurology.* 2000; 54(12): 2292-2298.

[40] Currie LJ, Harrison MB, Trugman JM, Bennett JP, Wooten GF. Postmenopausal estrogen use affects risk for Parkinson disease. *Arch Neurol.* 2004; 61(6): 886-888.

[41] Popat RA, Van Den Eeden SK, Tanner CM, McGuire V, Bernstein AL, Bloch DA, Leimpeter A, Nelson LM. Effect of reproductive factors and postmenopausal hormone use on the risk of Parkinson disease. *Neurology.* 2005; 65(3): 383-390.

[42] Kessler II. Epidemiologic studies of Parkinson's disease. II. A hospital-based survey. *Am J Epidemiol.* 1972;95(4):308-318.

[43] Paddison RM, Griffith RP. Occurrence of Parkinson's disease in black patients at Charity Hospital in New Orleans. *Neurology.* 1974; 24(7):688-690.

[44] Schoenberg BS, Osuntokun BO, Adeuja AO, Bademosi O, Nottidge V, Anderson DW, Haerer AF. Comparison of the prevalence of Parkinson's disease in black populations in the rural United States and in rural Nigeria: door-to-door community studies. *Neurology.* 1988; 38(4): 645-646.

[45] McInerney-Leo A, Gwinn-Hardy K, Nussbaum RL. Prevalence of Parkinson's disease in populations of African ancestry: a review. *J Natl Med Assoc.* 2004; 96(7): 974-979.

[46] Van Den Eeden SK, Tanner CM, Bernstein AL, Fross RD, Leimpeter A, Bloch DA, Nelson LM. Incidence of Parkinson's disease: variation by age, gender, and race/ethnicity. *Am J Epidemiol.* 2003; 157(11): 1015-1022.

[47] Tanner CM, Ottman R, Goldman SM, Ellenberg J, Chan P, Mayeux R, Langston JW. Parkinson disease in twins: an etiologic study. *JAMA.* 1999; 281(4): 341-346.

[48] Ward CD, Duvoisin RC, Ince SE, Nutt JD, Eldridge R, Calne DB. Parkinson's disease in 65 pairs of twins and in a set of quadruplets. *Neurology.* 1983; 33(7):815-824.

[49] Wirdefeldt K, Gatz M, Schalling M, Pedersen NL. No evidence for heritability of Parkinson disease in Swedish twins. *Neurology.* 2004; 63(2):305-311.

[50] Laihinen A, Ruottinen H, Rinne JO, Haaparanta M, Bergman J, Solin O, Koskenvuo M, Marttila R, Rinne UK. Risk for Parkinson's disease: twin studies for the detection of asymptomatic subjects using [18F]6-fluorodopa PET. *J Neurol.* 2000; 247 Suppl 2:II110-113.

[51] Piccini P, Burn DJ, Ceravolo R, Maraganore D, Brooks DJ. The role of inheritance in sporadic Parkinson's disease: evidence from a longitudinal study of dopaminergic function in twins. *Ann Neurol.* 1999; 45(5): 577-582.

[52] Golbe LI, Di Iorio G, Bonavita V, Miller DC, Duvoisin RC. A large kindred with autosomal dominant Parkinson's disease. *Ann Neurol.* 1990; 27(3): 276-282.

[53] Sveinbjornsdottir S, Hicks AA, Jonsson T, et al. Familial aggregation of Parkinson's disease in Iceland. *N Engl J Med* 2000; 343: 1765–1770.

[54] Maher NE, Golbe LI, Lazzarini AM, Mark MH, Currie LJ, Wooten GF, Saint-Hilaire M, Wilk JB, Volcjak J, Maher JE, Feldman RG, Guttman M, Lew M, Waters CH, Schuman S, Suchowersky O, Lafontaine AL, Labelle N, Vieregge P, Pramstaller PP, Martin ER, Scott WK, Nance MA, Watts RL, Hubble JP, Koller WC, Lyons K, Pahwa R, Stern MB, Colcher A, Hiner BC, Jankovic J, Ondo WG, Allen FH Jr, Goetz CG, Small GW, Masterman D, Mastaglia F, Laing NG, Stajich JM, Ribble RC, Booze MW, Rogala A, Hauser MA, Zhang F, Gibson RA, Middleton LT, Roses AD, Haines JL, Scott BL, Pericak-Vance MA, Vance JM. Association of single-nucleotide

polymorphisms of the tau gene with late-onset Parkinson disease. *JAMA*. 2001; 286(18): 2245-2250.

[55] Maraganore DM, Harding AE, Marsden CD. A clinical and genetic study of familial Parkinson's disease. *Mov Disord*. 1991; 6(3): 205-211.

[56] Rocca WA, Peterson BJ, McDonnell SK, Bower JH, Ahlskog JE, Schaid DJ, Maraganore DM. The Mayo Clinic family study of Parkinson's disease: study design, instruments, and sample characteristics. *Neuroepidemiology*. 2005; 24(3): 151-167.

[57] Rocca WA, McDonnell SK, Strain KJ, Bower JH, Ahlskog JE, Elbaz A, Schaid DJ, Maraganore DM. Familial aggregation of Parkinson's disease: The Mayo Clinic family study. *Ann Neurol*. 2004; 56(4): 495-502.

[58] Cummings JL. Understanding Parkinson disease. *JAMA*. 1999; 281(4): 376-378.

[59] Gasser T. Genetics of Parkinson's disease. *Curr Opin Neurol*. 2005; 18(4):363-369.

[60] Golbe LI. Is there a familial form of Parkinson's disease? In: Factor SA, Weiner WJ, eds. *Parkinson's Disease Diagnosis and Clinical Management*. New York, NY: Demos; 2002: 591-597.

[61] Polymeropoulos MH, Lavedan C, Leroy E, Ide SE, Dehejia A, Dutra A, Pike B, Root H, Rubenstein J, Boyer R, Stenroos ES, Chandrasekharappa S, Athanassiadou A, Papapetropoulos T, Johnson WG, Lazzarini AM, Duvoisin RC, Di Iorio G, Golbe LI, Nussbaum RL. Mutation in the alpha-synuclein gene identified in families with Parkinson's disease. *Science*. 1997; 276(5321): 2045-2047.

[62] Kruger R, Kuhn W, Muller T, Woitalla D, Graeber M, Kosel S, Przuntek H, Epplen JT, Schols L, Riess O. Ala30Pro mutation in the gene encoding alpha-synuclein in Parkinson's disease. *Nat Genet*. 1998; 18(2): 106-108.

[63] Zarranz JJ, Alegre J, Gomez-Esteban JC, Lezcano E, Ros R, Ampuero I, Vidal L, Hoenicka J, Rodriguez O, Atares B, Llorens V, Gomez Tortosa E, del Ser T, Munoz DG, de Yebenes JG. The new mutation, E46K, of alpha-synuclein causes Parkinson and Lewy body dementia. *Ann Neurol*. 2004; 55(2): 164-173.

[64] Singleton AB, Farrer M, Johnson J, Singleton A, Hague S, Kachergus J, Hulihan M, Peuralinna T, Dutra A, Nussbaum R, Lincoln S, Crawley A, Hanson M, Maraganore D, Adler C, Cookson MR, Muenter M, Baptista M, Miller D, Blancato J, Hardy J, Gwinn-Hardy K. alpha-Synuclein locus triplication causes Parkinson's disease. *Science*. 2003; 302(5646): 841.

[65] Ibanez P, Bonnet AM, Debarges B, Lohmann E, Tison F, Pollak P, Agid Y, Durr A,Brice A. Causal relation between alpha-synuclein gene duplication and familial Parkinson's disease. 2004; 364(9440): 1169-1171.

[66] Spillantini MG, Schmidt ML, Lee VM, Trojanowski JQ, Jakes R, Goedert M. Alpha-synuclein in Lewy bodies. *Nature*. 1997; 388(6645): 839-840.

[67] Lohmann E, Periquet M, Bonifati V, Wood NW, De Michele G, Bonnet AM, Fraix V, Broussolle E, Horstink MW, Vidailhet M, Verpillat P, Gasser T, Nicholl D, Teive H, Raskin S, Rascol O, Destee A, Ruberg M, Gasparini F, Meco G, Agid Y, Durr A, Brice A; French Parkinson's Disease Genetics Study Group; European Consortium on Genetic Susceptibility in Parkinson's Disease. How much phenotypic variation can be attributed to parkin genotype? *Ann Neurol*.; 54(2): 176-185.

[68] Funayama M, Hasegawa K, Kowa H, Saito M, Tsuji S, Obata F. A new locus for Parkinson's disease (PARK8) maps to chromosome 12p11.2-q13.1. *Ann Neurol.* 2002; 51(3): 296-301.

[69] Wszolek ZK, Pfeiffer RF, Tsuboi Y, Uitti RJ, McComb RD, Stoessl AJ, Strongosky AJ, Zimprich A, Muller-Myhsok B, Farrer MJ, Gasser T, Calne DB, Dickson DW. Autosomal dominant parkinsonism associated with variable synuclein and tau pathology. *Neurology.* 2004; 62(9): 1619-1622.

[70] Zimprich A, Biskup S, Leitner P, Lichtner P, Farrer M, Lincoln S, Kachergus J, Hulihan M, Uitti RJ, Calne DB, Stoessl AJ, Pfeiffer RF, Patenge N, Carbajal IC, Vieregge P, Asmus F, Muller-Myhsok B, Dickson DW, Meitinger T, Strom TM, Wszolek ZK, Gasser T. Mutations in LRRK2 cause autosomal-dominant parkinsonism with pleomorphic pathology. *Neuron.* 2004; 44(4):601-607.

[71] Smith WW, Pei Z, Jiang H, Moore DJ, Liang Y, West AB, Dawson VL, Dawson TM, Ross CA. Leucine-rich repeat kinase 2 (LRRK2) interacts with parkin and mutant LRRK2 induces neuronal degeneration. *Proc Natl Acad Sci U S A.* 2005 Dec 13; [Epub ahead of print]

[72] Neudorfer O, Giladi N, Elstein D, Abrahamov A, Turezkite T, Aghai E, Reches A, Bembi B, Zimran A. Occurrence of Parkinson's syndrome in type I Gaucher disease. *QJM.* 1996; 89(9): 691-694.

[73] Machaczka M, Rucinska M, Skotnicki AB, Jurczak W. Parkinson's syndrome preceding clinical manifestation of Gaucher's disease. *Am J Hematol.* 1999; 61(3):216-217.

[74] Tayebi N, Walker J, Stubblefield B, Orvisky E, LaMarca ME, Wong K, Rosenbaum H, Schiffmann R, Bembi B, Sidransky E Gaucher disease with parkinsonian manifestations: does glucocerebrosidase deficiency contribute to a vulnerability to parkinsonism? *Mol Genet Metab.* 2003; 79(2): 104-109.

[75] Aharon-Peretz J, Rosenbaum H, Gershoni-Baruch R. Mutations in the glucocerebrosidase gene and Parkinson's disease in Ashkenazi Jews. *N Engl J Med.* 2004; 351(19):1972-1977.

[76] Feany MB. New genetic insights into Parkinson's disease. *N Engl J Med.* 2004; 351(19): 1937-1940.

[77] Scott WK, Nance MA, Watts RL, Hubble JP, Koller WC, Lyons K, Pahwa R, Stern MB, Colcher A, Hiner BC, Jankovic J, Ondo WG, Allen FH Jr, Goetz CG, Small GW, Masterman D, Mastaglia F, Laing NG, Stajich JM, Slotterbeck B, Booze MW, Ribble RC, Rampersaud E, West SG, Gibson RA, Middleton LT, Roses AD, Haines JL, Scott BL, Vance JM, Pericak-Vance MA. Complete genomic screen in Parkinson disease: evidence for multiple genes. *JAMA.* 2001; 286(18): 2239-2244.

[78] Martin ER, Scott WK, Nance MA, Watts RL, Hubble JP, Koller WC, Lyons K,Pahwa R, Stern MB, Colcher A, Hiner BC, Jankovic J, Ondo WG, Allen FH Jr, Goetz CG, Small GW, Masterman D, Mastaglia F, Laing NG, Stajich JM, Ribble RC, Booze MW, Rogala A, Hauser MA, Zhang F, Gibson RA, Middleton LT, Roses AD, Haines JL, Scott BL, Pericak-Vance MA, Vance JM. Association of single-nucleotide polymorphisms of the tau gene with late-onset Parkinson disease. *JAMA.* 2001; 286(18): 2245-2250.

[79] Farrer M, Skipper L, Berg M, Bisceglio G, Hanson M, Hardy J, Adam A, Gwinn-Hardy K, Aasly J. The tau H1 haplotype is associated with Parkinson's disease in the Norwegian population. *Neurosci Lett.* 2002; 322(2): 83-86.

[80] Healy DG, Abou-Sleiman PM, Lees AJ, Casas JP, Quinn N, Bhatia K, Hingorani AD, Wood NW. Tau gene and Parkinson's disease: a case-control study and meta-analysis. *J Neurol Neurosurg Psychiatry.* 2004; 75(7): 962-965.

[81] Zhang J, Song Y, Chen H, Fan D. The tau gene haplotype h1 confers a susceptibility to Parkinson's disease. *Eur Neurol.* 2005; 53(1): 15-21. Epub 2004 Dec 27.

[82] Ishizawa T, Mattila P, Davies P, Wang D, Dickson DW. Colocalization of tau and alpha-synuclein epitopes in Lewy bodies. *J Neuropathol Exp Neurol.* 2003; 62(4):389-397.

[83] Mamah CE, Lesnick TG, Lincoln SJ, Strain KJ, de Andrade M, Bower JH, Ahlskog JE, Rocca WA, Farrer MJ, Maraganore DM. Interaction of alpha-synuclein and tau genotypes in Parkinson's disease. *Ann Neurol.* 2005; 57(3): 439-443.

[84] Strittmatter WJ, Saunders AM, Schmechel D, Pericak-Vance M, Enghild J, Salvesen GS, Roses AD. Apolipoprotein E: high-avidity binding to beta-amyloid and increased frequency of type 4 allele in late-onset familial Alzheimer disease. *Proc Natl Acad Sci USA.* 1993 1; 90(5):1977-1981.

[85] Treves TA, Chandra V, Korczyn AD. Parkinson's and Alzheimer's diseases: epidemiological comparison. 2. Persons at risk. *Neuroepidemiology.* 1993;12(6):345-349.

[86] Drory VE, Birnbaum M, Korczyn AD, Chapman J. Association of APOE epsilon4 allele with survival in amyotrophic lateral sclerosis. *J Neurol Sci.* 2001; 190(1-2): 17-20.

[87] Chapman J, Korczyn AD, Karussis DM, Michaelson DM. The effects of APOE genotype on age at onset and progression of neurodegenerative diseases. *Neurology.* 2001;57(8):1482-1485.

[88] Li YJ, Hauser MA, Scott WK, Martin ER, Booze MW, Qin XJ, Walter JW, Nance MA, Hubble JP, Koller WC, Pahwa R, Stern MB, Hiner BC, Jankovic J, Goetz CG, Small GW, Mastaglia F, Haines JL, Pericak-Vance MA, Vance JM. Apolipoprotein E controls the risk and age at onset of Parkinson disease. *Neurology.* 2004; 62(11): 2005-2009.

[89] Martinez M, Brice A, Vaughan JR, Zimprich A, Breteler MM, Meco G, Filla A, Farrer MJ, Betard C, Singleton A, Hardy J, De Michele G, Bonifati V, Oostra BA, Gasser T, Wood NW, Durr A. Apolipoprotein E4 is probably responsible for the chromosome 19 linkage peak for Parkinson's disease. *Am J Med Genet B Neuropsychiatr Genet.* 2005; 136(1): 72-74.

[90] Huang X, Chen PC, Poole C. APOE- [varepsilon] 2 allele associated with higher prevalence of sporadic Parkinson disease. *Neurology.* 2004; 62(12):2198-2202.

[91] Harhangi BS, de Rijk MC, van Duijn CM, Van Broeckhoven C, Hofman A, Breteler MM. APOE and the risk of PD with or without dementia in a population-based study. *Neurology.* 2000; 54(6): 1272-1276.

[92] Ghosh SS, Swerdlow RH, Miller SW, Sheeman B, Parker WD Jr, Davis RE. Use of cytoplasmic hybrid cell lines for elucidating the role of mitochondrial dysfunction in Alzheimer's disease and Parkinson's disease. *Ann N Y Acad Sci.* 1999;893:176-191.

[93]   Parker WD Jr, Parks JK. Mitochondrial ND5 mutations in idiopathic Parkinson's disease. *Biochem Biophys Res Commun.* 2005; 326(3):667-669.

[94]   Zhou Y, Gu G, Goodlett DR, Zhang T, Pan C, Montine TJ, Montine KS, Aebersold RH, Zhang J. Analysis of alpha-synuclein-associated proteins by quantitative proteomics. *J Biol Chem.* 2004; 279(37):39155-39164.

[95]   Beal MF. Mitochondria take center stage in aging and neurodegeneration. *Ann Neurol.* 2005; 58(4): 495-505.

[96]   Smigrodzki R, Parks J, Parker WD. High frequency of mitochondrial complex I mutations in Parkinson's disease and aging. *Neurobiol Aging.* 2004; 25(10):1273-1281.

[97]   Kahn HA. The Dorn study of smoking and mortality among U.S. veterans: report on eight and one-half years of observation. *Natl Cancer Inst Monogr.* 1966; 19: 1-125.

[98]   Hofman A, Collette HJ, Bartelds AI. Incidence and risk factors of Parkinson's disease in The Netherlands. *Neuroepidemiology.* 1989;8(6):296-299.

[99]   Stern M, Dulaney E, Gruber SB, Golbe L, Bergen M, Hurtig H, Gollomp S, Stolley P. The epidemiology of Parkinson's disease. A case-control study of young-onset and old-onset patients. *Arch Neurol.* 1991; 48(9):903-907.

[100] Grandinetti A, Morens DM, Reed D, MacEachern D. Prospective study of cigarette smoking and the risk of developing idiopathic Parkinson's disease. *Am J Epidemiol.* 1994; 139(12):1129-1138.

[101] Tzourio C, Rocca WA, Breteler MM, Baldereschi M, Dartigues JF, Lopez-Pousa S, Manubens-Bertran JM, Alperovitch A. Smoking and Parkinson's disease. An age-dependent risk effect? The EUROPARKINSON Study Group. *Neurology.* 1997 ;49(5):1267-1272.

[102] Allam MF, Campbell MJ, Hofman A, Del Castillo AS, Fernandez-Crehuet Navajas R. Smoking and Parkinson's disease: systematic review of prospective studies. *Mov Disord.* 2004 Jun; 19(6): 614-621.

[103] Hernan MA, Takkouche B, Caamano-Isorna F, Gestal-Otero JJ. A meta-analysis of coffee drinking, cigarette smoking, and the risk of Parkinson's disease. *Ann Neurol.* 2002; 52(3): 276-284.

[104] Benedetti MD, Bower JH, Maraganore DM, McDonnell SK, Peterson BJ, Ahlskog JE, Schaid DJ, Rocca WA. Smoking, alcohol, and coffee consumption preceding Parkinson's disease: a case-control study. *Neurology.* 2000; 55(9): 1350-1358.

[105] O'reilly EJ, McCullough ML, Chao A, Jane Henley S, Calle EE, Thun MJ, Ascherio A. Smokeless tobacco use and the risk of Parkinson's disease mortality. *Mov Disord.* 2005; 20(10): 1383-1384.

[106] Tanner CM, Goldman SM, Aston DA, Ottman R, Ellenberg J, Mayeux R, Langston JW Smoking and Parkinson's disease in twins. *Neurology.* 2002; 58(4): 581-588.

[107] Anderson C, Checkoway H, Franklin GM, Beresford S, Smith-Weller T, Swanson PD. Dietary factors in Parkinson's disease: the role of food groups and specific foods. *Mov Disord.* 1999; 14(1):21-27.

[108] Johnson CC, Gorell JM, Rybicki BA, Sanders K, Peterson EL. Adult nutrient intake as a risk factor for Parkinson's disease. *Int J Epidemiol.* 1999; 28(6):1102-1109.

[109] De Lau LM, Bornebroek M, Witteman JC, Hofman A, Koudstaal PJ, Breteler MM. Dietary fatty acids and the risk of Parkinson disease: the Rotterdam study. *Neurology.* 2005;64(12):2040-2045.

[110] Park M, Ross GW, Petrovitch H, White LR, Masaki KH, Nelson JS, Tanner CM, Curb JD, Blanchette PL, Abbott RD. Consumption of milk and calcium in midlife and the future risk of Parkinson disease. *Neurology.* 2005; 64(6):1047-1051.

[111] Hellenbrand W, Seidler A, Boeing H, Robra BP, Vieregge P, Nischan P, Joerg J, Oertel WH, Schneider E, Ulm G. Diet and Parkinson's disease. I: A possible role for the past intake of specific foods and food groups. Results from a self-administered food-frequency questionnaire in a case-control study. *Neurology.* 1996 Sep; 47(3):636-643.

[112] Fall PA, Fredrikson M, Axelson O, Granerus AK. Nutritional and occupational factors influencing the risk of Parkinson's disease: a case-control study in southeastern Sweden. *Mov Disord.* 1999 14(1): 28-37.

[113] Checkoway H, Powers K, Smith-Weller T, Franklin GM, Longstreth WT Jr, Swanson PD. Parkinson's disease risks associated with cigarette smoking, alcohol consumption, and caffeine intake. *Am J Epidemiol.* 2002; 155(8):732-738.

[114] Abbott RD, Ross GW, White LR, Sanderson WT, Burchfiel CM, Kashon M, Sharp DS, Masaki KH, Curb JD, Petrovitch H. Environmental, life-style, and physical precursors of clinical Parkinson's disease: recent findings from the Honolulu-Asia Aging Study. *J Neurol.* 2003; 250 Suppl 3:III30-39.

[115] Ascherio A, Zhang SM, Hernan MA, Kawachi I, Colditz GA, Speizer FE, Willett WC. Prospective study of caffeine consumption and risk of Parkinson's disease in men and women. *Ann Neurol.* 2001; 50(1): 56-63.

[116] Ascherio A, Weisskopf MG, O'Reilly EJ, McCullough ML, Calle EE, Rodriguez C, Thun MJ. Coffee consumption, gender, and Parkinson's disease mortality in the cancer prevention study II cohort: the modifying effects of estrogen. *Am J Epidemiol.* 2004; 160(10): 977-984.

[117] McGeer PL, Itagaki S, Boyes BE, McGeer EG. Reactive microglia are positive for HLA-DR in the substantia nigra of Parkinson's and Alzheimer's disease brains. *Neurology.* 1988; 38(8): 1285-1291

[118] Langston JW, Forno LS, Tetrud J, Reeves AG, Kaplan JA, Karluk D. Evidence of active nerve cell degeneration in the substantia nigra of humans years after 1-methyl-4-phenyl-1,2,3,6-tetrahydropyridine exposure. *Ann Neurol.* 1999; 46(4): 598-605.

[119] Zhang W, Wang T, Pei Z, Miller DS, Wu X, Block ML, Wilson B, Zhang W, Zhou Y, Hong JS, Zhang J. Aggregated alpha-synuclein activates microglia: a process leading to disease progression in Parkinson's disease. *FASEB J.* 2005; 19(6): 533-542.

[120] Nagatsu T, Sawada M. Inflammatory process in Parkinson's disease: role for cytokines. *Curr Pharm Des.* 2005; 11(8): 999-1016.

[121] Chen H, Jacobs E, Schwarzschild MA, McCullough ML, Calle EE, Thun MJ, Ascherio A Nonsteroidal antiinflammatory drug use and the risk for Parkinson's disease. *Ann Neurol.* 2005; 58(6):963-967.

[122] Martyn CN, Osmond C. Parkinson's disease and the environment in early life. *J Neurol Sci.* 1995; 132(2): 201-206.

[123] Sasco AJ, Paffenbarger RS Jr. Measles infection and Parkinson's disease. *Am J Epidemiol.* 1985; 122(6):1017-1031.

[124] Poskanzer DC, Schwab RC. Cohort analysis of Parkinson's syndrome: evidence for a single etiology related to subclinical infection about 1920. *J Chronic Dis.* 1963; 16:961-973.

[125] Takahashi M, Yamada T. A possible role of influenza A virus infection for Parkinson's disease. *Adv Neurol.* 2001; 86:91-104.

[126] Baldi I, Cantagrel A, Lebailly P, Tison F, Dubroca B, Chrysostome V, Dartigues JF, Brochard P. Association between Parkinson's disease and exposure to pesticides in southwestern France. *Neuroepidemiology.* 2003; 22(5): 305-310.

[127] Firestone JA, Smith-Weller T, Franklin G, Swanson P, Longstreth WT Jr, Checkoway H. Pesticides and risk of Parkinson disease: a population-based case-control study. *Arch Neurol.* 2005; 62(1): 91-95.

[128] Gorrel JM, Johnson CC, Rybicki BA, Peterson EL, Richardson RJ. The risk of Parkinson's disease with exposure to pesticides, farming, well water, and rural living. *Neurology.* 1998; 50(5):1346-1350.

[129] Hertzman C, Wiens M, Bowering D, Snow B, Calne D. Parkinson's disease: a case-control study of occupational and environmental risk factors. *Am J Ind Med.* 1990; 17(3): 349-355.

[130] Baldi I, Lebailly P, Mohammed-Brahim B, Letenneur L, Dartigues JF, Brochard P. Neurodegenerative diseases and exposure to pesticides in the elderly. *Am J Epidemiol.* 2003; 157(5):409-414.

[131] Rocca WA, Anderson DW, Meneghini F, Grigoletto F, Morgante L, Reggio A, Savettieri G, Di Perri R. Occupation, education, and Parkinson's disease: a case-control study in an Italian population. *Mov Disord.* 1996; 11(2):201-206.

[132] Koller W, Vetere-Overfield B, Gray C, Alexander C, Chin T, Dolezal J, Hassanein R, Tanner C. Environmental risk factors in Parkinson's disease. *Neurology.* 1990; 40(8): 1218-1221.

[133] Smargiassi A, Mutti A, De Rosa A, De Palma G, Negrotti A, Calzetti S. A case-control study of occupational and environmental risk factors for Parkinson's disease in the Emilia-Romagna region of Italy. *Neurotoxicology.* 1998; 19(4-5): 709-712.

[134] McCann SJ, LeCouteur DG, Green AC, Brayne C, Johnson AG, Chan D, McManus ME,Pond SM. The epidemiology of Parkinson's disease in an Australian population. *Neuroepidemiology.* 1998; 17(6):310-317.

[135] Racette BA, McGee-Minnich L, Moerlein SM, Mink JW, Videen TO, Perlmutter JS. Welding-related parkinsonism: clinical features, treatment, and pathophysiology. *Neurology.* 2001; 56(1): 8-13.

[136] Seidler A, Hellenbrand W, Robra BP, Vieregge P, Nischan P, Joerg J, Oertel WH, Ulm G, Schneider E. Possible environmental, occupational, and other etiologic factors for Parkinson's disease: a case-control study in Germany. *Neurology.* 1996; 46(5): 1275-1284.

[137] Semchuk KM, Love EJ, Lee RG. Parkinson's disease: a test of the multifactorial etiologic hypothesis. *Neurology.* 1993; 43(6):1173-1180.

[138] Olanow CW. Manganese-induced parkinsonism and Parkinson's disease. *Ann N Y Acad Sci.* 2004; 1012:209-223.

[139] Jankovic J. Searching for a relationship between manganese and welding and Parkinson's disease. *Neurology.* 2005; 64(12): 2021-2028.

[140] Pezzoli G, Canesi M, Antonini A, Righini A, Perbellini L, Barichella M, Mariani CB, Tenconi F, Tesei S, Zecchinelli A, Leenders KL. Hydrocarbon exposure and Parkinson's disease. *Neurology.* 2000; 55(5): 667-673.

[141] Ohlson CG, Hogstedt C. Parkinson's disease and occupational exposure to organic solvents, agricultural chemicals and mercury--a case-referent study. *Scand J Work Environ Health.* 1981;7(4):252-256.

[142] Okada K, Kobayashi S, Tsunematsu T. Prevalence of Parkinson's disease in Izumo City, Japan. *Gerontology.* 1990; 36(5-6): 340-344.

[143] Bharucha EP, Bharucha NE. Epidemiological study of Parkinson's disease in Parsis in India. *Adv Neurol.* 1993; 60: 352-354.

[144] Razdan S, Kaul RL, Motta A, Kaul S, Bhatt RK. Prevalence and pattern of major neurological disorders in rural Kashmir (India) in 1986. *Neuroepidemiology.* 1994;13(3):113-119.

[145] Tison F, Dartigues JF, Dubes L, Zuber M, Alperovitch A, Henry P. Prevalence of Parkinson's disease in the elderly: a population study in Gironde, France. *Acta Neurol Scand.* 1994; 90(2): 111-115.

[146] De Rijk MC, Breteler MM, Graveland GA, Ott A, Grobbee DE, van der Meche FG, Hofman A. Prevalence of Parkinson's disease in the elderly: the Rotterdam Study. *Neurology.* 1995; 45(12): 2143-2146.

[147] Giroud Benitez JL, Collado-Mesa F, Esteban EM. Prevalence of Parkinson disease in an urban area of the Ciudad de La Habana province, Cuba. Door-to-door population study. *Neurologia.* 2000; 15(7): 269-273.

[148] Milanov I, Kmetska K, Karakolev B, Nedialkov E. Prevalence of Parkinson's disease in Bulgaria. *Neuroepidemiology.* 2001; 20(3):212-214.

[149] Anca M, Paleacu D, Shabtai H, Giladi N. Cross-sectional study of the prevalence of Parkinson's disease in the Kibbutz movement in Israel. *Neuroepidemiology.* 2002;21(1):50-55.

[150] Taba P, Asser T. Prevalence of Parkinson's disease in Estonia. *Acta Neurol Scand.* 2002; 106 (5):276-281.

[151] Kis B, Schrag A, Ben-Shlomo Y, Klein C, Gasperi A, Spoegler F, Schoenhuber R, Pramstaller PP. Novel three-stage ascertainment method: prevalence of PD and parkinsonism in South Tyrol, Italy. *Neurology.* 2002; 58(12):1820-1825.

[152] Claveria LE, Duarte J, Sevillano MD, Perez-Sempere A, Cabezas C, Rodriguez F, de Pedro-Cuesta J. Prevalence of Parkinson's disease in Cantalejo, Spain: a door-to-door survey. *Mov Disord.* 2002; 17(2):242-249.

[153] Nicoletti A, Sofia V, Bartoloni A, Bartalesi F, Gamboa Barahon H, Giuffrida S, Reggio A. 1996; 15(4): 201-7. Prevalence of Parkinson's disease: a door-to-door survey in rural Bolivia. *Parkinsonism Relat Disord.* 2003; 10(1): 19-21.

[154] Benito-Leon J, Bermejo-Pareja F, Rodriguez J, Molina JA, Gabriel R, Morales JM; Neurological Disorders in Central Spain (NEDICES) Study Group. Prevalence of PD

and other types of parkinsonism in three elderly populations of central Spain. *Mov Disord.* 2003; 18(3):267-274.

[155] Woo J, Lau E, Ziea E, Chan DK. Prevalence of Parkinson's disease in a Chinese population. *Acta Neurol Scand.* 2004; 109(3): 228-331.

[156] Tan LC, Venketasubramanian N, Hong CY, Sahadevan S, Chin JJ, Krishnamoorthy ES, Tan AK, Saw SM. Prevalence of Parkinson disease in Singapore: Chinese vs Malays vs Indians. *Neurology.* 2004; 62(11): 1999-2004.

[157] Chan DK, Cordato D, Karr M, Ong B, Lei H, Liu J, Hung WT. Prevalence of Parkinson's disease in Sydney. *Acta Neurol Scand.* 2005; 111(1): 7-11.

[158] Hobson P, Gallacher J, Meara J. Cross-sectional survey of Parkinson's disease and parkinsonism in a rural area of the United Kingdom. *Mov Disord.* 2005 ; 20(8):995-998.

[159] Fall PA, Axelson O, Fredriksson M, Hansson G, Lindvall B, Olsson JE, Granerus AK. Age-standardized incidence and prevalence of Parkinson's disease in a Swedish community. *J Clin Epidemiol.* 1996; 49(6):637-641.

[160] Vines JJ, Larumbe R, Gaminde I, Artazcoz MT. Incidence of idiopathic and secondary Parkinson disease in Navarre. Population-based case registry. *Neurologia.* 1999; 14(1): 16-22.

RECOMMENDED FURTHER READING

1. Samii A, Nutt JG. Ransom BR. Parkinson's disease. *Lancet* 363(9423):1783-93, 2004
2. Nutt JG, Wooten GF. Clinical practice. Diagnosis and initial management of Parkinson's disease. *New England Journal of Medicine* 353(10):1021-7, 2005
3. Rascol O, Goetz C, Koller W, Poewe W, Sampaio C. Treatment interventions for Parkinson's disease: an evidence based assessment. *Lancet* 359(9317):1589-98, 2002
4. Pahwa R, Lyons KE (Editors). Handbook of Parkinson's Disease. 4th Edition, Informa Healthcare, 2007.

In: Handbook of Clinical Neuroepidemiology
Editors: V. L. Feigin and D. A. Bennett, pp. 557-572

ISBN 978-1-60021-511-7
© 2007 Nova Science Publishers, Inc.

Chapter 16

MULTIPLE SCLEROSIS

Gustavo C. Román and Patricia Castellanos-Mateus

University of Texas, Health Sciences Center at San Antonio, USA.

ABSTRACT

The neuroepidemiology of multiple sclerosis (MS) offers numerous interesting features including the peculiar distribution of this disease by age and sex, affecting predominantly women in young and middle-age adult age-groups, as well as a typical geographic pattern of occurrence with low prevalence in tropical regions and increasing prevalence in temperate regions. Although ethnic, racial, and genetic factors have been implicated, no definitive genetic markers have been identified and the mode of transmission remains unknown. Likewise, no single environmental factor has been demonstrated to cause MS. The recently proposed protective effect of sunlight exposure and vitamin D offers new hopes for the prevention and treatment of this potentially devastating condition. Finally, novel clinical trial methodologies have been proposed to determine in shorter and more efficient trials the effectiveness of future therapeutic agents in MS.

INTRODUCTION

Multiple sclerosis (MS) is a common demyelinating disease of unknown cause most frequently affecting young adults and characterized by the presence of islands of perivascular demyelination anywhere in the central nervous system (CNS) which give rise to intermittent or progressive neurological signs [1]. In 1835, Jean Cruveilhier provided the first neuropathological description of the disease and Jean-Martin Charcot described in 1868 its clinical features. Common symptoms include fatigue, visual and sensory disturbances, cerebellar symptoms and gait alterations, motor weakness, paralysis and spasticity, bladder and bowel incontinence, as well as subcortical cognitive impairment observed in about 50%

of patients [2]. Excluding trauma, MS is the leading cause of neurological disability among young and middle-age adults.

DIAGNOSTIC CRITERIA

The diagnosis of MS requires evidence of neurological dysfunction affecting the central nervous system disseminated in space and time. Despite the clinically heterogeneous nature of MS, the advent of accurate brain imaging techniques—in particular magnetic resonance imaging (MRI)—has resulted in a simplification of the diagnostic process reflected in an increase of incidence figures in many parts of the world. However, as emphasized by Poser [3], it is important to distinguish MS from other demyelinating disorders, in particular acute disseminated encephalomyelitis (ADEM) [4]. Clinical diagnostic criteria were first suggested by Schumacher et al [5] in 1965; these were followed in 1983 by the criteria of Poser et al [6] that have been widely used in epidemiological and clinical studies. Most recently, in 2001, the criteria of McDonald et al. [7] require evidence of two or more attacks and two or more lesions, particularly in cases with insidious neurological progression (Table 1).

PATHOGENESIS

It is generally accepted that MS is a cell-mediated autoimmune disease directed against antigens in myelin in the central nervous system (CNS). Weiner [10] hypothesized that the main pathogenetic mechanism is an inappropriate class of immune response against myelin antigens favoring pro-inflammatory Th1 versus anti-inflammatory Th2 or Th3 type responses. MS is a multifactorial disease influenced by environmental and genetic factors. The inflammatory demyelinating process in the CNS of the patient genetically determined to develop MS results in a pathognomonically unique lesion, the sharp-edged plaque (felicitously described by Ludo van Bogaert as *'découpée à l'emporte pièce'*) [4,11]. The sharp-edged plaque is a zone where oligodendrocytes and intact myelinated internodes abut demyelinated, gliotic, and oligodendrocyte-depleted parenchyma [11]. Axonal loss is an important component of MS, particularly in patients with permanent neurological deficits and secondary brain atrophy [12].

DESCRIPTIVE EPIDEMIOLOGY

There are marked differences in the prevalence of MS around the world suggesting interplay of racial versus environmental factors [13]. It is generally accepted that susceptibility genes can be modified by the environment to induce MS [14]. Rosati [15], in a recent update on the prevalence of MS, pointed out that a number of methodological problems complicate the interpretation of epidemiological studies of MS including variations regarding age distribution, size, sex, and ethnicity of the populations studied. Completeness of case ascertainment is determined by local factors such as public awareness of MS, access of patients to medical services, number of neurologists, and availability of diagnostic equipment such as MRI. Last but not least, the use of different diagnostic criteria and the interobserver variability when applying the same diagnostic criteria also influence the number of cases diagnosed as MS. Zavadinov et al [16] have recommended that crude incidence and prevalence rates in epidemiological studies on MS should be adjusted by age and sex to a common standard population using direct or indirect standardization methods in order to permit a more reliable comparison among studies performed in different countries.

Table 1. Diagnostic Criteria for Multiple Sclerosis (McDonald et al) [7]

Clinical Presentation	*Additional Data Needed for MS Diagnosis*
≥ 2 attacks; objective clinical evidence of ≥ 2 lesions	None.*
≥ 2 attacks; objective clinical evidence of 1 lesion	Dissemination in space (by MRI§) *or* ≥ 2 MRI-detected lesions consistent with MS *plus* positive CSF¶ *or* await further clinical attack implicating a different site
1 attack; objective clinical evidence of ≥2 lesions	Dissemination in time, demonstrated by MRI§ *or* second clinical attack
1 attack; objective clinical evidence of 1 lesion (mono-symptomatic presentation; clinically isolated syndrome)	Dissemination in space (by MRI§) *or* ≥ 2 MRI-detected lesions consistent with MS *plus* positive CSF¶ *and* dissemination in time, demonstrated by MRI§ *or* second clinical attack
Insidious neurological progression suggestive of MS	Positive CSF¶ *and* dissemination in space, demonstrated by: (1) ≥ 9 T2 MRI-detected brain lesions, *or* (2) ≥ 2 MRI-detected spinal cord lesions, *or* (3) 4-8 brain *plus* 1 spinal cord lesion *or* abnormal VEP** associated with 4-8 brain lesions, *or* < *4* brain lesions *plus* 1 spinal cord lesion demonstrated by MRI and dissemination in time, demonstrated by MRI§§ *or* continued progression for 1 year.

If criteria indicated are fulfilled, the diagnosis is MS; if the criteria are not completely met, the diagnosis is possible MS, if the criteria are fully explored and not met, the diagnosis is not MS.

*No additional tests are required; however, if tests MRI, CSF are undertaken and are negative, extreme caution should be taken before making a diagnosis of MS. Alternative diagnoses should be considered. There must be no better explanation for the clinical picture.

§ MRI demonstration of space dissemination must fulfill the criteria developed by Barkof et al [8] and Tintore et al [9].

¶ Positive CSF determined by oligoclonal bands detected by established methods (preferably isoelectric focusing) different from any such bands in serum or by a raised Ig index.

§§ MRI demonstration of time dissemination must fulfill the criteria listed above.

** Abnormal visual evoked potentials of the type seen in MS (delayed with a well-preserved wave form).

Geographic Distribution

Despite the above difficulties, epidemiological studies have shown significant variations in incidence, prevalence and mortality rates of MS according to latitude. In general, according to Kurtzke [13], higher prevalence rates (>30 per 100,000) occur in temperate regions including northern Europe, northern USA and Canada, as well as southern Australia and New Zealand. Regions of medium prevalence (5-30 per 100,000) include southern Europe, southern USA, and northern Australia. Low prevalence of MS (around 5/100,000) has been estimated for tropical areas of Asia, Africa, and South America. Recent prevalence studies indicate variations within neighboring countries, and often within regions of a single country.

Based on these recent data we suggest classifying the worldwide prevalence of MS according to the following categories: countries with *very high prevalence* of MS (≥130 cases per 100,000), *high prevalence* (80-129 per 100,000), *medium prevalence* (30-79 per 100,000), *low prevalence* (5-29 per 100,000), and *very low prevalence* (0-4 per 100,000). Figure 1 shows the worldwide prevalence of MS in different countries according to this classification.

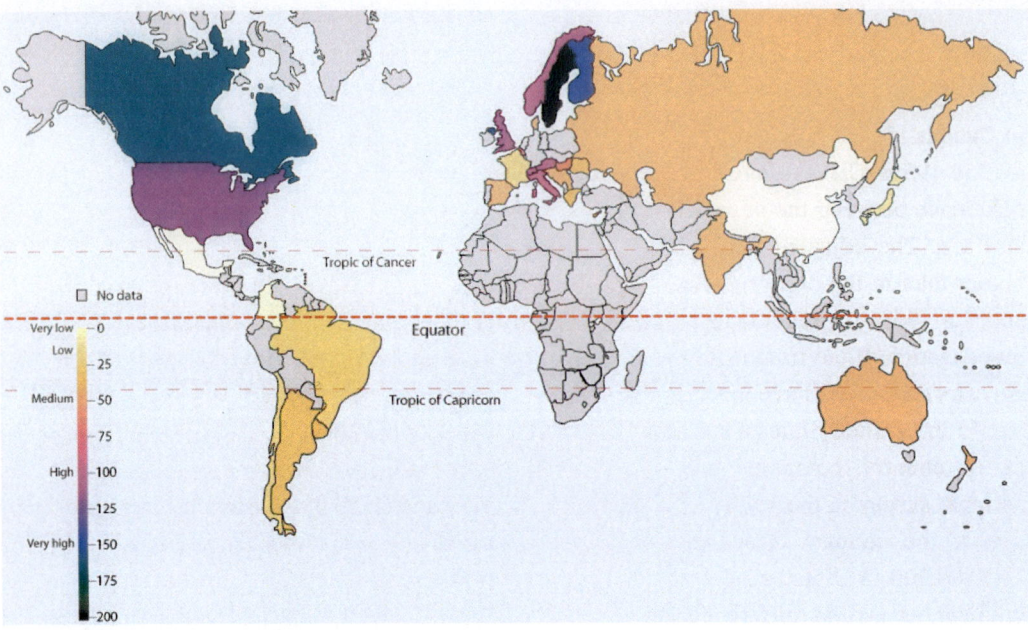

Figure 1. Worldwide prevalence of MS in different countries

Europe

Very high prevalences of MS, ranging from 145 to 193 per 100,000 [15] have been consistently documented in Scotland and its offshore islands including Shetland and Orkney islands, as well as in Northern Ireland (168 per 100,00). Likewise, very high prevalences are found in Scandinavian countries [15] including Norway (Oslo: 132), Denmark (112), Finland (93), Iceland (92) and Sweden (152). In Sweden, the highest prevalence rates for MS cluster around the two major lakes of south central Sweden, and the Bays of Bothnia and Stockholm

[17-19]. Although geographically separated from the latitudes above 60° North of the previously listed countries, the island of Sardinia (40° North) represents an exception to the distribution of MS in Italy and other Mediterranean countries since the prevalence of MS in Sardinia reaches 150 per 100,000 with an increasing trend in incidence [20]. This population is highly stable from the genetic viewpoint suggesting that possible exogenous risk factors may explain these figures [20].

European countries with *high prevalences* of MS (80-129 per 100,000) include Germany (range 85-108), Switzerland (Berne: 110), the Czech Republic (89), Slovenia (83), and Croatia (124). Most of the remaining countries in Europe (France, Italy, The Netherlands, Belgium, Austria, Russia, Ukraine, Baltic Republics, Poland, Hungary, Spain, Portugal, Bulgaria, Greece, Macedonia, and Cyprus) have *medium prevalences* ranging from 30 to 79 cases per 100,000 [15]. *Low prevalences* (5-29 per 100,000) have been reported in Armenia, Azerbaijan, Kurdistan, Uzbekistan, and Kyrgyzstan [15]. The lowest prevalence rates of MS in Europe have been documented in the island of Malta (4 per 100,000); although recent studies indicate an increase in incidence and prevalence [21].

The Americas

North America: Canada has a *very high prevalence* of MS (≥130 cases per 100,000), with a gradient of increasing frequency from east to west. The highest prevalence was 248/100,000 in Saskatoon [22]. A recent study [23] showed that the overall prevalence of MS in Canada is 240/100,000 (95% CI: 210-280), ranging from 180 (95% CI: 90-260) in Quebec to 350 (95% CI: 230-470) in Atlantic Canada. Logistic regression revealed no statistical difference between the odds of MS in Quebec, Ontario and British Columbia adjusted for age and sex. The adjusted odds of MS in the Prairies and Atlantic regions were significantly higher than in the other regions combined, with odds ratios of 1.7 (95%CI: 1.1-2.4, P <0.01) and 1.6 (95%CI: 1.1-2.4, P <0.05) respectively. These regional differences may facilitate investigation of environmental influences. Native Amerindians and the Hutterites (of German ancestry) appear to have low risk for MS [24].

In the United States a significant increase in MS prevalence is found in the northern tier of the country, compared with the southern tier [13]. This gradient was confirmed by a national survey in the 1970s [25] and probably reflects Scandinavian ancestry in the northern tier of the country. Prevalence rates have ranged from 22/100,000 in Los Angeles to 160/100,000 in Olmstead County [15]. Studies in Veterans have confirmed this north—south gradient, as well as differences by race and sex [26]. Among veterans, risk of MS is higher for all women, at 2.99 for whites, 2.86 for blacks, and 3.51 for other races. Residence at service entry in the northern tier had a relative risk of 2.02 versus the southern tier. These changes in geography, sex, and race strongly imply a primary environmental factor in MS [26].

Redelings et al [27] analyzed MS mortality rates in the United States from 1990 to 2001. The overall age-adjusted mortality rate from MS was 1.44/100,000 population. MS mortality rates were higher in whites than in any other racial/ethnic group. Observed mortality rates were more than 10 times lower in Asians and Pacific Islanders than in whites.

Latin America: A summary of recent epidemiological studies of MS in Latin America [28] indicates increased awareness of this condition, accompanied by a probable increase in prevalence. For instance, in Mexico the prevalence of MS in hospital-based and population-based studies increased from 1.6/100,000 in 1970 [29] to 13/100,000 in 2003 [30], confirming the *low prevalence* of MS (5-29 per 100,000) in this country. Other studies performed in central areas of Mexico have registered lower prevalences of about 5/100,000 at latitudes 16–20° north [31]. In Mexico, optic neuritis represents 12% of the patients referred to a specialized neuro-ophthalmology clinic and about 40% of them eventually develop MS [32,33].

In Latin-America, MS prevalences range from *low* to *medium:* Argentina (12 to 88/100,000) [34,35], Brazil (15) [36-38], Uruguay, (20.9) [39], Chile (11.7) [40,41], Colombia (1.48 to 4.98) [42]. There are no reliable data from the Caribbean with the exception of a careful study from the French West Indies [43]. Cabré et al [43] demonstrated higher prevalence of MS in Martinique than in Guadeloupe (21.0 vs. 8.5) and a higher MS incidence (2.0/100,000 vs. 0.7) suggesting an environmental factor in the emergence of MS in the French West Indies, either introduced by migrants from continental France and/or due to disappearance of protective environmental factors acting before age 15 years. The presence of epidemic optic myeloneuropathy in Cuba and tropical spastic paraparesis from HTLV-I infections of the nervous system in the Caribbean constitute complicating factors for prevalence studies of MS in this region.

Australia and New Zealand

Epidemiological studies have demonstrated a south-north gradient with prevalence rates ranging from 11/100,000 in north Queensland, Australia, to 69/100,000 in Otago, New Zealand [15]. A significant increase in MS prevalence has been documented in three Australian cities (Newcastle, Perth and Hobart) between 1950 and 1996 [44]. MS is reportedly rare among the native Maoris. Regional variation dependent on ambient ultraviolet radiation has been postulated [45].

Asia and Other Regions

MS appears to have *very low prevalences* (0-4 per 100,000) in Asia, including China, India, Japan, South East Asia, the Middle East, as well as in Africa and the Pacific Islands.

GENETIC EPIDEMIOLOGY

Rosati [15] concluded that racial and ethnic differences are important in explaining the worldwide distribution of MS. It seems clear that Scandinavian racial groups have increased susceptibility to MS. From the historical viewpoint, Poser [46] suggested that Viking voyages provide a likely explanation for the unexpectedly high prevalence rates of MS in some regions around the Mediterranean and Russia that otherwise are considered to have low risk.

Familial aggregation studies in siblings, twins, and adoption studies, also provide strong data in favor of the genetic susceptibility to MS. Identical twins with MS have relative risks of 100-190 compared to general population; siblings 20-40, half siblings 7-13, and offspring of an affected parent 5.5 [47].

Although the mode of inheritance is unclear, segregation analyses have shown evidence of a major MS susceptibility gene in the main histocompatibility complex (MHC) in some families. Class I human leukocyte antigen (HLA) and class II have been associated, in particular the HLA-DR2 haplotype, consistently found in Caucasians of northern European descent. Current research indicates consistent linkage for chromosome 6p21, the location of the MHC containing HLA. However, overall results of these studies have been disappointing.

ENVIRONMENTAL FACTORS

Alter and colleagues [48] were the first to point out that European migrants that traveled to Israel after the age of 15 years retained the high risk of the country of origin, whereas those traveling before age 15 had the lower risk found in the Mediterranean environment of Israel. These studies have been widely confirmed [14], and as mentioned above, most recently among Martinique migrants from continental France [43]. These studies suggest the existence of either a protective factor in areas with low prevalence or a risk factor in those with high risk. The following environmental factors have been postulated in MS.

Infection

The possible association of MS with viral diseases is based on the fact that infections may trigger autoimmune diseases. Only the most relevant ones will be reviewed here. Thacker et al [49] conducted a systematic review and meta-analysis of 14 case-control and cohort studies of infectious mononucleosis (IM) and MS. The relative risk of MS after IM was 2.3 (95% CI 1.7-3.0). These authors concluded that Epstein-Barr virus infection causing IM appears to be a risk factor for MS. Studies from Mexico, with isolation of the varicella-zoster virus during attacks of MS [50-52], suggest that this virus could be an etiological agent of MS. Risk factors such as decrease in breastfeeding in Mexico and an increased incidence of varicella and childhood eczema could predispose to activation of varicella-zoster virus during MS relapses [50-52].

The numerous agents of common childhood infections have been considered potential causal agents of MS. However, Bager et al [53], using information recalled in childhood from a large historical cohort of school children in Denmark, recently concluded that measles, rubella, mumps, varicella, pertussis and scarlet fever, even if acquired late in childhood, are not associated with increased risk of multiple sclerosis later in life.

Vaccination, particularly with hepatitis B [54] has been implicated as a causative factor for MS. However, large epidemiological studies failed to find an increased risk of MS after vaccination [55].

Sotgiu et al [56] have reviewed the "hygiene hypothesis" of MS, whereby the balance of immune responses between TH1 (defending host against bacterial and viral infections) and TH2 (defending against parasitic infections) is pivotal. The consequence of reducing infectious stressors during infancy would result in increased autoimmunity (TH1-mediated) and allergy (TH2-mediated). Epidemiological studies confirm that allergic and autoimmune diseases are significantly increased in "developed" countries and negatively associated with childhood infections. This factor could explain the low prevalence of MS in underdeveloped countries and the progressive increase associated with improved environmental conditions.

Physical Environment Factors

Low levels of ultraviolet (UV) radiation have been associated to the increased frequency of MS found at higher northern and southern latitudes, and to the low prevalence of tropical areas [57]. Vitamin D (cholecalciferol) is a lipid-soluble vitamin synthesized by conversion of 7-dehydrocholesterol to vitamin D in the skin by exposure to ultraviolet (UV) B radiation [58]. Vitamin D is converted by the liver to 25-hydroxyvitamin D or 25(OH)D. Serum levels of 25(OH)D are used to monitor vitamin D status. Vitamin D appears to have immunomodulatory effects. The metabolically active form, 1,25-dihydroxyvitamin D3 (calcitriol) protects mice from experimental autoimmune encephalomyelitis (EAE), an animal model for MS, compared with 100% incidence in the control group [59].

Munger et al [60] correlated dietary vitamin D intake with risk of MS in two large cohorts of US women: the Nurses' Health Study (n=92,253 women) and the NHS II (n=95,310 women). The pooled age-adjusted relative risk (RR) was 0.67 (95% CI = 0.40 to 1.12) comparing the highest quintile of vitamin D intake at baseline with those with the lowest intake; the RR was 0.59 comparing women with intake of $\geq$400 IU/day with women with no supplemental vitamin D intake. Long-term use of a multivitamin (>10 yrs) resulted in a 41% risk reduction compared with participants who had never used a multivitamin (95% CI 0.18 to 0.93) even after controlling for age, smoking, and geographic latitude at birth. These findings support a protective effect of vitamin D intake on risk of developing MS. Vitamin D may be effective in prevention and treatment of patients with MS.

CLINICAL TRIALS DESIGN IN MS

Despite the complexity of the pathogenesis and clinical presentation of MS, including the unpredictability of its clinical and radiological progression, a number of therapies have demonstrated beneficial effects on controlled clinical trials. Based on traditional double-blind placebo controlled randomized trials, the US Food and Drug Administration (FDA) approved the following drugs for the treatment of MS: three pharmaceutical forms of beta interferon, one peptide polymer (glatiramer acetate); and, mitoxantrone, an immunosuppressant agent. Natalizumab, a humanized monoclonal antibody to the $\alpha 4$ subunit of $\alpha_4\beta_1$-integrin, was initially approved but later recalled due to the unexpected development of fatal progressive multifocal leukoencephalopathy (PML) in 3 cases [61]. Natalizumab blocks integrin, a cellular adhesion molecule (CAM) crucial for adhesion and migration of immunocompetent T cells through its binding to vascular CAM1 on the surface of endothelial cells of the brain and spinal cord, allowing leucocytes to cross the blood–brain barrier into the CNS. In the animal model of EAE natalizumab blocks this interaction preventing the influx of activated leukocytes into the CNS. In patients with MS the addition of natalizumab to interferon beta-

1a was superior to added placebo in terms of both clinical measures (relapse rate, progression of disability), and MRI measures such as appearance of new or enhancing lesions (Table 2) [61]. In contrast, interferon beta and glatiramer acetate only reduced relapses by around a third [61].

Table 2. Main 2-year outcomes for the different treatments approved by the US Food and Drug Administration for MS [61]

| | Baseline EDSS | Clinical measures | | MRI measures | | |
		Mean attack rate	Progression	New T2 lesions	Gd+ or CU lesions	Disease burden
Interferon beta-1b, 250 µg, sc, qod	2.9	-34%***	-29% (ns)	-83%**	nr	-17%***
Interferon beta-1a, 30 µg, im, qw	2.4	-37%*	-37%*	-36%**	-42%*	-4% (ns)
Interferon beta-1a, 44 µg, sc, tiw	2.5	-30%*	-30%*	-78%***	-88%***	-15%***
Glatiramer acetate 20 mg, sc, qod	2.6	-12% (ns)	-12% (ns)	-38%**	-33%**	-8%**
Mitoxantrone 12 mg/m³, iv, q 3 mo	4.5	-75%*	-75%*	-79%*	-79% (ns)	nr
Natalizumab 300 mg, iv, q mo	2.3	-42%***	-42%***	-83%***	-92%***	-18%***

Percentage reductions (or increases) have been calculated by dividing the reported rates in the treated group by the comparable rates in the placebo group, apart from MRI disease burden, which was calculated as the difference in the median % change between the treated and placebo groups. Progression=1 point EDSS progression, sustained for 3 months (in the interferon beta-1a 30 µg qw trial, this change was sustained for 6 months; in the interferon beta-1b trial, this was sustained for more than 3 years). Different studies measured the MRI measures differently, making comparisons difficult (numbers for new T2 and Gd+ represent the best case scenario for each trial).
EDSS = expanded disability status score ; GD+ = gadolinium enhanced; CU = combined unique lesion; sc = subcutaneous; qod = every other day; im = intramuscular; qw = once per week; tiw = three times per week; iv = intravenous; q 3 mo = once every 3 months; q mo = once per month; ns = not significant; nr = not reported; *p≤0.05; **p≤0.01; ***p≤0.001.

The three fatal cases of PML were due to reactivation of the JC virus in patients treated with natalizumab (one patient had MS, one probably had migraine and infarcts, and one had Crohn's disease). The FDA initially discontinued natalizumab and encouraged physicians to report immediately any symptoms suggestive of PML. Later, the FDA allowed continuation of open-label natalizumab monotherapy trials in the same patients recruited for the initial double-blind trials [61,62]. The risk of PML in patients receiving natalizumab infusions over several years is unknown, but it is probably >1 per 1000. The presence of PML as a complication of treatment opens new questions for future MS trials with natalizumab and other integrin antagonists, as well as with immunomodulatory agents. The peculiar problems in designing controlled trials in MS will be briefly reviewed. The National Multiple Sclerosis Society Advisory Committee on Clinical Trials of New Agents in Multiple Sclerosis recently published the conclusions of a meeting on this topic [63].

Patient Selection

The first and foremost requirement for a valid trial in MS is the use of appropriate inclusion and exclusion criteria for recruitment of patients. This requirement is crucial for the selection of a homogeneous population that would allow the generalized application of the trial results. Langer-Gould and Steinman [62] correctly emphasized that entry criteria into clinical trials of relapsing-remitting MS must exclude patients with misdiagnosed migraine and cerebrovascular disease, as well as other conditions mimicking MS. A mandatory requirement for objective evidence of CNS inflammation and demyelination at some point in a patient's disease course, avoiding the exclusive reliance on imaging criteria, should defend against misdiagnosis [62]. In general, the Poser criteria [6] and the criteria of McDonald et al. [7] are adequate for patient selection in most studies.

From the clinical view point it is also important to limit the trials to a particular clinical form of MS since the prognosis changes with the clinical form. About 85% of patients develop the relapsing-remitting form (RRMS) with slowly accumulating disability. The remaining 15% develop from onset the primary progressive form (PPMS) with poor prognosis and reduced life-expectancy. The overall prognosis of MS is less disabling than generally acknowledged. Runmarker and Andersen [64] followed a population-based cohort and found that only 43% of the patients with MS required a cane or worse after 25 years of follow-up. The best predictors of disease severity are incomplete recovery from attacks and accumulation of disability in the first 2–5 years after onset [62].

Study Design

One major problem in MS trials design is the fact that any placebo-controlled trial withholding active therapy is consider unethical [63], despite the fact that available therapies for MS only provide partially effective symptomatic improvement. Furthermore, finding patients naïve to therapy is notoriously difficult and recruiting established patients for placebo controlled trials is no easy task.

Possible solutions include shorter clinical trials using multiple outcomes [63]. Traditionally, most studies have used the Kurtzke Expanded Disability Status Scale (EDSS) [65] as the main clinical outcome, despite the linearity of this scale and the emphasis on ambulation. The original DSS had steps from 0 (normal) to 10 (death due to MS). In the EDSS, each one of the former steps (1,2,3 . . . 9) is divided into two (1.0, 1.5, 2.0 . . . 9.5). The lower portion is obligatorily defined by Functional System (FS) grades including Pyramidal, Cerebellar, Brain Stem, Sensory, Bowel & Bladder, Visual, Cerebral, and Other. There have been some attempts to correlate the EDSS with diffusion tensor MRI (DT-MRI), a method that allows quantification of pathology in specific white matter tracts [66,67]. This method may increase the specificity of MRI in monitoring progression of motor and cognitive deficits in MS.

Other, more recently studied clinical end-point scales include the Multiple Sclerosis Impairment Scale (MSIS) [68,69] that was proposed following WHO's recommendation to quantify accumulated deficits (impairment) in MS patients. The items are obtained from the standard neurological examination, plus a short battery of cognitive tests. Normal findings are assigned a zero value, and the theoretical maximum score is 204. The MSIS is easy to use, has excellent interobserver kappa values, follows a monomodal univariate distribution and has a better discriminatory power than the EDSS, especially in the EDSS range 6-9 [68]. Also, the responsiveness of the MSIS is better than that of the EDSS in terms of both magnitude and stability [69]. Other scales recently proposed include the Multiple Sclerosis Impact Scale (MSIS-29) [70], the Multiple Sclerosis Spasticity Scale (MSSS-88) [71], and the Multiple Sclerosis Functional Composite (MSFC) that includes both clinical and MRI lesions [72]. However, regulatory agencies are not favorable to the use of a 'z score' composite reflecting combined endpoints for MS trials, and most of the above measures are yet to be used in controlled clinical trials.

Alternative trial designs in MS may include among others: (1) dose finding strategies for phase II or phase I/II studies where the placebo is replaced by a lowest dose arm expected to be minimally effective; (2) change from the usual 1:1 randomization scheme to a 2:1 schedule enrolling more patients in the active agent arm than in the placebo arm of the study; (3) deferred randomization; as well as (4) "add on" randomization in which all patients start treatment on a single therapy and after a pre-specified period are randomized the modeling of data to an "add on" an experimental therapy; and (5) use of a 'virtual' placebo group whereby the untreated patient group is modeled from patient data from extant clinical trials and natural history studies [63].

The use of validated surrogate endpoints to replace the traditional clinical outcomes has been suggested; for instance, gadolinium enhancing T1 lesions in the brain, brain atrophy and T2 burden of disease have been proposed as surrogates for clinical disease relapses [66]. However, the MRI T2 burden of disease appears to plateau for EDSS values >4.5 [73]. As mentioned earlier, DT-MRI may be a better method to quantify relevant white matter tract pathology [67]. Finally, use of alternative statistical techniques, such as the Bayesian approach [74] may allow a less rigid statistical analysis and may provide better definition of actual clinical outcomes.

Future trials may involve a different approach for MS treatment by using neuroprotective agents and drugs that enhance axonal and myelin repair [75]. With advent of these agents there will be a need to develop imaging and biological markers of protection and repair that will require formal validation as surrogates for clinical outcomes.

Despite significant controversy regarding the time and type of treatment to be used after a diagnosis of MS [76], there appears to be current agreement on the need for early treatment of MS at the time of diagnosis [77,78].

REFERENCES

[1]   Pryse-Phillips W: *Companion to Clinical Neurology.* Second Edition, Oxford: Oxford University Press, 2003.

[2]   Lensch E, Matzke M, Petereit H-F, Scherer P, Schramm S, Calabrese P: Identification and management of cognitive disorders in multiple sclerosis--a consensus approach. *J Neurol* 2006;253(Suppl 1):I29-31.

[3]   Poser CM: Multiple sclerosis. Observations and reflections—a personal memoir. *J Neurol Sci* 1992;107:127–140.

[4]   Poser CM, Brinar VV: The nature of multiple sclerosis. *Clin Neurol Neurosurg* 2004;106: 159–171.

[5]   Schumacher GA, Beebe G, Kibler RF, et al. Problems of experimental trials of therapy in multiple sclerosis: Report by the Panel on the Evaluation of Experimental Trials of Therapy in Multiple Sclerosis. *Ann NY Acad Sci* 1965;122:552-568.

[6]   Poser CM, Paty DW, Scheinberg L, et al. New diagnostic criteria for multiple sclerosis: Guidelines for research protocols. *Ann Neurol* 1983;13:227-231.

[7]   McDonald WI, Compston DAS, Edan G, et al. Recommended diagnostic criteria for multiple sclerosis: Guidelines from the International Panel on the Diagnosis of Multiple Sclerosis. *Ann Neurol* 2001;50:121-127.

[8]   Barkhof F, Filippi M, Miller DH, et al. Comparison of MRI criteria at first presentation to predict conversion to clinically definite multiple sclerosis. *Brain* 1997;120:2059-2069.

[9]   Tintore M, Rovira A, Martinez M, et al. Isolated demyelinating syndromes: comparison of different MR imaging criteria to predict conversion to clinically definite multiple sclerosis. AJNR *Am J Neuroradiol* 2000;21:702-706.

[10] Weiner HL: A 21 point unifying hypothesis on the etiology and treatment of multiple sclerosis. *Can J Neurol Sci* 1998;25:93-101.

[11] Frohman EM, Racke MK, Raine CS: Multiple sclerosis--the plaque and its pathogenesis. *N Engl J Med* 2006;354:942-955.

[12] Kuhlmann T, Lingfeld G, Bitsch A, et al. Acute axonal damage in multiple sclerosis is most extensive in early disease stages and decreases over time. *Brain* 2002;125: 2202-2212.

[13] Kutzke JF: Epidemiology and etiology of multiple sclerosis. *Phys Med Rehabil Clin N Am* 2005;16:327-349.

[14] Marrie RA: Environmental risk factors in multiple sclerosis aetiology. *Lancet Neurology* 2004;3:709-718.

[15] Rosati G: The prevalence of multiple sclerosis in the world: an update. *Neurol Sci* 2001;22: 117-139.

[16] Zavadinov R, Iona R, Monti-Bragadin L, et al. The use of standardized incidence and prevalence rates in epidemiological studies on multiple sclerosis. A meta-analysis study. *Neuroepidemiology* 2003;22:65-74.

[17] Landtblom AM, Riise T, Boiko A, Söderfeldt B. Distribution of multiple sclerosis in Sweden based on mortality and disability compensation statistics. *Neuroepidemiology* 2002;21:167–179.

[18] Landtblom AM, Riise T, Kurtzke JF: Further considerations on the distribution of multiple sclerosis in Sweden. *Acta Neurol Scand* 2005;111:238-246.

[19] Callender M, Landtblom A-M: A cluster of multiple sclerosis cases in Lysvik in the Swedish county of Varmland. *Acta Neurol Scand* 2004;110:14-22

[20] Pugliatti M, Riise T, Sotgiu MA, et al. Increasing incidence of multiple sclerosis in the province of Sassari, northern Sardinia. *Neuroepidemiology* 2005;25:129-134.

[21] Dean G, Elian M, de Bono AG, et al. Multiple sclerosis in Malta in 1999: an update. *J Neurol Neurosurg Psychiatry* 2002;73:256-260.

[22] Hader WJ. The incidence and prevalence of multiple sclerosis in Saskatoon, Saskatchewan: A reappraisal. *Neuroepidemiology* 1999;18:331.

[23] Beck CA, Metz LM, Stevenson LW, Patten SB. Regional variation of multiple sclerosis prevalence in Canada. *Mult Scler* 2005;11:516-519.

[24] Hader WJ, et al. The occurrence of multiple sclerosis in the Hutterites of North America. *Can J Neurol Sci* 1996;23:291-295.

[25] Baum HM, Rothschild BB. The incidence and prevalence of reported multiple sclerosis. *Ann Neurol* 1981;10:420-428.

[26] Wallin MT, Page WF, Kurtzke JF. Multiple sclerosis in US veterans of the Vietnam era and later military service: race, sex, and geography. *Ann Neurol* 2004;55:65-71.

[27] Redelings MD, McCoy L, Sorvillo F. Multiple sclerosis mortality and patterns of comorbidity in the United States from 1990 to 2001. *Neuroepidemiology* 2006;26:102-107.

[28] Corona T, Román GC. Multiple sclerosis in Latin America. *Neuroepidemiology* 2006;26:1-3.

[29] Alter M, Olivares O: Multiple sclerosis in México. *Arch Neurol* 1970:23;451–459.

[30] Velázquez M, Macias MA, Rivera OV, Lozano Z. Grupo Mexicano de estudio de la esclerosis múltiple. *Rev Neurol* 2003; 36: 1019–1022.

[31] Corona T, Rodríguez LJ, Otero E, Stopp L: Multiple sclerosis in México: hospital cases at the National Institute of Neurology and Neurosurgery. *Neurología* 1996;11:170–173.

[32] Corona T, Ruiz JL, Arriada N: Optic neuritis progressing to multiple sclerosis. *Acta Neurol Scand* 1997;95;85–89.

[33] Lazo M, Corona T: Neuritis óptica: seguimiento a largo plazo en población mexicana. *Rev Neurol* 2002;35:1190.

[34] Cristiano E, Patrucco L, Garcea O, et al. Prevalence of multiple sclerosis (MS) in Argentina using the capture-recapture method. *Neurology* 1999; 2(suppl):A438.

[35] Piedrabuena R, Giobellina R, Alvarez D, Abatedaga V. High prevalence of multiple sclerosis in the city of Oliva, Cordoba, Argentina. *Arq Neuropsiquiatr* 2004; 62: 13.

[36] Papais-Alvarenga R, Alves S, Miranda C, et al: Characteristics of multiple sclerosis in Brazil: multicentric study in a prevalence cohort – South Atlantic project phase 1. *J Neurol Sci* 1997;150:S229.

[37] Gama P, Trigo L, Andrade R, Sala C, on behalf of the Brazilian Committee for Treatment and Research in Multiple Sclerosis (BCTRIMS). Epidemiological study of multiple sclerosis in the city of Sorocaba, Brazil. *Arq Neuropsiquiatr* 2004;62:13.

[38] Callegaro D, Godbaum M, Morais L, et al. The prevalence of multiple sclerosis in the city of Sao Paulo, Brazil. *Acta Neurol Scand* 2001:104: 2208–2137.

[39] Ketzoian C, Oeninger C, Alcántaran J, et al: Estudio de la prevalencia de la esclerosis múltiple en Uruguay. *Acta Neurol Col* 1999;15:6.

[40] Alvarez G, Castillo J, Cárdenas M, et al. Multiple sclerosis in Chile. *Acta Neurol Scand* 1992; 85: 1–4.

[41] Barahona J, Montero A, Flores A: Multiple sclerosis in Chile. *Arq Neuropsiquiatr* 2004:62: 11.

[42] Sánchez JL, Aguirre C, Arcos OM, et. al: Prevalencia de la esclerosis múltiple en Colombia. *Rev Neurol* 2000;31:1101–1103.

[43] Cabré P, Signate A, Olindo S, et al. Role of return migration in the emergence of multiple sclerosis in the French West Indies. *Brain* 2005;128:2899-2910.

[44] Barnett MH, Williams DB, Day S, et al. Progressive increase in incidence and prevalence of multiple sclerosis in Newcastle, Australia: a 35-year study. *J Neurol Sci* 2003;213:1-6.

[45] van der Mei IA, et al. Regional variation in multiple sclerosis prevalence in Australia and its association with ambient ultraviolet radiation. *Neuroepidemiology* 2001;20:168-174.

[46] Poser CM. Viking voyages: the origin of multiple sclerosis? An essay in medical history. *Acta Neurol Scand Suppl* 1995;161:11-22.

[47] Kenealy SJ, Pericak-Vance MA, Haines JL. The genetic epidemiology of multiple sclerosis. *J Neuroimmunol* 2003;143:7-12.

[48] Alter M, Leibowitz U, Speer J. Risk of multiple sclerosis related to age of immigration to Israel. *Arch Neurol* 1966;15:234-237.

[49] Thacker EL, Mirzaei F, Ascherio A. Infectious mononucleosis and risk for multiple sclerosis: a meta-analysis. *Ann Neurol* 2006;59:499-503.

[50] Tartas R, Ordoñez G, Rios C, Sotelo J: Varicella, ephemeral breastfeeding and eczema as risk factors for multiple sclerosis in Mexicans. *Acta Neurol Scand* 2002; 105: 88–94.

[51] Ordoñez G, Pineda B, Garcia-Navarrete R, Sotelo J: Brief presence of varicella-zoster viral DNA in mononuclear cells during relapses of multiple sclerosis. *Arch Neurol* 2004;61:529–532.

[52] Perez-Cesari C, Saniger MM, Sotelo J. Frequent association of multiple sclerosis with varicella and zoster. *Acta Neurol Scand* 2005;112:417-419.

[53] Bager P, Nielsen NM, Bihrmann K, et al. Childhood infections and risk of multiple sclerosis. *Brain* 2004;127:2491-2497.

[54] DeStefano F, et al. Vaccinations and risk of central nervous system demyelinating diseases in adults. *Arch Neurol* 2003;60:504-509.

[55] Ascherio A et al. Hepatitis B vaccination and the risk of multiple sclerosis. *N Engl J Med* 2001;344:327-332.

[56] Sotgiu S, Pugliatti M, Sotgiu A, Sanna A, Rosati G. Does the "hygiene hypothesis" provide an explanation for the high prevalence of multiple sclerosis in Sardinia? *Autoimmunity* 2003;36:257-260.

[57] Acheson ED, Bachrach CA, Wright FM. Some comments on the relationship of the distribution of multiple sclerosis to latitude, solar radiation and other variables. *Acta Psychiatr Scand* 1960;35(Suppl 147):132.

[58] Brown SJ. The role of vitamin D in multiple sclerosis. *Ann Pharmacother* 2006;40: May 9 [e-publication]

[59] Cantorna MT, Hayes CE, DeLuca HF. 1,25-Dihydroxyvitamin D3 reversibly blocks the progression of relapsing encephalomyelitis, a model of multiple sclerosis. *Proc Natl Acad Sci U S A* 1996;93:7861- 7864.

[60] Munger KL, Zhang SM, O'Reilly E, et al. Vitamin D intake and incidence of multiple sclerosis. *Neurology* 2004;62:60–66.

[61] Goodin D. The return of natalizumab: weighing benefit against risk. *Lancet Neurol* 2006; 5:375-377.

[62] Langer-Gould A, Steinman L. What went wrong in the natalizumab trials? *Lancet* 2006; 367:1484-1485.

[63] McFarland HF, Reingold SC. The future of multiple sclerosis therapies: redesigning multiple sclerosis clinical trials in a new therapeutic era. *Multiple Sclerosis* 2005;11:669-676.

[64] Runmarker B, Andersen O. Prognostic factors in a multiple sclerosis incidence cohort with twenty-five years of follow-up. *Brain* 1993;116: 117–134.

[65] Kurtzke JF. Rating neurologic impairment in multiple sclerosis: an expanded disability status scale (EDSS). *Neurology* 1983;33:1444-1452.

[66] Li DK, Li MJ, Traboulsee A, et al. The use of MRI as an outcome measure in clinical trials. *Adv Neurol* 2006;98:203-26.

[67] Li X, Tench CR, Morgan PS, et al. 'Importance sampling' in MS: use of diffusion tensor tractography to quantify pathology related to specific impairment. *J Neurol Sci* 2005;237: 13-19.

[68] Ravnborg M, Gronbech-Jensen M, Jonsson A. The MS Impairment Scale: a pragmatic approach to the assessment of impairment in patients with multiple sclerosis. *Mult Scler* 1997;3:31-42.

[69] Ravnborg M, Blinkenberg M, Sellebgerg F et al. Responsiveness of the Multiple Sclerosis Impairment Scale in comparison with the Expanded Disability Status Scale. *Mult Scler* 2005;11:81-84.

[70] Hobart J, Lamping D, Fitzpatrick R et al. The Multiple Sclerosis Impact Scale (MSIS-29): a new patient-based outcome measure. *Brain* 2001;124:962-973.

[71] Hobart JC, Riazi A, Thompson AJ, et al. Getting the measure of spasticity in multiple sclerosis: the Multiple Sclerosis Spasticity Scale (MSSS-88). *Brain* 2006;129:224-234.

[72] Hobart J, Kalkers N, Barkhof F, et al. Outcome measures for multiple sclerosis clinical trials: relative measurement precision of the Expanded Disability Status Scale and Multiple Sclerosis Functional Composite. *Mult Scler* 2004;10:41-46.

[73] Li DK, Held U, Petkau D, et al. MRI T2 lesion burden in multiple sclerosis: a plateauing relationship with clinical disability. *Neurology* 2006;66:1384-1389.

[74] Thall PF, Wathen JK, Bekele BN, et al. Hierarchical Bayesian approaches to phase II trials in diseases with multiple subtypes. *Stat Med* 2003; 22: 763-780.

[75] Kapoor R. Neuroprotection in multiple sclerosis: therapeutic strategies and clinical trial design. *Curr Opin Neurol* 2006;19:255-259.

[76] Pittock SJ, Weinshenker BG, Noseworthy JH et al. Not every patient with multiple sclerosis should be treated at time of diagnosis. *Arch Neurol* 2006;63:611-614.

[77] Frohman EM, Havrdova E, Barkhof F, et al. Most patients with multiple sclerosis or a clinically isolated demyelinating syndrome should be treated at time of diagnosis. *Arch Neurol* 2006;63:614-619.

[78] Roach ES. Early multiple sclerosis. To treat or not to treat? *Arch Neurol* 2006;63:619.

RECOMMENDED FURTHER READING

1. Multiple Sclerosis 2. W. Ian McDonald and John H. Noseworthy, eds. Boston: Butterworth-Heinemann, 2003.

2. Multiple Sclerosis: a guide for the newly diagnosed. Nancy J. Holland, T. Jock Murray, Stephen C. Reingold. New York: Demos Vermande, 2002.

3. Multiple Sclerosis as a neuronal disease. Stephen G. Waxman, editor. Burlington, Mass.: Elsevier Academic Press, 2005.

4. Multiple Sclerosis: etiology, diagnosis, and new treatment strategies. Michael J. Olek, editor. Totowa, N.J.: Humana Press, 2005.

5. Multiple Sclerosis: immunology, pathology, and pathophysiology. Robert M. Herndon, editor. New York, N.Y.: Demos Medical Pub., 2003.

6. Multiple Sclerosis: diagnosis, medical management, and rehabilitation. Jack S. Burks and Kenneth P. Johnson, eds. New York, N.Y.: Demos Medical Pub., 2003.

7. Multiple Sclerosis in clinical practice. Aaron E. Miller, Fred D. Lublin and Patricia K. Coyle, editors. London; New York: Martin Dunitz, 2003.

8. Multiple Sclerosis : psychosocial and vocational interventions. Robert T. Fraser, David C. Clemmons, and Francie Bennett. New York: Demos Medical Pub., 2002.

9. Multiple Sclerosis: the guide to treatment and management. Chris H. Polman et al. for the Multiple Sclerosis International Federation. New York, N.Y.: Demos, 2006.

10. Multiple Sclerosis therapeutics. Jeffrey A. Cohen and Richard A. Rudick, editors. London: Martin Dunitz, 2003.

In: Handbook of Clinical Neuroepidemiology
ISBN 978-1-60021-511-7
Editors: V. L. Feigin and D. A. Bennett, pp. 573-593 © 2007 Nova Science Publishers, Inc.

Chapter 17

HUNTINGTON'S DISEASE

Nektarios K. Mazarakis[1] and Anthony J. Hannan[2]

[1]University Laboratory of Physiology, University of Oxford, Parks Road, Oxford, OX1 3PT, UK;
[2]Howard Florey Institute, National Neuroscience Facility, University of Melbourne, Parkville, VIC 3010, Australia

ABSTRACT

Huntington's disease (HD) is an autosomal dominant disorder involving progressive motor, cognitive and psychiatric symptoms. HD is caused by a trinucleotide (CAG) repeat expansion, encoding an extended polyglutamine tract in the huntingtin protein.

While there is an inverse relationship between CAG repeat length and age of onset, there is substantial recent evidence for both genetic and environmental modifiers which modulate age of onset and rate of progression. Research utilising transgenic mouse models of HD has made great progress in understanding mechanisms of pathogenesis and gene-environment interactions, and this information has led to promising preclinical and clinical trials, however there is not yet a proven treatment or cure for this fatal disease.

INTRODUCTION

Huntington's disease (HD) is one of an increasing number of neurodegenerative diseases known to be caused by expanded trinucleotide (CAG) repeats coding for extended polyglutamine tracts in the respective disease proteins. These include spinal and bulbar muscular atrophy (SBMA) [1], dentatorubral pallidoluysian atrophy (DRPLA) [2] and spinocerebellar ataxia (SCA) types 1, 2, 3, 6, 7 and 17 [3-6]. HD is the most common of these nine so-called 'polyglutamine neurodegenerative diseases', and has therefore been most intensively studied. In addition to these nine diseases, there are a range of other trinucleotide repeat diseases known to involve neurological symptomatology. Some of these, caused by trinucleotide repeats outside of protein-coding regions, consist of forms of ataxia. In contrast, long or medium-length CGG repeats in the non-coding region of the FMR1 gene are known to cause Fragile X syndrome, or a recently identified tremor-ataxia syndrome (FXTAS), respectively [7].

Trinucleotide repeats are just one of a large class of simple-sequence repeats, or microsatellites, which form the template of 'dynamic mutations' [8] contributing to a wide range of clinical disorders. These microsatellites are extremely common, and widely distributed, in the human genome, and show a high degree of polymorphism in the normal population, below threshold repeat lengths for disease. One reason for this may be that microsatellite polymorphisms provide a wider range of genotypes at a given locus, as opposed to 'binary' polymorphisms, such as single nucleotide polymorphisms (SNPs), which usually are limited to two genotypes at a given locus. Microsatellite diversity may thus increase the levels of phenotypic variability in a population which, in the context of 'brain and mind' phenotypes, could have substantial selective advantage [9].

HD takes its name from the American physician George Huntington who in 1872 described this hereditary brain disorder as "hereditary chorea" [10]. Chorea derives from the Greek word χορός (choros), which means dance. Chorea was used to describe the dramatic motor symptoms of the disease, which involve uncontrollable dance-like movements. Since those early days many descriptions of the clinical features, epidemiology and neuropathology of the disease have been made but a major breakthrough came 120 years after Huntington's first report when, through a collaborative effort [11], it was found that the cause of the disease was an expansion of a trinucleotide (CAG) repeat in exon 1 of the HD gene. Since this discovery there has been an explosion of research trying to elucidate the mechanisms of the disease at the molecular, cellular and systems levels both in animals and humans. The use of molecular biology in the production of transgenic mice carrying the mutant gene has been of great importance in gaining a deeper understanding of this complex disease. To date however no effective treatment or cure has been discovered for this fatal brain disease. Currently, treatment of HD is restricted to palliative care aiming to maintain quality of life as much as possible.

CLINICAL SYMPTOMATOLOGY

The typical age of onset varies significantly depending on the number of CAG repeats in the HD gene [12], as well as other genetic and environmental modifiers. Generally, the age of onset for HD patients falls in the range between 30 and 50 years old. However about 5-7% of HD sufferers, with longer CAG repeats, show the juvenile form of the disease, with onset as young as 2 years of age, more rapid progression and greater severity of symptoms [13].

Symptoms of adult-onset HD (the vast majority of cases) develop gradually and early symptoms are very difficult to distinguish from normal behaviour. HD manifests as a diverse spectrum of psychiatric, cognitive and motor symptoms. Early behavioural changes can be observed before the appearance of the characteristic motor symptoms. Psychiatric symptoms, which often precede the motor symptoms, include irritability, anxiety, depression, and sleep disorders [14-17]. Cognitive decline, which also occurs at early stages, commonly involves difficulties in concentration and retaining newly acquired information, decline in language skills, disorganised speech and perceptual impairments [17-19].

HD is better known for its obvious motor symptoms. Early symptoms involve clumsiness in fine motor movements and balance difficulties. As disease progresses, the patient develops chorea which is characterized by purposeless, involuntary, jerky "dance-like" movements [20]. At an early stage, chorea is restricted to the fingers or toes. However, as the disease progresses, choreatic movements extend to the arms, legs, face and trunk. Other motor symptoms involve difficulties in executing voluntary movements, eating and swallowing, speech production, as well as bradykinesia, rigidity and dystonia [21].

NEUROPATHOLOGICAL FEATURES

Although in advanced HD there is a reduction in overall brain weight, the most obvious neuropathological feature of the disease is a profound degeneration of the striatum [22]. De la Monte and colleagues [23] showed, using *post mortem* morphometric analysis, that the brains of HD patients on average were 30% lighter than control brains. Moreover they reported 21-29% volume shrinkage of the cerebral cortex, 28% shrinkage of the thalamus, 29-34% loss of the white matter and, strikingly, 57% shrinkage of the caudate and 64% of the putamen. Shrinkage was also observed in other regions, including the amygdala and the hippocampus. Structural magnetic resonance imaging studies have indicated that the volume of these brain regions, particularly the cortex and striatum, is shrinking at early stages, even in gene-positive HD family members prior to the onset of symptoms. Evidence from low Vonsattel grade cases of HD, in which the patients had died of HD yet few cells have been lost, as well as findings in accurate transgenic mouse models of HD [9], suggest that cell death occurs relatively late in the disease process and therefore molecular changes underlying early cell dysfunction provide the most promising therapeutic targets.

EPIDEMIOLOGY

As expected of an autosomal dominant disorder, both males and females are equally afflicted by HD. In Europe (South and North), 4 to 8 individuals in every 100,000 are affected [24]. However, there are important regional differences. For example, in Finland HD is extremely rare [25]. Prevalence within the above range has also been reported, albeit with great regional diversities, in North America, Australia and New Zealand, as detailed in a comprehensive review of HD epidemiology by Harper [26]. Interestingly, Japan has an exceptionally low prevalence (0.11-0.72/100000), although has a uniquely high prevalence of a related polyglutamine neurodegenerative disease, DRPLA. This may simply be due to the fact that there was a preponderance of huntingtin alleles with short CAG repeat length in ancestral populations, and the likelihood of CAG repeat expansion events in the germline are sufficiently low to ensure, in a population with historically low levels of immigration, that prevalence has remained low. However, the possibility that there may be selective pressure, either positive or negative, for huntingtin alleles with specific ranges of CAG repeat lengths, cannot be excluded.

In specific countries and regions, founder effects have been observed, the most extreme of which is found in Lake Maricabo, Venezuela, where as many as 1 in 4 of the population may be either symptomatic of presymptomatic carriers of the CAG repeat expansion [27]. The extremely high incidence of HD in Lake Maricabo was instrumental in providing a large set of kindreds which facilitated the genetic discovery of the HD mutation (Huntington's Disease Collaborative Research Group, 1993), as well as recent exploration of possible genetic and environmental modifiers (Wexler et al., 2004). Detailed information on HD prevalence for different countries and regions within a country has been collected by Harper and colleagues and can be found in the following University of Wales online database: http://archive.uwcm.ac.uk/uwcm/mg/fidd/search.html.

As well as founder effects, initial CAG repeat lengths in the huntingtin gene of specific populations, expansions and contractions of CAG repeats between generations (more common through the paternal germline) also impact on epidemiological findings. When the CAG repeat length in the huntingtin gene is around 40 or greater, the HD mutation exhibits complete penetrance (the probability of expressing a phenotype given a genotype), although there is a large degree of variability in age of onset for a given CAG repeat length. In the range of 35-39 repeats, incomplete penetrance is observed, presumably due to genetic and environmental modifiers (discussed subsequently). Nevertheless, germline expansions or contractions of CAG repeats which lead to a transition across the repeat length threshold for disease are sufficiently rare that the children of a symptomatic HD parent are approximately 50% at risk of inheriting a disease-causing *huntingtin* allele, as expected for an autosomal dominant disorder.

GENETIC FACTORS

The aetiology of HD involves an expansion of unstable trinucleotide CAG repeats in exon 1 of the HD gene (also known as gene *IT15*) located on chromosome 4. The HD gene encodes the protein huntingtin [11]. Each of the CAG repeats codes for the amino acid glutamine. Therefore in HD, the mutation in the HD gene encodes an expanded polyglutamine stretch at the N-terminal region of the huntingtin protein.

Normal asymptotic individuals have 35 or fewer CAG repeats in the *IT15* gene. Individuals manifesting HD symptoms exhibit 36 or more CAG repeats [12] although there have been cases of people with up to 39 CAG repeats who remained symptom-free [28]. It seems that within the range of 36-39 CAG repeats, which can cause HD, there are cases of incomplete penetrance [29,30]. A greater number of CAG repeats generally causes earlier onset of the motor symptoms of the disease [12]. HD individuals with more than 47 repeats, for example, have earlier onset of motor symptoms compared with HD patients with 37-46 repeats [31]. However, there is no apparent correlation between CAG length and psychiatric symptoms [32,33]. A range of 40-55 repeats is usually correlated with the adult-onset form of the disease. As part of this inverse correlation, HD patients with 55 or more repeats generally have the juvenile-onset form of HD, and up to 250 repeats have been reported to induce onset as early as 1-2 years of age. Although the inverse correlation between the number of CAG repeats and the age of HD onset is quite strong, repeat length is only a partial predictor of onset age, generally accounting for 50-70% of the variation in age of onset, suggesting that other factors (presumably genetic or environmental modifiers) might also account for this variability [12,34,35]. Additionally, the predicative value of the CAG repeats length is further reduced at the lower range of lengths (<52 repeats) [34].

Interestingly, part of this variation (13%) could be explained by a TAA repeat polymorphism in close linkage to a kainate receptor gene, GluR6 [36,37]. The association between the GluR6 polymorphism and HD is of particular importance given the evidence suggesting that the selective damage occuring in HD could be attributed to abnormal neurotransmission of the excitatory amino acid, glutamate, a process known as excitotoxicity [38-40]. Other genes influencing age of onset have been identified. Recent findings show that the genes encoding the NR2A and NR2B regulatory subunits of the NMDA receptor can act as genetic modifiers[82], providing additional support for a glutamate receptor-mediated excitotoxic model of HD pathogenesis. Interestingly, a specific apoE genotype [41], also implicated in defining onset age of Alzheimer's disease (AD), has been identified as a genetic modifier in HD, suggesting that this gene has a general role in neurodegenerative disease. The transcription factor CA150, containing a polymorphism in the polyglutamine tract also influences age of onset in HD, possibly via direct interaction with mutant huntingtin [42]. The role of environmental factors and associated gene-environment interactions as modulators of disease onset and progression will now be discussed.

ENVIRONMENTAL FACTORS AND GENE-ENVIRONMENT INTERACTIONS

HD was until recently considered to be the epitome of genetic determinism, a monogenic autosomal dominant disorder with complete penetrance. However, data generated in recent years, first in mouse models of the disease and later in clinical populations, has revolutionised our view of the aetiology and epidemiology of HD. The first evidence for environmental modifiers in HD came from studies using transgenic mouse models. Environmental enrichment has been shown to dramatically delay the onset and progression of HD in transgenic mice [43-46]. Environmental enrichment involves providing the mice with environments containing complex, stimulating objects, which are changed regularly. Compared to standard-housed HD mice, the environmentally enriched HD mice had delayed onset and progression of motor symptoms, and ameliorated loss of cerebral volume [43]. Environmental enrichment is thought to induce enhanced sensory, cognitive and motor stimulation. The mechanisms by which the beneficial effects of enrichment are mediated in HD mice are as yet unknown, though there are several plausible possibilities. Enrichment is known to affect synaptic plasticity and this effect could potentially counteract some of the deficits in synaptic plasticity known to occur in HD [47,48]. Enrichment is associated with increased synaptic signaling and the resultant traffic across a synapse is known to promote its efficacy as well as stimulating second messenger systems within the cell and encouraging intra-neuronal protein trafficking. Enrichment also has a direct effect on neuronal morphology, with enrichment being associated with an increased spine density, although the HD mutation may disrupt aspects of this experience-dependent synaptic plasticity (Spires et al., 2004b).

Enrichment also increases transcription of specific genes, presumably through activity-dependent intra-neuronal signaling pathways. Many of these genes found to be upregulated by environmental stimulation are linked to neuronal structure (including its cytoskeletal modulation) and synaptic plasticity. We have recently shown that enrichment does indeed rescue striatal BDNF protein levels in HD mice, possibly via amelioration of corticostriatal protein trafficking abnormalities [45]. The rescue of HD-induced gene expression deficits was also demonstrated for the pivotal intra-neuronal signaling protein, DARPP-32 [45]. Changes in the phosphorylation state of DARPP-32, abundantly expressed in the medium spiny neurons of the striatum, reinforce the behavioural effects of stimulation or inhibition of the cAMP pathway because of its key role in dopamine and adenosine transmission. The restoration of BDNF levels could also have either a neuromodulatory or direct neurotrophic effect, given BDNF's postulated role in synaptic signaling and plasticity. BDNF appears to play a significant role in protecting vulnerable neurons from excitotoxic insults, through the TrkB receptor and interactions with PKA.

Finally, enrichment has been shown to have an effect on neurogenesis, increasing the endogenous production of neurons in the hippocampus of adult rodents [49]. However, it is not clear whether these cells can indeed migrate to diseased areas of the brain, such as the cortex and striatum, as well as subsequently functionally integrate, unless generated in response to the death of specific cell populations. Recent evidence for altered neurogenesis in HD mice [50,51] and a postmortem HD brain region adjacent to cell loss [52] has opened up experimental possibilities for testing therapeutic approaches which target neurogenesis.

The effects of environmental enrichment can be analysed in the context of discrete components, including enhanced sensory and cognitive stimulation, reduced anxiety and increased motor activity. An increase in both fine motor activity as well as an increase in overall gross motor activity is seen. At present, it is unclear exactly which component of enrichment exhibits the greatest neuroprotective effect and we are currently actively exploring such questions. Furthermore, there is recent evidence that dietary factors can also impact upon the disease [53,54], opening up the spectrum of possible environmental modulators affecting HD. What is not clear is whether the beneficial effects of enrichment are specific to HD in relation to its pathogenesis or reflect a broader neuroprotective effect that is equally as applicable to other neurodegenerative diseases. It is likely that the latter is the case, given the role for altered synaptic plasticity in other neurodegenerative disorders and a general neuroprotective effect of increased neurotrophin expression, such as BDNF. Environmental enrichment has been postulated to confer general protection against cerebral insults through induction of glial derived neurotrophic factor (GDNF) as well as BDNF.

ENVIRONMENTAL FACTORS AND EPIDEMIOLOGY

Although CAG repeat length is known to inversely relate to disease onset, there is in fact a wide variation in age of onset for a given CAG repeat length in the *huntingtin* gene [11,12], suggesting possible modulatory effects of genetic and environmental modifiers on pathogenesis and subsequent disease manifestation. While the putative genetic modifiers described above may contribute to variance in age of onset that is not explained by CAG repeat length, a recent study of a large group of Venezuelan HD kindreds by Wexler and colleagues [27] has confirmed the previous evidence from transgenic mouse models of HD [43-46], that environmental factors can modulate disease onset and progression. However the Venezuelan kindred study [27] is not able to identify what these environmental factors may be, and clearly retrospective and prospective epidemiological studies need to be conducted to reveal the nature of environmental modifiers in clinical HD.

The beneficial effects of environmental stimulation in some HD patients have been demonstrated in a clinical setting through the use of remotivation therapy [55]. The provision of a more stimulating environment improved physical, mental and social function even in patients with late stage disease. Whether such results are due to increased motor, cognitive or sensory stimulation is unclear, and further research involving larger cohorts is required in order to elucidate the components of enrichment that can exert the greatest reduction in disease onset and progression. Interestingly, clinical studies have also underscored the wider applicability of environmental enrichment in other neurodegenerative conditions, for example the association between a higher level of educational attainment and a reduced risk of Alzheimer's and Parkinson's Disease, as reviewed recently [56]. By understanding some of the underlying molecular mechanisms, the tantalising potential for the pharmacological induction of an 'enrichment-like effect' may become reality, possibly through triggering synaptic plasticity, adult neurogenesis, or other protective mechanisms.

The 'silver bullet' treatment for HD, which is yet to be found, would be a pharmacological agent capable of hindering or reversing the disease process. Some promising therapeutic targets, logically following from the proposed mechanisms of pathogenesis we have outlined above include: inhibition of polyglutamine-mediated protein folding and aggregation; protein cleavage and protein-protein interactions; transcriptional regulation and histone deacetylase inhibitors; glutamate release and glutamate receptors; dopamine, adenosine and cannabinoid receptors; trophic factors; antioxidants and mitochondrial modulators. These therapeutic possibilities as well as screening strategies in animal models have recently been extensively reviewed elsewhere [57,58]. Overall, however, the small number of drug therapies clinically trialled in HD have so far proved to be ultimately disappointing.

The nature of HD, with a complex mixture motor and cognitive deficits, complicates the measurement of therapeutic efficacy, with the possibility that specific treatments have a predominant effect on one aspect of the disease rather than globally. The multiple molecular pathways which become abnormal as the disease progresses suggest that the use of multiple drugs ('polypharmacy'), differentially administered at different stages of the disease, may be required. Once we understand the mechanisms underlying the beneficial effects of environmental enrichment, the development of 'enviromimetics' may be facilitated; drugs which might mimic or enhance the beneficial effects of environmental stimulation [58,59].

EVIDENCE-BASED MANAGEMENT

In the present section we will review recent double-blind, randomised control trials (RCT) of agents used therapeutically in HD. Our aim is to provide the clinician with an overview of the best designed clinical studies in which a double-blind randomized controlled methodology has been applied. It has to be emphasised that so far there has been no effective treatment or cure demonstrated for the disease, although a great deal of recent progress has been made in preclinical trials, involving novel therapeutics [58]. The majority of the agents currently used in HD are useful only in reducing some of the motor symptoms of the disease. The reason for this, as in many (if not most) brain diseases, is the lack of a full understanding of the underlying pathophysiological mechanisms of the disease, and novel therapeutics based on some of this recently acquired knowledge are currently in preclinical and clinical trials.

Modulators of Glutamatergic Neurotransmission

The suggestion that NMDA receptors are involved in excitotoxicity, in addition to the hypothesis that NMDA receptor sensitisation in neurons might be factors involved in HD has led to the plausible suggestion that NMDA antagonists might be a very good candidate to combat certain symptoms of the disease. Murman and colleagues [60] carried out a double-blind RCT to examine the effects of the NMDA receptor antagonist ketamine on HD patients. In the trial 10 HD patients were enrolled and all of them received both the placebo and ketamine treatments separated by 1 week to ensure complete clearance of ketamine and no progression of the disease. Ketamine was administered at a dose of 0.1, 0.4 and 0.6 mg/kg/hr (i.v.). The results revealed that ketamine was well tolerated at doses of 0.1 and 0.4 mg/kg/hr. Ketamine induced significant impairments in certain neuropsychological measurements such as verbal memory, fluency and reaction time. There was no significant improvement in the ketamine-treated group in terms of chorea. Ketamine actually induced worsening of eye movements when the patient received the highest dose. At these high doses ketamine also increased certain behavioural symptoms such as thought disturbance and anergia.

In a relatively small RCT study involving 24 HD patients Verhagen Metman and colleagues [61] showed that administration of amantadine, an NMDA antagonist, reduced chorea in HD patients without causing any adverse effect such as parkinsonism. Moreover, no effects of the drugs were observed in the cognitive performance of the patients. However, there was significant variability in individual patient responses to the drug and the study was short-term, therefore no conclusions could be made concerning long-term use, tolerability and side effects.

Similarly, Lucetti and colleagues [62] showed that both acute (2-hour, i.v.) and chronic (up to 1-year) administration of amantadine resulted in a significant decrease in choreic dyskinesias without any effect on cognitive performance. However, Heckmann and colleagues [63] suggested that amantadine does not reduce choreic dyskinesias. In another double-blind RCT, O'Suilleabhain and Dewey [64] examined the effects of a 2-week treatment of amantadine using a dose of 300 mg/day in total. The outcome of the study revealed no difference between experimental and placebo groups in chorea and proprioception. Interestingly, HD patients on amantadine reported some improvements in subjective measures of HD.

In another double-blind RCT the Huntington Study Group [65] examined the effect of riluzole, an anti-glutamatergic agent, in 63 patients with HD for a period of 8 weeks. They reported a reduction in choreic dyskineseas in a dose-dependent fashion with higher doses of the drug (200 mg/d) being more effective. Interestingly, a lower dose (100 mg/d) had a beneficial effect in the first 4 weeks but then there was a complete gradual reversal of any beneficial effect. On the contrary in the higher dose group (200 mg/d) the beneficial effect, in term of chorea reduction, was evident even at the end of the trial (8th week). As in the case of amantadine, riluzole had no effect on cognitive performance. However, side effects of riluzole administration included elevated levels of alanine aminotranferase, muscle weakness and fatigue. The above effect would significantly limit the utility of riluzole as an antichoreic agent.

Modulators of Dopamine and Cannabinoid Receptors

Bassi and colleagues [66] examined the effects of transdihydrolisuride (TDHL) in HD. TDHL is a drug that has a dual effect on dopaminergic receptors with both a partial agonistic and antagonistic effect. 10 HD patients were recruited for this double-blind RCT (note that the first part of the study was an open-labelled one). The TDHL group received 1 mg/d of the drug for a period of 3 months. The results, interestingly, revealed a 41% reduction in chorea and a 32% decrease in disease severity in the TDHL group. Both decreases reached statistical significance. There was no difference in cognitive performance between TDHL and placebo groups. These are very promising results however, to the best of our knowledge there has not been another double-blind RCT to date to replicate these results in a larger sample of patients.

Albanese and colleagues [67] examined the effects of acute administration of apomorphine in HD patients. Apomorphine is a dopamine agonist which shows high affinity for D_4, D_3, D_2 and low affinity for D_5 and D_1 receptors and has been used in the treatment of parkinsonian patients. For this double-blind randomised crossover study 9 HD patients were recruited who received subcutaneous doses of apomorphine (1.5 mg or 3 mg) or placebo. Neurological features were assessed every 15 min for 2 hours following the administration of the drug. A dose of 1.5 mg of apomorphine resulted in a 38.5% reduction in neurological symptoms (including chorea) of HD patients and a dose of 3 mg resulted in a 30.4% reduction 50 min following the administration of apomorphine. Both these effects reached statistically significant levels. This promising study suggests that a moderate dose of apomorphine (1.5 mg) is useful in acutely reducing neurological symptoms of HD.

In another double-blind trial Consroe and colleagues [68] examined the effects of cannabidiol on HD. 18 HD patients were recruited but only 15 completed the trial. Cannabidiol was administered for a period of 6 weeks at a dose of 10 mg/kg/day. The total duration of the trial was 15 weeks (crossover design). The results of the study failed to provide any statistically significant evidence that cannabidiol reduces choreic symptoms or improves cognitive performance.

Modulators of GABAergic Neurotransmission

In a double-blind RCT Scigliano and colleagues [69] examined the effects of gamma-vinyl GABA, an irreversible inhibitor of GABA-transaminase in HD. The basic assumption behind the study was that the lowered levels of GABA due to the disease would be elevated by the administration of gamma-vinyl GABA and this might reduce the severity of the symptoms. 6 HD patients received 2 g/d of gamma-vinyl GABA in a crossover design for a period of two weeks. Analysis of the results failed to show any protective role of gamma-vinyl GABA. Similarly, an older double-blind RCT by Shoulson and colleagues [70] used dipropylacetic acid (DPA), an anticonvulsant that raises the levels of GABA in the brain, on 8 HD patients. DPA was administered either alone or in combination with GABA. As in the study of Scigliano and colleagues [69], DPA (alone or with GABA) failed to decrease the severity of motor symptoms in HD patients although 2 patients reported subjective improvement when DPA was combined with GABA.

Shoulson and colleagues [71] in a double-blind RCT involving 49 HD patients examined the effects of baclofen, a $GABA_B$ agonist, in the progression of HD. The drug was used at a dose of 60mg/day and the duration of the trial was up to 42 months. The results showed no statistical differences between the baclofen and placebo groups in terms of total functional capacity.

In another study Manyam and colleagues [72] examined the effects of isoniazid in HD patients. Isoniazid is an inhibitor of GABA aminotranferase (GABA-T). The hypothesis was that administration of isoniazid would elevate GABAergic levels which are depleted in HD. In this double-blind RCT 8 HD patients were recruited but only 6 completed the trial. The patients in a crossover design received in total 900 mg/d of isoniazid and 100 mg of pyridoxine for a period of 6 weeks. Statistical analysis revealed that isoniazid significantly reduced chorea assessed with Abnormal Involuntary Movement Scale (AIMS). However, in a clinical context, this result should be interpreted with caution because only 2 out of 6 patients (30%) actually showed clinical improvement. On the contrary, one patient even displayed worsening of the symptoms while on isoniazid. Finally, 2 out of 6 patients on isoniazid reported improved mnemonic performance. Although an encouraging study it is obviously very difficult to draw any conclusions concerning the therapeutic potential of isoniazid because the number of patents involved in the study was low and also because the effects of isoniazid were evident in a minority of patients. A similar study failed to show any protective role of isoniazide in HD [73].

Antipsychotics and Antidepressants

Clozapine is an atypical neuroleptic drug which has few extrapyramidal side effects compared to typical neuroleptics such as haloperidol. Van Vugt and colleagues [74] in a double-blind RCT examined the hypothesis that clozapine might be effective in reducing choreic symptoms in HD patients. 33 HD patients were enrolled for the study but 26 actually completed the trial. The study lasted for a period of 31 days and the scheduled dose of clozapine was 150 mg/day but due to side effects much lower doses were practically used. The results of the study revealed that clozapine produced a borderline significant reduction of chorea measured by the AIMS and a tendency (which did not reach significance) of reduced chorea measured with UHDRS only in HD patients who were *not* on some form of neuroleptic treatment. In HD patients already receiving neuroleptic treatment clozapine had no effect on choreic symptoms which were similar to those on the placebo group. It is important to note that the frequent occurrence of side effects associated with the use of clozapine restricts its use as a potential medication for the reduction of chorea in HD patients.

In another double-blind RCT Como and colleagues [75] examined the effects of fluoxetine on non-depressed HD patients. Fluoxetine is a selective serotonin re-uptake inhibitor which is used as an antidepressant drug. For the trial 30 non-depressed early HD patients were enrolled. The dose of fluoxetine used was 20 mg/day for a period of 4 months. The results of the trial failed to display any protective role of fluoxetine as there was no difference between the fluoxetine-treated group and the placebo group in motor symptoms (e.g. chorea and eye movement) and cognitive performance. Patients on fluoxetine showed a significant reduction in agitation. Grote and colleagues [51] have recently demonstrated that fluoxetine rescues a deficit of hippocampal neurogenesis, as well as cognitive and affective symptoms, in a mouse model of HD.

Antioxidants

In the context of the theory that oxidative stress may be partially involved in HD, Peyser et al. (1995) examined the effects of the antioxidant d-α-tocopherol on 81 HD patients (73 completed the trial). In this double-blind RCT that lasted 1 year, patients received 3000 I.U of d-α-tocopherol (plus vitamins A and C). The overall results showed no difference between the d-α-tocopherol and the placebo groups. However post hoc analyses revealed that in patients with early HD and a score on the Quantified Neurological Examination of <45 showed significant improvement on d-α-tocopherol whereas those patients with late HD and a score >45 showed worsening of the symptoms with d-α-tocopherol. These interesting results suggest that the antioxidant d-α-tocopherol may play a protective role in HD patients with early symptoms. Further studies are required to confirm these results. Additionally, it would be very important to examine the possible neuroprotective effects of d-α-tocopherol in pre-symptomatic HD patients.

Ranen and colleagues [77] attempted to examine the effects of idebenone on the progression of HD. Idebenone is an agent with antioxidant properties that also increases oxidative metabolism and in terms of this the assumption behind this double-blind RCT was that it might play a protective role against excitotoxicity. 100 HD patients were recruited but 91 completed the trial which lasted for a period of 1 year. In the experimental group the HD patients received in total 90 mg of idebenone daily. Following the completion of the trial, statistical analysis revealed no significant differences in any of the clinical measures between the idebenone group and the placebo group. Clinical measures included the HD Activities Daily Living (ADL) and the Quantitative Neurologic Examination (QNE) which consists of eye movements, chorea and impairment scales. Finally, there were no differences in any of the neuropsychological measurements.

In a double-blind RCT the Huntington Study Group [78] using a sample of 347 early HD patients examined the effects of the antioxidant coenzyme Q_{10} (involved in mitochondrial electron transport) and remacemide hydrochloride (a non-competitive NMDA receptor antagonist) for a period of 30 months. The outcome of this study suggested a failure of both coenzyme Q_{10} and remacemide to alter the functional progress of the disease. In the case of the patients receiving Q_{10} there was a trend towards decreased progression which nevertheless did not reach statistically significant levels. An early double-blind RCT study by Kieburtz and colleagues [79] in which remacemide was also used, showed a trend in reduction of chorea in patients receiving 200mg of remacemide but this effect did not reach statistical significance either.

In another double-blind RCT, The Huntington Study Group [80] examined the effects of the free radical scavenger OPC-14117 in HD patients. For the purposes of the study 64 HD patients (56 completed the trial) were enrolled and the duration of the study was 20 weeks. The dose of OPC-14117 was 60, 120 or 240 mg/day. The results showed that OPC-14117 was well tolerated with few side effects (such as elevated transaminases) but there was no difference in UHRDS and cognitive performance between the OPC-14117 and placebo groups.

Mitochondrial Modulators

Creatine is important in energy metabolism and in animal models of HD it has been shown to decrease motor impairment, protect the brain from atrophy and prolong survival [81,82]. In a double-blind controlled study (but not fully randomised), Verbessem and colleagues [83] examined the effects of creatine supplementation at a dose of 5 mg/day in the progression of HD on 42 patients for a period of 12 months. The trial failed to show any improvement in the creatine group compared to the placebo group in the Unified Huntington's Disease Rating Scale (UHDRS), cardiovascular fitness, muscle strength, bimanual coordination and cognitive performance. Therefore this clinical study failed to confirm the animal studies. Certainly some benefits of creatine could arise from a longer-term study. However a recent small open-label study by Tabrisi and colleagues [84] failed to show any promising effects of creatine in a 2-year long study.

In another double-blind RCT Kremer and colleagues [85] examined the effects of lamotrigine on progression of early HD. Lamotrigine is an anti-epileptic drug that blocks voltage-gated sodium channels and inhibits glutamate release. The hypothesis behind this study was that lamotrigine-induced glutamate blockage will decrease the progression of HD.

For this study, 64 patients with early HD were examined for a period of 30 months. The dose of the drugs used reached progressively 400 mg/day. The results showed no significant difference between the lamotrigine group and the placebo group in Total Functional Capacity (TFC) although there was a trend for slower deterioration in the lamotrigine group. Additionally, 26 patients underwent brain imaging scanning using positron emission tomography (PET). Although there was a significant metabolic activity decrease in the basal ganglia, the frontal cortex, the temporal cortex and thalamus there was no significant differences in metabolic activity between the lamotrigine and placebo groups. Moreover, there was no significant statistical difference in neurological measurements such as eye movements, motor performance and chorea (although lamotrigine displayed some anti-choreic action). Interestingly, 54% of HD patients on lamotrigine reported a subjective improvement of symptoms compared to 15% in the placebo group. This difference in subjective experience reached statistical significance. Finally, lamotrigine did not improve cognitive performance.

Fatty Acids

Highly unsaturated fatty acids (HUFAs) which are found in cellular membranes are important in the structure of membrane-bound proteins and affect the function of receptors, ion channels, enzymes and intracellular signalling. In this context, Vaddadi and colleagues [86] examined the possibility that HUFAs might play a protective role in 19 HD patients. HUFAs were administered for a period of 19-20 months to a dose of 8 mg/day. This double-blind RCT clinical trial was initially designed to last for 2 years. However, results from another clinical trial in the meantime provided evidence that HUFAs play a protective role in HD, so the authors terminated the trials and the results were reported to that point. The results revealed a borderline significant improvement in UHDRS motor and functional scores and significant improvement in the Dyskinesia Rating Scale in the experimental group compared to the controlled group. No difference was observed in cognitive performance. These interesting results were supported by another double-blind RCT study published at the same time by Puri and colleagues [87]. These researchers examined for a period of 6 months the effects of eicosapentaenoic acid (EPA), an unsaturated fat known to inhibit phospholipase A_2 which has been implicated in neurodegeneration in HD patients with severe chorea (stage III). The dose of EPA used was 2 mg/day. The results showed a significant improvement in the orofacial component of UHDRS in HD patients who received EPA compared to placebo patients. MRI scans in two placebo patients revealed increased ventricular size suggesting progressive neurodegeneration, as expected. Interestingly, in 2 patients on EPA there was an overall decrease in ventricular size, consistent with therapeutic efficacy. Note that only 4 patients (2 placebo, 2 on EPA) were utilised for scanning. These exciting results raise the possibility that EPA protects the brain from, or could even reverse, neurodegeneration. However, it is crucial to replicate the above results in a double-blind RCT using a much larger sample of patients.

Other Drugs Clinically Trialled in Huntington's Disease Patients

In a relatively older study Shults and colleagues [88] examined the effects of cysteamine in HD. Cysteamine is a drug that depletes the brain of the neuropeptide somatostatin. In HD the levels of cysteamine are elevated and the hypothesis of Shults and colleagues was that administration of cysteamine, by lowering the levels of somatostatin, might reduce the symptoms of the disease. For this double-blind crossover study 5 HD patients were recruited. The patients gradually received a maximum dose of 4 g/d (except two patients who received 1.5 g/d & 2.5 g/d) for a period of two weeks. The results showed no statistical difference between the cysteamine group and the placebo group in both motor symptoms and cognitive performance.

In another double-blind RCT study published by Mateo & Gimenez-Roldan [89] the effects of piracetam on HD were examined. Piracetam is a nootropic thought to increase mental capabilities. 11 HD patients randomly received either piracetam or placebo and the main outcome of the study was a significant increase in choreic movements in the piracetam group. This suggests that the administration of piracetam to combat cognitive decline associated with HD is not an appropriate medication.

In a recent double-blind RCT [90], the effects of minocycline on 60 HD patients was examined for a period of 8-weeks. Minocycline is an antibiotic that may block pro-apoptotic pathways and reactive microgliosis. Although the antibiotic was well tolerated, the principal outcome of this study was that there was no difference between the experimental and placebo groups in the HD rating scale. Interestingly, the placebo group performed significantly better in the Stroop test. A longer-term study examining the effects of minocycline is currently underway.

CONCLUSION

The above studies, summarized in Table, highlight the apparent lack of an effective treatment in HD. Some agents seem to moderately reduce motor symptoms and improve cognitive performance but, then again, even more failed to show any protective effect. Moreover, there are always methodological problems and limitations that require further examination of those agents that show some promising results. It is clear that we need to learn a lot more about the underlying pathophysiological mechanisms involved in the disease. Only then there is a chance to design drugs that might have a widespread beneficial effect. In this context the emerging therapeutic technologies of gene therapy, RNA interference and neural stem cell therapy might provide promising possibilities and, in tandem with ongoing drug development, provide the answers for a definite treatment of HD.

The discovery of environmental factors which modulate onset and progression of HD, and the gene-environment interactions which mediate these effects, has revolutionised our understanding of this fatal brain disease which was once considered the 'epitome of genetic determinism'. While recent epidemiology is beginning to provide support for the original research in mouse models, detailed retrospective and prospective epidemiological studies are required to define exactly what the environmental factors are which induce clinically therapeutic effects. One implication of these findings is that occupational therapies, or related approaches which enhance levels of mental and physical activity, may provide some benefit in delaying disease onset and slowing progression. Once sufficient epidemiological evidence is obtained, systematically organised environmental interventions within health systems (e.g. medical guidelines or 'environmentally-orientated' HD clinics) could be particularly useful for clinicians, especially those involved in primary healthcare, as they would provide a useful framework for long-term management of HD patients. Any interventions aimed at increasing levels of environmental stimulation could naturally be combined with drug administration, and the dual interventions might even have a synergistic effect. Furthermore, increased knowledge of how environmental stimulation can induce beneficial effects may lead to development of a new class of drugs which mimic or enhance this therapeutic actions: 'enviromimetics' [58,59].

Table. Double-blind randomized controlled clinical trials on Huntington's disease

AUTHORS	DRUG	CHOREA	COGNITION
Huntington Study Group, 2004 [90]	Minocycline	-	-
Heckmann et al., 2004 [63]	Amantadine	-	-
Lucetti et al., 2003 [62]	Amantadine	↓	-
Huntington Study Group, 2003 [65]	Riluzole	↓	-
Verbessem et al., 2003 [83]	Creatine	-	-
O'Suilleabhain & Dewey, 2003 [64]	Amantadine	-	n/a
Verhagen Metman et al., 2002 [61]	Amantadine	↓	-
Vaddadi et al., 2002 [86]	HUFAs	↓	-
Puri et al., 2002 [87]	HUFAs	↓	n/a
Huntington Study Group, 2001 [78]	Q_{10} & remacemide	-	-
Kremer et al., 1999 [85]	Lamotrigine	-	-
Huntington Study Group, 1998 [80]	OPC-14117	-	-
Murman et al., 1997 [60]	Ketamine	-	↓
van Vugt et al., 1997 [74]	Clozapine	↓	n/a
Como et al., 1997 [75]	Fluoxetine	-	-
Ranen et al., 1996 [77]	Idebenone	-	-
Kieburtz et al., 1996 [79]	Remacemide	-	-
Mateo & Gimenez-Roldan, 1996 [89]	Piracetam	↑	n/a
Albanese et al., 1995 [67]	Apomorphine	↓	n/a
Peyser et al., 1995 [76]	d-α-tocopherol	↓ (see text)	-
Consroe et al., 1991 [68]	Cannabidiol	-	-
Manyam et al., 1981 [72]	Isoniazid	↓	n/a
Shoulson et al., 1989 [71]	Baclofen	-	n/a
Shults et al., 1986 [88]	Cysteamine	-	-
Bassi et al., 1986 [66]	Transdihydrolisuride	↓	-
Scigliano et al., 1984 [69]	Gamma-vinyl GABA	-	n/a
Shoulson et al., 1976 [70]	Dipropylacetic acid	-	n/a

REFERENCES

[1]   La Spada, A.R., Wilson, E.M., Lubahn, D.B., Harding, A.E. & Fischbeck, K.H. (1991). Androgen receptor gene mutations in X-linked spinal and bulbar muscular atrophy. *Nature, 352*: 77-79.

[2]   Koide R, Ikeuchi T, Onodera O et al. (1994) Unstable expansion of CAG repeat in hereditary dentatorubral-pallidoluysian atrophy (DRPLA). *Nat Genet., 6*:9-13.

[3]   Orr, H.T., Chung, M.Y., Banfi, S. et al. (1993). Expansion of an unstable trinucleotide CAG repeat in spinocerebellar ataxia type 1. *Nature Genetics, 4*: 221-226.

[4]   Imbert, G., Saudou, F., Yvert, G. et al. (1996). Cloning of the gene for spinocerebellar ataxia 2 reveals a locus with high sensitivity to expanded CAG/glutamine repeats. *Nature Genetics, 14*: 285-291.

[5]   Kawaguchi, Y., Okamoto, T., Taniwaki, M. et al. (1994). CAG expansions in a novel gene for Machado-Joseph disease at chromosome 14q32.1. *Nat. Genet., 8*: 221-228.

[6]   Zhuchenko, O., Bailey, J., Bonnen, P. et al. (1997). Autosomal dominant cerebellar ataxia (SCA6) associated with small polyglutamine expansions in the alpha 1A-voltage-dependent calcium channel. *Nature genetics, 15*: 62-69.

[7]   Hagerman, P. J., Hagerman, R. J. (2004). Fragile X-associated tremor/ataxia syndrome (FXTAS). *Ment Retard Dev Disabil Res Rev., 10*:25-30.

[8]   Richards, R. I., Sutherland, G.R. (1992) Dynamic mutations: a new class of mutations causing human disease. *Cell 70*:709-12.

[9]   van Dellen, A., Grote, H.E. and Hannan, A.J. (2005) Gene-environment interactions, neuronal dysfunction and pathological plasticity in Huntington's disease. *Clin. Exp Pharmacol Physiol 32*:1007-19.

[10] Huntington, G. (1872). On Chorea. *Med Surg Rep., 26*:317-321.

[11] Huntington's Disease Collaborative Research Group. (1993). A novel gene containing a trinucleotide repeat that is expanded and unstable on Huntington's disease chromosomes. *Cell, 72*:971-983.

[12] Snell, R. G., MacMillan, J. C., Cheadle, J. P. et al. (1993). Relationship between trinucleotide repeat expansion and phenotypic variation in Huntington's disease. *Nat Genet., 4*:393-7.

[13] Nance, M. A. and Myers, R. H. (2001). Juvenile onset Huntington's disease--clinical and research perspectives. *Ment Retard Dev Disabil Res Rev., 7*:153-7.

[14] Berrios, G. E., Wagle, A. C., Markova, I. S. et al. (2001). Psychiatric symptoms and CAG repeats in neurologically asymptomatic Huntington's disease gene carriers. *Psychiatry Res., 102*:217-25.

[15] Craufurd, D., Thompson, J. C. & Snowden, J. S. (2001). Behavioral changes in Huntington Disease. *Neuropsychiatry, neuropsychology, and behavioral neurology, 14*: 219-226.

[16] Berrios, G. E., Wagle, A. C., Markova, I. S., Wagle, S. A., Rosser, A. and Hodges, J. R. (2002). Psychiatric symptoms in neurologically asymptomatic Huntington's disease gene carriers: a comparison with gene negative at risk subjects. *Acta Psychiatr Scand., 105*:224-30.

[17] Craufurd, D & Snowden, J. (2002). Neuropsychological and neuropsychiatric aspects of Huntington's disease. In *Huntington's disease.* 3rd Edition. Bates, G., Harper, P. S. & Jones, L. (Eds). Oxford University Press, pp. 62-94.

[18] Butters, N., Wolfe, J., Martone, M., Granholm, E. and Cermak, L. S. (1985). Memory disorders associated with Huntington's disease: verbal recall, verbal recognition and procedural memory. *Neuropsychologia 23*: 729-43.

[19] Ho, A. K., Sahakian, B. J., Robbins, T. W., Barker, R. A., Rosser, A. E. & Hodges, J.R. (2002). Verbal fluency in Huntington's disease: a longitudinal analysis of phonemic and semantic clustering and switching. *Neuropsychologia, 40*: 1277-1284.

[20] Harper, P. S. (1996). *Huntington's disease.* London: Saunders.

[21] Kremer, B. (2002). Clinical neurology of Huntington's disease. In *Huntington's disease.* 3rd Edition. Bates, G., Harper, P. S. & Jones, L. (Eds). Oxford University Press, pp. 28-61.

[22] Vonsattel, J.P., DiFiglia M. (1998) Huntington disease. *J Neuropathol Exp Neurol., 57*:369-84.

[23] De-la-Monte, S. M., Vonsattel, J. P. and Richardson, E. P., Jr. (1988). Morphometric demonstration of atrophic changes in the cerebral cortex, white matter, and neostriatum in Huntington's disease. *J Neuropathol Exp Neurol., 47*:516-25.

[24] Harper, P. S. (1992). The epidemiology of Huntington's disease. *Hum Genet., 89*:365-76.

[25] Palo, J., Somer, H., Ikonen, E., Karila, L. and Peltonen, L. (1987). Low prevalence of Huntington's disease in Finland. *Lancet, 2*:805-6.

[26] Harper, P. S. (2002). The epidemiology of Huntington's disease. In *Huntington's disease.* 3rd Edition. Bates, G., Harper, P. S. & Jones, L. (Eds). Oxford University Press, pp. 159-197.

[27] Wexler, N.S., Lorimer J, Porter J et al.; U.S.-Venezuela Collaborative Research Project. (2004) Venezuelan kindreds reveal that genetic and environmental factors modulate Huntington's disease age of onset. *Proc Natl Acad Sci USA, 101*:3498-503

[28] Rubinsztein, D. C., Leggo, J., Coles, R. et al. (1996). Phenotypic characterization of individuals with 30-40 CAG repeats in the Huntington disease (HD) gene reveals HD cases with 36 repeats and apparently normal elderly individuals with 36-39 repeats. *Am J Hum Genet., 59*:16-22.

[29] Brinkman, R. R., Mezei, M. M., Theilmann, J., Almqvist, E. and Hayden, M. R. (1997). The likelihood of being affected with Huntington disease by a particular age, for a specific CAG size. *Am J Hum Genet., 60*:1202-10.

[30] McNeil, S. M., Novelletto, A., Srinidhi, J. et al. (1997). Reduced penetrance of the Huntington's disease mutation. *Hum Mol Genet., 6*:775-9.

[31] Brandt, J., Bylsma, F. W., Gross, R., Stine, O. C., Ranen, N. and Ross, C. A. (1996). Trinucleotide repeat length and clinical progression in Huntington's disease. *Neurology, 46*:527-31.

[32] MacMillan, J. C., Snell, R. G., Tyler, A. et al. (1993). Molecular analysis and clinical correlations of the Huntington's disease mutation. *Lancet, 342*: 954-958.

[33] Weigell-Weber, M., Schmid, W. and Spiegel, R. (1996). Psychiatric symptoms and CAG expansion in Huntington's disease. *Am J Med Genet., 67*: 53-57.

[34] Duyao, M., Ambrose, C., Myers, R. et al. (1993). Trinucleotide repeat length instability and age of onset in Huntington's disease. *Nat Genet, 4*:387-92.

[35] Andrew, S. E., Goldberg, Y. P., Kremer, B. et al. (1993) The relationship between trinucleotide (CAG) repeat length and clinical features of Huntington's disease. *Nat Genet, 4*:398-403.

[36] Rubinsztein, D. C., Leggo, J., Chiano, M. et al. (1997). Genotypes at the GluR6 kainate receptor locus are associated with variation in the age of onset of Huntington disease. *Proc Natl Acad Sci U S A, 94*:3872-6.

[37] MacDonald, M.E., Vonsattel, J.P., Shrinidhi, J. et al. (1999) Evidence for the GluR6 gene associated with younger onset age of Huntington's disease. *Neurology 53*:1330-2.

[38] Feigin, A. (1998). Advances in Huntington's disease: implications for experimental therapeutics. *Curr Opin Neurol., 11*:357-62.

[39] Zeron, M. M., Chen, N., Moshaver, A., Lee, A. T., Wellington, C. L., Hayden, M. R. and Raymond, L. A. (2001). Mutant huntingtin enhances excitotoxic cell death. *Mol Cell Neurosci., 17*:41-53.

[40] Zeron, M. M., Hansson, O., Chen, N. et al. (2002). Increased sensitivity to N-methyl-D-aspartate receptor-mediated excitotoxicity in a mouse model of Huntington's disease. *Neuron, 33*:849-60.

[41] Kehoe, P., Krawczak, M., Harper, P.S. et al. (1999)Age of onset in Huntington disease: sex specific influence of apolipoprotein E genotype and normal CAG repeat length. *J. Med. Genet. 36*:108-11.

[42] Holbert, S., Denghien, I., Kiechle, T. et al. (2001) The Gln-Ala repeat transcriptional activator CA150 interacts with huntingtin: neuropathologic and genetic evidence for a role in Huntington's disease pathogenesis. *Proc Natl Acad Sci USA. 98*:1811-6.

[43] Van Dellen, A., Deacon, R., York, D., Blakemore, C. and Hannan, A.J. (2000a) Delaying the onset of Huntington's in mice. *Nature 404*:721-2.

[44] Hockly, E., Cordery, P. M., Woodman, B. et al. (2002) Environmental enrichment slows disease progression in R6/2 Huntington's disease mice. *Ann Neurol. 51*:235-42.

[45] Spires, T.L. Grote HE, Varshney NK, Cordery PM, van Dellen A, Blakemore C, Hannan AJ. (2004a) Environmental enrichment rescues protein deficits in a mouse model of Huntington's disease, indicating a possible disease mechanism. *J Neurosci. 24*:2270-6.

[46] Van Dellen, A. and Hannan, A.J. (2004) Genetic and environmental factors in the pathogenesis of Huntington's disease. *Neurogenetics 5*:9-17.

[47] Spires, T. L., Grote, H. E., Garry, S., Cordery, P. M., Van Dellen, A., Blakemore, C., Hannan, A. J. (2004b) Dendritic spine pathology and deficits in experience-dependent dendritic plasticity in R6/1 Huntington's disease transgenic mice. *Eur J Neurosci. 19*:2799-807.

[48] Mazarakis, N. K., Cybulska-Klosowicz, A., Grote, H. et al. (2005) Deficits in experience-dependent cortical plasticity and sensory-discrimination learning in presymptomatic Huntington's disease mice. *J Neurosci. 25*:3059-66.

[49] van Praag, H., Kempermann, G., Gage, F.H. (2000) Neural consequences of environmental enrichment. *Nat Rev Neurosci. 1*:191-8.

[50] Lazic, SE, Grote H, Armstrong RJ, Blakemore C, Hannan AJ, van Dellen A, Barker RA. (2004). Decreased hippocampal cell proliferation in R6/1 Huntington's mice. *Neuroreport. 15*:811-3.

[51] Grote, H.E, Bull, N.D., Howard, M.L. et al. Cognitive disorders and neurogenesis deficits in Huntington's disease mice are rescued by fluoxetine. *Eur. J. Neurosci. 22*:2081-8.

[52] Curtis, M. A., Penney, E. B., Pearson, A. G. et al. (2003) Increased cell proliferation and neurogenesis in the adult human Huntington's disease brain. *Proc Natl Acad Sci USA 100*:9023-7.

[53] Clifford JJ, Drago J, Natoli AL *et al.* (2002) Essential fatty acids given from conception prevent topographies of motor deficit in a transgenic model of Huntington's disease. *Neuroscience 109*: 81-8.

[54] Duan, W., Guo, Z., Jiang, H., Ware, M., Li, X.J., Mattson, M.P. (2003). Dietary restriction normalizes glucose metabolism and BDNF levels, slows disease progression, and increases survival in huntingtin mutant mice. *Proc. Natl Acad. Sci. USA 100*:2911-6.

[55] Sullivan, F. R., Bird, E. D., Alpay, M., Cha, J. H. (2001) Remotivation therapy and Huntington's disease. *J. Neurosci. Nurs. 33*: 136-42.

[56] Spires, T.L. and Hannan, A.J. (2005) Nature, nurture and neurology: Gene-environment interactions in neurodegeneration. *FEBS J. 272*:2347-61.

[57] Beal, M.F. and Ferrante, R.J. (2004) Experimental therapeutics in transgenic mouse models of Huntington's disease. Nat Rev Neurosci. *5*:373-84.

[58] Hannan, A.J. (2005) Novel therapeutic targets for Huntington's disease. *Exp Opin Therapeutic Targets 9*:639-50.

[59] Hannan, A.J. (2004) Huntington's disease: Which drugs might help patients. *IDrugs 7*:351-8.

[60] Murman, D. L., Giordani, B., Mellow, A. M. et al. (1997). Cognitive, behavioral, and motor effects of the NMDA antagonist ketamine in Huntington's disease. *Neurology, 49*:153-61.

[61] Verhagen Metman L, Morris MJ, Farmer C, Gillespie M, Mosby K, Wuu J, Chase TN. (2002). Huntington's disease: a randomized, controlled trial using the NMDA-antagonist amantadine. *Neurology, 59*:694-9.

[62] Lucetti, C., Del Dotto, P., Gambaccini, G. et al. (2003). IV amantadine improves chorea in Huntington's disease: an acute randomized, controlled study. *Neurology, 60*:1995-7.

[63] O'Suilleabhain, P., Dewey, R. B. Jr. (2003). A randomized trial of amantadine in Huntington disease. *Arch. Neurol., 60*:996-8.

[64] Heckmann, J. M., Legg, P., Sklar, D., Fine, J., Bryer, A., Kies, B. (2004). IV amantadine improves chorea in Huntington's disease: an acute randomized, controlled study. *Neurology, 63*:597-8.

[65] Huntington Study Group. (2003). Dosage effects of riluzole in Huntington's disease: a multicenter placebo-controlled study. *Neurology, 61*:1551-6.

[66] Bassi, S., Albizzati, M.G., Corsini, G.U. et al. (1986). Therapeutic experience with transdihydrolisuride in Huntington's disease. Neurology, *36*:984-6.

[67] Albanese, A., Cassetta, E., Carretta, D., Bentivoglio, A. R., Tonali, P. (1995). Acute challenge with apomorphine in Huntington's disease: a double-blind study. *Clin Neuropharmacol, 18*:427-34.

[68] Consroe, P., Laguna, J., Allender, J. et al. (1991). Controlled clinical trial of cannabidiol in Huntington's disease. *Pharmacol. Biochem. Behav. 40*:701-8.

[69] Scigliano G, Giovannini P, Girotti F, Grassi MP, Caraceni T, Schechter PJ. (1984). Gamma-vinyl GABA treatment of Huntington's disease. *Neurology, 34*:94-6.

[70] Shoulson, I., Kartzinel, R., Chase, T. N. (1976). Huntington's disease: treatment with dipropylacetic acid and gamma-aminobutyric acid. *Neurology, 26*:61-3.

[71] Shoulson, I., Odoroff, C., Oakes, D. et al. (1989). A controlled clinical trial of baclofen as protective therapy in early Huntington's disease. *Ann Neurol, 25*:252-9.

[72] Manyam, B. V., Katz, L., Hare, T. A., Kaniefski, K., Tremblay, R. D. (1981). Isoniazid-induced elevation of CSF GABA levels and effects on chorea in Huntington's disease. *Ann Neurol., 10*:35-7.

[73] Perry, T. L., Wright, J. M., Hansen, S. et al. (1982). A double-blind clinical trial of isoniazid in Huntington disease. *Neurology, 32*:354-8.

[74] van Vugt JP, Siesling S, Vergeer M, van der Velde EA, Roos RA. (1997). Clozapine versus placebo in Huntington's disease: a double blind randomised comparative study. *J Neurol Neurosurg Psychiatry, 63*:35-9.

[75] Como, P. G., Rubin, A. J., O'Brien, C. F. et al. (1997). A controlled trial of fluoxetine in nondepressed patients with Huntington's disease. *Mov. Disord. 12*:397-401.

[76] Peyser, C. E., Folstein, M., Chase, G. A. et al. (1995). Trial of d-alpha-tocopherol in Huntington's disease. *Am J Psychiatry, 152*:1771-5.

[77] Ranen, N. G., Peyser, C. E., Coyle, J. T. et al. (1996). A controlled trial of idebenone in Huntington's disease. *Mov Disord, 11*:549-54.

[78] Huntington Study Group. (2001). A randomized, placebo-controlled trial of coenzyme Q10 and remacemide in Huntington's disease. *Neurology, 57*:397-404.

[79] Kieburtz, K., Feigin, A., McDermott, M. et al. (1996). A controlled trial of remacemide hydrochloride in Huntington's disease. *Mov Disord, 11*:273-7.

[80] Huntington Study Group. (1998). Safety and tolerability of the free-radical scavenger OPC-14117 in Huntington's disease. The Huntington Study Group. *Neurology, 50*:1366-73.

[81] Andreassen OA, Dedeoglu A, Ferrante RJ et al. (2001). Creatine increase survival and delays motor symptoms in a transgenic animal model of Huntington's disease. *Neurobiol Dis, 8*:479-91.

[82] Ferrante, R. J., Andreassen, O. A., Jenkins, B. G. et al. (2000). Neuroprotective effects of creatine in a transgenic mouse model of Huntington's disease. *J Neurosci., 20*:4389-97.

[83] Verbessem P, Lemiere J, Eijnde BO et al. (2003). Creatine supplementation in Huntington's disease: a placebo-controlled pilot trial. *Neurology, 61*:925-30.

[84] Tabrizi, S. J., Blamire, A. M., Manners, D. N., Rajagopalan, B., Styles, P., Schapira, A. H., Warner, T. T. (2005). High-dose creatine therapy for Huntington disease: a 2-year clinical and MRS study. *Neurology, 64*:1655-6.

[85] Kremer, B., Clark, C.M., Almqvist, E.W. et al. (1999). Influence of lamotrigine on progression of early Huntington disease: a randomized clinical trial. *Neurology*, *53*:1000-11.

[86] Vaddadi KS, Soosai E, Chiu E, Dingjan P. (2002). A randomised, placebo-controlled, double blind study of treatment of Huntington's disease with unsaturated fatty acids. *Neuroreport*, *13*:29-33.

[87] Puri, B. K., Bydder, G. M., Counsell, S. J. et al. (2002). MRI and neuropsychological improvement in Huntington disease following ethyl-EPA treatment. *Neuroreport*, *13*:123-6.

[88] Shults, C., Steardo, L., Barone, P. et al. (1986). Huntington's disease: effect of cysteamine, a somatostatin-depleting agent. *Neurology*, *36*:1099-102.

[89] Mateo D, Gimenez-Roldan S. (1996). The effect of piracetam on involuntary movements in Huntington's disease. A double-blind, placebo-controlled study. *Neurologia* (Spanish), *11*:16-9.

[90] Huntington Study Group. (2004). Minocycline safety and tolerability in Huntington disease. *Neurology*, *63*:547-9.

RECOMMENDED FURTHER READING

1. Bates G, Harper PS, Jones L. *Huntington's disease*, 3rd ed. Oxford: Oxford University Press, 2002.

2. Bertram L, Tanzi RE. The genetic epidemiology of neurodegenerative disease. *J Clin Invest* 2005; 115:1449-57.

3. Everett CM, Wood NW. Trinucleotide repeats and neurodegenerative disease. *Brain* 2004; 127:2385-405.

4. Mayeux R. Epidemiology of neurodegeneration. *Annu Rev Neurosci* 2003; 26:81-104.

5. Spires TL, Hannan AJ. Nature, nurture and neurology: Gene-environment interactions in neurodegeneration. *FEBS J* 272:2347-61.

6. van Dellen A, Hannan AJ. Genetic and environmental factors in the pathogenesis of Huntington's disease. *Neurogenetics* 2004; 5:9-17.

HEALTH MEASUREMENTS SCALES IN NEUROEPIDEMIOLOGY

In: Handbook of Clinical Neuroepidemiology   ISBN 978-1-60021-511-7
Editors: V. L. Feigin and D. A. Bennett, pp. 597-619   © 2007 Nova Science Publishers, Inc.

Chapter 18

GENERAL HEALTH MEASUREMENT SCALES IN NEUROLOGY

Ian McDowell

Department of Epidemiology & Community Medicine, University of Ottawa,
451 Smyth Rd., Ottawa, Ontario K1H 8M5, Canada

ABSTRACT

Therapeutic trials in neurology traditionally record the results of treatment in terms of physical indicators of disease process, supplemented by measures of disability tailored to the disease in question. This chapter reviews further options in outcome measurement for clinical trials in neurology. It proposes to extend the current measurement repertoire to include measures of participation, showing the impact of disease on patients' daily roles. Such measures involve a degree of subjectivity that characterizes the theme of quality of life. Several illustrations of established scales are given, covering body functioning measures, psychological well-being, anxiety and depression and pain.

INTRODUCTION

There never can, and never will, be an ideal all-purpose health measure. Basic differences contrast the design and content of measures used in diagnosing a condition and those used in rating its severity, or in evaluating the outcomes of treatment [1]. And measurement instruments continue to evolve in each of these areas. This chapter reviews some of the measurement options in clinical trials of neurological treatment and outlines some of the directions in which this field may progress.

Traditionally, clinical research in neurology has focused on objective measures of disease process (e.g., recording the severity of seizures in epilepsy), supplemented by ratings of function and overall clinical impression, such as the Glasgow, Rankin, or Oxford scales [2].

These describe the proximal effects of disease, but provide limited coverage of the broader consequences of disease: what the patient can actually do despite their condition. To extend this measurement repertory, many trials have included measures of disability, which refers to the impact of an impairment on daily function [3]. Most studies use disease-specific measures of disability: for Parkinson's disease [4], multiple sclerosis [5,6], stroke [7,8] or epilepsy [9-11]. These measures have been reviewed by Wade [2] and, more briefly, by Bowling [12]. The advantages of disease-specific instruments are that they focus on the issues most relevant to each disorder, and they can offer sensitive measures of improvement following treatment. A disadvantage is that the specific measures are all different, complicating comparisons of treatments across diseases. This becomes relevant, for example, in allocating resources among specialties according to the benefits of therapy, which requires a common yardstick for recording improvement. A deeper concern is that disease-specific measures may be tailored to highlight areas in which a particular treatment has its greatest effect, perhaps concealing limitations and possible side-effects of the therapy. This is the purpose of generic health measures, which cover a wide range of common symptoms and functions to give a comprehensive summary of treatment effectiveness. Generic measures permit comparisons across treatments and across medical conditions. In turn, the disadvantage of generic measures is that their breadth of coverage comes at the expense of depth: with fewer questions on each topic they cannot provide the fine-grained information of the disease-specific measure. Two resolutions have been tried. First, some studies have recorded the severity of common syndromes that may arise secondary to a neurological disorder, such as pain [13], depression [14,15] or anxiety [16]. Second, hybrid measures combine a generic assessment that covers a wide range of topics applicable to many conditions, plus disease-specific supplements. Examples include the QLQ-C30 Quality of Life Questionnaire [17,18] and the World Health Organization's WHOQOL [19,20]. These have rarely seen application in neurological studies.

A further possible extension of the generic activity or disability measures is to cover functioning in society. Ultimately, a health problem is rated in terms of what the patient desires to do that they cannot do because of the condition. But this is not standard for all patients: a slight visual deficit holds different implications for an active airline pilot and for a retired teacher. This is the WHO's conception of handicap, recently reformulated as participation in society [21,22]. In this perspective, function is viewed as a dynamic interaction between the health condition and the patient's expectations and the context in which they live (including physical environment and cultural norms relevant to their disease). Reflecting this approach, health measures have broadened considerably, as summarized by the rubric "health-related quality of life measures". These include the patient's subjective judgments of the impact of health problems on their daily function, usual activities and normal social roles. Over the past ten or so years, measures of quality of life have been used in studies of Parkinson's disease [23], multiple sclerosis [24], stroke [25,26] and epilepsy [27]. Quality of life measures are intended to supplement objective and specific measures of bodily function, not to replace them. They lie at the distal end of a logical sequence of outcome indicators, running from measures of physical function, through disability measures, to measures of impact on a patient's life. These are deliberately subjective: quality of life represents "the importance of people's subjective perceptions of their current ability to function, as compared with their own internalised standards of what is possible or ideal" [28]. Such measures describe the quality rather than merely the extent of function and capture the variation between patients in response to similar diagnoses. Subjective measures give insights into matters of human concern such as pain, suffering or depression that could not be inferred solely from physical measurements or laboratory tests. They focus the assessment on those aspects of function that are most relevant to the patient: the actual problem caused by the disease.

This chapter reviews some of the options for extending the scope of routine neurological assessment to incorporate some of the existing wide range of patient-assessed measures. The chapter is divided into five fields of measurement: general health and quality of life, physical function, psychological well-being, depression and anxiety, and pain. It cannot present an exhaustive review of measures, but focuses on a small selection of leading scales in each field to illustrate some of the variety of measures available and to illustrate some of the issues to be considered in choosing a measurement instrument. The measures are ordered from the general to the specific.

GENERIC HEALTH STATUS AND QUALITY OF LIFE

Measures in this class divide into health profiles, which score several dimensions of health separately, and health indexes, which combine the dimensions into a single, weighted summary score. Among the many representatives of the health profiles, such as the Sickness Impact Profile, the Nottingham Health Profile or the Short-Form-36 Health Survey, we can describe the latter as the most commonly used generic health status measure.

Health Profiles

The Short-Form-36 includes 36 questions derived from a longer instrument; hence its name. It was designed as a broad-ranging indicator of health status that is applicable to almost any type or severity of condition. It can be used in population surveys and in policy research; in conjunction with disease-specific measures, it can also be used as an outcome measure in clinical practice and research [29]. The SF-36 scores eight aspects of health: Physical functioning; Pain; Vitality, energy or fatigue; General mental health; Social functioning; Role limitations due to physical health problems; Role limitations due to emotional problems, and General health perceptions. The questions generally take five to ten minutes to complete. The eight section scores can be presented as a profile, or two summary scores may be used, covering physical and mental health.

Extensive testing in a range of settings has demonstrated good reliability of this measure. Validity testing has concentrated on comparing the SF-36 with other, similar measures, and on the internal structure of the instrument. The correlational evidence suggests that the SF-36 performs as well as, or better than other measures. It is also capable of detecting change in health status, which is indispensable for use as an outcome measure and there are population norms that allow users to relate a patient's score to the percentile distribution on a population reference distribution [30].

The SF-36 has been developed over 10 years in a number of countries; its development is managed by a non-profit organization. The take-home messages are that developing a good quality health measure requires extensive work over a period of years. It requires a high level of organizational support and careful promotion to ensure its standard administration. Too many good instruments in the past were simply published and then left to researchers to use freely. Over time this leads to the uncoordinated creation of variants that, after a while, erode the goal of achieving comparable results across studies. While the SF-36 is freely available, permission to use it has to be obtained from a corporation that provides information on its administration, scoring, and interpretation, presented in a user's manual [30]. An international consortium has been developed to translate and adapt the SF-36 for use outside the USA [31]; this project evaluates the psychometric properties of the instrument, gathers general population norms and summarizes findings.

Health Indexes

Among the leading health indexes, the EuroQol EQ-5D was developed in Europe; the Health Utilities Index was developed in Canada, while the Quality of Well-Being scale was developed in the United States. Of these measures, the European Quality of Life (EuroQol) illustrates the simultaneous development of a measure in several countries as an international effort. As subjective reactions to sickness may vary from culture to culture, the earlier approach to developing a measure in one country and then translating it for use elsewhere is now generally regarded as inadequate. Health indexes express health status in a single score and are intended for use in evaluative studies such as drug trials, and in policy research [32]. The crucial contrast with health profile measures is that indexes accept the challenge of combining separate dimensions of health into a single score, permitting direct comparisons to be drawn between, say, the effectiveness of drug management of Alzheimer's disease and neurosurgical treatment for stroke.

The EQ-5D was developed simultaneously in several languages by an international collaboration among European countries, the USA, Canada and Japan, as a standard instrument for use in international studies [33]. It is very brief, with just five generic quality of life ratings that can be supplemented for particular disease applications. The EQ-5D was designed as a self-completed questionnaire suited for use in postal surveys and that would represent health status as a single aggregated index value. The current version, the EQ-5D, covers Mobility, Self-care, Usual activities, Pain and discomfort, and Anxiety/depression. Each dimension is scored to indicate no problem, moderate, or severe problems. There is also a self-rating of overall health on a 0-to-100 scale.

In scoring the EQ-5D, a person's health state is first summarized by a 5-digit profile, indicating their score on each dimension. Thus, a profile of 12311 would represent no difficulties with mobility, pain, and anxiety/depression, but some problems with self-care and severe difficulty in performing usual activities. The resulting profile can be graphed or it can be converted into a summary index using a scoring system that weights each of the five dimensions differentially. The weights either use the respondent's own judgment, or standard utility weights may be used, derived from responses to large surveys [34]. Utility weights have been derived in several countries, including the USA and Japan; the EuroQol web site lists 21 sets of scoring weights at www.euroqol.org.

Several studies have reported on the reliability of the EuroQol [35,36], and in validation studies scores correlate highly with the Health Utilities Index [37], the SF-36 [38], among others. Shortcomings of the EuroQol include its rather coarse scale that is well suited to patients with major morbidity, but is relatively insensitive to variations in well-being at the upper ends of the health continuum [39]. The SF-36 appears to be less affected by this problem [32]. Estimates of the EQ-5D's sensitivity to detecting change in health status vary, some studies reporting positive results [40,41], perhaps more sensitive than the SF-36 [42], while other studies show it to be less so [43,44].

As with the SF-36, the EuroQol was developed by a well-organized team that promotes its continued development and testing. The EuroQol Foundation disseminates information on the instrument and a Business Management center in Rotterdam coordinates development work.

Single-Item Health Measures

The SF-36 and the EQ-5D illustrate measures of general health developed through long-term collaborative research efforts. At the same time, it is somewhat humbling that remarkably good results may be obtained in a far simpler fashion, by asking patients a single overall question such as "In general, would you say your health is: Excellent, Very Good, Good, Fair, Poor?" A surprising finding is that this simple, low-tech question correlates reasonably highly with the more detailed health indexes or profiles, sometimes as highly as the more detailed scales correlate among themselves [45]. Furthermore, patients can report their health very accurately and numerous longitudinal studies have confirmed remarkably strong associations between the simple self-rating score and subsequent mortality, even after controlling for age, socioeconomic status and a range of standard risk factors [46,47]. Naturally, with only five steps on the response scale, the summary question cannot be as sensitive to subtle changes in health as the SF-36 or the EQ-5D, but its value as a predictor of subsequent health status has led to its routine inclusion as part of a measurement battery, as in the SF-36.

DISABILITY AND PHYSICAL FUNCTION

Assessments of physical function have evolved in a way that reflects the distinctions between impairment, disability and handicap. Formal measurements of physical function began in the 1930s and 1940s with impairment scales covering capacities such as balance, sensory abilities, or range of motion. Most of these scales were designed for elderly or chronically ill patients and were rating scales applied by a clinician; examples include the PULSES Profile [48]. Later, as the goals of care (especially rehabilitation) were expanded to include restoring patients to their independent life, assessing impairments was no longer sufficient and it became important to measure disability and handicap as well. Assessment methods were broadened to consider the activities a patient could or did perform at his level of physical capacity, the classic example being Katz's 1957 scale of independence in Activities of Daily Living (ADL) [49]. This summarizes the patient's independence in bathing, dressing, using the toilet, moving around the house, and eating–topics that Katz selected to represent "primary biological functions." ADL scales are concerned with severe levels of disability, relevant mainly to institutionalized patients and to the elderly. In 1969, Lawton and Brody extended the ADL concept to consider problems more typically experienced by those living in the community: mobility, difficulty in shopping, cooking, or managing money, a field that came to be termed "Instrumental Activities of Daily Living" or "Performance Activities of Daily Living" [50]. Instrumental activities are more complex and demanding than basic ADLs; they offer indicators of "applied" problems that include elements of the handicap concept. More recently, the 2001 WHO International Classification of Functioning, Disability and Health (ICF) extended the earlier notions of disability and handicap to describe outcomes in terms of body functioning, activities (the activities undertaken by an individual), participation (their involvement in a life situation), and environment [22]. One of the most widely used IADL measures is the Functional Independence Measure. More recently, measures have been developed to assess handicap via fulfillment of social roles or working ability, as proposed in the ICF; a recent example is the SMAF.

The Functional Independence Measure (FIM)

The FIM assesses physical and cognitive disability in terms of the care a patient will require. It is used to monitor progress and to assess the outcomes of rehabilitation. It is a rating scale comprising 18 ratings of independence in self-care, sphincter control, mobility, locomotion, communication, and cognition [51]. It takes about 30 minutes to administer and score. A summary of administration procedures is available at www.sci-queri.research.med.va.gov/fim.htm.

The FIM is very widely used in rehabilitation facilities in the United States, where a 1983 national task force established a Uniform Data System to standardize measurements of disability; the FIM is the central measurement of this scheme [52]. Because of its widespread use, extensive evidence has accumulated for its validity and reliability; often based on very large samples [53]. From the UDS, reference scores have been derived from tens of thousands of patients at admission and discharge for various categories of rehabilitation patients [51].

As a measure developed for use in rehabilitation settings, FIM scores are intended to suggest the amount of time that will be required to care for a patient. Applied to multiple sclerosis patients, for example, scores predicted the time required for assistance with personal care ($R^2 = 0.77$). This result improved to $R^2 = 0.99$ when patients with visual impairments were omitted from the analyses, indicating that the FIM did not capture the additional time required to care for someone with vision problems. Hence, FIM scores can be translated into expected minutes of care per day [54]; similar analyses have been applied to stroke patients [55]. As with all ADL scales, the FIM is best suited to patients with severe disabilities. A more recent measure, the SMAF, extends coverage to patients living independently at home.

The Système de mesure de l'autonomie fonctionnelle (SMAF)

The SMAF is a 29-item clinical rating scale that measures the functional autonomy of elderly patients [56]. It was developed in Quebec to guide decisions about allocating home care or in deciding on institutional admission [57]. It records both the patient's functional disabilities and the available material and social resources that may compensate for the disabilities. It assesses activities of daily living, mobility, communication, mental function and instrumental activities of daily living. The SMAF integrates disability and handicap in a single instrument. Where a disability is identified, the assessor asks whether human resources (family members, volunteers, or paid staff) are available to compensate for the disability. If so, the handicap score is set at zero, but otherwise the handicap score equals the disability score. The stability of support is also rated, adding a prognostic dimension. The ratings of support make the SMAF a family-level measure, reflecting research on caregiving and family-centered care. As with the FIM, scores can be translated into an estimate of the time required to care for a patient [58]. The SMAF can also be used as an outcome measure, and responsiveness appears somewhat better than that of the FIM [59,60].

By identifying disabilities that are not alleviated by the family's resources, the SMAF records unmet needs and, by extension, is used in needs-based health care planning, evaluation and cost-benefit analyses [61,62]. The SMAF conceptualizes handicap as the shortfall between a patient's disability and the social or material resources they have to manage their condition [63,64]. But a handicap need not only be due to illness: Hébert noted that "a man who cannot perform domestic tasks, regardless of the reason, is disabled and must rely on his social resources, usually represented by his wife, to compensate for the disabilities. These social and cultural disabilities are real, since with the loss of the resource, the handicaps generated are often sufficient to justify admission to an institution" [63]. The SMAF is also innovative in focusing on a profile of disability scores, rather than the conventional overall score. This led to the identification of patterns of disability that hold similar implications for the need for care: the so-called ISO-SMAF patient profiles [64]. These comprise groups of people with perhaps different types of disability, but who require similar types of care. Fourteen such groups were identified, running from people with loss of IADL abilities in group 1, to bedridden people who require total care in group 14. Groups 2 to 13 form intermediate steps, at each of which roughly equivalent resources are required, and average costs of care for each profile have been calculated for various care settings [65]. Finally, studies recorded the typical disability profiles that each level of institution could manage, so that the clinician can judge which level of care would suit a particular client.

PSYCHOLOGICAL WELL-BEING

Generic health measures all include a brief overview of psychological well-being, but several instruments cover this theme in greater depth. Measures evolved from check-lists of symptoms of distress developed in the 1940s as screens for psychiatric disorders, toward self-report scales that could also cover positive aspects of adjustment. This led to an interest in recording morale and life satisfaction, but these measures proved less useful in screening for psychiatric distress. Newer scales, such as those developed by Goldberg or Dupuy, combine the check-list approach with questions on subjective well-being and may offer the best of both worlds. They can identify emotional disorders and can also be used in studies of the protective impact of positive mental health and in studies of "wellness." There have been many attempts to specify what is being measured, to distinguish, for example, between "distress" and "disorder," between "feelings", "mood" and "affect," and between "psychological," "emotional," and "mental" well-being. But many of the measures form indicators of the very general concept of "non-specific psychological distress" [66]. Considerable attention has been paid to the structure of these concepts, debating their distinctness and whether positive and negative feelings lie at opposite ends of one continuum or form separate continua [67,68].

The General Health Questionnaire (GHQ)

This measure, developed by Goldberg, illustrates the category of measures that screen for potentially treatable psychological distress. The GHQ is a self-administered questionnaire that may be used in surveys or in clinical settings to identify potential cases, leaving the task of diagnosing actual disorder to a subsequent psychiatric interview [69]. It covers relatively mild levels of depression, anxiety, social impairment, and hypochondriasis. The original version covered 60 symptoms (including organic symptoms, abnormal feelings or thoughts) and behaviors; 28- and 12-item abbreviations are commonly used [70]. A single score is produced, and Goldberg paid close attention to establishing cutting-points to identify possible psychiatric disorder [71]. The GHQ has been used across the world, and innumerable studies have reported on its validity and reliability [69,71,72]. To give just one example, Goldberg studied the validity of the 12-item version in 15 cities (and 11 languages), documenting how the relative sensitivity and specificity of the questions varied from place to place. He found that there was no question that could be discarded as each proved highly valid somewhere in the world [73].

The GHQ has become a benchmark against which other scales are compared. It was well founded on a clear conceptual approach, the initial item selection and item analyses were fully documented, and the questions have not been altered by subsequent users. It has seen widespread use in general practice for screening for mental disorders and is potentially well suited to extend the coverage of psychological distress in the generic health measures described above for use in neurology research.

The General Well-Being Schedule (GWB)

This scale was developed by Dupuy in 1977 and offers a brief but broad indicator of subjective feelings of psychological well-being and distress. It was originally designed for use in community surveys [74]. Eighteen self-report questions represent common feelings, including anxiety, depression, positive well-being, vitality and general health during the past month. The validation studies of the GWB have followed the approach typical for survey research instruments, focusing on the internal structure of the measure via factor analysis, and secondarily covering its correlations with other scales; reference values have also been produced [74]. The validity results are good, and strong correlations have been shown with most of the leading depression and anxiety scales. The GWB also appears capable of discriminating between patient and non-patient samples [75], but we have little information on its sensitivity to change following treatment. A 22-item version is named the Psychological General Well-Being Index [74], and a ten-question abbreviated version is called the Psychological Mental Health Index. This offers an alternative to purpose-built depression or anxiety scales when a brief rating is appropriate. The set of GWB scales illustrate the existence of instruments that may hold potential for clinical outcome studies, especially with patients with low levels of psychological distress. They cover positive and negative aspects of well-being, are brief, and have a broad coverage. However, as they have chiefly been used in non-clinical studies, they need to be tested in neurological research studies.

DEPRESSION AND ANXIETY

Depression Measures

As an alternative to general psychological well-being scales, purpose-built anxiety or depression scales are available. These may be similar in length to the general scales, but have a narrower focus. In terms of clinical interpretation, the advantage lies in their greater specificity, but as outcome measures this narrower scope may make them less sensitive to the possibly broad range of emotional responses to a chronic neurological disorder. Among depression scales, the second version of the Beck Depression Inventory (the BDI-II) is extremely well-established. It includes 21 symptoms of depression and is designed to reflect DSM-IV criteria [76,77]. It has been used as a community screening instrument and in clinical research [78] and its validity and reliability have been widely tested. An example of an instrument with a less clinical orientation is the Center for Epidemiologic Studies Depression Scale (CES-D) which was developed to identify depression in general population studies [79]. With 20 self-report items, it provides a score that indicates the probability that the respondent would receive a diagnosis of depression if evaluated clinically. Sensitivity and specificity have been tested many times and can be very high [80]. As a screening instrument, however, we know less about how sensitive it is to detecting *change* in level of depression.

Anxiety Measures

There are likewise several well-established anxiety measures. Beck's self-report Anxiety Inventory (BAI) is again a leading method; it measures the severity of self-reported anxiety and was designed to minimize confounding with symptoms of depression [81,82]. It is a 21-item measure in which 14 items cover somatic symptoms and seven reflect subjective aspects of anxiety or panic. An overall score is provided with cutting-points to identify clinically significant anxiety; validity is well-established. Beyond the Beck instrument, perhaps the best-known anxiety measure is the State-Trait Anxiety Inventory developed by Spielberger [83]. This self-report measure indicates the intensity of feelings of anxiety; it distinguishes between state anxiety (a temporary condition experienced in specific situations) and trait anxiety (a general tendency to perceive situations as threatening) [84]. It was originally developed as a research instrument to study anxiety in normal adult population samples, but it can also be used to screen for anxiety disorders and can be used with patient samples [85]. The STAI has also received extensive validity and reliability testing; correlations with the Beck anxiety scale typically range from 0.45 to 0.68 [86,87]. Of the two dimensions, the 20-item state anxiety scale is the more relevant for use as an evaluative instrument as it is more sensitive to short-term variations in anxiety.

Combined Depression and Anxiety Scales

Because anxiety and depression share overlapping symptoms that are difficult to distinguish and that frequently occur together, several scales cover both. Many authors have debated the interrelations of depression and anxiety, illustrating contrast between categorical and dimensional traditions in health measurement. The medical approach to disorders such as anxiety and depression is categorical; to receive a diagnosis, a patient must meet specified criteria such as those in the DSM-IV [88]. The categorical approach is practical and provides a basis for deciding whether or not to treat a patient. The underlying assumption is that there is a qualitative distinction between those who are well and those who are sick; sickness can vary in severity, but cases do not lie on the same continuum as non-cases, or at least form a distinct cluster at one end of the continuum. This conception is widely challenged, however, and psychologists generally take a dimensional approach that treats anxiety as a continuum of severity with no intrinsic threshold (the same debate occurs with cognitive impairment and dementia). The arguments for a dimensional conception point out that there does not seem to be a bimodal distribution of scores representing well and sick groups in the population, and there seems to be no clear threshold beyond which rising anxiety scores would indicate an anxiety disorder. Clark and Watson have been leading contributors to distinguishing between anxiety and depression from a dimensional perspective [67].

This distinction between categorical and dimensional models of disorders is also relevant to the differing purposes of making measurements. Where the intention is diagnostic, to classify a person as a case or non-case, the categorical approach works well; where the purpose is to evaluate progress following treatment, the finer gradients implied by a dimensional model is more suitable. These distinctions also connect to perspectives on the overlap between anxiety and depression, for measurements based in the categorical tradition seek to make clinically relevant distinctions between anxiety and depression; the Hospital Anxiety and Depression scale is an example. By contrast, within the dimensional tradition the Depression Anxiety Stress Scales were designed to record disease severity rather than to distinguish and classify the disorders.

The Hospital Anxiety and Depression Scale (HADS)

The Hospital Anxiety and Depression scale (HADS) is a self-assessment instrument designed to detect clinically significant depression and anxiety in patients attending outpatient medical clinics, and to discriminate between the two conditions. The HADS originated from a request for a test to identify those seemingly depressed patients who would benefit from antidepressant medication [89]. Existing instruments, such as the General Health Questionnaire, were inadequate as they did not indicate the nature of any disorder identified [90]. As it was intended for use with general medical patients, the HADS focused on relatively mild degrees of disorder (items on suicidal thoughts were excluded), and somatic items such as dizziness or headaches were deliberately not used. It has been widely used as a screening instrument outside of the hospital setting, and for rating psychiatric patients [91]. Of the 14 items, seven cover anxiety and seven cover depression. Reliability has been described in at least 18 studies [92], and several studies have reviewed the independence of the ratings of anxiety and depression. Nineteen studies, for example, have reported separation between the two concepts using factor analysis [92], although the two scores correlate positively. The HADS has been compared to the GHQ and the BDI in several studies [93,94]. The overall impression is that the GHQ performs best in detecting depression, but the HADS is superior in identifying anxiety. Sensitivity figures for depression, for example, were 72% for the HADS and 79% for the GHQ. Sensitivity and specificity results have been summarized from 24 studies, showing mean values of about 80% for both [92].

The HADS has become widely used, and the general consensus is that it achieves its purpose. It is brief and simple to administer, it does seem to separate anxiety from depression, and scores are not confounded by physical illness. Convergent correlations with other scales appear good: it performs as well as the longer Beck or GHQ instruments. Developed for use in the hospital setting, the HADS would seem appropriate for use with neurology patients. It should not be considered as a general screening instrument, for which the GHQ would be more appropriate [95]. The extensive information available on the validity and reliability of this scale illustrates the amount of effort that goes into testing a health measurement of this type. This takes a period of years (the HADS was originally developed in 1983); indeed, most of the leading health measures have been in existence for over ten years.

The Depression Anxiety Stress Scales

Also originally published in 1983, the Depression Anxiety Stress Scales (DASS) were designed to assess the severity of core symptoms of depression, anxiety, and stress. Together, three scales provide a broad-spectrum measure of psychological distress, indicating the range and frequency of symptoms. Originally developed for use with population samples, this instrument can also be used to characterize an emotional disturbance as part of a broader clinical assessment. It was derived from empirical analyses of items, selecting those that measured anxiety and depression separately, plus other items to reflect a tripartite conceptual model proposed by Clark and Watson [67]. The third dimension was termed 'stress' because of its focus on symptoms of tension. Lovibond argued that the differences between depression, anxiety and stress are matters of degree and not of quality, and underlies the observed correlations between measures of anxiety and depression. The DASS includes 42 negative symptoms, with 14 covering each theme. Evidence for reliability and validity is less extensive than that for the HADS, but the results suggest high quality. Correlations with the Beck Depression Inventory, for example, are typically in the range 0.7 to 0.8 [96,97], while correlations with the STAI range from 0.65 to 0.70 [97]. Correlations between the DASS and HADS depression scores range from 0.65 to 0.75, while those between the two anxiety scales run from 0.53 to 0.60 [98,99].

Reviews of anxiety and depression scales illustrate the considerable measurement challenge that these topics pose. Although the syndromes can be distinguished conceptually, their co-occurrence makes it difficult to discriminate between them. There is an inherent tension between the goals of discriminating between anxiety and depression, versus providing comprehensive coverage of the breadth of their symptoms, since these overlap. Thus the DASS includes symptoms such as tension, irritability that are not included in instruments such as the Beck anxiety or depression scales, because they discriminate. But equally, the DASS omits several common anxiety and depression symptoms that may be useful in screening or case-detection because they are not specific to one or the other condition. Lovibond attributed the relatively low correlation between the DASS and Beck depression scales to the inclusion of items on the Beck scale (such as disturbance of appetite, weight loss, sleeping difficulties, tiredness or lack of energy) that are sensitive, but not specific, to depression [96]. Thus, for use in identifying and characterizing the *type* of psychological sequelae of neurologic disorders, an instrument such as the DASS may be suitable, while for use as an outcome measure to show change it may be that the broader scope of an instrument such as the Beck is better. By contrast to the general health measures, however, there has been very little emphasis on sensitivity to change in the validity studies of anxiety and depression scales. Another characteristic of this measurement field is the relative absence of an emphasis on developing internationally-applicable instruments. This in part reflects the existence of differing diagnostic traditions in different countries, and in part the reality that there is more cultural variation in expressions of psychiatric disorders than of physical disability.

PAIN

There are especial challenges in measuring pain. Like depression or anxiety, pain is a private and internal sensation that cannot be directly observed or measured, and whose measurement depends on the subjective response of the person experiencing it. By contrast, physical disabilities can be measured more directly: we both define and measure them in terms of observable behavior such as walking ability. Pain is also multidimensional; intensity alone will not adequately reflect the contrast between, say, a toothache and a burn. Finally, pain measurement is, *par excellence*, the area in which subjective reports represent a blend of the strength of the underlying stimulus and of the person's emotional response to it. This is relevant because in measuring pain we try to infer pain (as a stimulus) from the sufferer's subjective response, which can be influenced by biological, social, and psychological factors [100].

The majority of pain questionnaires concentrate on intensity and use adjectives or a numerical scale to represent the intensity continuum. A variant uses visual analog scales to represent intensity by a plain line without verbal or numerical guides. Extending the questionnaire approach to cover more than the intensity and duration of pain, Melzack's McGill Pain Questionnaire gives both a qualitative description and a quantification of the pain and of the patient's affective response to pain.

The McGill Pain Questionnaire (MPQ)

The MPQ consists of a set of 78 adjectives that reflect three aspects of the pain experience. Severity scores are also assigned to each adjective, so the measure provides both qualitative and quantitative profiles of the "sensory", "affective" and "evaluative" dimensions of pain [101]. Melzack based the instrument on a cognitive and neurological model of pain that he has subsequently reformulated as a "neuromatrix model" [102]. The MPQ was originally used in evaluating pain therapies, but it has also been used as a diagnostic aid. Much of the validation of the MPQ has focused on its internal structure. While results seem to differ according to the types of pain being studied, there is reasonably strong support for the existence of the three dimensions of pain proposed by Melzack [80]. Correlations between MPQ scores and visual analogue intensity scales typically range from 0.45 to 0.65 [103]. The MPQ has been widely used and sections have been incorporated into several other leading scales. A 15-word short-form MPQ has been developed [104], and there have also been several extensions to the MPQ: the McGill Comprehensive Pain Questionnaire [105], the Dartmouth Pain Questionnaire [106], and a computer animated version [107]. As a candidate for use in studies of neurological outcomes, the MPQ offers a well-established measure that provides sufficient descriptive detail that it would permit a classification of the types of pain experienced by the patient. However, if a rating of pain intensity is all that is required, a visual analogue or numerical rating scale is much more easily administered.

Visual Analogue Scales (VAS)

Visual Analogue Scales (VAS) provide a simple way to record subjective estimates of pain intensity [108]. Visual analogue scales involve the respondent placing a mark a certain distance along a line to represent the intensity of a stimulus. They have long been used in many areas of psychology [109]; their application in health measurement began with pain but has extended to general health assessments. Huskisson popularized the application of visual analogue scales to measuring pain during the 1970s [110,111]. Conventionally, VAS use a straight line 10 cm long, marked at each end with labels such as "pain as bad as it could be" and "no pain." There are, however, numerous variants, including computer administration, the use of colors and curved lines [80]. A score simply records the distance in mm. from the lower end of the scale. In recording pain relief as an outcome, the VAS may be set up to run from no relief to complete relief of pain. The VAS typically takes less than 30 seconds to complete, but some patients may require instruction to grasp the metaphor of the line; reliability of using the scale improves with the educational level of the respondent [112]. Visual analogue scales appear to be more sensitive to change than verbal rating scales and so require smaller sample sizes in evaluative studies [113]. The comparison between visual analogue and numerical rating scales is less clear, however, and the correlations between them are high, typically around 0.85. In theory there is much greater precision in a VAS than in a 10- or a 12-point numerical rating scale, but the precision is likely not translated into reliable variance. Hence, Guyatt et al. showed that VAS and numerical scales showed similar responsiveness when standardized to the same scale range and so, given its greater simplicity, they recommended the numerical rating [114].

Pain intensity ratings may be extended to add a time dimension by using diaries or pain charts that record variations in pain over the course of a day, also recording the medications taken. Cumulative scores representing the duration of pain at each intensity level may be derived from the chart [115]. As an alternative to a visual analog scale, a physical analog can be used. This requires the patient to match her clinical pain with various levels of experimentally induced pain, typically radiant heat or an electric shock. Once a match is found, the clinical pain is described in terms of the strength of the stimulus used to induce the experimental pain. Alternatively, the patient may be asked to apply a physical effort (such as squeezing a pressure bulb) at an intensity that matches his pain level; Peck had patients match the intensity of their pain with the intensity of a sound produced by an audiometer [116]. All of these approaches, however, record only the intensity of pain; an instrument such as the McGill Questionnaire is required to cover qualitative aspects of pain.

CONCLUSION

The focus in this review has been on broadening the scope of outcome measures used in clinical trials of neurological cases. Many of these measures are termed "general health status measures" or "measures of health-related quality of life." Of the two, quality of life measures are broader, including the dimensions of physical, mental and social well-being covered by general health measures, but extending these to include other topics such as work and role performance or spiritual well-being and use of transportation [117]. Beyond being broad in scope, there is still a lack of a clear consensus over what dimensions of quality of life are relevant to health studies. There is, however, consensus that health-related quality of life is assessed subjectively: it is the perception of the respondent that is important, and not just an objective judgment of their status. This represents something of a departure from the original approach to assessing quality of life in the social sciences, where "quality of life" generally referred to the adequacy of people's material circumstances and to their feelings about these circumstances. It was distinguished from the more subjective concepts of life satisfaction, morale, or happiness [118]. The benefits of quality of life measures in health research lie in broadening the scope of outcome measures, and in providing a formal means for the patient's judgment to influence treatment. There is an implicit hierarchy of measurement, and quality of life measures complement, rather than supplant, more objective measures. They are helpful in distinguishing between treatments that have been found equivalent in terms or morbidity and mortality: lumpectomy versus radiation for Stage I and II breast cancers, for example [119]. They may also be used in involving the patient in reaching decisions over whether or not to use therapy at all, or how to judge a treatment that has survival advantages but at the cost of significant side effects. Here, an innovative procedure for illustrating the pay-off has been to incorporate the subjective quality of life judgments into a metric that balances treatment efficacy against its side effects called the Quality-adjusted Time Without Symptoms and Toxicity method (Q-TWiST) [120]. This is used, for example, in choosing between short- or long-duration adjuvant chemotherapy, which entails weighing the possible delayed remission of the latter against the longer duration of experiencing treatment side-effects. The Q-TWiST moves beyond the traditional cross-sectional perspective of health measures and uses the metaphor of an investment in which contrasting patterns of advantage to different treatment options unfold over time, offering a more dynamic perspective than that provided by summative population health measures such as disability-adjusted life years.

A potential disadvantage of invoking quality of life measures include possibly deliberate attempts to direct attention away from the limited success of some therapies when measured by more objective indicators. Patients may be grateful to any attempt to help them, but this gratitude should not remove the need for solid evidence of effectiveness. Hence, a combination of objective measures and quality of life appears ideal. A further challenge in using subjective quality of life assessments lies in their very subjectivity: there is no guarantee that each dimension of QoL considered important by the researcher will have the same salience to the respondent, or even that the questions asked are relevant. This has led some investigators to include patient-specific items in measurement tools. For example, the Asthma Quality of Life Questionnaire asks the patient to identify and to rate five activities that are relevant to their quality of life [121], while the Schedule for the Evaluation of Quality of Life (SEIQOL [122]) and the Patient Generated Index (PGI [123]) have no pre-set questions but instead ask patients to choose the areas of life that are important to them, then to rate their current status in each area and also to rate their relative importance in forming an overall score. These instruments illustrate what is currently the opposite extreme to objective measures of disease process that form the mainstay of evaluative measures in most neurological studies. The question is not which is better, but what blend should be established between the various types of instrument. A review of this type can only set out some of the many possibilities.

REFERENCES

[1]   Streiner DL, Norman GR. *Health measurement scales: a practical guide to their development and use*. 3rd ed. New York: Oxford, 2003.

[2]   Wade DT. *Measurement in neurological rehabilitation*. Oxford: Oxford University Press, 1992.

[3]   World Health Organization. International classification of impairments, disabilities, and handicaps. *A manual of classification relating to the consequences of disease*. Geneva: World Health Organization, 1980.

[4]   Jenkinson C, Fitzpatrick R, Peto V, Greenhall R, Hyman N. The Parkinson's Disease Questionnaire (PDQ-39): development and validation of a Parkinson's disease summary index score. *Age Ageing* 1997; 26:353-377.

[5]   Cella DF, Dineen K, Arnason B, Reder A, Webster KA, karabatsos G et al. Validation of the functional assessment of multiple sclerosis quality of life instrument. *Neurology* 1996; 47:129-139.

[6]   Lankhorst GJ, Jelles F, Smits RC, Polman CH, Kuik DJ, Pfennings LE et al. Quality of life in multiple sclerosis: the disability and impact profile (DIP). *J Neurol* 1996; 243:469-474.

[7]   Goldstein LB, Bertels C, Davis JN. Interrater reliability of the NIH stroke scale. *Arch Neurol* 1989; 46:660-662.

[8]   Harwood RH, Gompertz P, Ebrahim S. Handicap one year after a stroke: validity of a new scale. *J Neurol Neurosurg Psychiatry* 1994; 57:825-829.

[9]   Abetz L, Jacoby A, Baker GA, NcNulty P. Patient-based assessments of quality of life in newly diagnosed epilepsy patients: validation of the NEWQOL. *Epilepsia* 2000; 41:1119-1128.

[10]   Cramer JA, Perrine K, Devinsky O, Bryant-Comstock L, Meador K, Hermann B. Development and cross-cultural translations of a 31-item quality of life in epilepsy inventory. *Epilepsia* 1998; 39:81-88.

[11]   Vickrey BG, Hays RD, Graber J. A health-related quality of life instrument for patients evaluated for epilepsy surgery. *Med Care* 1992; 30:299-319.

[12]   Bowling A. *Measuring disease: a review of disease-specific quality of life measurement scales*. 2nd. ed. Buckingham, England: Open University Press, 2001.

[13]   Torenbeek M, Caulfield B, Garrett M, van Harten W. Current use of outcome measures for stroke and low back pain rehabilitation in five European countries: first results of the ACROSS project. *Int J Rehabil Res* 2001; 24:95-101.

[14]   Avasarala JR, Cross AH, Trinkaus K. Comparative assessment of Yale single question and Beck Depression Inventory scale in screening for depression in multiple sclerosis. *Multiple Sclerosis* 2003; 9:307-310.

[15] Marinus J, Leentjens AF, Visser M, Stiggelbout AM, van Hilten JJ. Evaluation of the hospital anxiety and depression scale in patients with Parkinson's disease. *Clin Neuropharmacol* 2002; 25:318-324.

[16] Schramke CJ, Stowe RM, Ratclif G, Goldstein G, Condray R. Poststroke depression and anxiety: different assessment methods result in variations in incidence and severity estimates. *J Clin Exp Neuropsychol* 1998; 20:723-737.

[17] Aaronson NK, Cull A, Kaasa S, Sprangers MAG. The EORTC modular approach to quality of life assessment in oncology. *Int J Mental Health* 1994; 23:75-96.

[18] Fayers PM, Aaronson NK, Bjordal K, Groenvold M, Curran D, Bottomley A. *The EORTC QLQ-C30 scoring manual* (3rd. edition). 2001. Brussels, European Organisation for Research and Treatment of Cancer.

[19] Skevington SM, Sartorius N, Amir M, WHOQOL Group. Developing methods for assessing quality of life in different cultural settings. *Soc Psychiatry Psychiatr Epidemiol* 2004; 39:1-8.

[20] WHOQOL Group. The World Health Organization Quality of Life Assessment (WHOQOL): development and general psychometric properties. *Soc Sci Med* 1998; 46:1569-1585.

[21] Simeonsson RJ, Lollar D, Hollowell J, Adams M. Revision of the International Classification of Impairments, Disabilities and Handicaps. Developmental issues. *J Clin Epidemiol* 2000; 53:113-124.

[22] Üstün TB, Chatterji S, Kostansjek N, Bickenbach J. WHO's ICF and functional status information in health records. *Health Care Financing Review* 2003; 24(3):77-88.

[23] Siderowf A, Ravina B, Glick HA. Preference-based quality-of-life in patients with Parkinson's disease. *Neurology* 2002; 59:103-108.

[24] Nortvedt MW, Riise T, Myhr K-M, Nyland HI. Performance of the SF-36, SF-12, and RAND-36 summary scales in a multiple sclerosis population. *Med Care* 2000; 38:1022-1028.

[25] Anderson C, Laubscher S, Burns R. Validation of the Short Form 36 (SF-36) health survey questionnaire among stroke patients. *Stroke* 1996; 27:1812-1816.

[26] Dorman PJ, Waddell F, Slattery J, Dennis M, Sandercock P. Are proxy assessments of health status after stroke with the EuroQol questionnaire feasible, accurate, and unbiased? *Stroke* 1997; 28:1883-1887.

[27] Stavem K, Bjornaes H, Lossius MI. Properties of the 15D an the EQ-5D utility measures in a community sample of people with epilepsy. *Epilepsy Res* 2001; 17944:189.

[28] Cella DF, Tulsky DS. Measuring quality of life today: methodological aspects. *Oncology* 1990; 4:29-38.

[29] Ware JE, Sherbourne CD. The MOS 36-Item Short-Form Health Survey (SF-36). I. Conceptual framework and item selection. *Med Care* 1992; 30:473-483.

[30] Ware JE, Jr., Kosinski M, Gandek B. SF-36 *Health Survey: manual and interpretation guide.* Lincoln,R.I.: QualityMetric Inc., 2002.

[31] Ware JE, Jr., Gandek B. Overview of the SF-36 Health Survey and the International Quality of Life Assessment (IQLA) project. *J Clin Epidemiol* 1998; 51:903-912.

[32] Brazier J, Jones N, Kind P. Testing the validity of the Euroqol and comparing it with the SF-36 health survey questionnaire. *Qual Life Res* 1993; 2:169-180.

[33] EuroQol Group. EuroQol: a new facility for the measurement of health-related quality of life. *Health Policy* 1990; 16:199-208.

[34] Brooks R. EuroQol: the current state of play. *Health Policy* 1996; 37:53-72.

[35] van Agt HME, Essink-Bot M-L, Krabbe PFM, Bonsel GJ. Test-retest reliability of health state valuations collected with the EuroQol questionnaire. *Soc Sci Med* 1994; 39:1537-1544.

[36] Luo N, Chew LH, Fong KY, Koh DR, Ng SC, Yoon KH et al. Validity and reliability of the EQ-5D self-report questionnaire in English-speaking Asian patients with rheumatic diseases in Singapore. *Qual Life Res* 2003; 12:87-92.

[37] Oostenbrink R, Moll HA, Essink-Bot M-L. The EQ-5D and the Health Utilities Index for permanent sequelae after meningitis: a head-to-head comparison. *J Clin Epidemiol* 2002; 55:791-799.

[38] Myers C, Wilks D. Comparison of Euroqol EQ-5D and SF-36 in patients with chronic fatigue syndrome. *Qual Life Res* 1999; 8:9-16.

[39] Anderson RT, Aaronson NK, Wilkin D. Critical review of the international assessments of health-related quality of life. *Qual Life Res* 1993; 2:369-395.

[40] Conner-Spady B, Cumming C, Nabholtz J-M, Jacobs P, Stewart D. Responsiveness of the EuroQol in breast cancer patients undergoing high dose chemotherapy. *Qual Life Res* 2001; 10:479-486.

[41] Conner-Spady B, Suarez-Almazor ME. Variation in the estimation of quality-adjusted life-years by different preference-based instruments. *Med Care* 2003; 41:791-801.

[42] Tidermark J, Bergström G, Svensson O, Törnqvist H, Ponzer S. Responsiveness of the EuroQol (EQ 5-D) and the SF-36 in elderly patients with displaced femoral neck fractures. *Qual Life Res* 2003; 12:1069-1079.

[43] Wu AW, Jacobson DL, Frick KD, Clark R, Revicki DA, Freedberg KA et al. Validity and responsiveness of the EuroQol as a measure of health-related quality of life in eople enrolled in an AIDS clinical trial. *Qual Life Res* 2002; 11:273-282.

[44] Hurst NP, Kind P, Ruta D, Hunter M, Stubbings A. Measuring health-related quality of life in rheumatoid arthritis: validity, responsiveness, and reliability of EuroQol (EQ-5D). *Br J Rheumatol* 1997; 36:551-559.

[45] Bosch JL, Hunink MGM. Comparison of the Health Utilities Index Mark 3 (HUI3) and the EuroQol EQ-5D in patients treated for intermittent claudication. *Qual Life Res* 2000; 9:591-601.

[46] Idler EL, Benyami Y. Self-rated health and mortality: a review of twenty-seven community studies. *J Health Soc Behav* 1997; 38:21-37.

[47] Idler EL, Angel RJ. Self-rated health and mortality in the NHANES-I Epidemiologic Follow-up Study. *Am J Public Health* 1990; 80(4):446-452.

[48] Granger CV, Albrecht GL, Hamilton BB. Outcome of comprehensive medical rehabilitation: measurement by PULSES Profile and the Barthel Index. *Arch Phys Med Rehabil* 1979; 60:145-154.

[49] Katz S, Downs TD, Cash HR, Grotz RC. Progress in development of the Index of ADL. *Gerontologist* 1970; 10:20-30.

[50] Lawton MP, Brody EM. Assessment of older people: self-maintaining and instrumental activities of daily living. *Gerontologist* 1969; 9:179-186.

[51] Granger CV, Hamilton BB. The Uniform Data System for Medical Rehabilitation report of first admissions for 1991. *Am J Phys Med Rehabil* 1993; 72:33-38.

[52] Hamilton BB, Granger CV, Sherwin FS, Zielezny M, Tashman JS. A uniform national data system for medical rehabilitation. In: Fuhrer MJ, editor. *Rehabilitation outcomes: analysis and measurement.* Baltimore, Maryland: Paul H. Brookes, 1987: 137-147.

[53] Stineman MG, Jette A, Fiedler R, Granger C. Impairment-specific dimensions within the Functional Independence Measure. *Arch Phys Med Rehabil* 1997; 78:636-643.

[54] Granger CV, Cotter AC, Hamilton BB, Fiedler RC, Hens MM. Functional assessment scales: a study of persons with multiple sclerosis. *Arch Phys Med Rehabil* 1990; 71:870-875.

[55] Granger CV, Cotter AC, Hamilton BB, Fiedler RC. Functional assessment scales: a study of persons after stroke. *Arch Phys Med Rehabil* 1993; 74:133-138.

[56] Hébert R, Carrier R, Bilodeau A. Le système de mesure de l'autonomie fonctionnelle (SMAF). *Revue de Gériatrie* 1988; 13:161-167.

[57] Hébert R, Carrier R, Bilodeau A. The Functional Autonomy Measurement System (SMAF): description and validation of an instrument for the measurement of handicaps. *Age Ageing* 1988; 17:293-302.

[58] Hébert R, Dubuc N, Buteau M, Desrosiers J, Bravo G, Trottier L et al. Resources and costs associated with disabilities of elderly people living at home and in institutions. *Can J Aging* 2001; 20:1-22.

[59] Hébert R, Spiegelhalter DJ, Brayne C. Setting the minimal metrically detectable change on disability rating scales. *Arch Phys Med Rehabil* 1997; 78:1305-1308.

[60] Mercier L, Audet T, Hébert R, Rochette A, Dubois M-F. Impact of motor, cognitive, and perceptual disorders on ability to perform activities of daily living after stroke. *Stroke* 2001; 32:2602-2608.

[61] Hébert R, Brayne C, Spiegelhalter D. Factors associated with functional decline and improvement in a very elderly community-dwelling population. *Am J Epidemiol* 1995; 150:501-510.

[62] Robichaud L, Hébert R, Roy P-M, Roy C. A preventive program for community-dwelling elderly at risk of functional decline: a pilot study. *Arch Gerontol Geriatr* 2000; 30:73-84.

[63] Hébert R. Functional decline in old age. *Can Med Assoc J* 1997; 157:1037-1045.

[64] Hébert R, Guilbeault J, Desrosiers J, Dubuc N. The Functional Autonomy Measurement System (SMAF): a clinical-based instrument for measuring disabilities and handicaps in older people. *Geriatrics Today: J Can Geriatrics Soc* 2001; 4:141-147.

[65] Tousignant M, Hébert R, Dubuc N, Simoneau F, Dieleman L. Application of a case-mix classification based on the functional autonomy of the residents for funding long-term care facilities. *Age Ageing* 2003; 32:60-66.

[66] Dohrenwend BP, Shrout PE, Egri G, Mendelsohn FS. Nonspecific psychological distress and other dimensions of psychopathology. *Arch Gen Psychiatry* 1980; 37:1229-1236.

[67] Clark LA, Watson D. Tripartite model of anxiety and depression: psychometric evidence and taxonomic implications. *J Abnorm Psychol* 1991; 100:316-336.

[68] Russell JA, Carroll JM. On the bipolarity of positive and negative affect. *Psychol Bull* 1999; 125:3-30.

[69] Goldberg DP. *The detection of psychiatric illness by questionnaire.* London: Oxford University Press (Maudsley Monograph No. 21), 1972.

[70] Goldberg DP, Hillier VF. A scaled version of the General Health Questionnaire. *Psychol Med* 1979; 9:139-145.

[71] Goldberg D. *Manual of the General Health Questionnaire.* Windsor, England: NFER Publishing, 1978.

[72] Vieweg BW, Hedlund JL. The General Health Questionnaire (GHQ): a comprehensive review. *J Operat Psychiatry* 1983; 14:74-85.

[73] Rost K, Burnam MA, Smith GR. Development of screeners for depressive disorders and substance disorder history. *Med Care* 1993; 31:189-200.

[74] Dupuy HJ. The Psychological General Well-Being (PGWB) Index. In: Wenger NK, Mattson ME, Furberg CD, Elinson J, editors. *Assessment of quality of life in clinical trial of cardiovascular therapies.* New York: Le Jacq, 1984: 170-183.

[75] Edwards DW, Yarvis RM, Mueller DP, Zingale HC, Wagman WJ. Test-taking and the stability of adjustment scales: can we assess patient deterioration? *Eval Q* 1978; 2:275-291.

[76] Beck AT, Ward CH, Mendelson M, Mock J, Erbaugh J. An inventory for measuring depression. *Arch Gen Psychiatry* 1961; 4:561-571.

[77] Beck AT, Steer RA, Brown GK. BDI-II. *Beck Depression Inventory - second edition.* San Antonio, Tx. Psychological Corporation, 1996.

[78] Beck AT, Steer RA, Garbin MG. Psychometric properties of the Beck Depression Inventory: twenty-five years of evaluation. *Clin Psychol Rev* 1988; 8:77-100.

[79] Radloff LS. The CES-D Scale: a self-report depression scale for research in the general population. *Appl Psychol Measurement* 1977; 1:385-401.

[80] McDowell I, Newell C. Measuring health: a guide to rating scales and questionnaires. 2nd. ed. New York: Oxford University Press, 1996.

[81] Beck AT, Epstein N, Brown G, Steer RA. An inventory for measuring clinical anxiety: psychometric properties. *J Consult Clin Psychol* 1988; 56:893-897.

[82] Beck AT, Steer RA. *Beck Anxiety Inventory manual.* 1st. ed. San Antonio, Texas: Psychological Corporation, 1990.

[83] Spielberger CD. Anxiety: state-trait-process. In: Spielberger CD, Sarason IG, editors. *Stress and anxiety, vol. I.* Washington, DC: Hemisphere Publishers, 1975: 115-143.

[84] Spielberger CD. Assessment of state and trait anxiety: conceptual and methodological issues. *Southern Psychologist* 1985; 2:6-16.

[85] Spielberger CD, Gorsuch RL, Lushene RE. *Test manual for the State Trait Anxiety Inventory.* Palo Alto, California: Consulting Psychologists Press, 1970.

[86] Kabacoff RI, Segal DL, Hersen M, van Hasselt VB. Psychometric properties and diagnostic utility of the Beck Anxiety Inventory and the State-Trait Anxiety Inventory with older adult psychiatric outpatients. *J Anx Disord* 1997; 11:33-47.

[87] Creamer M, Foran J, Bell R. The Beck Anxiety Inventory in a non-clinical sample. *Behav Res Ther* 1995; 33:477-485.

[88] American Psychiatric Association. *Diagnostic and statistical manual of mental disorders (DSM-IV).* Washington, DC: American Psychiatric Association, 1994.

[89] Aylard PR, Gooding JH, McKenna PJ, Snaith RP. A validation study of three anxiety and depression self-assessment scales. *J Psychosom Res* 1987; 31:261-268.

[90] Zigmond AS, Snaith RP. The Hospital Anxiety and Depression Scale. *Acta Psychiatr Scand* 1983; 67:361-370.

[91] Flint AJ, Rifat SL. Factor structure of the Hospital Anxiety and Depression Scale in older patients with major depression. *Int J Geriatr Psychiatry* 2002; 17:117-123.

[92] Bjelland I, Dahl AA, Haug TT, Neckelmann D. The validity of the Hospital Anxiety and Depression Scale. An updated literature review. *J Psychosom Res* 2002; 52:69-77.

[93] Clarke DM, Smith GC, Herrman HE. A comparative study of screening instruments for mental disorders in general hospital patients. *Int J Psychiatry Med* 1993; 23:323-337.

[94] Lewis G, Wessely S. Comparison of the General Health Questionnaire and the Hospital Anxiety and Depression Scale. *Br J Psychiatry* 1990; 157:860-864.

[95] Snaith RP. The GHQ and the HAD. *Br J Psychiatry* 1991; 158:433.

[96] Lovibond PF, Lovibond SH. The structure of negative emotional states: comparison of the Depression Anxiety Stress Scales (DASS) with the Beck Depression and Anxiety Inventories. *Behav Res Ther* 1995; 33:335-343.

[97] Antony MM, Bieling PJ, Cox BJ, Enns MW, Swinson RP. Psychometric properties of the 42-item and 21-item versions of the Dperession Anxiety Stress scales in clinical groups and a community sample. *Psychol Assess* 1998; 10:176-181.

[98] Nieuwenhuijsen K, de Boer AEGM, Verbeek JHAM, Blonk RWB, van Dijk FJH. The Depression Anxiety Stress Scales (DASS): detecting anxiety disorder and depression in employees absent from work because of mental health problems. *Occup Environ Med* 2003; 60 (Suppl 1):i77-i82.

[99] Crawford JR, Henry JD. The Depression Anxiety Stress Scales (DASS): normative data and latent structure in a large non-clinical sample. *Br J Clin Psychol* 2003; 42:111-131.

[100] Chapman CR. Pain perception, affective mechanisms, and conscious experience. In: Hadjistavropoulos T, Craig KD, editors. *Pain: psychological perspectives.* Mahwah, New Jersey: Lawrence Erlbaum, 2004: 59-85.

[101] Melzack R. The McGill Pain Questionnaire: major properties and scoring methods. *Pain* 1975; 1:277-299.

[102] Melzack R, Katz J. The gate control theory: reaching for the brain. In: Hadjistavropoulos T, Craig KD, editors. *Pain: psychological perspectives.* Mahwah, New Jersey: Lawrence Erlbaum, 2004: 13-34.

[103] Taenzer P. Postoperative pain: relationships among measures of pain, mood, and narcotic requirements. In: Melzack R, editor. *Pain measurement and assessment.* New York: Raven Press, 1983: 111-118.

[104] Melzack R. The short-form McGill Pain Questionnaire. *Pain* 1987; 30:191-197.

[105] Monks R, Taenzer P. A comprehensive pain questionnaire. In: Melzack R, editor. *Pain measurement and assessment.* New York: Raven Press, 1983: 233-237.

[106] Corson JA, Schneider MJ. The Dartmouth Pain Questionnaire: an adjunct to the McGill Pain Questionnaire. *Pain* 1984; 19:59-69.

[107] Swanston M, Abraham C, Macrae WA, Walker A, Rushmer R, Elder L et al. Pain assessment with interactive computer animation. *Pain* 1993; 53:347-351.

[108] Ho K, Spence J, Murphy MF. Review of pain-measurement tools. *Ann Emerg Med* 1996; 27:427-432.

[109] McCormack HM, Horne DJ, Sheather S. Clinical applications of visual analogue scales: a critical review. *Psychol Med* 1988; 18:1007-1019.

[110] Huskisson EC. Measurement of pain. *Lancet* 1974; 2:1127-1131.

[111] Scott J, Huskisson EC. Graphic representation of pain. *Pain* 1976; 2:175-184.

[112] Scott J, Huskisson EC. Vertical or horizontal visual analogue scales. *Ann Rheum Dis* 1979; 38:560.

[113] Sriwatanakul K, Kelvie W, Lasagna L, Calimlim JF, Weis OF, Mehta G. Studies with different types of visual analog scales for measurement of pain. *Clin Pharmacol Ther* 1983; 34:234-239.

[114] Guyatt GH, Townsend M, Berman LB, Keller JL. A comparison of Likert and visual analogue scales for measuring change in function. *J Chronic Dis* 1987; 40:1129-1133.

[115] Elton D, Burrows GD, Stanley GV. Clinical measurement of pain. *Med J Aust* 1979; 1:109-111.

[116] Peck RR. A precise technique for the measurement of pain. *Headache* 1967; 7:189-194.

[117] WHOQOL Group. The World Health Organization quality of life assessment (WHOQOL): position paper from the World Health Organization. *Soc Sci Med* 1995; 41:1403-1409.

[118] Horley J. Life satisfaction, happiness, and morale: two problems with the use of subjective well-being indicators. *Gerontologist* 1984; 24:124-127.

[119] de Haes JCJM, van Knippenberg FCE. The quality of life of cancer patients: a review of the literature. *Soc Sci Med* 1985; 20:809-817.

[120] Gelber S, Gelber RD, Cole BF, Goldhirsch A. Using the Q-TWIST method for treatment comparisons in clinical trials. In: Staquet MJ, Hays RD, Fayers PM, editors. *Quality of life assessment in clincial trials: methods and practice.* Oxford: Oxford University Press, 1998: 281-296.

[121] Juniper EF, Buist AS, Cox FM, Ferroe PJ, King DR. Validation of a standardized version f the Asthma Quality of Life Questionnaire. *Chest* 1999; 115:1265-1270.

[122] Joyce CRB, Hickey A, McGee HM, O'Boyle CA. A theory-based method for the evaluation of individual quality of life: the SEIQoL. *Qual Life Res* 2003; 12:275-280.

[123] Ruta DA, Garratt AM, Leng M, Russell IT, MacDonald LM. A new approach to the measurement of quality of life: The Patient-Generated Index. *Med Care* 1994; 32:1109-1126.

RECOMMENDED FURTHER READING

1.   Streiner DL, Norman GR. *Health measurement scales: a practical guide to their development and use.* 3rd edition, Oxford University Press, New York, 2003.

2. Bowling A. *Measuring disease: a review of disease-specific quality of life measurement scales.* Open University Press, Buckingham, 1995.

3. Feinstein AR. *Clinimetrics.* Yale University Press, New Haven, 1987.

4. Staquet MJ, Hays RD, Fayers PM. *Quality of life assessment in clinical trials: methods and practice.* Oxford University Press, New York, 1998.

5. McDowell I. *Measuring health: a guide to rating scales and questionnaires.* 3rd. edition, Oxford University Press, New York, 2006.

In: Handbook of Clinical Neuroepidemiology   ISBN 978-1-60021-511-7
Editors: V. L. Feigin and D. A. Bennett, pp. 621-648   © 2007 Nova Science Publishers, Inc.

Chapter 19

NEUROPSYCHOLOGICAL ASSESSMENT

Suzanne Barker-Collo and Dianne McCarthy

Department of Psychology, University of Auckland, Private Bag 92019, Auckland,
New Zealand.

ABSTRACT

This chapter provides the practitioner with an overview of information that will
assist in understanding Neuropsychological Reports and engaging Neuropsychological
services. The chapter begins with a definition of neuropsychological assessment and
identification of the three main questions that can be addressed by neuropsychological
assessments, as well as identification of the type of questions a neuropsychological
assessment cannot answer. The remainder of the chapter examines three common areas
of deficit that are assessed as part of any neuropsychological assessment: memory,
executive functioning, and language. For each area, the following are provided: (1)
definitions/models and related physiology, (2) prevalence in relation to specific
disorders/diagnoses, and (3) an overview of rehabilitation strategies.

INTRODUCTION

According to Lezak [1] neuropsychology involves examination of the brain through
assessment of its behavioural correlates, where neuropsychological assessment may be
defined as "Intensive study of behavior by means of interviews and standardized, scaled tests
and questionnaires that provide relatively precise and sensitive indices of behavior....it is
neuropsychological so long as the questions that prompt it, the central issues, the findings, or
the inferences drawn from them ultimately relate to brain function "(p.18).

Many referrals to neuropsychologists simply state 'Please see Mr. Jones for assessment'.
As a practitioner, the question that must then be asked by the neuropsychologist is Why? In
order to accurately address the questions of the referrer, the referral question must be

specified. For example, is it that the referral source wants to know if Mr. Jones is able to live independently?, or is it that his CT scan was clear, but that Mr. Jones may have suffered a mild brain injury?

In practice, referral for neuropsychological assessment may be required for any one of three main purposes: (1)*Diagnosis*: With recent advances in scanning technologies the issue of diagnosis is a less common prompt to referral than in the past. However, neuropsychological assessment can still provide useful discrimination in areas where scanning technologies are less helpful, such as dementia and Mild Traumatic Brain Injury (mild TBI) where scan results are often unclear. Neuropsychological assessment can also be of use in determining whether the behavioural profile of an individual is consistent with a particular diagnosis or pattern of brain insult. (2) *Management and care planning*: Once a person has been identified as having a neurological condition, it is important for the person and those who care for him/her to know his/her capabilities and limitations. Neuropsychological assessment can assist in the development of management and care plans by identifying an individual's cognitive strengths and weaknesses, determining his or her level of awareness and adjustment to changes in cognitive functioning, as well as the contribution of other factors, such as emotional issues to his or her functioning. For example, the neuropsychologist may be asked to comment on the likelihood of an individual being able to return to full-time employment, or on an individual's ability to follow a structured self-care regimen. Neuropsychological assessment can also provide information on the extent to which medication either enhances or compromises an individual's cognitive functioning, and on changes in functioning inherent in neurological recovery or progression of neurological disease (3). *Evaluation of treatment:* "careful, sensitive, broad-gauged, and accurate neuropsychological assessment is a necessary foundation on which appropriate treatment of organic brain dysfunctions can be based" (p.13) [1]. With increasing emphasis on accountability to funding authorities, neuropsychological assessment results can provide evidence of treatment efficacy, and can also guide the clinician or clinical team in adapting treatment to an individual's changing care needs. A neuropsychological assessment can provide a team of professionals working with an individual with not only an indication of that individual's areas of deficit but, through examination of qualitative aspects of test performance, can also provide some insight into the reasons an individual cannot perform certain tasks [1].

Having identified some of the main ways in which neuropsychological assessment can aid in the provision of care, it is important to note that because neuropsychological assessment focuses on assessing the behaviours that result from damage to particular brain areas, neuropsychological assessment cannot answer some referral questions. The most common such scenario is to be faced with a referral to provide differential diagnosis of two conditions that cause similar behavioural profiles. For example, both schizophrenia and frontal brain injury are known to produce behaviours of executive dysfunction, such as perseveration, difficulties with initiation, and reduced awareness. If a referral is made to determine the extent to which an individual's problems are due to a brain injury and not the presence of schizophrenia, a neuropsychological assessment may only be able to state that the individual's performance is consistent with executive dysfunction. Because neuropsychology focuses on the behavioural correlates of brain disturbance, and because the two disorders can present with similar behavioural profiles it would be impossible to state whether that dysfunction is due to brain injury or to schizophrenia.

The remainder of this chapter examines three common areas of cognitive functioning that are assessed as part of any neuropsychological assessment: memory, executive functioning, and language.

MEMORY

Memory is "the mental processes of retaining information for later use and retrieving such information, and the mental storage system that allows this retention and retrieval" (p.10) [2]. There is some consensus as to the different memory components contributing to memory processes, which may be roughly viewed as either time-related or content-related. Typically, the neuropsychological assessment will make reference to time-related aspects of memory, and discrepancies in performance in time-related forms of memory are used to make inferences about the different processes that underlie memory performance. References to memory content in neuropsychological assessments are usually limited to whether stimuli to be remembered are either verbal/auditory or nonverbal/visual.

Memory Definitions

If one examines memory as a set of related processes that occur over time, memory may be divided into four broad subsystems/stages: sensory memory, working memory, short-term memory, and long-term memory. Within each of these, memory is typically divided into verbal/auditory and non-verbal/visual, a division meant to reflect the specialization of the cerebral hemispheres with the left or dominant hemisphere associated with language/verbal and the right or non-dominant hemisphere associated with non-language/visual materials. It should be noted, however, that in most cases, verbal material can be processed both verbally and visually, and that visual information can be processed both visually and verbally. Table 1 presents the four time-related stages of memory and their definitions, as well as content-related definitions of memory type.

Ashcraft provides the following example of the flow of information over time in the creation of a memory. When the question is asked, "What is 6x3?" the sound waves heard are encoded into auditory sensory/echoic memory for a brief period of time, where encode means "to take in information and convert it to a usable mental form" (p.47) [2]. As the question is attended to, the encoded stimulus is immediately passed on to the short-term store or short-term memory/working memory system where further mental processing of the information occurs, that is in your conscious awareness. To provide an answer to the problem, the system is aware that it needs to call on long-term memory so one of the control processes in working memory initiates this search. Following the memory search, long-term memory "sends" the answer 18 to short-term memory, where the final answer is prepared to output to the appropriate device (e.g., as speech). In the case of learning new information such as times tables, sensory and attentional processes operate, so the stimulus is put into short-term memory and a consolidation process, such as repetition, operates to ensure the problem is moved to long-term memory for permanent storage.

Table 1.Time-related and content-related definitions of memory

Memory Type	Definition
Time-Related Memory Definitions	
Sensory Memory	How an individual first gains access to information. Visual sensory or iconic memory is a very brief ($^{1/}_4$ to ½ second) visual store designed to receive and hold visual stimulation. Auditory sensory or echoic memory is a very brief (2 to 3 second for speech sounds) sensory store that receives auditory stimulation
Working Memory	Sometimes considered part of short-term memory, WM involves temporary storage and manipulation of small amounts of information. It is where verbal rehearsal and other conscious processing take place.
Short-Term / Immediate memory	The "memory buffer or register that holds current or recently attended information"; receives information from the internal, mental world; and "encodes information from sensory memory and from long-term memory" (Ashcraft, 1989, p.53). Duration is 15 to 20 second, longer if rehearsal occurs.
Long-Term / Delayed memory	Characterized by an unlimited capacity and a very slow rate of decay that is responsible for storing information on a relatively permanent basis, from minutes to years
Content-Related Memory Definitions	
Declarative/Explicit	Memory for facts, events, & conceptual knowledge. It is acquired through learning, accessible to consciousness, & can be verbalised. There are 2 types: (1) episodic - memory for personally experienced & remembered events. Recall requires awareness of specific learning incidents; and (2) semantic – memory for general world knowledge relating concepts/ ideas to one another, facts, & knowledge of the rules of language. Learning takes place over many occasions, therefore no temporal landmarks or reference is made to particular events.
Non-declarative or Procedural Memory	The ability to learn motor skills & sequences, classical conditioning, perceptual learning tasks, & solving perceptual/ reasoning problems that do not require verbalization or conscious awareness of information as a 'memory'. It is independent of episodic memory and can accumulate information but not access and identify specific episodes. Procedural memory is spared in globally amnesic patients and in other neurological conditions such as Alzheimer's disease.

Processing Stages of Memory

The memory system performs three functions, "it must allow information to be fed into the system, the input or learning stage; it must be able to maintain information, storage; and it must be able to access information when appropriate, the process of retrieval" (p.19) [3]. These functions involve "four sequential, interrelated processes or stages, including *attending* to the information; *encoding*, organising and maintaining the information in working (short-term) memory; *storing* or consolidating the information into long-term memory; and *retrieving* consolidated information as needed" (p.18) [4]. Memory difficulties may reflect impairment in one or more of these stages. These stages and their relationship to the 4 parts of memory are presented in figure 1.

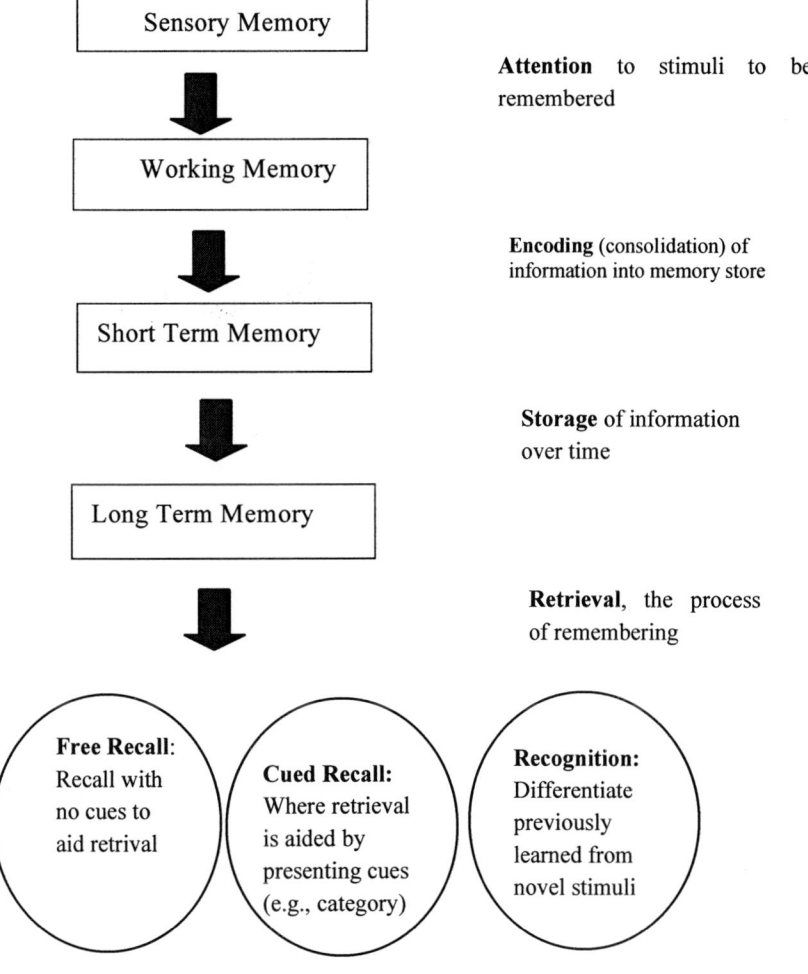

Figure 1. A simple model of memory.

Attention

An individual must pay attention if he/she wants to learn. Attention is "responsible for the transfer of information from sensory memory to short-term/working memory, and is also assumed to be a critical mental resource necessary for the operation of any conscious or partly conscious process" (p.64) [2]. According to Wood learning relies upon attention, which is a major "control process in the passage of information into, and out of, memory" (p.220) [5]. *Selective attention* involves selectively attending to certain environmental stimuli in preference to others, while avoiding distractions [5]. Selective attention can be divided into focused and divided attention. *Focused attention* is where attention is centred on one kind of information in preference to others (e.g., listening to the phone while ignoring other conversations. *Divided attention* is a level of awareness that is "broad enough to be divided, or shared, between two or more sources of information"; several objects or sets of stimuli; or two or more mental operations (p.226) [5]. *Sustained attention* is the ability to pay attention to a stimulus, source of information, or mental operation for a long period of time. *Alternating attention* involves switching attention from one stimulus, source of information, or mental operation, to another.

Encoding

The initial processing of information to be remembered/learned is called 'encoding'. Encoding is a manner of learning new material involving categorisation and organisation of information in relation to what is already known, and may be described as the laying down of information for future recall [5]. A large part of encoding occurs involuntarily, though it may also occur at a conscious level, for example studying for an exam [5]. Encoding occurs within working memory and short-term memory. A number of factors have been found to impact on depth of encoding, including organisation of information; distribution of practice; levels of processing; and rehearsal of information.

Organisation is an important part of encoding that sets up memories that are accessible to retrieval [6]. Organisation by category (e.g., animal, vegetable), or by subjectively defined clusters or chunks (e.g., dog, food, house; linked in a sentence: "The dog ate his food in the house") improves memory by storing information securely, and providing a structure to assist retrieval [2]. *Distribution of practice* involves being presented with small amounts of information often [3]. Material can be handled at differing *levels of processing,* and the deeper the processing or encoding the better the retention [3]. Deep processing involves elaboration (relating detail of new material to what one already knows); compatibility (it is easier to learn material that is either neutral or consistent with existing knowledge); and self-reference (learning is more efficient if material is judged in relation to the person themselves) [3]. *Rehearsal* "maintains information in the short-term store, preventing it from being lost or displaced by other information", and the "longer an item is held in short-term memory by rehearsal, the greater the probability that the rehearsal will also store the item in long-term memory" (p.204) [2].

Storage

Information is registered and encoded in memory and then stored until needed. The important variables in storage are organisation, rehearsal, and visual imagery. Organisation and rehearsal are described above. As noted above well-organised material can be accurately stored and retrieved, and the more rehearsal the stronger the memory, allowing increased access for retrieval [2]. Visual imagery, involves mentally picturing a stimulus, which aids in later recall or recognition [2]. To be useful, information stored in long-term memory must be accessible. The process of accessing stored information is termed retrieval.

Retrieval, or the 'remembering' of information can occur at both a conscious level (e.g., trying to remember someone's name), or at an unconscious level (e.g., becoming aware of certain memories whilst having a discussion [5]). Retrieval can take two main forms: Recall and Recognition; where recall tasks can be free and cued recall. Free recall tasks are where one recalls information with no cues to aid retrieval whereas cued recall tasks are easier as cues serve as a guide to retrieval. For example, in learning word lists, being asked to say all the words you remember, would be considered free recall. If you were asked to remember all the furniture items from the list, the cue 'furniture' would aid in recall and it would be a cued recall condition. Recognition tasks can be performed at even more shallow levels of processing as accurate recognition involves identifying a previously experienced stimulus from an array. In the previous example, you may be asked which of two words, Table or Apple, was on a list of words you had previously seen.

Failure to recall memories does not necessarily mean the memory has been destroyed, it may represent difficulty in accessing or retrieving the memory. Recognition typically leads to a higher rate of responses than recall because the information that has been learned facilitates access to its memory trace [6]. Within months, recall performances tends to decline, whereas, recognition memory for information acquired across a prolonged period is accurate across many years [2].

Neurophysiology of Memory

The processes involved in the creation and accessing of memories are complex and involves numerous structures. While it is beyond the scope of this chapter to review all that is known about the neurophysiology of memory, it is important for practitioners to be aware of those structures to which damage is likely to result in memory impairment. The areas of the brain involved in memory functioning are the medial temporal lobes (particularly the hippocampal system, including the hippocampus, amygdala, and adjoining entorhinal and parrahippocampal gyri), the midline diencephalic region (specifically the dorsomedial nucleus of the thalamus and mammillary bodies of the hypothalamus), frontal lobes, and basal forebrain [7].

At the level of *attention*, memory problems may occur following damage to the pre-frontal cortex, which also plays a role in working memory [8]. Damage to the frontal lobes frequently results in memory impairment when conducting complex tasks such as memory of temporal order or recall of information where strategies are required to aid recall. Frontal lobe damage may also impact working memory and thereby, episodic memory [7]. The hippocampal formations are thought to be central to the *encoding or consolidation* of new declarative memories with the left hippocampal complex involved in verbal material and the right complex specialised for nonverbal material (i.e., melodies, spatial information, faces, geographical routes) [9]. Damage to the medial-temporal lobes and diencephalic structures severely affect episodic memory [10]. The thalamus and hypothalamus are also thought to have involvement in this process [4]. However, these structures do not store memories, nor do they have much involvement in the retrieval of previously learned information. Those individuals with a consolidation deficit may, however, have intact attentional capacity and working memory [4].

While *declarative memory* is impaired when amnesia results from damage to the medial-temporal structures, including the diencephalic structures and the hippocampus [10], types of nondeclarative or procedural learning (i.e., habits, learning motor skills) are independent of hippocampal function [9]. Since *procedural memory* is often spared in amnesia, structures other than the diencephalic and medial temporal regions are thought to be involved [10]. It has been proposed that the basal ganglia and the cerebellum (motor related structures) are involved in forms of non-declarative memory, in particular procedural learning and memory [9].

The areas involved in short-term memory and learning include the fornix, temporal lobes, mamillary bodies, temporal lobes, thalamus, hypothalamus, and the hippocampus [11], with *storage functions* being distributed throughout the neocortex [7]. For example, memory for the visual aspects of a particular event may be stored in visual processing areas, while verbal elements are stored in language areas. *Retrieval* of previously learned information is impacted by damage to structures in the non-medial temporal region (i.e., structures in anterior, inferior, and lateral portions of the temporal lobe), which are involved in retrograde memory [9]. The basal forebrain plays a key role in the "binding together of different modal components of a particular memory" such as linking pieces of information related to one episode (e.g., someone's name, their accent, what they were doing, who their family is) [9].

Prevalence of Memory Dysfunction

While memory impairment is synonymous with the presence of dementia, and is indeed a required symptom for diagnosis of dementia of the Alzheimer's type, memory impairment can be caused by a wide range of neurological disorders. Below is a brief summary of memory problems experienced by persons with stroke, TBI, and Multiple Sclerosis. While any disorder that impacts those brain areas associated with memory may cause memory deficit, specific disorders not reviewed here that may involve medial temporal lobe damage causing memory dysfunction include herpes simplex encephalitis, hypoxic ischemia, and bilateral electroconvulsive therapy. Two further disorders that commonly lead to memory dysfunction due to midline diencephalic damage are Korsakoff's disease, and third-ventricle tumours.

Stroke

Stewart investigated the incidence and nature of memory impairment late after stroke and found that "on the basis of RBMT (Rivemead Behavioural Memory Test) performance and relatives ratings, more than a third of the patients assessed appeared to have significant memory problems in everyday life" (p.376) [12]. Similarly, Lincoln conducted one-month and seven-month follow-ups of 78 patients under 80 years of age who had memory impairment following a stroke and who were not severely dysphasic [13]. They found that compared to orthopaedic controls, those with stroke experienced significantly more frequent everyday memory failures, and on RBMT 49% of the patients were impaired.

Traumatic Brain Injury (TBI)

As with stroke, memory deficits following TBI are linked to the areas of the brain that have been affected. Impaired memory functioning is the most marked and persistent problem following closed TBI, which often persists beyond the period of immediate recovery [14-16]. Following a severe TBI, 36% of people will have permanent and significant memory impairments [17]. McKinlay reported memory deficits in 73% of the cases at three months post-injury [18]. These figures reflect over 1000 new cases each year in the United States, and about 2500 new cases in the United Kingdom [17]. Severity of the TBI is related to the degree and persistence of the resulting memory deficit, with more severe injuries producing greater deficits [15]. "The more severe the injury, the more severe the retrograde amnesia (loss of memory for events that occurred prior to the TBI), with events experienced years before the injury often being retained better than events experienced weeks or months just prior to the injury" (p.18) [4]. Individuals with TBI also experience problems in new learning and retrieval of information [4,17]. For the majority of individuals with a mild to moderate brain injury, memory difficulties result from a disruption at the attentional level, the retrieval level, or a combination of both [4]. Following severe brain injury, working memory and/or consolidation deficits are also likely, and individuals evidence "greater difficulty recalling information related to declarative memory than to procedural memory" (p.18) [4].

Multiple Sclerosis (MS)

In a review of memory impairment it has been reported that cognitive impairment will impact between 40% and 60% of individuals with MS; with decline in memory the most frequently reported area of deficit [19]. It has been suggested that the disease differentially affects different aspects of memory. It has been suggested that, of three clusters of MS patients (i.e., no memory impairment, mild to moderate memory impairment, and severe memory impairment), 53% of the sample had severe impairment suggestive of impairments in retrieval [20]. Short-term memory storage was thought to remain relatively intact [21], whereas substantial deficits are typical in the on-line processing or working memory aspects of performance [22]. Recently, this views has been challenged. For example, it has been reported that while MS patients require more trials to learn new information, they retrieved information as well as controls if learning was complete [23].

In terms of disease related factors, small lesions at the juxtacortical boundary correlate with impaired retention of information in memory tasks, which is characteristic of cognitive problems in patients with MS [24]. A recent review of studies on memory in MS suggests significant impairment across all memory domains and failed to support a retrieval-based account of memory dysfunction [19]. In addition, robust associations were found between clinical features of MS and memory impairment. Specifically, chronic-progressive MS, greater neurological disability, and longer disease duration were related to more pronounced memory impairments. The findings suggest a more global pattern of memory deficits in MS than has been previously believed, with deficits clearly associated with neurological disability and disease course.

Rehabilitation of Memory

Memory impairment is one of the most debilitating or handicapping of cognitive deficits [25], often preventing returning to work or independent living [26], and other aspects of treatment [11]. Rehabilitation strategies for memory impairment range from drills and practice (including computer-based tasks), to internal strategies (mnemonic techniques) and external aids (memory notebooks).

Direct Retraining /Repetitive Drills

Historically, memory rehabilitation has focused on restoring underlying capacities using exercises that provide repetitive practice and drills recalling target stimuli [4,27]. Direct retraining involves "practice in the basic skill with feedback and reinforcement so that the individual improves in the use of that skill" (p.36) [11]. For example, training a patient to learn lists by using repetitive rehearsal with the goal of generalization toward remembering a daily schedule [11]. According to Harris these tasks are "based on the assumption that memory responds like a "mental muscle" and that exercising it on one task will strengthen it for use on other tasks" (p.208) [28]. Empirical research has demonstrated that this approach is not successful in improving memory in everyday life outside the laboratory or clinical settings [27,29-32], that is, improvement does not generalize [33].

Alternate Functioning Systems

Using alternate functioning system "may involve teaching visual encoding strategies to an individual with verbal encoding deficits in order to concentrate on spared skill areas and thereby compensate for relative deficit skill areas" (p.36) [11]. The most common application of this is in the substitution of verbal skills for deficient visual skills, and vice versa.

Compensatory Strategies

In more recent years the focus of rehabilitative efforts has shifted to compensatory strategies, optimizing residual abilities, and/or overcome related cognitive problems contributing to the memory deficit [4]. Compensatory strategies seek to directly improve performance on daily activities. Compensatory behaviours are more successfully employed if the patient (1) recognizes their memory problem; (2) is young; (3) has good executive skills to enable coping with the difficulties; (4) has shorter length of coma (for those following TBI); and (5) used compensatory strategies prior to neurological insult [34]. Wilson further notes that most memory-impaired people will not use memory strategies spontaneously [35]. Compensatory strategies include environmental adaptation, external aids, and internal/mnemonic strategies.

Environmental adaptations. Arranging or structuring the environment to reduce reliance on memory is a simple way to help people with memory impairment cope. Fewer memory lapses will result if the proximal environment (layout of a vehicle or room) is tidy and well structured [36]. For example, labeling doors, cupboards in the kitchen, or drawers in the bedroom; drawing colored lines or arrows to indicate a route from one place to another; putting objects in a position so they are not forgotten or missed; or positioning material in places where it is most likely to be seen and sign-posting [17,34]. For individuals with severe intellectual impairment, environmental adaptations are particularly useful. It is important to categorize items that are to be stored for later retrieval, for example allocating separate storage units to each category (e.g., alphabetizing cupboard contents).

External memory aids. According to Wilson external memory aids are the most likely to be used in the long run and are most useful with the greatest number of people and are defined as "anything outside of the individual that serves to aid memory" (p.491) [25]. These aids are designed to help utilize, organize, and recall information to meet daily living needs, and to prevent everyday memory lapses from occurring in the first place. For prospective memory, external aids are particularly beneficial (e.g., remembering to attend an appointment) [37]. There are two main kinds of external aids (1) aids that enable access to internally stored information (e.g., a timer to remind us to look at a diaries/notebook); and (2) aids used to record or store information externally such as alarm clocks, notebooks, post-it pads, diaries, watches, calendars/wall charts, address tags/labels that help items to be identified, reminders from other people, address books, and lists [27,36-38]. Diaries in particular facilitate a number of functional tasks, including initiating household chores, keeping appointments, carrying out errands, and recalling important events [39,40]. Recently electronic devices have become common memory aids, including electronic count-down timers, electronic organizers/reminders; dictating machines or tape recorders, telephone memory aid (stores and retrieves telephone numbers); and computers and computer software (have diary and alarm functions). Pill blister packs or boxes can be used to organize the correct dosage of pills into compartments that correspond to the time of day or day of the week. External aids are portable, and they should be readily accessible and visible to encourage use. Other forms of external aids include asking people to remember things for you, and putting things in unusual places or the same place all the time to act as a reminder.

Memory impaired people often find it difficult to use external memory aids efficiently or successfully, as remembering to use the aids is in itself a task involving memory [34,41]. Examples of problems experienced with the use of external memory aids include forgetting to record the required information, forgetting where information has been recorded; using aids in a disorganized or unsystematic way; being unable to programme the (electronic) aid; and being embarrassed when using them [42].

Internal strategies. Internal strategies can be divided into two groups, those that are learned naturally, and artificial aids/mnemonics employed to assist learning [17,38]. These strategies have been found to be more successful with those whose memory is not severely impaired[17]. Strategies that are learned naturally include the tendency to recall the last few items first when asked for free recall of a word list, and concentrating on items not recalled previously when attempting to learn a list of words [17]. Training the use of mnemonic strategies is a common memory rehabilitation approach, used to assist encoding and/or organization of information to ease recall [27]. Mnemonic strategies can be divided into three categories: verbal techniques, visual imagery-based techniques and operant self/instructional techniques [43].

Visual Imagery involves "the formation of a mental picture of information to aid remembering" (p.101) [44], and is useful if the memory deficit primarily involves verbal memory. Two well-known visual techniques are peg-word mnemonics and method of loci. The peg-word mnemonic "is a system that associates images of objects with the items to be remembered" (p.130) [27], while the method of loci involves "visually linking items of information to be recalled with specific locations, such as the path of a familiar route, body parts etc. whereby locations trigger the recall of information" (p.909) [26]. Though useful for non-impaired individuals, for memory-impaired people these two methods have limited application to every day living [26].

For remembering names face-name association is used whereby a unique link is made between the person's face and name (e.g., Angela Webster becomes an angel, a web and a star, where the individual's distinctive hair makes up the web) [44]. The mental image (e.g., drawing) may need to be provided for the memory-impaired person. Another method that helps you to remember people's names and recognize their faces involves studying the person's face to find an unusual feature, changing their name into something meaningful; then associating the two with a ridiculous image. For example, "red-bearded Mr. Hills could be imagined with hills growing out of his beard" (p.62) [38].

Verbal Strategies. Verbal strategies appear to be most effective for those with a reasonably intact language dominant (left) hemisphere and whose memory problems are of a nonverbal nature [35]. These strategies require "the creation of a word or sentence to serve as a verbal mediator or verbal cue" (p.487) [37], and include organizing words in categories according to sound or meaning; adding verbal links; and forming a story which links the words or items together. One type of verbal strategy is a first letter mnemonic where the first letters of the words in the sentence are also the first letters of the words you want to remember. For example, the first letters of the words in the sentence: "Richard of York Gained Battles In Vain…are also the first letters of the colours of the rainbow, and they are in order: Red, Orange, Yellow, Green, Blue, Indigo, Violet" (p.63) [38]. Rhymes can be used to remember information, for example, a rhyme can be used to remember the number of days in each calendar month (Thirty days has September, April, June and November…etc).

A simple verbal strategy is two-word association where verbal mediators are developed to "meaningfully connect the target word and its paired cue word in paired associate learning" (e.g., 'tiger' and 'monkey' would be associated by 'jungle'; p.488) [37]. Another strategy, verbal elaboration, involves formulating or expanding a sentence in a meaningful way to aid recall (e.g., "Robin West" is remembered by "The robin is flying west in the winter") [37]. Similarly, remembering a random sequence of words, can be done by making up a story that connects the words, while maintaining them in order. Individuals experiencing other non-verbal memory difficulties such as remembering the way from one place to another, may be taught techniques to make the task more a verbal one by verbalizing the steps required.

Operant/self-instructional techniques incorporate learning techniques such as the PQRST method ('PQRST' is an acronym for 'Preview, Read, Question, State, and Test'), which has been designed to facilitate memory for prose material [27,44]. This technique encourages individuals to process written material more thoroughly [4], and is superior to rote rehearsal for almost all patients with memory problems, particularly for recall after a delay.

When teaching memory strategies, Wilson and colleague [35] outlined the following guidelines: (1) "Internal strategies can be used to teach some new information although they will not be taken on board and used spontaneously" (p.142); (2) "Dual coding is better than single coding" (p. 142). When trying to learn and retain information, there is a greater chance of success if two methods of remembering are used (e.g., mnemonics, repetition) rather than one; (3) "Teaching should proceed one step at a time" (p.142); (4) Rather than rely on mental imagery it is better to draw images for visual imagery procedures. Those with moderately and severely impaired memory showed superior performance with drawn images; (5) "Material to be learned should be realistic and relevant to the needs of the patient" (p.143); and (6) "Therapists should also recognize that individual patients have individual styles and preferences when it comes to learning" (p.143).

EXECUTIVE DYSFUNCTION

"When executive functions are impaired, the individual may no longer be capable of satisfactory self-care . . . or of maintaining normal relationships regardless of how well preserved the cognitive capacities (to perform these activities) are or how high the person scores on tests of skills, knowledge, and abilities" (p. 43) [1].

Executive functions are important for problem-solving and carrying out goal-directed actions and involving many different abilities such as attention, organisation, planning and abstract thinking. Individuals with executive dysfunction are often described by their carers as having undergone a change to pre-existing personality, for example the previously meek individual may become explosive and unpredictable, while the previously gregarious individual may become apathetic. Executive functions are integrated with mood and emotion, and executive functions are mediated primarily by the frontal lobes (more specifically the prefrontal cortex) of the brain [45,46]. Indeed, "It is nearly impossible to find a discussion of the prefrontal lobes that does not make reference to disturbances of executive functioning" (p.1) [47]. Executive functions impact our lives in relation to practical activities, having meaningful relationships, controlling our impulses, keeping appointments and learning new material. Below, the behavioural indices of executive function and dysfunction are reviewed, followed by a brief account of the anatomy of the frontal lobes.

Defining Executive Dysfunction

The term dysexecutive syndrome is a functional definition that refers to those deficits arising from prefrontal lobe damage, and has replaced terms such as "frontal lobe syndrome" to avoid the potentially misleading linking of a syndrome to a particular anatomical region [48]. Behavioural changes associated with executive dysfunction (ED) include problems with planning, problem solving, attention, impulsivity, disinhibition, initiating action, abstract thinking and being overly rigid or concrete [45,49]. Mateer [49] provides a comprehensive list of the five overlapping categories of behaviour problems commonly demonstrated by people with executive dysfunction that are summarised in Table 2. Additional difficulties associated with ED are outlined below.

Table 2. Mateer's (1999) five types of behaviour associated with Executive Dysfunction

Problem Area	Mateer (1999)
Problems starting	involves reduced initiation and spontaneity of behaviour. For example, verbalising an intention to act but failing to do so without cues or prompts
Problems stopping	involving disinhibition, impulsivity, and unpredictable shifts in behaviour and emotion. This failure to inhibit responses may also create difficulties with problem-solving and planning. For example, acting in an unrestrained manner with unpredictable outbursts, where the individual is unable to stop him or herself from saying or doing something inappropriate
Difficulty making mental or behavioral shifts	leading to behaviours that are rigid or perseverative (repeated without benefit), and a concrete attitude with diminished ability to think abstractly. This may limit spontaneous and meaningful social interaction, the ability to think of alternative solutions to problems, or to learn from mistakes
Poor awareness of self and others	Having limited insight into one's own behaviour and how this behaviour impacts other people. Problems with social awareness may occur as frontal and limbic association cortices may mediate the feelings and emotions associated with social stimuli. Thus, a related problem is difficulty empathising or identifying with others.
Problems with attention	Being easily distracted, suffering from impaired attention which is poorly selective or inappropriately divided. This has negative implications for concentration and the ability to process several sources of information being delivered at the same time. It can make learning/following instructions confusing, particularly in busy environments such as the classroom or workplace.

Lezak [1] provides a similar listing of five overlapping behaviours associated with ED that roughly equate to those of Mateer. Of note is the additional concept of *"stimulus boundedness"* (roughly equivalent to Mateer's Problem's Stopping and Problems making mental/behavioural shifts). When experiencing stimulus boundedness, the individual is driven by external stimuli and cannot easily shift from one element in the environment to another. This is explained by Lezak as an information-processing deficit that reduces sensitivity to novel stimuli. A particular form of stimulus boundedness, 'utilization behaviour' is where an individual is compelled to use objects near them when not asked to, or even when they are told not to. Some authors now include this behaviour as a specific form of ED [47,50].

Memory disorders may also accompany ED. Working memory, the temporary holding of information that is being processed, can be affected by prefrontal damage. This may result from the person's inability to resist interference with what they are keeping in mind, which can make initial holding of information difficult [1]. Alternatively, "frontal amnesia" can occur where information may be stored, but the person is unable to generate search strategies/structures to aid retrieval [51]. *Confabulation* (the production of erroneous material on being questioned about the past) is often seen in people with prefrontal lesions/ED and may accompany the amnesia associated with a wide variety of pathological disorders. Walsh and Darby [46] point out that confabulation is not caused by memory loss alone and the majority of amnesiac patients do not confabulate. He notes that lack of self-awareness with an inability to inhibit responses, both of which have been identified as parts of ED, are a precondition for confabulation.

It is important to mention that cognitive and intellectual abilities, such as knowledge of factual information, are often preserved in people with ED [52]. Lezak [1] describes executive functions as asking "how or whether" a person goes about doing something, whereas questions about "what or how much" a person knows or does is a function of other cognitive systems.

The Prefrontal Cortex and Executive Functioning

An anatomical view of the brain, including an indication of the main aspects of the frontal lobes' is presented in Figure 2.

The frontal lobes lie anterior to the central sulcus and above the temporal gyrus, making up about one third of the mass of the cerebral hemispheres with the prefrontal cortex making up the largest area [46]. It is agreed that the prefrontal cortex has rich incoming and outgoing connections with most other areas of the cortex. Examples of these connections are the ones between the prefrontal cortex and the limbic system (such as connections between the prefrontal cortex and the thalamus, or mediodorsal nucleus of the thalamus). These connections are important as they are thought to mediate the involvement of the prefrontal cortex with mood, motivation and emotion [52]. Through these connections, executive functions become integrated with mood, impulse control, interpersonal relationships, monitoring of our own and other's behaviour, and self-awareness [49]. Cummings [53] suggests five parallel but independent circuits between the frontal lobe and subcortical structures (including the thalamus), each with separate cognitive and behavioural profiles. These circuits are presented in figure 3 and are called the cortical-striate circuits.

Cummings suggests three circuits emanating from the three separate regions of the prefrontal cortex: (1) the dorsolateral prefrontal cortex and its associated circuits were proposed to mediate verbal and non-verbal fluency and problem solving, as well as retrieval of learned material, which is hypothesised to have connections with the limbic memory system[1]; (2) the lateral orbital cortex and its associated circuits were proposed to mediate inhibition and impulse control; and (3) the medial frontal/anterior singular cortex circuit was proposed to mediate initiation.

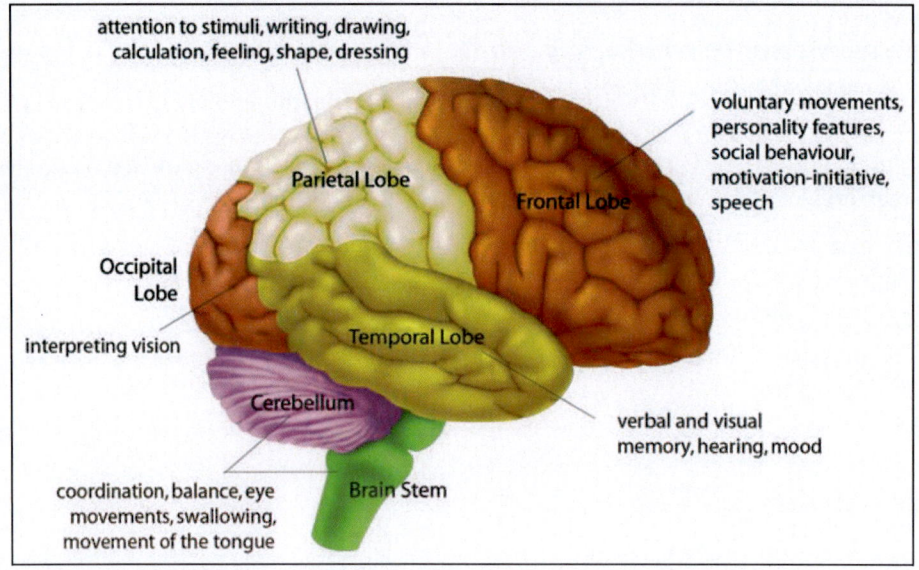

Figure 2. A lateral view of the brain's surface. Adopted from V Feigin "When Lightning Strikes. An Illustrated Guide to Stroke Prevention and Recovery" HarperCollins Publishers (New Zealand) Limited, Auckland 2004, with permission.

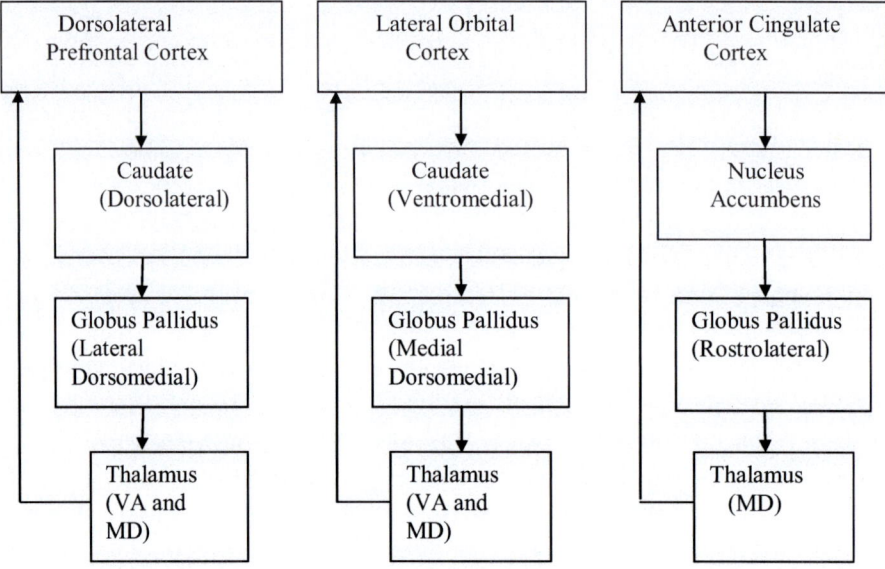

Figure 3 Cortical-Striate Circuits proposed by Cummings (1993).

The same anatomical disruption to the prefrontal lobes can result in different ED behaviours in different people. Indeed, any localized model of executive dysfunction has limitations. One limitation is that the most complex behaviours require that all three prefrontal cortical-striate circuits act together [53]. Therefore damage to any one of the circuits can manifest as disruption, and damage to different areas of the frontal lobe can result in similar problems. A second limitation is that naturally occurring lesions often damage multiple subsystems [1]. As such, it is difficult to determine the extent to which a particular circuit is responsible for a particular pattern of behavioural dysfunction. A third limitation is that some deficits described as being part of ED can result from either frontal *or* non-frontal lesions (e.g., abstract reasoning is susceptible to injury of frontal systems, but is not specific to frontal injury) [54]. Indeed, the behaviours associated with ED may also result from damage to other areas such as limbic damage resulting from anoxia [55], or inhalation of solvents [56].

Prevalence

ED is "probably the most common neuropsychological symptom cluster in the neurological populations" (p142) [45], and is associated with a number of clinical disorders including closed head injury, obsessive-compulsive disorder, schizophrenia, Tourette syndrome, Attention Deficit Hyperactivity Disorder, Autistic Spectrum disorders (ASD), Parkinson's and Huntington's disease, HIV infection, phenylketonuria, and those with focal frontal lobe damage following stroke, penetrating head injury or tumor.

Further, there are a number of environmental agents to which early exposure can contribute to ED, such as prenatal and birth complications or childhood exposure to neurotoxins [57]. In addition it has been proposed that ED type behaviours may result from environmental deprivation. Specifically, more complex areas of the brain (such as the frontal lobes) are not fully developed from birth. The prefrontal cortex, and therefore ED, is thought to reach full maturity between the ages of 15 and 19 [58]. A key neurodevelopmental factor determining an individual's capacity to moderate reactions and impulses is that the brain develops in a "use" dependant fashion - while all nerve cells are present at birth, the connections between them are not [58,59]. Thus, childhood experiences have an impact on the development of ED in that any deprivation of optimal developmental experiences may lead to the underdevelopment of neural systems in cortical areas such as the prefrontal lobe.

Reported frequencies of specific executive deficits in children with *ASD* and *severe TBI,* respectively, are as follows: Inhibition (46% and 32%); shifting (69% and 21%); emotional control (44% and 24%); initiation (50% and 32%); planning (70% and 44%); organising materials (35% and 18%); and monitoring (65% and 38%) [60]. Of 256 patients with *ischemic stroke,* 40.6% had ED [61]. Also, it has been reported that approximately 64% of persons with *Dementia of the Alzheimer's Type* (DAT) can be classified as having ED [62]. Further, it has been reported [62] that DAT individuals with ED performed worse on tests of cognition, dementia severity, and activities of daily living and have more frequent symptoms of psychosis with greater emergence during a 12-month interval when compared with patients with normal executive function. Although motor impairment is the hallmark of, *Parkinson's disease* (PD), *multisystem atrophy* (MSA), and *progressive supranuclear palsy* (PSP) the earliest and most evident cognitive findings in all three conditions are impaired executive function [63]. Portin and Rinne [64] found that 70% of their patients with PD deteriorated significantly on cognitive evaluation over an 8 to 10 year period.

Rehabilitation

Essentially, treatment of ED may involve several components. These include pharmacologic treatment, behavioural strategies, and education and support of the family.

Pharmacologic Treatments

Treatment can focus on particular aspects of ED, such as dyscontrol, aggression, or mood disturbances using certain medications. It has been reported that those individuals with ED following TBI who experience heightened disorganisation/agitation when under stress may benefit from neuroleptic treatment, though the benefits of this must be weighted against possible side effects [65]. Poor impulse control/aggressive behaviour has also been successfully treated with anticonvulsants, mood stabilizers (e.g., lithium, valproic acid), beta-adrenergic receptor blockers, and seratonin re-uptake inhibitors [66-68]. Where initiation/arousal is impaired tricyclic antidepressants [69] and dopaminergic agents [70] have been used.

Behavioural Interventions

The patient with ED often losses his ability to control or monitor his own behaviour, but will respond well when a consistent external structure is set up. Providing the individual with a structured environment, such as a regular schedule of daily events, and consistency in caregiver responses to difficult behaviours can often have a dramatic impact upon coping and independence. The management of the individual's environment can also involve organization of the physical space in order to reduce the need for executive control. For example, reducing clutter, using highly visible planning calendars, and organising and labelling drawers, cupboards and file cabinets all reduce the need for internal organisation strategies. Similarly, providing lists of steps in common activities can assist difficulties with initiating tasks or with remaining on task. For example, an individual's morning routine may be broken down into a small list of tasks and posted above the sink (e.g., flush toilet, brush teeth, shave, turn off light).

Having noted the importance of environmental manipulation in reducing behaviour difficulties in individuals with ED, it must be noted that a thorough review of behaviour management techniques is beyond the scope of this chapter. For more detailed information, a number of behavioural rehabilitation manuals are available (e.g., The Behaviour Management Handbook - A Practical Approach to Patients with Neurological Disorders [71]). Further, a concise summary of interventions for ED and self-awareness is provided by Turner and Levine (p. 241 – 246) [72].

LANGUAGE

Language deficits (or *aphasias*) are one of the most common outcomes of neurological insult. Aphasias are abnormalities in the production or understanding of spoken language caused by insult (e.g., vascular damage, trauma, tumour, etc) to specific regions of the brain typically in the left hemisphere. They can be distinguished from other disorders of speech such as *dysarthria* (a disturbance in articulation) or *dysphonia* (a disturbance in vocalisation) in that these types of speech disorders do not affect the comprehension of language or the central processes of expression. By contrast, *aphasias* are a disturbance in language ability; either in production or comprehension or both, that is not the result of a mechanical impediment.

The assessment and rehabilitation of language disorders is a task that is often shared by Neuropsychologists and Speech Language Therapists (SLT). Neuropsychological assessments often include tests used to assess an individual's ability to produce and comprehend speech, naming ability, and verbal abstract reasoning.; with interpretation of performance placed within the broader context of other areas of cognition. In contrast, the SLT is more likely to include a thorough screening for all forms of aphasia, including tasks of verbal repetition, reading, writing, and assessment of the motor mechanisms of speech. As a result, rehabilitative efforts employed by neuropsychologists are limited with the SLT typically the primary language therapist.

Neurophysiology and Definitions of Language

Verbal behaviour is a literalised function in that in almost all right-handers, and in a small majority of left handers, linguistic abilities are concentrated in the left hemisphere. Support for this conclusion comes from numerous clinical observations of patients with various types of brain lesions, studies of electrical and metabolic activity in the cerebral hemispheres of normal brains, and studies of "split-brain" patients whose corpus callosum has been sectioned to control epilepsy.

Language deficits following brain injury can occur with different severity and in different patterns, resulting in a number of distinct subtypes of aphasia, with each subtype displaying a distinct set of neuropsychological manifestations and a typical site of neural dysfunction [73].

Two areas of the brain are especially important in producing and understanding speech: *Broca's area* is involved in speech production, and lies in the frontal lobe just rostral to the region of the primary motor cortex that controls the speech muscles. *Wernicke's area* is involved in speech perception, and is situated in the posterior superior temporal lobe. The paragraphs that follow provide general descriptions of the various aphasias and their anatomical correlates, which are summarised for the reader in Table 3.

Broca's aphasia results from damage to Broca's area in the inferior left frontal lobe disrupting the ability to produce fluent speech. This disorder is characterised by slow, laborious, nonfluent speech, but comprehension of aural and written forms of language usually remains intact. Generally speaking, while non-fluent aphasias result in effortful and scant speech production, the contents of speech are appropriate; whereas in fluent aphasias speech is abundant and melodic, yet meaningless. Patients with Broca's aphasia often display three major speech deficits depending upon location and severity of the lesion. One is *agrammatism*, or a difficulty in using grammatical constructions. Patients have difficulty with 'function' words which contain important grammatical meaning, such as *a, the, in,* etc. 'Content' words that convey meaning, such as nouns, verbs, adjectives, and adverbs, are usually unimpaired. Also, grammatical markers, such as *–ed,* or auxiliaries, such as *have* are often absent in their speech. A second is *anomia,* or a word-finding difficulty, which, although a characteristic of all subtypes of aphasia, is somewhat more pronounced in Broca's aphasia because of the lack of speech fluency in this disorder. The third speech deficit characteristic of Broca's aphasia is an *articulation difficulty* resulting in the mispronunciation of words.

   Wernicke's aphasia results from damage to Wernicke's area in the left posterior superior temporal gyrus disrupting the ability to express thoughts in meaningful speech and to comprehend aural or written forms of language. In contrast to Broca's aphasia, Wernicke's aphasia is fluent and unlaboured. Patients use function words, but few content words such that the sentences they utter just do not make sense. Most people with Wernicke's aphasia seem remarkably unaware of their deficit; they appear not to notice that their speech is faulty nor do they acknowledge that they cannot understand the speech of others.

There is a direct anatomical connection between Broca's area and Wernicke's area (see Figure 4) in the form of a bundle of axons called the *arcuate fasciculus.* A third subtype of aphasia, namely **Conduction aphasia**, results from damage to the inferior parietal lobe that extends into the subcortical white matter and damages the arcuate fasciculus.

Table 3. Types of aphasias and their characteristics

Aphasia Type	Site of Lesion	Speech Fluency	Compre-hension	Repetition	Naming	Other
Broca's	Left posterior frontal cortex	Non-fluent; effortful	Preserved for single words and simple sentences	Impaired	Impaired	Right sided hemiparesis; aware of deficit
Wernicke's	Left posterior, superior and middle temporal cortex	Fluent; abundant "Word Salad"	Impaired	Impaired	Impaired	No motor signs; poor awareness of deficit
Conduction	Between left temporal and parietal lobes (Left superior temporal and supramarginal gyri)	Fluent; some articulation problems	Largely preserved or intact	Impaired	Good	Possible sensory loss, weakness of right arm
Global	Widespread left perisylvian damage	Non-fluent and scant	Impaired	Impaired	Impaired	Right sided hemiparesis
Transcortical Motor	Anterior or superior to Broca's area	Non-fluent; explosive	Largely preserved or intact	Largely preserved or intact	Difficult	Some right side weakness
Transcortical Sensory	Posterior or inferior to Wernicke's area	Fluent but scant	Impaired	Largely preserved or intact	Impaired	No motor signs

Conduction aphasia is characterised by meaningful, fluent speech, relatively good comprehension, but a severe deficit in verbatim repetition. Naming is usually impaired and the patient is often unable to write in response to dictation, but can usually copy the written word. Difficulty in reading aloud is often evident.

Two other subtypes of aphasia result from damage to regions just adjacent to Broca's and Wernicke's areas. *Transcortical motor aphasia* results from an *anterior* lesion that disconnects Broca's area from the motor cortex. The lesion results in a *nonfluent aphasia* in which the patient cannot produce creative speech. They will attempt conversation but only utter a few syllables. They are typically able to repeat words and phrases well. *Transcortical sensory aphasia* results from a posterior lesion which disconnects Wernicke's area from the posterior parietal-temporal association area. This produces a fluent aphasia with impaired comprehension, but the patient can repeat what they hear.

Global aphasia is a combination of Broca, Wernicke, and Conduction aphasias. It results from lesions in the entire perisylvian region, thereby compromising both Broca and Wernicke's area, and the arcuate fasciculus. Patients are unable to comprehend language, formulate speech, and repeat sentences; at best, speech is reduced to a few words.

With few exceptions, aphasias are accompanied by writing impairments (*agraphia*) that resemble the speech production deficits, and by reading impairments (*alexia*) that resemble the speech comprehension deficits. This is hardly surprising given reading and writing are closely linked to listening and talking and thus these abilities share many brain mechanisms [74].

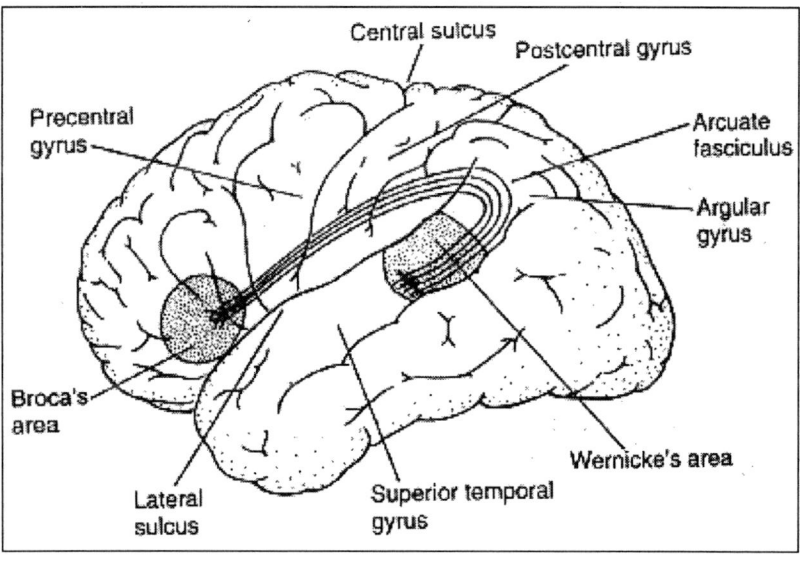

Figure 4. Lateral view of the left hemisphere with language areas identified.

Pure alexia (sometimes also referred to as *pure word blindness* or *alexia without agraphia*) describes an inability to read resulting from lesions that prevent visual information from reaching the extrastriate cortex of the left hemisphere. Although patients with pure alexia cannot read, they are able to recognize words that are spelled aloud to them. *Dyslexia*, or "faulty reading", may be *acquired* (i.e., caused by brain damage to those who already know how to read), or *developmental* as in the case of reading difficulties that become apparent when children are learning to read. Neurological insults can also produce *dysgraphia*, or writing deficits. Such writing disorders may take two forms; one involves difficulty in motor control and hence in forming letters and words; the other involves problems in spelling.

Prevalence

Our understanding of the neurobiology of language has largely been acquired through the study of people's verbal behaviour patterns following traumatic head injury, brain tumours or infections, brain surgery, or stroke. Of these, the most prevalent are focal brain lesions resulting from head injury or stroke. A high incidence of language disorders has also been found for children with focal epilepsy [75].

Stroke is thought to account for the largest proportion of aphasias. Post-stroke observations of the frequency of aphasia range from 21% to 38% [76-78], and there are estimated to be approximately 80 000 new cases of aphasia per annum in the United States [79]. In examined incidence of aphasia in a group of 881 stroke survivors, it has been reported that 38% had aphasia (11.5% mild aphasia, 6.4% moderate aphasia, and 19.6% severe aphasia) at admission to hospital, and 19% had aphasia at the time of discharge [77].

In a study of 308 consecutive stroke patients, 207 (67.2%) had aphasia in the acute phase, of whom 50% had global aphasia or nonclassified aphasias, 22 (10.6%) had Broca's aphasia, 30 (14.5%) Wernicke's, 17 (8.2%) Transcortical Motor, 7 (3.3%) each had Transcortical Sensory or conduction aphasias, and 5 (2.4%) had anomia [80].

Rehabilitation of Language Disorders

As indicated by Sohlberg and Mateer [81] "poor communication skills... present a serious handicap and a major barrier to community reintegration; they are the probable cause of social isolation and decrease in vocational ability"(p. 10). As noted at the beginning of the section on language, the assessment and rehabilitation of language and language related difficulties is a role that is usually shared by SLTs and neuropsychologists. While the SLT's typical focus is on the aphasia itself, the neuropsychologist is more typically involved in addressing commonly associated problems. The goals of rehabilitation for individuals with aphasia are not only to improve the ability to speak, comprehend speech, read, and write; but also to develop strategies that compensate for communication deficits; address associated psychological problems that compromise communication; and help the family and community members interact effectively with the patient.

For the neuropsychologist, intervention may involve providing cognitive rehabilitation strategies to reduce the impact of cognitive deficits that may reduce effectiveness of speech therapy. Feelings of frustration at the inability to communicate can lead to anger and depression. Thus, it may be necessary to provide individual therapy for the client to address issues of depression, grief, and adjustment following illness and/or provide individual therapy and/or behaviour management strategies to address low frustration tolerance and aggression. Provision of individual treatment to assist in increasing awareness/insight may also be a focus of therapy.

Family members may also feel strong emotions such as anxiety, anger, confusion, depression, and despair. It is natural to go through a grieving process when a family member develops aphasia, and family members need to be helped through this process. In addition to provision of psychological support to family members, the neuropsychologist often takes a leading role in supporting the SLT by assisting in educating and managing the behaviours of those who interact with the client. For example, educating staff and family members about (i) the need to be patient and not speak for the client; (ii) the need to support and encourage attempts to communicate; (iii) the need to encourage the use of gestures; (iv) speak simple, using simple 'yes' and 'no' questions if this is consistent with the clients' ability level; (v) the usefulness of pictureboards and other alternative means of communication; (vi) the need to avoid giving incorrect feedback (i.e., avoid conveying that you understand something if you do not); and (vii) the need to avoid assuming that an individual who cannot speak cannot hear or understand.

CONCLUSION

Cognitive deficits are a common consequence of many neurological and psychiatric conditions. As such, neuropsychological assessments are often sought as part of addressing clinical issues in these populations. However, it is often unclear to the general practitioner what role(s) this assessment might fulfill, and interpretation of the findings may be hampered by assumptions of common language/understandings across professional groups. To address these issues this chapter begins with identification of the three main questions that can be addressed by neuropsychological assessments. To provide a common language for interpreting neuropsychological assessments the chapter then provides an overview of commonly used definitions/models for specific disorders and areas of deficit and an overview of commonly used rehabilitation strategies. It is hoped that the above will increase other clinicians' confidence in understanding Neuropsychological Reports and engaging Neuropsychological services.

REFERENCES

[1]   Lezak, M. D. (1995). *Neuropsychological Assessment (3rd edition)*. New York, NY: Oxford University Press.

[2]   Ashcraft, H. M. (1989) *Human memory and cognition*. NY: Harper Collins.

[3]   Baddeley, A. D. (1992) Memory theory and memory therapy. In B. A. Wilson & N. Moffat (Eds.) *Clinical management of memory problems* (2nd ed., pp.1-31). California: Singular Publishing Group Inc.

[4]   Raymond, M. J., Bewick, K. C., Malia, B., & Bennett, T. L. (1996). A comprehensive approach to memory rehabilitation following brain injury. *The Journal of Cognitive Rehabilitation, 14(2),* 18-23.

[5]   Wood, R. Ll. (1991). *Neurobehavioural sequelea of traumatic brain injury.* The New York: Psychology Press.

[6]   Baddeley, A. D., Wilson, B. A., Watts, F. N. (Eds.) (1995). *Handbook of memory disorders.* Chichester England: Wiley.

[7]   Glisky, E. L. (2004). Disorders of memory. In J Ponsford, (ed.) *Cognitive and Behavioral Rehabilitation. From Neurobiology to Clinical Practice.* New York: The Guilford Press. p 100-128.

[8]   Shimamura, A. P., & Squire, L. R. (1991). The relationship between fact and source memory: Findings from amnesic patients and normal subjects. *Psychobiology, 19,* 1-10.

[9]   Tranel, D., Damasio, A. R. (1995). Neurobiological foundations of human memory. In A. D. Baddeley and B. A. Wilson (Eds). *Handbook of memory disorders.* Oxford, England: John Wiley & Sons. (pp.27 –50).

[10]   Reeves, D., & Wedding, D. (1994). *The clinical assessment of memory: A practical guide.* New York: Springer Publishing Company.

[11]   Franzen, M.D., & Haut, W. M. (1991). The psychological treatment of memory impairment: A review of empirical studies. *Neuropsychological Review, 2(1),* 29 – 63.

[12]   Stewart, F. M., Sunderland, A., & Sluman, S. M. (1996). The nature and prevalence of memory disorders late after stroke. *British Journal of Clinical Psychology, 35,* 369-379.

[13]   Lincoln, N. B., & Tinson, D.J. (1989). The relation between subjective and objective memory impairment after stroke. *British Journal of Clinical Psychology. 28(1) 61-65.*

[14]   Kapur, N. (1988)..*Memory disorders in clinical practice.* Boston, MA, England: Butterworth Publishers.

[15]   Levin, H.S. (1989). Memory deficit after closed head injury. *Journal of Clinical and Experimental Neuropsychology, 12(1),* 129-153.

[16]   Richardson, J. T. E., & Sanpe, W. (1984). The effects of closed head injury upon human memory: An experimental analysis. *Cognitive Neuropsychology, 1(3),* 217-231.

[17]   Wilson, B. A. (1995). Management and remediation of memory problems in brain injured adults. In A.D. Baddeley, B.A. Wilson, and F.N. Watts (eds.) *Handbook of Memory Disorders* .Chichester: John Wiley & Sons.

[18]   McKinlay, W. W., Brooks, D. N., Bond, M. R., Martinage, D. P., & Marshall, M. M. (1981). The short-term outcome of severe blunt head injury as reported by relatives of the injured person. *Journal of Neurology, Neurosurgery, and Psychiatry, 44,* 527-533.

[19]   Thornton A.E., Raz N. (1997) Memory impairment in multiple sclerosis: a quantitative review. *Neuropsychology.11(3):*357-366.

[20]   Beatty, WW; Paul, RH; Wilbanks, SL; et al. 1995. Identifying multiple sclerosis patients with mild or global cognitive impairment using the Screening Examination for Cognitive Impairment (SEFCI). *Neurology 45:*718-723.

[21]   Rao, S.M., Leo, G.J., Haughton, V.M. et al. (1989). Correlation of magnetic resonance imaging with neuropsychological testing in multiple sclerosis. *Neurology 39:*161-6.

[22] Grigsby J, Ayarbe SD, Kravcisin N, Busenbark D. (1994). Working Memory Impairment Among Persons With Chronic/Progressive Multiple Sclerosis *Journal of Neurology, 241(3):*125-31

[23] DeLuca, J., Barbieri-Berger, S., Johnson, S. K. (1994). The nature of memory impairments in multiple sclerosis: Acquisition versus retrieval *Journal of Clinical & Experimental Neuropsychology. Vol 16(2)*, 183-189.

[24] Moriarty, D. M, Blackshaw, A. J., Talbot, P. R., Griffiths, H. L., Snowden, J. S., Hillier, V. F., Capener, S., Laitt, R. D., & Jackson, A. (1999). Memory Dysfunction in Multiple Sclerosis Corresponds to Juxtacortical Lesion Load on Fast Fluid-Attenuated Inversion-Recovery MR Images. *American Journal of Neuroradiology 20*:1956-1962

[25] Wilson, B. A. (1991). Long-term prognosis of patients with severe memory disorders. *Neuropsychological Rehabilitation, 1(2),* 117-134.

[26] Tate, R.L. (1997). Beyond one-bun, two-shoe: Recent advances in the psychological rehabilitation of memory disorders after acquired brain injury. *Brain Injury, 11,* 907-918.

[27] Sohlberg, M. M., White, O., Evans, E., & Mateer, C. A. (1992). An investigation into the effects of prospective memory training. *Brain Injury, 6(2),* 139-154.

[28] Harris, J. E., & Sunderland, A. (1981). A brief management of memory disorders in rehabilitation units in Britain, *International Rehabilitation Medicine, 3,* 206 – 209.

[29] Gasparrini, B., & Satz, P. (1979). A treatment for memory problems in left hemisphere CVA patient *Journal of Clinical Psychology, 1,* 137-150.

[30] Godfrey, H.P.D., & Knight, R.G. (1985). Cognitive rehabilitation of memory functioning in amnesic alcoholics. *Journal of Consulting and Clinical Psychology. 53,* 555-557.

[31] Prigatano, GP, Fordyce, DJ, Zeiner, HK, Roueche, RR, Pepping, M, and Wood, BC (1984). Neuropsychological rehabilitation after closed head injury in young adults. *Journal of Neurology, Neurosurgery, and Psychiatry, 47,* 505- 513.

[32] Schacter, D. L., Rich, S. A., & Stampp, M. S. (1985). Remediation of memory disorders: Experimental evaluation of the spaced-retrieval technique. *Journal of Clinical and Experimental Neuropsychology, 7,* 79-96.

[33] Ryan T. V., & Ruff, R. M. (1988). The efficacy of structured memory retraining in a group comparison of head trauma patients. *Archives of Clinical Neuropsychology, 3,* 165-179.

[34] Wilson, B. A. (1996). Rehabilitation and management of memory problems. *Acta Neurological Belgica, 96,* 51-54.

[35] Wilson, B., & Moffat, N. (1992). The development of group memory therapy. In B. A. Wilson and N. Moffat (Eds.) C*linical Management of memory Problems.* San Diego, Calif.: Singular Publishing Group, Inc. (pp. 240- 270).

[36] Kapur, N. (1993). Focal retrograde amnesia in neurological disease: A critical review. *Cortex, 29,* 217-234.

[37] West, R. L. (1995). Compensatory strategies for age-associated memory impairment. In A.D. Baddeley, B. A. Wilson, & F. N. Watts (Eds.), *Handbook of memory disorders* (pp. 481-500). West Sussex: John Wiley & Sons Ltd.

[38] Harris, R. J. (ed). (1992). Cognitive processing in bilinguals. *Advances in psychology; 83*. Amsterdam: North-Holland Publishing Co.

[39] Fluharty, G. and Priddy, D. (1993) Methods of increasing client acceptance of a memory book, *Brain Injury, 7(1),* 85-88.

[40] Sohlberg, M. M., & Mateer, C. A. (1989*). Introduction to cognitive rehabilitation, theory and practice.* New York: Guilford Press.

[41] Wilson, B. A. (1987). *Rehabilitation of Memory.* New York: Guilford Press.

[42] Intons-Peterson, M.J. & Fourrier, J. 1986. External and internal memory aids: when and how often do we use them? *Journal of Experimental Psychology: General, 115,* 267-280.

[43] Ruff R.M., & Niemann H. (1990).Cognitive rehabilitation versus day treatment in head-injured adults: Is there an impact on emotional and psychosocial adjustment? *Brain Injury. 4(4),* 339-47.

[44] Moffat, N. (1992). Strategies of memory therapy. In B. A. Wilson and N. Moffat (Eds.) *Clinical Management of memory Problems.* San Diego, Calif.: Singular Publishing Group, Inc. (pp. 83 –116).

[45] Ogden, J.A. (1996). *Fractured minds. A case-study approach to clinical neuropsychology.* New York: Oxford University Press.

[46] Walsh K.W., & Darby D.G. (1999) *Neuropsychology: a clinical approach* (4th edition). Churchill Livingstone.

[47] Tranel, D., Anderson, S. W., & Benton, A. (1994). Development of the concept of 'executive function" and its relationship to the frontal lobes. In F. Boller & J. Grafman (eds.) *Handbook of Neuropsychology.* Amsterdam: Elsevier (Vol 9, p. 125-148).

[48] Wilson, B. A., Evans, J.J., Emslie, H., Alderman, N., & Burgess, P. (1998). The development of an ecologically valid test for assessing patients with dysexecutive syndrome.] *Neuropsychological Rehabilitation, 8(3), 213-228.*

[49] ateer, C. A. (1999). The rehabilitation of executive disorders. In D. T. Stuss, G. Wincour, & I. Robertson (eds.), *Cognitive neurorehabilitation.* Cambridge, UK: Cambridge University Press. (pp. 314-332).

[50] Lhermitte, F., & Signoret, J. L. (1972). Analyse neuropsychologique et differentiation des syndromes amnesiques. *Revue Neurologique, 126,* 161-178.

[51] Luria AR. (1973). *The Working Brain. An Introduction to Neuropsychology.* New York: Basic Books

[52] Darling, S., Della Sala, S., Gray, C., & Trivelli, C. (1998). Putative functions of the prefrontal cortex: Historical perspectives and new horizons. In G. Mazzoni & T. O. Nelson (Eds.), *Metacognition and cognitive neuropsychology: Monitoring and control processes.* New York: Erlbaum. pp. 53 - 95.

[53] Cummings, J. L. (1993). Frontal-Subcortical circuits and human behavior. *Archives of Neurology, 50,* 873-879.

[54] Malloy, P. F., & Richardson, E. D. (1994). Assessment of frontal lobe functions. *Journal of Neuropsychiatry and Clinical Neuroscience, 6,* 399-410

[55] Falicki Z., & Sep-Kowalik, B. (1969). Psychic disturbances as a result of cardiac arrest. *Polish Medical Journal, 8(1),* 200-206.

[56] Hawkins, J. D., Catalano, R.F., Gillmore, M.R., & Wells, E. A. (1989). Skills training for drug abusers: Generalization, maintenance, and effects on drug use. *Journal of Consulting & Clinical Psychology. 57(4),* 559-563.

[57] Kandel, E., & Jessel, T. (1991). Early experience and the fine tuning of synaptic connections. In E. R. Kandel, J. H. Schwartz, & T. M. Jessell (Eds.), *Principles of neural science* (pp. 945-958). New York: Elsevier.

[58] Huttenlocker, P. R. (1979). Synaptic density in human frontal cortex - Developmental changes and effects of aging *Brain Research, 163 (2)*, 195-205.

[59] Perry, B. D. (2000). Trauma and Terror in Childhood: The neuropsychiatric impact of childhood trauma. In I. Schulz, S. Carella & D.O. Brady (Eds.), *Handbook of Psychological Injuries: Evaluation, Treatment and Compensable Damages.* Washington, D.C.: American Bar Association Publishing.

[60] Gioia, G.A., Isquith, P. K., Kenworthy, L., & Barton, R. M. (2002). Profiles of everyday executive function in acquired and developmental disorders. *Child Neuropsychology. 8(2),* 121-137.

[61] Pohjasvaara, T, Leskelae, M., Vataja, R., Kalska, H., Ylikoski, R., Hietanen, M., Leppaevuori, A., Kaste, M., Erkinjuntti, T. (2002). Post-stroke depression, executive dysfunction and functional outcome. *European Journal of Neurology. 9(3),* 269-275.

[62] Swanberg, M. M., Tractenberg, R. E., Mohs, R., Thal, L. J., & Cummings, J. L. (2004) Executive Dysfunction in Alzheimer's disease. *Archives of Neurology 61(4)*, 556-560.

[63] Soliveri, P., Monza, D., Paridi, D., Carella, F., Genitrini, S., Testa, D., & Girotti, F. (2000) Neuropsychological follow up in patients with Parkinson's disease, striatonigral degeneration-type multisystem atrophy, and progressive supranuclear palsy *J* Neurol Neurosurg Psychiatry, *69*:313-318.

[64] Portin R, Rinne UK. Neuropsychological responses of parkinsonian patients to long-term levodopa treatment. In: Rinne UK, Klinger M, Stamm G, eds. *Parkinson's disease-current progress, problems and management.* Amsterdam: Elsevier, 1980;271-304.

[65] Campbell, J. J., Duffy, J. D., & Salloway, S. P. (1994). Treatment strategies for patients with dysexecutive syndrome. *Journal of Neuropsychiatry and Clinical Neuroscience, 6,* 411-418.

[66] Anderson,, K & Silver, J. M. (1998). Modulation of anger and aggression. *Seminars in Clinical Neuropsychiatry, 3*, 232-241.

[67] Glenn, M. B., Wroblewski, B., & Parziale, J. (1989). Lithium carbonate for aggressive behaviour or affective instability in ten brain injured patients. *American Journal of Physical and Medical Rehabilitation, 68*, 221-226.

[68] McAllister, T. W. (1985). Carbamazepine in mixed frontal lobe and psychiatric disorders. *Journal of Clinical Psychiatry, 46*, 393-394.

[69] Reinhard, D. L., Whyte, J., & Sandel, M. E. (1996). Improved arousal and initiation following tricyclic antidepressant use in severe brain injury. *Archives of Physical and Medical rehabilitation, 7*, 80-83.

[70] Van Reekum, R., Bayley, M., Garner, S., Burke, I. M., Fawcett, S., Hart, A., & Thompson, W. (1995). N of 1 study: amantadine for the amotivational syndrome in a patient with traumatic brain injuty. *Brain Injury, 9*, 49-53.

[71] Matthies, B., Kreutzer, J., & West, D. (1998). *The behavior management handbook: A practical approach to patients with neurological disorders.* San Antonio, TX: Psychological Corporation.

[72] Turner, G. R., & Levine, B. (2004). Disorders of executive functioning and self-awareness. In J. Ponsford (Ed). *Cognitive and behavioural rehabilitation. From Neurobiology to clinical practice.* New York: The Guilford Press.

[73] Dronkers, N., Pinker, S., & Damasio, A. (2000) Language and the aphasias. In E. R. Kandel, J. H. Schwartz, & T. M. Jessell (Eds.), *Principles of Neural Science Fourth Edition.* New York: McGraw Hill.

[74] Carlson, N. R. (2003). *Physiology of Behaviour 8th Edition. Chapter 15: Human Communication.* Allyn & Bacon.

[75] Parkinson, G. M. (2002). High incidence of language disorder in children with focal epilepsies. *Developmental Medicine and Child Neurology, 44,* 533-537.

[76] Brust, J. C. M., Shafer, S. Q., Richter, R. W., & Bruun, B. (1976). Aphasia in acute stroke. *Stroke, 7,* 167-174.

[77] Pedersen, P. M., Jorgensen, H. S., Nakayama, H., Raaschou, H. O., & Olsen, (1995). Aphasia in acute stroke: Incidence, determinants, and recovery. *Annals of Neurology, 38(4),* 659-666.

[78] Wade, D. T., Hewer, R. L., David, R. M., & Enderby, P. M. (1986). Aphasia after stroke: natural history and associated deficits. *Journal of Neurology, Neurosurgery, and Psychiatry, 49,* 11-16.

[79] Holland, A. L., Fromm, D. S., DeRuyter, F., & Stein, M. (1996). Treatment efficacy: aphasia. *Journal of Speech hearing Research, 39,* S27-S36.

[80] Godefroy, O., Dubois, C., Debachy, B., Lecllerc, M., & Kreisler, A (2002). Vascular aphasias. Main characteristics of patients hospitalised in acute stroke units. *Stroke, 33,* 702-711.

[81] Sohlberg, M. M., & Mateer, C. A. (2001). *Cognitive Rehabilitation. An integrative neuropsychological approach.* New York: The Guilford Press.

RECOMMENDED FURTHER READING

1. Wilson, B. A., & Moffat, N. (eds.) *The clinical management of memory problems.* San Diego, CA: Singular Publishing Group.
2. Ponsford, J. (ed.) (2004). *Cognitive and Behavioral Rehabilitation. From Neurobiology to Clinical Practice.* New York: The Guilford Press.
3. Sohlberg, M. M., & Mateer, C. A. (2001). *Cognitive Rehabilitation. An Integrative Neuropsychological Approach.* New York: The Guilford Press.
4. Matthies, B., Kreutzer, J., & West, D. (1998). The behaviour management handbook: A practical approach to patients with neurological disorders. San Antonio, TX: Psychological Corporation

INDEX

B

C

E

F

H

J

K

L

N

O

Q

S

T

W